Critical Dietary Factors in Cancer Chemoprevention

Mohammad Fahad Ullah • Aamir Ahmad
Editors

Critical Dietary Factors in Cancer Chemoprevention

Springer

Editors
Mohammad Fahad Ullah
Prince Fahd Research Chair
Department of Medical Laboratory Technology
FAMS, University of Tabuk
Tabuk, Saudi Arabia

Aamir Ahmad
Department of Pathology
Karmanos Cancer Institute
Wayne State University
Detroit, Michigan
USA

ISBN 978-3-319-21460-3 ISBN 978-3-319-21461-0 (eBook)
DOI 10.1007/978-3-319-21461-0

Library of Congress Control Number: 2015952214

Springer Cham Heidelberg New York Dordrecht London

Printed on acid-free paper

Springer International Publishing AG Switzerland is part of Springer Science+Business Media (www.springer.com)

Foreword

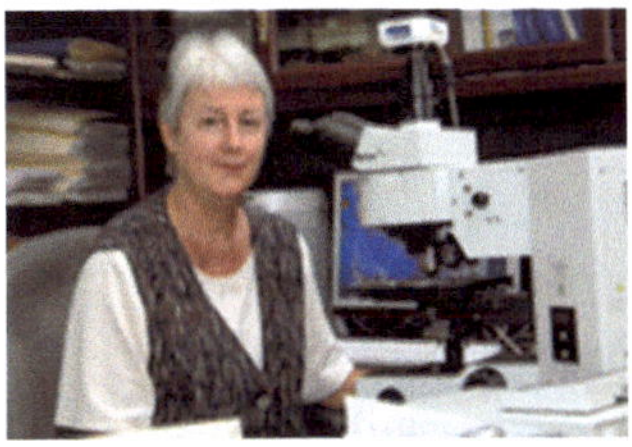

This book entitled "Critical dietary factors in cancer chemoprevention" is a comprehensive attempt to highlight novel opportunities for the prevention of neoplastic diseases by dietary means. Recently emerging evidence has revealed that long-term lifestyle factors including dietary habits significantly influence cancer development, progression, and response to therapy. Modification of dietary habits to include dietary factors with evidence of chemopreventive properties via the modulation of intracellular signaling pathways as regular components of diet has thus been conceived to be a potential strategy to lower the risk and burden of cancer incidence. Furthermore, these dietary factors also provide leads to potent therapeutic drugs with elevated margins of safety. This book provides an update on contemporary research in this field with an impressive group of authors. A unique feature of the book is that along with regular chapters, there are expert opinions from renowned authors, a strategy that enhances the impact of the knowledge and information emanating from this compilation.

I commend the editors, Dr. Mohammad Fahad Ullah and Dr. Aamir Ahmad and all the contributors, for this significant piece of work that encourages the engagement of dietary factors as an effective paradigm in cancer prevention.

Knoxville, TN, USA　　　　　　　　Hildegard M. Schuller, D.V.M., Ph.D

Preface

The success of scientific research on the ladder of validation is perfected when the idea traverses the untrodden path and delivers the desired benefit to the community of people. This book "Critical dietary factors in cancer chemoprevention" is an attempt of archiving a few such ideas in scientific and public domain. We commend Springer Publishers in providing the foundation for this endeavor and entrusting us with the task of managing and editing the current volume of the compilation that we present before the audience.

Precisely, the volume contains two sections. Section I introduces the importance of the topic of this book through the opinion of three renowned experts who have immensely contributed to the area of dietary factors in prevention of cancer for more than four decades. This is followed by Section II which has 15 chapters that are intended to highlight the significance of dietary factors in the premises of cancer chemoprevention as part of prophylactic, therapeutic, or adjuvant interventions.

Section I: Curcumin, a constituent of turmeric which is used as spice in food and anti-inflammatory agent in traditional medicines, has been known for long to possess anticancer properties. In the first expert opinion, Dr. Sarkar provides an update on a novel synthetic analogue of curcumin, CDF, with regard to its enhanced efficacy against cancer. This reflects that the dietary agents have the potential to not only provide preventive strategy as part of regular consumption but also have the potential to act as lead compound for the development of therapeutic interventions. The second opinion comes from Dr. Mukhtar, which advocates the synergism of bioactive compounds as a cocktail in the development of personalized approach to cancer chemoprevention. Dr. Hadi contributes the third expert opinion whereon he explains the delicate balance of the contrasting properties of bioactive molecules acting as both the antioxidants and prooxidants and how these could be utilized in their potential against cancer.

Section II: Chapter "Phytocomplexity: the key to rational chemoprevention" provides an excellent presentation of a concept that links the significance of phytocomplexity of whole fruits or vegetables in harvesting the desired chemopreventive efficacy in cancer prevention. Chapter "The ketogenic diet as an adjuvant therapy for brain tumors and other cancers" precisely deals with metabolic therapy where the authors suggest the application of ketogenic diet as an adjuvant therapy in starving the cancer cells of energy. Chapter "The role of organosulfur compounds derived from Allium vegetables in cancer prevention and therapy" explores the anticancer potential of bioactive compounds of organosulfur nature, emerging as a promising cancer chemopreventive strategy. Chapter "Epigenetic Impact of Bioactive Dietary Compounds in Cancer Chemoprevention" deliberates the influence of dietary factors in reversing the epigenetic events following the process of neoplastic transformation. Chapters "Potential for sesame seed-derived factors to prevent colorectal cancer" and "Progress in the development of black seed derived anticancer agents" present an overview of the anticancer potential of the bioactive constituents of sesame seed and black seed, respectively, and provide mechanism-based insights. Chapters "Soy isoflavones in the breast cancer risk: from preclinical findings to clinical strategy" and "Pharmacological role of dietary polyphenols in prostate cancer chemoprevention" focus on certain dietary agents with critical value in the prevention of breast cancer and prostate cancer, respectively. Chapter "Effects of garcinol from kokum (Garcinia indica) on the prevention and treatment of cancer" gives an account of nutraceutical garcinol and its chemopreventive efficacy against cancer. Chapters "Modulation of key signaling pathways in cancer cells by dietary factors" and "Pivotal role of chemokine receptor signaling axis and natural bioactive chemopreventive agents in metastasis of breast cancer" demonstrate the complex nature of cellular signaling in cancer cells and the ability of dietary compounds to interfere with these pathways. Chapter "Dietary factors may influence the clinical outcome of chemotherapy in cancer multidrug resistance" discusses the current interest in dietary molecules with respect to their potential role in addressing the drug resistance in cancer. Chapter "The role of energy balance in cancer prevention" points to the need of energy-balanced dietary intake in reducing the risk of cancer. Chapter "Dietary/environmental factors and breast cancer" reviews the significance of dietary fats and Mediterranean diet in relation to breast cancer risk. Finally, chapter "Probiotic bacteria in patients treated with chemotherapy and radiation therapy" addresses the emerging role of probiotics in the management of toxic responses associated with chemo- and radiation therapy in cancer patients.

We express our gratitude to all the authors for valuable contribution from around the globe. It is their willingness to share their onerous experiences which has empowered us to bring forth this piece of scientific literature. We appreciate the support of Dr. Beatrice Menz (Senior Editor, Springer Basel) for working out the procedural framework of our book proposal. Fortunately, we had Ms. Kay Stoll (Springer Production), as an excellent project coordinator, who provided the basic skeleton of strength that is required for any attractive and meaningful academic production. We are indeed honored to have Prof. Hildeguard M. Schuller introducing the substance of the book in the foreword.

Lastly, we wish that the audience will like the contents of this book and it will take us a step forward in understanding the critical nature of lifestyle issues vis–àvis dietary habits in reducing the risk of chronic diseases such as cancer.

Tabuk, Saudi Arabia — Mohammad Fahad Ullah
Detroit, MI, USA — Aamir Ahmad

Book Description

The poor survival statistics of fatal cancer diseases highlight the need for multiple alternative treatment options along with effective prophylactic strategies. Worldwide geographical variation in cancer incidence indicates a correlation between dietary habits and cancer risk. Moreover, an impressive embodiment of evidence supports the concept that dietary factors are key modulators of cancer. A number of action mechanisms have been reported for these dietary factors to retard, block, or reverse carcinogenesis.

Lifestyle issues including poor dietary habits are major impediment in the prevention of cancer. In addition, in recent past there has been an unprecedented surge of evidence implicating a large number of dietary agents in the prevention of cancer. A well-orchestrated campaign is thus required to highlight the clinical relevance of these factors in diet among the global population. The four distinct advantages of these agents are their diverse structure, pleiotropic action mechanism to simultaneously influence multiple targets, significantly lower toxicity, and selective killing of cancer cells (by certain dietary agents). Most of these agents are derived from fruits, vegetables, and grains and can easily be incorporated as routine dietary regimen. Further, their clinical potential might also be exploited as adjuvant therapy in the management of the disease along with conventional treatment to enhance the clinical outcome.

This book presents a *prophylactic approach* to primary prevention of cancer disease by highlighting the translational potential of diet-derived factors from epidemiological, laboratory, and clinical studies, as *prevention strategy* in normal/risk populations through routine inclusion of specific dietary regimens and as *therapeutic strategy* for better management through adjuvant interventions in cancer treatment.

The volume shares the experiences of highly reputed experts working in the area of dietary agents and cancer chemoprevention to promote the significance of dietary factors and elevate the dietary habits as an elite priority for containing the cancer disease.

Contents

About the Editors

Mohammad Fahad Ullah is an Assistant Professor of biochemistry in the Faculty of Applied Medical Sciences and a Research scientist at Prince Fahd Research Chair, University of Tabuk, Saudi Arabia. He received his academic degrees along with a gold medal in M.Sc. (biochemistry) from Aligarh Muslim University, India. Further he worked as a research associate at Experimental Oncology laboratory, Department of Biomedical and Diagnostic Sciences, University of Tennessee, USA, where he received an excellence in research award on studies related to cancer cell signaling in cellular and animal models of lung and pancreatic cancer. His research interest is in the field of novel plant- or diet-derived chemopreventive compounds for assessing the mechanism of action and examining their translational potential. He is member of the editorial/reviewer board of a number of scientific journals.

Aamir Ahmad is a Research Scientist at the Wayne State University, Department of Pathology, and Barbara Ann Karmanos Cancer Institute, Detroit, MI. His research interests include elucidating novel targets for therapy in aggressive breast cancers with special focus on key signaling pathways and microRNA-mediated regulation of metastases and drug resistance. Dr. Ahmad has authored more than 120 scientific publications and also serves as a section editor for the journal PLOS One.

Part I
Expert Opinion

Updates on the Promising Anticancer Activity of CDF, a Synthetic Curcumin Analogue

Kevin R. Ginnebaugh, Aamir Ahmad, and Fazlul H. Sarkar

Abstract In the last few decades we have witnessed an increased interest in nutraceuticals research for their putative use as anticancer therapeutics. A major drawback of nutraceuticals is their poor bioavailability. A few years back we synthesized a difluorinated analogue of curcumin, named CDF, which showed promise during our initial studies by being more bioavailable. This prompted us to investigate the anticancer mechanism(s) of this promising compound in detail, with the ultimate goal of taking this compound to the clinical setting. In this expert opinion, we provide a succinct overview of all the biological effects of CDF that we have discovered in the last few years. These include the ability of CDF to regulate epigenetic factors, miRNAs, and the cancer stem cell markers. Development and characterization of CDF is a good example of how natural chemical structures can be modified for better efficacy and activity against cancer cells, although such agents require further development for clinical studies.

1 Introduction

Cancer is a disease characterized by a few key events: division of cells containing mutations, unlimited replication potential, and invasion and growth of these cells in surrounding and distant organs through the assistance of the circulatory or

K.R. Ginnebaugh
Department of Pathology, Karmanos Cancer Institute, Wayne State University School of Medicine, 740 HWCRC Bldg, 4100 John R. Street, Detroit, MI 48201, USA

A. Ahmad
Department of Pathology, Karmanos Cancer Institute, Wayne State University-740 HWCRC, Detroit, Michigan, USA

F.H. Sarkar, Ph.D. (✉)
Department of Pathology, Karmanos Cancer Institute, Wayne State University School of Medicine, 740 HWCRC Bldg, 4100 John R. Street, Detroit, MI 48201, USA

Department of Oncology, Karmanos Cancer Institute, Wayne State University School of Medicine, 740 HWCRC Bldg, 4100 John R. Street, Detroit, MI 48201, USA
e-mail: fsarkar@med.wayne.edu

M.F. Ullah, A. Ahmad (eds.), *Critical Dietary Factors in Cancer Chemoprevention*,
DOI 10.1007/978-3-319-21461-0_1

lymphatic systems. These cells can arise through mutations accumulating due to the normal aging process and genetic predisposition or through the influence of environmental factors such as exposure to carcinogenic insults. In the year 2015, it has been predicted that 1,658,370 new cancer cases and 589,430 cancer deaths will occur in the United States alone (Siegel et al. 2015). Current drug and chemotherapy options contain many harmful side effects to the individual affected by the disease. Nutraceuticals, the therapeutic agents of natural origin, have shown promise to combat the harmful side effects of current treatment options. Nutraceuticals have been shown to help combat diseases like CVDs, obesity, GI tract disorders, as well as cancer (Gul et al. 2015). Nutraceuticals have been shown to have pleiotropic effects and the ability to target multiple cellular signaling pathways which has been one of the greatest attributes of natural agents, and is not achievable through current cancer therapeutics. Nutraceuticals have also been found to be effective in helping to resensitize drug-resistant cancers to conventional agents (Ahmad et al. 2015a). An example of the benefits found with nutraceuticals is in the chemoprevention of human cancers. For example, prostate cancer which typically impacts the aging population has been found to be heavily influenced by dietary habits (Syed et al. 2008). With increased dietary intake of chemopreventive substances, one could hope to possibly prevent or slow down the development and progression of prostate cancer. Pleiotropic effects of nutraceuticals have been found to be active in the regulation of miRNA–cancer stem cells nexus among many other biological effects of nutraceuticals (Ahmad et al. 2014). In the subsequent section, we will limit our discussion on curcumin and its analogues.

Curcumin, the active chemical found in the spice turmeric, is a yellow substance belonging to the polyphenols superfamily. Curcumin, through a variety of mechanisms, has been shown to exhibit anticancer effects (Shanmugam et al. 2015). Anticancer effects of curcumin are predominantly mediated through its negative regulation of growth factors, inflammatory cytokines, protein kinases, oncogenic molecules, and transcription factors (Shanmugam et al. 2015). One example of how this nutraceutical targets these processes was reported in bladder cancer, where it functions to increase miR-203 expression, ultimately decreasing levels of Akt2 and Src which were found to be elevated in untreated bladder cancer (Ahmad et al. 2014). Two other signaling pathways which have been associated with cancer development and progression are NF-kB and STAT3. Curcumin has been shown to inhibit these pathways resulting in the inhibition of either the development cancer and/or by inducing apoptosis of cancer cells (Vallianou et al. 2015). One of the reasons why curcumin has shown to be such a promising area of research is due to its documented lack of systemic toxicity. Multiple studies on a variety of mammals such as monkeys, horses, and rodents have provided great evidence in support of its superior safety profile and lack of systemic toxicity to the organism(s) (Howells et al. 2014). This has led to recent clinical trials with disappointing outcome in general. Besides cancer, curcumin is also being researched in pro-inflammatory diseases including cardiovascular disease, arthritis, ulcerative diseases, and Crohn's disease (Gupta et al. 2013a). Given orally, curcumin has been found to inhibit cancers including lung, skin, head and neck, oral, and many others in preclinical models (Gupta et al. 2013b; Rahmani et al. 2014). Sustained tissue concentrations have been reached using subcutaneous delivery, including one instance where mice liver was shown to contain curcumin a month after treatment (Gupta et al. 2013b). Despite all of these proven benefits of curcumin, curcumin has failed in clinical settings. This failure can be partly attributed to curcumin's poor bioavailability. When a subject takes an oral dose of curcumin, it undergoes complex metabolism rendering it inactive or rapid clearance via enzymatic processes. One way the bioavailability of curcumin could be improved is through generation of newly synthesized curcumin analogs; one such analogue is CDF (difluorinated curcumin) as described by our group (Padhye et al. 2009a, b). CDF has also been found to cause a marked decrease in NF-kB transcription and shows more pronounced effect at lower doses when compared with curcumin (Padhye et al. 2010). CDF also showed increased bioavailability after oral administration which was due to multiple beneficial attributes of CDF (Sarkar et al. 2010). In addition to studies on CDF, we have also synthesized CDF with β-cyclodextrin and this formulation was observed to enhance CDF's delivery to the pancreas, thus showcasing its improved bioavailability (Dandawate et al. 2012). In the following sections, we will summarize the various signaling pathways, factors, and therapeutic targets that are affected by CDF. Research investigations over past several years in our laboratory have focused on elucidating the mechanism(s) of antitumor activity of CDF, and thus we will provide a brief overview of this promising anticancer compound in this expert review.

2 Signaling Pathways

2.1 AR/TMPRSS2-ERG/Wnt Signaling

In patients suffering from prostate cancer, the progression to castrate-resistant prostate cancer (CRPC) after anti-androgen ablation therapy is driven in part by deregulated functions of the androgen receptor (AR), which is required for sustained growth of CRPC cells. Our lab discovered that AR activation resulted in greater ERG expression through the fusion of TMPRSS2-ERG (Li et al. 2011). ERG overexpression was also linked to Wnt signaling activation (Wu et al. 2013). CDF was found to inhibit signal transduction of the AR/TMPRSS2-ERG/Wnt signaling pathways, inhibiting invasion of prostate cancer cells and cellular proliferation. CDF was also linked to increased cancer cell apoptosis, underlying its potential application in the fight against prostate cancer (Li et al. 2011).

2.2 NF-κB Signaling

The role of NF-κB in the progression of human cancers has been well documented (Ben-Neriah and Karin 2011; Sarkar and Li 2008; Sarkar et al. 2008; Bao et al. 2012a; Ahmad et al. 2013; Tkach et al. 2014). Our lab looked at the levels of expression of NF-κB in pancreatic cancer cells BxPC-3 and MIAPaCa-epithelial (E)/mesenchymal(M) phenotypic cells (Ali et al. 2010). After the cells treated with CDF for 72 h, we reported a decrease in the DNA binding activity of NF-kB when compared to untreated cells. Such decrease in NF-κB activity was correlated with increased apoptotic cell death as well as resulted in the inhibition of cancer-associated signaling pathways. CDF's proven greater retention and bioavailability compared to curcumin have also been established in our lab. We have demonstrated that the inhibition of the DNA binding activity of NF-kB by CDF was far superior compared to curcumin (Padhye et al. 2009b).

3 The Biological Significance of microRNAs

The emerging role of small noncoding microRNAs (miRNAs) in human diseases, especially in cancer, is non-refutable (Xue et al. 2014; Hata and Lieberman 2015; Vidigal and Ventura 2015; Chan et al. 2015). Our own laboratory has been on the forefront of studies aimed at elucidating the mechanistic involvement of several miRNAs in human cancers which can serve as the basis of targeted anticancer therapies (Ali et al. 2011; Sethi et al. 2013, 2014; Ahmad et al. 2014). In the next few subsections, we will briefly discuss our published studies that documented deregulation of miRNAs by CDF.

3.1 miR-21 and miR-210

miR-21 is a miRNA that has been found to be associated with several cancers (Sheedy 2015; Pan et al. 2010; Gao et al. 2012; Liu et al. 2014; Fu et al. 2011). Being an oncogenic miRNA, its major targets are tumor suppressor genes, and it has been found to be expressed at higher levels in cancer cells than normal cells, potentially making it a biomarker for cancer diagnosis and prognosis as well as a target of the development of novel therapeutics. Upregulation of miR-21 has been found in colon cancer cells which could serve as a marker for potential recurrence of colon cancer in patients. PTEN, a target of miR-21, is a tumor suppressor gene responsible for the regulation of self-renewal in stem cells. Increased expression of PTEN has been found to be associated with decreased metastatic potential of tumor cells. Increased expression of miR-21 resulted in decreased expression of PTEN which was in part responsible for increased invasiveness and metastatic potential of colon cancer cells. Aggressive colon as well as pancreatic cancer cells treated with CDF showed re-expression of PTEN, which was mediated through downregulation in the expression of miR-21 (Roy et al. 2013; Bao et al. 2011; Ali et al. 2010).

Hypoxia causes prostate and pancreatic cancer cells to become much more aggressive. This aggression is in part due to increased expression of miRNAs, such as miR-21 and miR-210, and activation of many transcription factors. Increased expression of miR-21 has been found to be associated with increased mesenchymal transition of tumor cells, and upon treatment with CDF, resulted in decreased expression of these pro-metastatic genes which led to decreased cell proliferation and invasion, as well as increased apoptosis (Bao et al. 2012b, c).

Another consequence of miR-21 in pancreatic cancer is increased Ras GTPase activity (Ali et al. 2012). Such increased Ras activity causes increases in tumor aggressiveness and increased cell proliferation. CDF, when introduced in vitro to pancreatic cancer cells, showed decreased miR-21 levels which was correlated with decreased Ras activity.

3.2 miR-200, let-7s, miR-101, and miR-143

In addition to being regulated by miR-21, as discussed above, increased Ras GTPase activity in pancreatic cancer cells is also regulated by let-7s and miR-143. Forced re-expression of these miRNAs in pancreatic cancer cells showed marked reduction in GTPase activity as analyzed by western blot analysis (Ali et al. 2012). CDF treatment of pancreatic cancer cells resulted in decreased cell survival, invasion cell migration, and cancer stem cell function as well as decreased drug resistance. These decreases in tumor aggressiveness characteristics can be attributed to increased levels in the expression of tumor suppressor miRNAs such as miR-101, miR-143, miR-200, and the let-7 family, all of which were found to be upregulated by CDF treatment (Bao et al. 2011, 2012c, d; Ali et al. 2010, 2012).

Let-7 and miR-101 are also associated with the regulation of histone methyltransferase EZH2. EZH2 is a regulator of cell survival, proliferation, and cancer stem cell function. Due to its increased level of expression in human cancers, such as pancreatic cancer, it is associated with increased aggressive behavior of tumors. Let-7 and miR-101 when expressed in high concentration were able to inhibit these effects of EZH2. CDF positively regulates let-7 and miR-101, thus resulting in decreased pancreatic cancer cell survival, invasiveness, and cancer stem cell function by decreasing EZH2 expression (Bao et al. 2012d).

3.3 miR-874

In a recent study (Ahmad et al. 2015b), we compared the direct effect of curcumin vs. CDF on the inhibition of MMP-2 (matrix metalloproteinase-2). We focused on MMP-2 because of its reported role in invasion and metastasis of cancer cells. Through a number of approaches such as *in silico* docking, gelatin zymography, invasion assays, and ELISA, we observed a significantly more inhibition of MMP-2 by CDF, compared to its inhibition by curcumin in lung cancer cells (A549 and H1299 cells). As a mechanism, we noted an upregulation of miR-874, an MMP-2

Table 1 miRNA targets of CDF

miRNA	Up/downregulated by CDF	Reference(s)
Let-7s	Upregulated	Ali et al. (2012) and Bao et al. (2012d)
miR-21	Downregulated	Roy et al. (2013), Bao et al. (2011, 2012b, c) and Ali et al. (2010, 2012)
miR-101	Upregulated	Bao et al. (2012d)
miR-143	Upregulated	Ali et al. (2012)
miR-200	Upregulated	Bao et al. (2011, 2012d) and Ali et al. (2010)
miR-210	Downregulated	Bao et al. (2012c)
miR-874	Upregulated	Ahmad et al. (2015b)

targeting miRNA, by CDF. Thus, CDF induced the expression of miR-874 which resulted in the downregulation of its target MMP-2. These results provided another mechanism by which CDF could exert its anticancer effects.

In summary, detailed investigations reported by our laboratory have established a miRNA-modulating effect of CDF, which defines an important mechanism of action of CDF for the inhibition of cell growth of human cancer cells (Table 1). As discussed in this section, regulation of different miRNAs by CDF has been demonstrated in colon, prostate, pancreatic, as well as lung cancer cells. Given the versatility of CDF function, it will not be surprising to observe such effects of CDF in other cancer models as well, an idea that is under active investigation in our laboratory.

4 Cancer Stem Cells

Cancer stem cells, due to their resistance to chemotherapy, are currently thought to be the cause of recurrence in all human cancers. In order to fight cancer, these cells need to be eradicated. In a study conducted in colon cancer model (Kanwar et al. 2011), treatment with CDF resulted in increased levels of apoptosis and decreased cellular growth. CDF, due to its ability to downregulate cancer stem cell properties and induce apoptosis, along with conventional chemotherapeutics could prove to be effective in reducing reemergence of tumor growth.

Under hypoxic conditions, maintenance of cancer stem cell functions occurs through hypoxia-inducing factor (HIF) signaling (Bao et al. 2012c). In mouse models, in response to hypoxia-induced aggressiveness, cancer stem cell signatures were decreased in pancreatic cancer after administration of CDF. Moreover, CDF downregulated the expression of CD44 and EpCAM cell surface markers, which are usually the hallmark of cancer stem cells (Kanwar et al. 2011). One way by which CDF targets cancer stem cells is that it inhibits the formation of pancreatospheres. Inhibiting the formation of pancreatospheres was consistent with gradual decrease in the expression of CD44 and EpCAM cancer stem cell markers, which led to the inhibition of tumor growth (Bao et al. 2011).

5 Sensitization of Drug-Resistant Cells by CDF

Drug resistance is a major clinical problem. CDF has been found to be effective against chemotherapy-resistant colorectal cancer cells which was in part due to the ability of CDF to restore the levels of tumor suppressor PTEN (Roy et al. 2013). PTEN is an anti-metastatic/tumor suppressing protein, responsible for self-renewal of stem cells. This restoration of tumor suppressor PTEN was accompanied by downregulation of miR-21 which is typically increased during drug resistance due to the inhibition in the expression of tumor suppressor genes.

CDF was also able to resensitize pancreatic cancer cells to gemcitabine (Ali et al. 2010). Gemcitabine resistance appears to be in part associated with downregulation of miR-200 and increased miR-21 levels in pancreatic cancer cells. Treatment of pancreatic cancer cells with CDF led to increased expression of miR-200 and decreased expression of miR-21 which resulted in the gemcitabine-resistant cells sensitive to gemcitabine, and thus induced cell growth inhibition and increased apoptotic cell death.

6 Epigenetics

EZH2 is an enzyme that is highly expressed in numerous human cancers. EZH2 uses epigenetic programming to regulate cancer stem cell function, proliferation of cancer cells, and cellular survival. Treating pancreatic cancer cells with CDF, we were able to decrease the expression of EZH2; CDF also seemed to increase the expression of tumor suppressor miRNAs, including let-7s, miR-101, and miR-200 which were previously discussed. By targeting the EZH2-miRNA regulatory circuit, CDF inhibited pancreatic tumor growth and decreased the aggressiveness of tumors (Bao et al. 2012d).

7 Conclusions and Perspectives

Curcumin has been widely investigated and has been proven to be a potent anti-inflammatory, as well as an antioxidant agent with antitumor activity in preclinical studies. However, it has been shown to possess low bioavailability, which has rendered it clinically unacceptable. The bioavailability concerns led us to synthesize CDF among many other analogues that we had synthesized. We were able to demonstrate that CDF accumulates at a greater concentration in blood and in many other organs, for example, the pancreas. It has now been well accepted that cancer is difficult to treat which is, in part, due to deregulated expression of multiple signaling pathways supporting rapid cell proliferation and evasion of apoptosis. Therefore, cancer is a disease of multi-gene defects, and thus a multipronged approach is expected to be a better approach for the eradication of cancer. To that end, it is important to note that CDF is a multi-targeted agent whose antitumor activity is mediated through deregulation of a variety of signal transduction cascades including miRNAs, NF-κB, AR/TMPR552/Wnt signaling, epigenetic reprograming, and attenuating the many cellular attributes of cancer stem cells. Through these mechanisms, treatment of cancer cells with CDF causes cancer cells to undergo apoptosis, decrease their replicative potential, and also reduce "stemness" characteristics of cancer stem cells, thus resulting in the inhibition of tumor growth. Moreover, CDF could serve as a powerful agent for overcoming drug resistance, a major problem in cancer treatment. In addition, the superior bioavailability of CDF together with potential of its systemic nontoxic attributes could become clinically attractive for further development of CDF as a new anticancer drug for the treatment of human malignancies with better therapeutic outcome. In conclusion, CDF and other nutraceuticals or their synthetic analogues may open new horizon in the discovery of newer anticancer drugs toward achieving the goal to eradicate cancers.

References

Ahmad A, Biersack B, Li Y, Kong D, Bao B, Schobert R et al (2013) Targeted regulation of PI3K/Akt/mTOR/NF-kappaB signaling by indole compounds and their derivatives: mechanistic details and biological implications for cancer therapy. Anticancer Agents Med Chem 13(7): $32#1002–1013

Ahmad A, Li Y, Bao B, Kong D, Sarkar FH (2014) Epigenetic regulation of miRNA-cancer stem cells nexus by nutraceuticals. Mol Nutr Food Res 58(1):79–86. doi:10.1002/mnfr.201300528

Ahmad A, Ginnebaugh KR, Li Y, Padhye SB, Sarkar FH (2015a) Molecular targets of naturopathy in cancer research: bridge to modern medicine. Nutrients 7(1):321–334. doi:10.3390/nu7010321

Ahmad A, Sayed A, Ginnebaugh KR, Sharma V, Suri A, Saraph A et al (2015b) Molecular docking and inhibition of matrix metalloproteinase-2 by novel difluorinatedbenzylidene curcumin analog. Am J Transl Res 7(2):298–308

Ali S, Ahmad A, Banerjee S, Padhye S, Dominiak K, Schaffert JM et al (2010) Gemcitabine sensitivity can be induced in pancreatic cancer cells through modulation of miR-200 and miR-21 expression by curcumin or its analogue CDF. Cancer Res 70(9):3606–3617. doi:10.1158/0008-5472.CAN-09-4598

Ali AS, Ali S, Ahmad A, Bao B, Philip PA, Sarkar FH (2011) Expression of microRNAs: potential molecular link between obesity, diabetes and cancer. Obes Rev 12(12):1050–1062. doi:10.1111/j.1467-789X.2011.00906.x

Ali S, Ahmad A, Aboukameel A, Bao B, Padhye S, Philip PA et al (2012) Increased Ras GTPase activity is regulated by miRNAs that can be attenuated by CDF treatment in pancreatic cancer cells. Cancer Lett 319(2):173–181. doi:10.1016/j.canlet.2012.01.013

Bao B, Ali S, Kong D, Sarkar SH, Wang Z, Banerjee S et al (2011) Anti-tumor activity of a novel compound-CDF is mediated by regulating miR-21, miR-200, and PTEN in pancreatic cancer. PLoS One 6(3):e17850. doi:10.1371/journal.pone.0017850

Bao B, Thakur A, Li Y, Ahmad A, Azmi AS, Banerjee S et al (2012a) The immunological contribution of NF-kappaB within the tumor microenvironment: a potential protective role of zinc as an anti-tumor agent. Biochim Biophys Acta 1825(2):160–172. doi:10.1016/j.bbcan.2011.11.002

Bao B, Ahmad A, Kong D, Ali S, Azmi AS, Li Y et al (2012b) Hypoxia induced aggressiveness of prostate cancer cells is linked with deregulated expression of VEGF, IL-6 and miRNAs that are attenuated by CDF. PLoS One 7(8):e43726. doi:10.1371/journal.pone.0043726

Bao B, Ali S, Ahmad A, Azmi AS, Li Y, Banerjee S et al (2012c) Hypoxia-induced aggressiveness of pancreatic cancer cells is due to increased expression of VEGF, IL-6 and miR-21, which can be attenuated by CDF treatment. PLoS One 7(12):e50165. doi:10.1371/journal.pone.0050165

Bao B, Ali S, Banerjee S, Wang Z, Logna F, Azmi AS et al (2012d) Curcumin analogue CDF inhibits pancreatic tumor growth by switching on suppressor microRNAs and attenuating EZH2 expression. Cancer Res 72(1):335–345. doi:10.1158/0008-5472.CAN-11-2182

Ben-Neriah Y, Karin M (2011) Inflammation meets cancer, with NF-kappaB as the matchmaker. Nat Immunol 12(8):715–723. doi:10.1038/ni.2060

Chan B, Manley J, Lee J, Singh SR (2015) The emerging roles of microRNAs in cancer metabolism. Cancer Lett 356(2 Pt A):301–308. doi:10.1016/j.canlet.2014.10.011

Dandawate PR, Vyas A, Ahmad A, Banerjee S, Deshpande J, Swamy KV et al (2012) Inclusion complex of novel curcumin analogue CDF and beta-cyclodextrin (1:2) and its enhanced in vivo anticancer activity against pancreatic cancer. Pharm Res 29(7):1775–1786. doi:10.1007/s11095-012-0700-1

Fu X, Han Y, Wu Y, Zhu X, Lu X, Mao F et al (2011) Prognostic role of microRNA-21 in various carcinomas: a systematic review and meta-analysis. Eur J Clin Invest 41(11):1245–1253. doi:10.1111/j.1365-2362.2011.02535.x

Gao W, Xu J, Liu L, Shen H, Zeng H, Shu Y (2012) A systematic-analysis of predicted miR-21 targets identifies a signature for lung cancer. Biomed Pharmacother 66(1):21–28. doi:10.1016/j.biopha.2011.09.004

Gul K, Singh AK, Jabeen R (2015) Nutraceuticals and functional foods: the foods for future world. Crit Rev Food Sci Nutr. doi:10.1080/10408398.2014.903384

Gupta SC, Kismali G, Aggarwal BB (2013a) Curcumin, a component of turmeric: from farm to pharmacy. Biofactors 39(1):2–13. doi:10.1002/biof.1079

Gupta SC, Patchva S, Aggarwal BB (2013b) Therapeutic roles of curcumin: lessons learned from clinical trials. AAPS J 15(1):195–218. doi:10.1208/s12248-012-9432-8

Hata A, Lieberman J (2015) Dysregulation of microRNA biogenesis and gene silencing in cancer. Sci Signal 8(368):re3. doi:10.1126/scisignal.2005825

Howells LM, Mahale J, Sale S, McVeigh L, Steward WP, Thomas A et al (2014) Translating curcumin to the clinic for lung cancer prevention: evaluation of the preclinical evidence for its utility in primary, secondary, and tertiary prevention strategies. J Pharmacol Exp Ther 350(3): 483–494. doi:10.1124/jpet.114.216333

Kanwar SS, Yu Y, Nautiyal J, Patel BB, Padhye S, Sarkar FH et al (2011) Difluorinated-curcumin (CDF): a novel curcumin analog is a potent inhibitor of colon cancer stem-like cells. Pharm Res 28(4):827–838. doi:10.1007/s11095-010-0336-y

Li Y, Kong D, Wang Z, Ahmad A, Bao B, Padhye S et al (2011) Inactivation of AR/TMPRSS2-ERG/Wnt signaling networks attenuates the aggressive behavior of prostate cancer cells. Cancer Prev Res 4(9):1495–1506. doi:10.1158/1940-6207.CAPR-11-0077

Liu J, Zhu H, Yang X, Ge Y, Zhang C, Qin Q et al (2014) MicroRNA-21 is a novel promising target in cancer radiation therapy. Tumour Biol 35(5):3975–3979. doi:10.1007/s13277-014-1623-8

Padhye S, Yang H, Jamadar A, Cui QC, Chavan D, Dominiak K et al (2009a) New difluoro Knoevenagel condensates of curcumin, their Schiff bases and copper complexes as proteasome inhibitors and apoptosis inducers in cancer cells. Pharm Res 26(8):1874–1880. doi:10.1007/s11095-009-9900-8

Padhye S, Banerjee S, Chavan D, Pandye S, Swamy KV, Ali S et al (2009b) Fluorocurcumins as cyclooxygenase-2 inhibitor: molecular docking, pharmacokinetics and tissue distribution in mice. Pharm Res 26(11):2438–2445. doi:10.1007/s11095-009-9955-6

Padhye S, Chavan D, Pandey S, Deshpande J, Swamy KV, Sarkar FH (2010) Perspectives on chemopreventive and therapeutic potential of curcumin analogs in medicinal chemistry. Mini Rev Med Chem 10(5):372–387

Pan X, Wang ZX, Wang R (2010) MicroRNA-21: a novel therapeutic target in human cancer. Cancer Biol Ther 10(12):1224–1232

Rahmani AH, Al Zohairy MA, Aly SM, Khan MA (2014) Curcumin: a potential candidate in prevention of cancer via modulation of molecular pathways. Biomed Res Int 2014:761608. doi:10.1155/2014/761608

Roy S, Yu Y, Padhye SB, Sarkar FH, Majumdar AP (2013) Difluorinated-curcumin (CDF) restores PTEN expression in colon cancer cells by down-regulating miR-21. PLoS One 8(7):e68543. doi:10.1371/journal.pone.0068543

Sarkar FH, Li Y (2008) NF-kappaB: a potential target for cancer chemoprevention and therapy. Front Biosci 13:2950–2959

Sarkar FH, Li Y, Wang Z, Kong D (2008) NF-kappaB signaling pathway and its therapeutic implications in human diseases. Int Rev Immunol 27(5):293–319. doi:10.1080/08830180802276179

Sarkar FH, Li Y, Wang Z, Padhye S (2010) Lesson learned from nature for the development of novel anti-cancer agents: implication of isoflavone, curcumin, and their synthetic analogs. Curr Pharm Des 16(16):1801–1812

Sethi S, Li Y, Sarkar FH (2013) Regulating miRNA by natural agents as a new strategy for cancer treatment. Curr Drug Targets 14(10):1167–1174

Sethi S, Ali S, Sethi S, Sarkar FH (2014) MicroRNAs in personalized cancer therapy. Clin Genet 86(1):68–73. doi:10.1111/cge.12362

Shanmugam MK, Rane G, Kanchi MM, Arfuso F, Chinnathambi A, Zayed ME et al (2015) The multifaceted role of curcumin in cancer prevention and treatment. Molecules 20(2):$32#2728–2769. doi:10.3390/molecules20022728

Sheedy FJ (2015) Turning 21: Induction of miR-21 as a Key Switch in the Inflammatory Response. Front Immunol 6:19. doi:10.3389/fimmu.2015.00019

Siegel RL, Miller KD, Jemal A (2015) Cancer statistics, 2015. CA Cancer J Clin 65(1):5–29. doi:10.3322/caac.21254

Syed DN, Suh Y, Afaq F, Mukhtar H (2008) Dietary agents for chemoprevention of prostate cancer. Cancer Lett 265(2):167–176. doi:10.1016/j.canlet.2008.02.050

Tkach KE, Oyler JE, Altan-Bonnet G (2014) Cracking the NF-kappaB code. Sci Signal 7(313):e5. doi:10.1126/scisignal.2005108

Vallianou NG, Evangelopoulos A, Schizas N, Kazazis C (2015) Potential anticancer properties and mechanisms of action of curcumin. Anticancer Res 35(2):645–651

Vidigal JA, Ventura A (2015) The biological functions of miRNAs: lessons from in vivo studies. Trends Cell Biol 25(3):137–147. doi:10.1016/j.tcb.2014.11.004

Wu L, Zhao JC, Kim J, Jin HJ, Wang CY, Yu J (2013) ERG is a critical regulator of Wnt/LEF1 signaling in prostate cancer. Cancer Res 73(19):6068–6079. doi:10.1158/0008-5472.CAN-13-0882

Xue J, Niu J, Wu J, Wu ZH (2014) MicroRNAs in cancer therapeutic response: friend and foe. World J Clin Oncol 5(4):730–743. doi:10.5306/wjco.v5.i4.730

Prostate Cancer Chemoprevention by Dietary Agents: Advocating a Personalized Multi-agent Approach

Vaqar Mustafa Adhami and Hasan Mukhtar

Abstract Cancer chemoprevention research is rapidly evolving and our knowledge about the disease constantly updated. There is increasing acceptance of the fact that cancer is as diverse as the individual is and therefore needs a personalized rather than a generalized approach. This is true for chemoprevention but is also valid for chemotherapeutic intervention. Chemoprevention refers to the use of agents to intervene in the process of carcinogenesis with the intention to delay or inhibit the progression of cancer. Of all cancers, prostate cancer (PCa) is considered an ideal disease for chemopreventive intervention because its long latency provides a substantial opportunity to delay the onset of clinically detectable disease. Chemopreventive interventions need to be widely accepted and nontoxic since they would run over long periods of time and in usually healthy populations. In search for safe and nontoxic chemopreventive agents, many naturally occurring bioactive food components, capable of affording protection against carcinogenesis, have been defined. While laboratory studies with these agents have been promising, clinical trials have not yielded desired results. Considering the fact that carcinogenesis is a multistep process, it is unlikely that single-agent approach could prove effective in preventing cancer in individuals. We support the need to build an armamentarium of mechanism-based naturally occurring chemopreventive substances that could prevent or slow down the development and progression of cancer in general and use their tailored combination in different populations based on identified risk factors. Thus, the new effective approach for cancer chemoprevention prevention "building a customized mechanism-based chemoprevention cocktail of naturally occurring substances" is advocated.

V.M. Adhami • H. Mukhtar (✉)
University of Wisconsin, School of Medicine and Public Health, Medical Sciences Center-4385, 1300 University Avenue, Madison, WI 53706, USA
e-mail: hmukhtar@wisc.edu

M.F. Ullah, A. Ahmad (eds.), *Critical Dietary Factors in Cancer Chemoprevention*,
DOI 10.1007/978-3-319-21461-0_2

1 Introduction

Prostate cancer (PCa) is the second leading cause of cancer-related deaths among males in the United States (Siegel et al. 2015). According to estimates of the American Cancer Society, in the year 2015, approximately 220,800 new cases of PCa and 27,540 PCa-related deaths are predicted (Siegel et al. 2015). From a practical point of view, the most effective means of controlling PCa or the morbidity associated with its treatment is to establish effective chemopreventive approaches to block, reverse, or delay the process of carcinogenesis (Mukhtar 2012; Adhami and Mukhtar 2013). Whereas the diagnosis and treatment of patients with early-stage disease have markedly improved, the prognosis of patients with advanced stages of disease is still very poor. The concept of reduction of PCa occurrence by means of dietary intervention is gaining popularity and wide acceptance as PCa patients are increasingly using botanical supplements (Adhami and Mukhtar 2013). For a variety of reasons, the most important of which is human acceptance, dietary substances for chemoprevention are preferred (Adhami and Mukhtar 2013).

It is important to note that studies around the world have indicated a positive association of dietary agents in prevention and possibly cure of PCa. In recent years, much progress has been made in this direction, which has led to the identification of novel PCa chemopreventive agents (Lall et al. 2015). However, the prevailing approach for cancer chemoprevention has been "Find effective agents, with none to acceptable adverse effects and use them in relatively healthy individuals or in people stated for high risk for cancer development." This wisdom has not yielded desired results because clinical trials of single agents have ended with disappointing results. We argue that the lesson from these trials is that "One-size-fits-all approach is inappropriate." This is understandable since the process of carcinogenesis is multistep and multifactorial.

We advocate a three-step new approach for cancer chemoprevention under which there is a need to (1) establish the signature of defects in the individuals for whom chemoprevention is sought, (2) build an armamentarium of chemopreventive substances that could ameliorate defined biochemical defect(s) that occur in the carcinogenesis process, and (3) develop a customized cocktail, preferably dietary in nature, that the individual could be persuaded to consume (Fig. 1). At first thought this goal appears simple; however, it also raises many issues related to effectiveness and toxicity of each selected agent in a cocktail. However, in years to come, these issues could be resolved.

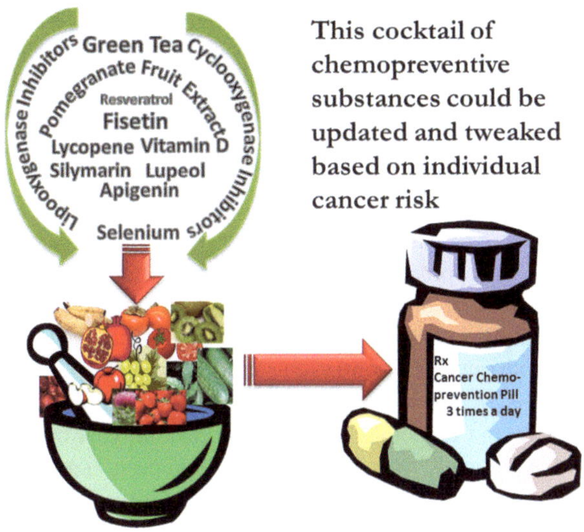

Fig. 1 Developing a prostate cancer chemoprevention cocktail. Cancer is as diverse as the individual is and therefore needs a personalized rather than a generalized approach. Also, carcinogenesis is a multistep process; it is unlikely that single-agent approach could prove effective in preventing cancer. In search for safe and nontoxic chemopreventive agents, many naturally occurring bioactive food components, capable of affording protection against carcinogenesis, have been defined. Thus, the new effective approach for cancer prevention "building a customized mechanism-based chemoprevention cocktail of naturally occurring substances" is advocated

2 Diet in Causation and Prevention of Cancer

Diet is a complex mixture of chemicals and thus for cancer risk is a mixed bag of bad and good stuff, carcinogens and anticarcinogens, respectively. Current evidence for the involvement of diet in cancer etiology is based on convincing laboratory data where dietary manipulations in rodent tumor bioassay protocols have established a definite link. Much of the knowledge of the role of diet in human cancer outcome however is based on indirect relationships between the consumption of selected food constituents and dietary habits and incidence of cancer at various sites. The indirect evidence, most often referred to, is the suggested correlation between the complex of fats-meat-egg-animal protein and the risk for cancer of various organs (Modan 1977). Carcinogenic agents identified include food additives, plant toxicants, aflatoxins, polycyclic hydrocarbons, nitrosamines, and certain normal major food constituents (Modan 1977). A synergistic action of ingested or metabolized carcinogens and a co-carcinogenic function of certain dietary components are suggested. Abundant epidemiological, observational, and metabolic biomarker studies have provided convincing evidence that nutrition plays an important causative role in the initiation, promotion, and progression stages of several types of human cancers [(Mukhtar and Ahmad 1999) and the references therein]. It has become clear that, in addition to substances that pose a cancer risk, the human diet also contains agents which are capable of affording protection against some forms of cancer.

Over last two decades there has been a constant increase in the awareness and utilization of diet as complementary and alternative medicine for cancer control. This increase is in part due to the fact that anything "natural" is considered inherently safe. Chemoprevention, by definition, is "*the use of drugs, vitamins, or other agents to try to reduce the risk of, or delay the development or recurrence of, cancer.*". A recent task force on chemoprevention defines the approach as "*the prevention of cancer or treatment of identifiable precancers*" (Kelloff et al. 2006; Herberman et al. 2006). The expectation of chemoprevention at the cellular level is regulation of growth and differentiation, at the tissue level is the reversal of premalignant lesions, and at the clinical level it is nothing less than reduction of cancer development and outcome. Thus, the achievable goal of chemoprevention could be defined as "slowing the process of carcinogenesis" (Adhami and Mukhtar 2013). Chemoprevention of cancer thus differs from cancer treatment in that the goal of this approach is to lower the rate of cancer incidence. Chemopreventive agents are often, but erroneously, also called as anticarcinogens. Chemoprevention in recent years is increasingly realized as a promising approach for cancer control because the therapy and surgery have not been fully effective against the high incidence or low survival rate of most of the cancer types including PCa (Herberman et al. 2006; Santillo and Lowe 2006). Micronutrients present in edible plants are regarded as the most desirable class of chemopreventive agents (Santillo and Lowe 2006). This information is supported by the fact that epidemiological studies suggest that consumption of fresh fruits and yellow-green vegetables reduces the cancer incidence and mortality due to stomach, colon, breast, lung, bladder, esophageal, prostate, and other cancers (Adhami et al. 2003; Khan et al. 2009; Wattenberg et al. 1990; Kellof et al. 1994). A wide range of such micronutrients present in plants consumed by humans has been shown to possess potential chemopreventive effects. Some of the well-identified chemopreventive agents, in addition of possessing preventive effects, are also showing therapeutic potential (Ames 1983; Greenwald 2002), and often they enhance the therapeutic efficacy of established chemotherapeutic agents. At the present time, about 30 classes of chemicals with such effects have been described, many of which may have practical implications in reducing cancer incidence at least in high-risk individuals (Tsao et al. 2004; Ren and Lien 1997; Surh 2003). Among the large list of chemopreventive agents, the polyphenolic antioxidants present in a variety of plant foods and beverages consumed by the human population are receiving increasing attention for human consumption (Lall et al. 2015; Mukhtar and Ahmad 1999; Santillo and Lowe 2006; Ren and Lien 1997; Surh 2003).

3 Prostate Cancer: An Ideal Disease for Chemoprevention

PCa represents an excellent candidate disease for chemoprevention because it is a unique malignancy which generally grows very slowly, likely for decades, before symptoms arise and a diagnosis is finally established. It is typically diagnosed in elderly men and, therefore, even a modest delay in the neoplastic development achieved through pharmacological or therapeutical intervention could result in substantial reduction in the incidence of the clinically detectable disease (Surh 2003; Klein and Thompson 2004). Consistent with this assumption, there is intense activity in defining chemopreventive agents and molecular targets for PCa chemoprevention [(Adhami et al. 2003) and references therein]. Among many such agents, for a variety of reasons naturally occurring nontoxic dietary substances are preferred. Our studies supported by the data from other laboratories worldwide suggest that there are multiple targets for PCa chemoprevention by naturally occurring agents and therefore highlight the need for further studies to identify novel pathways that may be modulated by dietary agents that could be further exploited for prevention and treatment of PCa.

It will be important to investigate which nutritional intervention could lead to a reduction in the incidence of PCa in what population and in what stage of the disease. Thus, efforts are under way to define agents that can delay the conversion of prostatic intra-epithelial neoplasia to well-differentiated adenocarcinoma, a delay in the conversion of well-differentiated adenocarcinoma to moderately differentiated adenocarcinoma, or a delay in the conversion of moderately differentiated adenocarcinoma to poorly differentiated adenocarcinoma (Brawley and Parnes 2000). Below we describe our experience with some of the agents and define the molecular targets of observed preventive effects.

4 ODC and Prostate Cancer

The enzyme ornithine decarboxylase (ODC) is a homodimer of 461 amino acids that catalyzes the decarboxylation of ornithine, producing as a result diamine putrescine. This is the first step and the rate-limiting step in humans for the production of polyamines which is required for cell growth, proliferation, and differentiation (Abrahamsen et al. 1991; Auvinen et al. 1992). Convincing evidence is there to provide the role of polyamines in tumor cell growth and in biological response of tumor promoters and growth factors (Pegg et al. 1995; Meyskens and Gerner 1999). Various rodent studies have established the importance of ODC in tumor progression [(Meyskens and Gerner 1999) and references therein; (Lan et al. 2000)].

In humans, among all tissues, the highest concentration of polyamines and polyamine synthesis enzymes, especially ODC, occurs in the prostate (Mohan 1999). We, thus, hypothesized that ODC could serve as a biomarker for the diagnosis or monitoring the therapeutic efficacy of PCa in human, and possibly as a target for intervention of the disease through chemoprevention. In our first set of experiments, we demonstrated that as compared to benign tissue ODC enzyme activity is elevated 2.7-fold in PCa tissue, PCa tissue has highly expressed ODC protein, and ODC enzyme activity is highly elevated in prostatic fluids of patients with PCa (Mohan 1999). In one of our subsequent study, we observed that ODC is upregulated in *tr*ansgenic *a*denocarcinoma of the *m*ouse *p*rostate (TRAMP) prostate model (Gupta et al. 2000a). TRAMP is an excellent mouse model of PCa that mimics progressive forms of human disease inasmuch as 100 % of males develop histological PIN by 8–12 weeks of age that progresses to adenocarcinoma with distant site metastases by 24–28 weeks of age. We then found that oral feeding of α-difluoromethylornithine (DFMO), a suicide substrate inhibitor of ODC, results in the inhibition of prostate carcinogenesis and its metastasis in TRAMP mice (Gupta et al. 2000a). DFMO has repeatedly been suggested to play a key role in the prevention of PCa in both in vivo and in vitro situations [(Kadmon 1992) and the references therein]. Clinical trials with ODC inhibitors in PCa patients have yielded encouraging results (Simoneau et al. 2001). A large clinical study has demonstrated that the administration of oral DFMO for 4 weeks reduces the levels of putrescine, spermidine, and spermine in a statistically significant manner in human prostate tissue (Hikosaka et al. 2004). Many dietary chemopreventive agents are known to inhibit ODC induction in various test systems. A recent study observed that the inhibitory effects of soy isoflavones on rat prostate carcinogenesis induced by PhIP are mediated by downregulation of ODC (Hikosaka et al. 2004). Thus, some of the dietary substances could be explored for their role in inhibiting PCa development by inhibiting ODC activity.

5 COX-2 and Prostate Cancer

Prostaglandin (PG) endoperoxidase synthase, commonly referred to as cyclo-oxygenase (COX), is a key enzyme involved in the conversion of arachidonic acid to PGs and other eicosanoids. COX exists in two isoforms, namely, COX-1 and COX-2 with distinct tissue distribution and physiological functions. COX-1 is the housekeeping enzyme, constitutively expressed in many tissues and cell types and is involved in normal cellular physiological functions, whereas COX-2 is the inducible isoform, is pro-inflammatory in nature, and is inducible by mitogens, cytokines, tumor promoters, and growth factors. Under laboratory conditions, induction of COX-2 has been shown to promote cell growth, inhibit apoptosis, and enhance motility and adhesion (Williams et al. 1999; Cao and Prescott 2002). Although there has not been a common consensus on the association of COX-2 with disease stage, it is generally agreed that COX-2's overexpression is associated with development of various cancers including cancers of prostate and colon. In several types of cancer, overexpression of Cox-2 is correlated with advanced diseases and poor prognosis (Hikosaka et al. 2004; Williams et al. 1999; Cao and Prescott 2002). In the search for agents that will prevent or delay the inception of cancer, it is realized that COX-2 is a promising therapeutic target (Pruthi 2004). We, in a study, have shown that COX-2 mRNA and protein levels were overexpressed in PCa tissue compared with paired benign tissue. Immunohistochemical analysis also verified COX-2 overexpression in cancer tissues (Gupta et al. 2000b). Many other studies have verified this initial observation and reported that as compared to normal tissue, COX-2 is overexpressed in human PCa. In this scenario, it has been suggested that selective inhibition of COX-2 may be useful for prevention and/or therapy of PCa [(Gupta et al. 2004) and the references therein].

Epidemiological studies and clinical observations suggest that nonsteroidal anti-inflammatory drugs (NSAIDs) and certain selective COX-2 inhibitors may reduce the relative risk of clinically evident PCa. NSAIDs are amongst the most commonly used medications worldwide. They are considered as effective anti-inflammatory, antipyretic, and analgesic drugs. Studies involving NSAIDs and PCa suggest that NSAIDs have a preventive effect on PCa. A multicentric cohort of over 90,000 men demonstrated a 24 % reduction in the risk for PCa in patients receiving aspirin daily in year prior to the study (Habel 2002). Other relatively large case–control studies demonstrated even more significant reduction in the risk of PCa (Roberts et al. 2002; Leitzmann et al. 2002; Irani et al. 2002; Royle and Ross 2004). NSAIDs, in spite of being effective against PCa have limited application due to severe toxic side effects on normal cells [(Irani et al. 2002) and the references therein]. Therefore, novel nontoxic COX-2-specific inhibitors that have the ability to spare normal cells from their cytotoxic effects are required for cancer chemoprevention. The efficacy of celecoxib, a selective COX-2 inhibitor which reduces inflammation and side effects associated with traditional NSAIDs, was tested in TRAMP mice on the progression of PCa by measuring the growth of primary tumor and effects on distant site metastases, the intermediate, and end point markers of PCa progression (Gupta et al. 2004). Celecoxib supplementation in the diet to TRAMP mice resulted in significant reduction in tumor development with no signs of metastasis. Celecoxib fed animals showed reduced proliferation and downmodulation of COX-2 and prostaglandin E2 levels in dorsolateral prostate and plasma. These results correlated with retention of anti-metastasis markers, viz., E-cadherin, and α- and β-catenin along with significant decrease in VEGF protein expression. Celecoxib supplementation also resulted in enhanced in vivo apoptosis in prostate as monitored by ^{99m}Tc-labeled annexin V in live animals followed by phosphor imaging. It is noteworthy that many other diet-based cancer chemopreventive agents also inhibit COX-2 induction. Hussain et al. (2005) recently demonstrated that EGCG inhibits COX-2 without affecting COX-1 expression at both the mRNA and protein levels, in androgen-sensitive LNCaP and androgen-insensitive PC-3 human prostate carcinoma cells. More studies are also needed for the identification of signaling pathways and specific genes being modulated by the Cox-2-derived prostaglandins in tumorigenesis. These studies will shed light on prostate cancer development and will also help design new targeted therapy for this disease.

6 Green Tea and Prostate Cancer

Various epidemiological studies have indicated that people who regularly consume tea have a decreased risk of PCa (Heilbrun 1986; Jain et al. 1998; Jian et al. 2004). A case–control study in southeast China suggested that green tea is protective against PCa (Jian et al. 2004). According to the study, the incidence rate of PCa per 100,000 is 104.33 in the USA and 75.97 in Australia but only 1.74 in China possibly because of use of green tea and other natural products. In a recent clinical trial, Bettuzzi et al. (2006a) observed that green tea catechins (GTC) when given to patients with high-grade prostate intra-epithelial neoplasia significantly decreased the tumor incidence to ~3 % in GTC-treated men as compared to 30 % in placebo-treated men.

More than a decade ago, our lab initiated a program to assess whether green tea consumption could afford chemopreventive effects against PCa development. Since then we have been able to assess multiple targets by which tea affords PCa chemopreventive effects. At first, we showed that ODC, a rate-controlling enzyme in the polyamine biosynthesis pathway, is overexpressed in prostate cancer and prostate fluid in humans (Gupta et al. 1999). High testosterone levels are known to mediate the induction of ODC activity and exposure of PCa cells to Epigallo-catechin-3-Gallate (EGCG), and infusion of green tea to Cpb: WU rats caused a downregulation of ODC activity. Green tea and its individual components have been found to modulate a variety of pathways involved in the pathogenesis of PCa.

Studies from ours and other laboratories have shown that EGCG results in an induction of apoptosis in PCa cells (Ahmad et al. 1997; Gupta et al. 2000c; Paschka et al. 1998). One of the additional study from our laboratory demonstrated that EGCG-induced apoptosis in human prostate carcinoma cells is mediated via modulation of two related pathways: p53 and NF-κB (Hastak et al. 2003). Yu et al. (Yu et al. 2004) demonstrated that the addition of EGCG and Cu^{2+} to the growth medium decreased the relative viability of human PCa cells. In a study from our laboratory, EGCG was also found to increase the expression of cell cycle regulatory molecules p21, p16, and p18 while downmodulating the protein levels of cyclin D1, cyclin E, cdk2, cdk4, and cdk6 (Gupta et al. 2003).

We then reasoned that the preclinical studies should be carried out in a model system that mimics the PCa development in a similar fashion to human disease. TRAMP is one such model and we have provided convincing evidence that oral infusion of green tea polyphenols (GTP) (equivalent to six cups of green tea human consumption) to the TRAMP mice inhibits prostate carcinogenesis through the modulation of IGF/IGFBP-3 signaling pathway (Gupta et al. 2001). In a subsequent study, we demonstrated that IGF/IGFBP-3 signaling is the prime pathway for GTP-mediated inhibition and metastasis of PCa in TRAMP mice that limits the progression of cancer through inhibition of metastasis and angiogenesis markers, most notably vascular endothelial growth factor (VEGF), urokinase plasminogen activator (uPA), and matrix metalloproteinases (MMPs) (Adhami et al. 2004).

Studies have also demonstrated the effects of tea and its polyphenols on the growth of prostate tumor xenografts. Subsequent to the work of Liao et al. (1995), we in a recent study demonstrated that GTP, black tea extract, EGCG, and the aflavin (polyphenol found in black tea) administration resulted in a significant inhibition in the growth and development of PCa cells implanted in nude mice and that this inhibition was accompanied with reduced serum prostate specific antigen (PSA) levels and an induction of apoptosis and inhibition of angiogenesis (Siddiqui 2006).

Green tea has been explored in the clinic for its anticancer effects. Studies that recruited patients at an advanced stage of the disease reported limited effect, suggesting that green tea could be more effective if given to patients at high risk for developing cancer. Bettuzzi et al. (2006b) observed that after a year of green tea administration, only one man in a group of 32 with high-grade PIN developed prostate cancer compared with 9 of 30 in the placebo group. A 24-month follow-up of patients from the same study suggested that the effects of green tea supplementation were long lasting (Brausi et al. 2008).

7 Pomegranate and Prostate Cancer

The fruit pomegranate, derived from the tree *Punica granatum*, has been shown to possess strong antioxidant, anti-inflammatory, antiatherogenic, and anti-tumorigenic properties (Gil et al. 2000; Afaq et al. 2005; Aviram and Dornfeld 2001). In fact, the antioxidant activity of pomegranate fruit is shown to be higher than that of red wine and green tea, two dietary substances, which are showing promise in preclinical PCa models and in PCa patients (Gil et al. 2000).

In a recent study, employing highly aggressive human PCa cells, we observed that pomegranate fruit extract (PFE) treatment resulted in inhibition of cell growth mediated through induction of apoptosis (Malik et al. 2005). We also observed a significant inhibition in the growth and development of PCa cells implanted in nude mice which was also accompanied with concomitant reduction in serum PSA levels.

A phase II clinical trial study with pomegranate juice was completed for 48 men with rising PSA levels after surgery or radiotherapy. Patients drank eight ounces of pomegranate juice daily. The outcome of the study showed that by pomegranate juice drinking the mean PSA doubling time increased from 15 to 54 months (Pantuck et al. 2006). In vitro assays comparing pretreatment and posttreatment patient serum on the growth of LNCaP showed a 12 % decrease in cell proliferation and a 17 % increase in apoptosis, a 23 % increase in serum nitric oxide, and significant reductions in oxidative state and sensitivity to oxidation of serum lipids after versus before pomegranate juice consumption. In another study, pomegranate extracts were found to potently suppress proliferation, xenograft growth, and invasion of human prostate cancer cells (Albrecht et al. 2004).

8 Lupeol and Prostate Cancer

Lupeol, a triterpene found in many fruits like mango, olives, grapes, strawberry, figs, and many vegetables, is found to have antioxidant, antimutagenic, and anti-inflammatory effects in in vitro and in vivo systems (Saleem et al. 2001; Geetha and Varalakshmi 2001). Lupeol has been found to induce differentiation and inhibit the cell growth of mouse melanoma and human leukemia cells (Hata et al. 2002; Aratanechemuge et al. 2004). Our laboratory recently demonstrated the antitumor promoter activity of lupeol in mouse skin carcinogenesis (Saleem et al. 2004). In a subsequent study, we demonstrated that lupeol induces Fas-mediated apoptotic death of prostate cancer cells and inhibits tumor growth in a xenograft model of PCa (Saleem et al. 2005). Lupeol treatment to prostate cancer cells was found to cause cell growth inhibition, induction of apoptosis, induction in the expression of PARP protein, and decrease in mitochondrial pathway proteins procaspase-6, -8, and -9. Lupeol was also found to significantly inhibit the growth and development of PCa cells implanted in nude mice which was also accompanied with concomitant reduction in serum PSA levels.

9 Selenium and Vitamin E Cancer Prevention Trial and Prostate Cancer

Vitamin E is the most popular supplement used by men (Boon et al. 2003; Beebe-Dimmer et al. 2004). Foods rich in plant-derived oils like avocadoes, nuts, eggs, soybeans, etc., are good source of vitamin E (Fleshner 2002). Many in vitro studies have shown that vitamin E can have beneficial impact on carcinogenesis. Vitamin E has been found to be an antioxidant, detoxifying free radicals that interfere with the cellular mechanisms important in cell growth and differentiation including the mechanisms involved in PCa (Fleshner 2002). Other roles of vitamin E include as an anti-prostaglandin; prostaglandins are believed to have some role in prostate carcinogenesis (Badawi 2000). Vitamin E has also been shown to induce cell cycle arrest as well as an upregulation in cell cycle regulatory molecules (Venkateswaran et al. 2002).

Selenium is a trace element found in seafood, meat, and grains. An excess of selenium results in decrease of natural killer cell activity, modulation in synthesis of thyroid hormones, nail and hair loss, and dermatitis (Vinceti et al. 2001). On the other hand, selenium is also known to be acting as an antioxidant, antiproliferative agent and it also results in induction of apoptosis and modulation of androgen levels (Klein and Thompson 2004; Zhao et al. 2004).

Two studies that looked at preventing other cancers suggest that selenium and vitamin E might prevent PCa. In a study conducted in the United States by Clark et al. (Clark et al. 1996), PCa incidence was found to be reduced by two-thirds among men taking selenium on a daily basis. In the Alpha-Tocopherol, Beta-

Carotene Study (Heinonen et al. 1998), there was a one-third reduction in PCa incidence and a 40 % reduction in PCa deaths in men taking vitamin E. But neither of these studies focused directly on PCa. So the National Cancer Institute, USA, came up with **Sel**enium and Vitamin **E**Cancer Prevention **T**rial (SELECT), the first study to look directly at the effect of selenium (200 mcg from L-selenomethionine) and/or vitamin E (400 mg of racemic alpha-tocopheryl acetate) on the risk of PCa. This study was undertaken to find out if selenium and/or vitamin E can really prevent PCa. The SELECT trial reached its full complement of 32,400 men in April 2004 and after 2 years the study concluded that Selenium or vitamin E, alone or in combination at the doses and formulations used, did not prevent prostate cancer in this population of relatively healthy men (Lippman et al. 2009).

The beneficial effects of many other dietary polyphenols have been examined in other studies. Although there are inconsistencies and variability in the outcome of results from these studies, there is a broad consensus that diet-derived polyphenols hold great promise for the management of prostate cancer (Lall et al. 2015).

10 Custom Tailoring of Chemopreventive Regimen for Prostate Cancer

The fact that cancer arises as a result of several genetic mutations resulting in defects in multiple signaling pathways, it is unlikely that any single agent may prove to be totally effective and beneficial on a long-term basis. To achieve greater and long-lasting effects, it is recommended that naturally occurring agents could be combined in a manner that could be more beneficial and at the same time do not exhibit toxicity. It is of interest that several dietary agents that are effective chemopreventive agents in one experimental setting can enhance or have no effects on carcinogenesis in another experimental setting. Thus, custom tailoring of chemopreventive regimens with known mechanisms targeted to individual need is advocated. This concept of combining chemopreventive agents to achieve greater benefits is being increasingly appreciated and studies are being conducted utilizing a combination of natural agents and chemotherapeutic drugs. There is also a need to understand genetic, environmental, and lifestyle factors that influence carcinogenesis in humans and to use this information to help in the selection of an appropriate cancer chemopreventive regimen in individuals with a high risk for cancer development. This approach could be extremely important when a promising chemopreventive agent demonstrates significant efficacy but may produce toxic effects at higher doses. A combined treatment with drugs having different mechanisms is most attractive since they could attack the carcinogenesis process at more than one site or pathway. This could result in the treatment having an additive or a synergistic effect against cancer growth and development. Combined growth inhibitory effects of GTP and COX-2 inhibitor on growth of prostate cancer cells in vivo and in vitro situations were determined (Adhami et al. 2007). This study reported an increased efficacy of selective COX-2 inhibitors in combination with polyphenols from green tea for inhibition of growth of human prostate cancer cells both in vitro and in vivo. The effect was mainly observed due to increased apoptosis following increased activation of caspases 6 and 9. A recent study demonstrated that combined treatment with lycopene and vitamin E, at 5 mg/kg BW each, suppressed orthotopic growth of PC-346C prostate tumors by 73 % and increased median survival time by 40 % (Limpens et al. 2006). In another study, Venkateswaran et al. demonstrated that selenium potentiates vitamin E-induced inhibition of LNCaP cells and this inhibition was demonstrated by a reduction of cells in the S-phase of cell cycle (Venkateswaran et al. 2004). A study by Tokar et al. (2006) examined the effects of synthetic retinoid N-(4-hydroxyphenyl)retinamide (4-HPR) in combination with cholecalciferol (vitamin D3) on growth, and on the expression of vimentin, matrix metalloproteinase-2 (MMP-2), and retinoid and vitamin D receptor (VDR) expression, using the non-tumorigenic, human prostate epithelial cell line RWPE-1. Treatment with 4-HPR and cholecalciferol resulted in synergistic growth inhibition when compared to that caused by each agent alone. Also a decrease in vimentin expression and MMP-2 activity and upregulation of VDR and some of the retinoid-X (RXRs) and retinoic acid receptor (RARs) subtypes were observed. These results suggest that combined treatment with 4-HPR and cholecalciferol, at doses lower than what might be effective with single agents, increase anticancer efficacy. In light of the observations suggesting more beneficial effects with a combination of chemopreventive agents at low doses (Wang et al. 2014; Vyas et al. 2013; Harper et al. 2009; Venkateswaran et al. 2009; McCormick et al. 2007), it is rational and appropriate to design experiments containing a mixture of substances that target multiple signaling pathways. Although a combinatorial approach sounds more rational and realistic, it may need to be carefully monitored for any unwanted side effects.

11 Future Perspectives

The prevailing approach of cancer chemoprevention has been to find effective agents, with acceptable or no toxicity and use them in relatively healthy people or individuals at high risks for cancer development. This concept has not provided the desired because of the fact that single agents, in spite of being effective in highly optimized laboratory conditions, have yielded disappointing results in clinical trials. They differ genetically and in lifestyle, dietary habits, and environmental exposures to name a few. Moreover, most of the single agents tested under laboratory conditions have been found to be effective against only one or few targets making it impossible for a single agent to thwart the menace of cancer.

We, through our extensive studies with different dietary agents, have come up with a three-step approach. In the first step of the approach, we need to identify the defects at genomic and proteomic levels through which particular cancer could occur in humans, and we then need to establish the signature of defects in the individuals for whom chemoprevention is sought. Keeping in mind the outcome of the first step, in the next two steps of the approach, a chemopreventive scientist could custom design a cocktail using an armamentarium of diet-based substances which could ameliorate the biochemical defect(s) that result in the course of action of carcinogenesis (Fig. 1). Regular follow-up might be needed to ensure the repair of aberrant expression of genes and proteins that resulted in cancer onset or development. Keeping this new approach in mind, novel agents and targets are being developed worldwide. Since our approach is relatively inexpensive, simple to use, and possibly nontoxic, studies to assess its role in PCa are accessible and will be of interest. As many in vitro and in vivo studies assessing the role of dietary agents on PCa have shown significant effects against multiple targets, an in-depth analysis of our approach with the chemopreventive cocktail is warranted.

References

Abrahamsen MS, Morris DR (1991) Regulation of expression of the ornithine decarboxylase gene by intracellular signal transduction pathways. In: Inouye M, Campisi J, Cunningham DD, Riley M (eds) Perspectives on cell regulation: from bacteria to cancer. Wiley-Liss Inc., New York, pp 107–119

Adhami VM, Mukhtar H (2013) Human cancer chemoprevention: hurdles and challenges. Top Curr Chem 329:203–220

Adhami VM, Ahmad N, Mukhtar H (2003) Molecular targets for green tea in prostate cancer prevention. J Nutr 133(7 Suppl):2417S–2424S

Adhami VM, Siddiqui IA, Ahmad N, Gupta S, Mukhtar H (2004) Oral consumption of green tea polyphenols inhibits insulin-like growth factor-I-induced signaling in an autochthonous mouse model of prostate cancer. Cancer Res 64:8715–8722

Adhami VM, Malik A, Zaman N, Sarfaraz S, Siddiqui IA, Syed DN, Afaq F, Pasha FS, Saleem M, Mukhtar H (2007) Combined inhibitory effects of green tea polyphenols and selective cyclooxygenase-2 inhibitors on the growth of human prostate cancer cells both in vitro and in vivo. Clin Cancer Res 13(5):1611–1619

Afaq F, Saleem M, Krueger C, Reed J, Mukhtar H (2005) Anthocyanin- and hydrolyzable tannin-rich pomegranate fruit extract modulates MAPK and NF-kappaB pathways and inhibits skin tumorigenesis in CD-1 mice. Intl J Cancer 113:423–433

Ahmad N, Feyes DK, Nieminen AL, Agarwal R, Mukhtar H (1997) Green tea constituent epigallocatechin-3-gallate and induction of apoptosis and cell cycle arrest in human carcinoma cells. J Natl Cancer Inst 89:1881–1886

Albrecht M, Jiang W, Kumi-Diaka J, Lansky EP, Gommersall LM, Patel A, Mansel RE, Neeman I, Geldof AA, Campbell MJ (2004) Pomegranate extracts potently suppress proliferation, xenograft growth, and invasion of human prostate cancer cells. J Med Food 7:274–283

Ames BN (1983) Dietary carcinogens and anticarcinogens. Science 221:1256–1264

Aratanechemuge Y, Hibasami H, Sanpin K, Katsuzaki H, Imai K, Komiya T (2004) Induction of apoptosis by lupeol isolated from mokumen (Gossampinusmalabarica L. Merr) in human promyelotic leukemia HL-60 cells. Oncol Rep 11:289–292

Auvinen M, Paasinen A, Andersson LA, Holtta E (1992) Ornithine decarboxylase activity is critical for cell transformation. Nature (London) 360:355–358

Aviram M, Dornfeld L (2001) Pomegranate juice consumption inhibits serum angiotensin converting enzyme activity and reduces systolic blood pressure. Atherosclerosis 158:195–198

Badawi AF (2000) The role of prostaglandin synthesis in prostate cancer. BJU Int 85:451–462

Beebe-Dimmer JL, Wood DP Jr, Gruber SB, Douglas JA, Bonner JD, Mohai C, Zuhlke KA, Shepherd C, Cooney KA (2004) Use of complementary and alternative medicine in men with family history of prostate cancer: a pilot study. Urology 63:282–287

Bettuzzi S, Brausi M, Rizzi F, Castagnetti G, Peracchia G, Corti A (2006a) Chemoprevention of human prostate cancer by oral administration of green tea catechins in volunteers with high-grade prostate intraepithelial neoplasia: a preliminary report from a one-year proof-of-principle. Cancer Res 66:1234–1240

Bettuzzi S, Brausi M, Rizzi F, Castagnetti G, Peracchia G, Corti A (2006b) Chemoprevention of human prostate cancer by oral administration of green tea catechins in volunteers with high-grade prostate intraepithelial neoplasia: a preliminary report from a one-year proof-of-principle study. Cancer Res 66(2):1234–1240

Boon H, Westlake K, Stewart M, Gray R, Fleshner N, Gavin A, Brown JB, Goel V (2003) Use of complementary/alternative medicine by men diagnosed with prostate cancer: prevalence and characteristics. Urology 62:849–853

Brausi M, Rizzi F, Bettuzzi S (2008) Chemoprevention of human prostate cancer by green tea catechins: two years later. A follow-up update. Eur Urol 54(2):472–473

Brawley OW, Parnes H (2000) Prostate cancer prevention trials in the USA. Eur J Cancer 36:1312–1315

Cao Y, Prescott SM (2002) Many actions of cyclooxygenase-2 in cellular dynamics and in cancer. J Cell Physiol 190:279–286

Clark LC, Combs GF Jr, Turnbull BW, Slate EH, Chalker DK, Chow J, Davis LS, Glover RA, Graham GF, Gross EG, Krongrad A, Lesher JL Jr, Park HK, Sanders BB Jr, Smith CL, Taylor JR (1996) Effects of selenium supplementation for cancer prevention in patients with carcinoma of the skin. A randomized controlled trial Nutritional Prevention of Cancer Study Group. JAMA 276:1957–1963

Fleshner NE (2002) Vitamin E and prostate cancer. Urol Clin North Am 29:107–113

Geetha T, Varalakshmi P (2001) Anti-inflammatory activity of lupeol and lupeollinoleate in rats. J Ethnopharmacol 76:77–80

Gil MI, Tomas-Barberan FA, Hess-Pierce B, Holcroft DM, Kedar AA (2000) Antioxidant activity of pomegranate juice and its relationship with phenolic composition and processing. J Agric Food Chem 10:4581–4589

Greenwald P (2002) Cancer chemoprevention. BMJ 324:714–718

Gupta S, Ahmad N, Mohan RR, Husain MM, Mukhtar H (1999) Prostate cancer chemoprevention by green tea: in vitro and in vivo inhibition of testosterone-mediated induction of ornithine decarboxylase. Cancer Res 59:2115–2120

Gupta S, Ahmad N, Marengo SR, MacLennan GT, Greenberg NM, Mukhtar H (2000a) Chemoprevention of prostate carcinogenesis by alpha-difluoromethylornithine in TRAMP mice. Cancer Res 60:5125–5133

Gupta S, Srivastava M, Ahmad N, Bostwick DG, Mukhtar H (2000b) Over-expression of cyclooxygenase-2 in human prostate adenocarcinoma. Prostate 42:73–78

Gupta S, Ahmad N, Nieminen AL, Mukhtar H (2000c) Growth inhibition, cell-cycle dysregulation, and induction of apoptosis by green tea constituent (-)-epigallocatechin-3-gallate in androgen-sensitive and androgen-insensitive human prostate carcinoma cells. Toxicol Appl Pharmacol 164:82–90

Gupta S, Hastak K, Ahmad N, Lewin JS, Mukhtar H (2001) Inhibition of prostate carcinogenesis in TRAMP mice by oral infusion of green tea polyphenols. Proc Natl Acad Sci U S A 98:10350–10355

Gupta S, Hussain T, Mukhtar H (2003) Molecular pathway for (-)-epigallocatechin-3-gallate-induced cell cycle arrest and apoptosis of human prostate carcinoma cells. Arch Biochem Biophys 410:177–185

Gupta S, Adhami VM, Subbarayan M, MacLennan GT, Lewin JS, Hafeli UO, Fu P, Mukhtar H (2004) Suppression of prostate carcinogenesis by dietary supplementation of celecoxib in transgenic adenocarcinoma of the mouse prostate model. Cancer Res 64:3334–3343

Habel LA, Zhao W, Stanford JL (2002) Daily aspirin use and prostate cancer risk in a large, multiracial cohort in the US. Cancer Causes Control 13:427–434
Harper CE, Cook LM, Patel BB, Wang J, Eltoum IA, Arabshahi A, Shirai T, Lamartiniere CA (2009) Genistein and resveratrol, alone and in combination, suppress prostate cancer in SV-40 tag rats. Prostate 69(15):1668–1682
Hastak K, Gupta S, Ahmad N, Agarwal MK, Agarwal ML, Mukhtar H (2003) Role of p53 and NF-kappaB in epigallocatechin-3-gallate-induced apoptosis of LNCaP cells. Oncogene 22:4851–4859
Hata K, Hori K, Takahashi S (2002) Differentiation- and apoptosis-inducing activities by pentacyclictriterpenes on a mouse melanoma cell line. J Nat Prod 65:645–648
Heilbrun LK, Nomura A, Stemmermann GN (1986) Black tea consumption and cancer risk: a prospective study. Br J Cancer 54:677–683
Heinonen OP, Albanes D, Virtamo J, Taylor PR, Huttunen JK, Hartman AM, Haapakoski J, Malila N, Rautalahti M, Ripatti S, Maenpaa H, Teerenhovi L, Koss L, Virolainen M, Edwards BK (1998) Prostate cancer and supplementation with alpha-tocopherol and beta-carotene: incidence and mortality in a controlled trial. J Natl Cancer Inst 90:440–446
Herberman RB, Pearce HL, Lippman SM, Pyenson BS, Alberts DS (2006) Cancer chemoprevention and cancer preventive vaccines—a call to action: leaders of diverse stakeholder groups present strategies for overcoming multiple barriers to meet an urgent need. Cancer Res 66:11540–11549
Hikosaka A, Asamoto M, Hokaiwado N, Kato K, Kuzutani K, Kohri K, Shirai T (2004) Inhibitory effects of soy isoflavones on rat prostate carcinogenesis induced by 2-amino-1-methyl-6-phenylimidazo[4,5-b]pyridine (PhIP). Carcinogenesis 25:381–387
Hussain T, Gupta S, Adhami VM, Mukhtar H (2005) Green tea constituent epigallocatechin-3-gallate selectively inhibits COX-2 without affecting COX-1 expression in human prostate carcinoma cells. Int J Cancer 113:660–669
Irani J, Ravery V, Pariente JL, Chartier-Kastler E, Lechevallier E, Soulie M, Chautard D, Coloby P, Fontaine E, Bladou F, Desgrandchamps F, Haillot O (2002) Effect of nonsteroidal anti-inflammatory agents and finasteride on prostate cancer risk. J Urol 168:1985–1988
Jain MG, Hislop GT, Howe GR, Burch JD, Ghadirian P (1998) Alcohol and other beverage use and prostate cancer risk among Canadian men. Int J Cancer 78:707–711
Jian L, Xie LP, Lee AH, Binns CW (2004) Protective effect of green tea against prostate cancer: a case-control study in southeast China. Int J Cancer 108:130–135
Kadmon D (1992) Chemoprevention in prostate cancer: the role of difluoromethylornithine (DFMO). J Cell Biochem Suppl 16H:122–127
Kellof GJ, Boone CW, Crowell JA, Steele VE, Lubet R, Doody LA (1994) Chemopreventive drug development: perspective and progress. Cancer Epidemiol Biomarkers Prev 3:85–98
Kelloff GJ, Lippman SM, Dannenberg AJ, Sigman CC, Pearce HL, Reid BJ, Szabo E et al (2006) AACR task force on cancer prevention. Progress in chemoprevention drug development: the promise of molecular biomarkers for prevention of intraepithelial neoplasia and cancer—a plan to move forward. Clin Cancer Res 12:3661–3697
Khan N, Adhami VM, Mukhtar H (2009) Review: green tea polyphenols in chemoprevention of prostate cancer: preclinical and clinical studies. Nutr Cancer 61(6):836–841
Klein EA, Thompson IM (2004) Update on chemoprevention of prostate cancer. Curr Opin Urol 14:143–149
Lall RK, Syed DN, Adhami VM, Khan MI, Mukhtar H (2015) Dietary polyphenols in prevention and treatment of prostate cancer. Int J Mol Sci 16(2):3350–3376
Lan L, Trempus C, Gilmour SK (2000) Inhibition of ornithine decarboxylase (ODC) decreases tumor vascularization and reverses spontaneous tumors in ODC/Ras transgenic mice. Cancer Res 60:5696–5703
Leitzmann MF, Stampfer MJ, Ma J, Chan JM, Colditz GA, Willett WC, Giovannucci E (2002) Aspirin use in relation to risk of prostate cancer. Cancer Epidemiol Biomarkers Prev 11:1108–1111

Liao S, Umekita Y, Guo J, Kokontis JM, Hiipakka RA (1995) Growth inhibition and regression of human prostate and breast tumors in athymic mice by tea epigallocatechingallate. Cancer Lett 96:239–243

Limpens J, Schroder FH, de Ridder CM, Bolder CA, Wildhagen MF, Obermuller-Jevic UC, Kramer K, van Weerden WM (2006) Combined lycopene and vitamin E treatment suppresses the growth of PC-346C human prostate cancer cells in nude mice. J Nutr 136:1287–1293

Lippman SM, Klein EA, Goodman PJ, Lucia MS, Thompson IM, Ford LG, Parnes HL, Minasian LM, Gaziano JM, Hartline JA, Parsons JK, Bearden JD 3rd, Crawford ED, Goodman GE, Claudio J, Winquist E, Cook ED, Karp DD, Walther P, Lieber MM, Kristal AR, Darke AK, Arnold KB, Ganz PA, Santella RM, Albanes D, Taylor PR, Probstfield JL, Jagpal TJ, Crowley JJ, Meyskens FL Jr, Baker LH, Coltman CA Jr (2009) Effect of selenium and vitamin E on risk of prostate cancer and other cancers: the Selenium and Vitamin E Cancer Prevention Trial (SELECT). JAMA 301(1):39–51

Malik A, Afaq F, Sarfaraz S, Adhami VM, Syed DN, Mukhtar H (2005) Pomegranate fruit juice for chemoprevention and chemotherapy of prostate cancer. Proc Natl Acad Sci 102:14813–14818

McCormick DL, Johnson WD, Bosland MC, Lubet RA, Steele VE (2007) Chemoprevention of rat prostate carcinogenesis by soy isoflavones and by Bowman-Birk inhibitor. Nutr Cancer 57 (2):184–193

Meyskens FL Jr, Gerner EW (1999) Development of difluoromethylornithine (DFMO) as a chemoprevention agent. Clin Cancer Res 5:945–951

Modan B (1977) Role of diet in cancer etiology. Cancer 40(4 Suppl):1887–1891

Mohan RR, Challa A, Gupta S, Bostwick DG, Ahmad N, Agarwal R, Marengo SR, Amini SB, Paras F, MacLennan GT, Resnick MI, Mukhtar H (1999) Overexpression of ornithine decarboxylase in prostate cancer and prostatic fluid in humans. Clin Cancer Res 5:143–147

Mukhtar H (2012) Chemoprevention: making it a success story for controlling human cancer. Cancer Lett 326(2):123–127

Mukhtar H, Ahmad N (1999) Cancer chemoprevention: future holds in multiple agents: contemporary issues in toxicology. Toxicol Appl Pharmacol 158:207–210

Pantuck AJ, Leppert JT, Zomorodian N, Aronson W, Hong J, Barnard RJ, Seeram N, Liker H, Wang H, Elashoff R, Heber D, Aviram M, Ignarro L, Belldegrun A (2006) Phase II study of pomegranate juice for men with rising prostate-specific antigen following surgery or radiation for prostate cancer. Clin Cancer Res 12:4018–4026

Paschka AG, Butler R, Young CY (1998) Induction of apoptosis in prostate cancer cell lines by the green tea component, (-)-epigallocatechin-3-gallate. Cancer Lett 130:1–7

Pegg AE, Shantz LM, Coleman CS (1995) Ornithine decarboxylase as a target for chemoprevention. J Cell Biochem 22:132–138

Pruthi RS, Derksen E, Gaston K, Wallen EM (2004) Rationale for use of cyclooxygenase-2 inhibitors in prevention and treatment of bladder cancer. Urology 64:637–642

Ren S, Lien EJ (1997) Natural products and their derivatives as cancer chemopreventive agents. Prog Drug Res 48:147–171

Roberts RO, Jacobson DJ, Girman CJ, Rhodes T, Lieber MM, Jacobsen SJ (2002) A population-based study of daily nonsteroidal anti-inflammatory drug use and prostate cancer. Mayo Clin Proc 77:219–225

Royle JS, Ross JA, Ansell I, Bollina P, Tulloch DN, Habib FK (2004) Nitric oxide donating nonsteroidal anti-inflammatory drugs induce apoptosis in human prostate cancer cell systems and human prostatic stroma via caspase-3. J Urol 172:338–344

Saleem M, Alam A, Arifin S, Shah MS, Ahmed B, Sultana S (2001) Lupeol, a triterpene, inhibits early responses of tumor promotion induced by benzoyl peroxide in murine skin. Pharmacol Res 43:127–134

Saleem M, Afaq F, Adhami VM, Mukhtar H (2004) Lupeol modulates NF-kappaB and PI3K/Akt pathways and inhibits skin cancer in CD-1 mice. Oncogene 23:5203–5214

Saleem M, Kweon MH, Yun JM, Adhami VM, Khan N, Syed DN, Mukhtar H (2005) A novel dietary triterpeneLupeol induces fas-mediated apoptotic death of androgen-sensitive prostate cancer cells and inhibits tumor growth in a xenograft model. Cancer Res 65:11203–11213

Santillo VM, Lowe F (2006) Role of vitamins, minerals and supplements in the prevention and management of prostate cancer. Int Braz J Urol 32:3–14

Siddiqui IA, Zaman N, Aziz MH, Reagan-Shaw SR, Sarfaraz S, Adhami VM, Ahmad N, Raisuddin S, Mukhtar H (2006) Inhibition of CWR22Rν1 tumor growth and PSA secretion in athymic nude mice by green and black teas. Carcinogenesis 27:833–839

Siegel RL, Miller KD, Jemal A (2015) Cancer statistics, 2015. CA Cancer J Clin 65(1):5–29

Simoneau AR, Gerner EW, Phung M, McLaren CE, Meyskens FL Jr (2001) Alpha-difluoromethylornithine and polyamine levels in the human prostate: results of a phase IIa trial. J Natl Cancer Inst 93:57–59

Surh YJ (2003) Cancer chemoprevention with dietary phytochemicals. Nat Rev Cancer 3:768–780

Tokar EJ, Ablin RJ, Webber MM (2006) Cholecalciferol (vitamin D3) and the retinoid N-(4-hydroxyphenyl)retinamide (4-HPR) are synergistic for chemoprevention of prostate cancer. J Exp Ther Oncol 1.5:323–333

Tsao AS, Kim ES, Hong WK (2004) Chemoprevention of cancer. CA Cancer J Clin 54:150–180

Venkateswaran V, Fleshner NE, Klotz LH (2002) Modulation of cell proliferation and cell cycle regulators by vitamin E in human prostate carcinoma cell lines. J Urol 168:1578–1582

Venkateswaran V, Fleshner NE, Klotz LH (2004) Synergistic effect of vitamin E and selenium in human prostate cancer cell lines. Prostate Cancer Prostatic Dis 7:54–56

Venkateswaran V, Klotz LH, Ramani M, Sugar LM, Jacob LE, Nam RK, Fleshner NE (2009) A combination of micronutrients is beneficial in reducing the incidence of prostate cancer and increasing survival in the Lady transgenic model. Cancer Prev Res (Phila) 2(5):473–483

Vinceti M, Wei ET, Malagoli C, Bergomi M, Vivoli G (2001) Adverse health effects of selenium in humans. Rev Environ Health 16:233–251

Vyas AR, Hahm ER, Arlotti JA, Watkins S, Stolz DB, Desai D, Amin S, Singh SV (2013) Chemoprevention of prostate cancer by d, l-sulforaphane is augmented by pharmacological inhibition of autophagy. Cancer Res 73(19):5985–5995

Wang P, Vadgama JV, Said JW, Magyar CE, Doan N, Heber D, Henning SM (2014) Enhanced inhibition of prostate cancer xenograft tumor growth by combining quercetin and green tea. J Nutr Biochem 25(1):73–80

Wattenberg LW (1990) Inhibition of carcinogenesis by naturally occurring and synthetic compounds. In: Kuroda Y, Shankel DM, Waters MD (eds) Antimutagenesis and anticarcinogenesis mechanisms II. Plenum press, New York, pp 155–166

Williams CS, Mann M, DuBois RN (1999) The role of cyclooxygenases in inflammation, cancer, and development. Oncogene 18:7908–7916

Yu HN, Yin JJ, Shen SR (2004) Growth inhibition of prostate cancer cells by epigallocatechingallate in the presence of Cu2+. J Agric Food Chem 52:462–466

Zhao H, Whitfield ML, Xu T, Botstein D, Brooks JD (2004) Diverse effects of methylseleninic acid on the transcriptional program of human prostate cancer cells. Mol Biol Cell 15:506–519

Making Sense of Antioxidant–Pro-oxidant Conundrum in Anticancer Research

SM Hadi and Mohd Farhan

Abstract Plant-derived dietary antioxidants have attracted considerable interest in recent past for their ability to induce apoptosis and regression of tumors in animal models. While it is believed that the antioxidant properties of these agents may contribute to lowering the risk of cancer induction by impeding oxidative injury to DNA, it could not account for apoptosis induction and chemotherapeutic observations. We have provided a number of evidence that dietary antioxidants can alternatively switch to a pro-oxidant action in the presence of transition metals such as copper. Such a pro-oxidant action leads to strand breaks in cellular DNA and growth inhibition in cancer cells.

1 Introduction

The term antioxidant is applied to small molecules and enzymes that are generally of biological origin and are capable of scavenging or eliminating oxygen radicals such as superoxide anion and the hydroxyl radical. Such metabolites are both endogenous and exogenous in origin. Some chemically synthesized molecules also exhibit antioxidant activity. The metabolites of endogenous origin include glutathione, vitamin E, ascorbic acid, and enzymes such as superoxide dismutase, glutathione peroxidase, etc. The exogenous molecules are essentially secondary metabolites that are synthesized by plants as a defense mechanism against attack by bacteria, fungi, and viruses. These include various classes of plant polyphenols such as flavonoids (quercetin), stilbenes (resveratrol), and curcuminoids (curcumin). Epidemiological studies have suggested that human consumption of fruits, vegetables. and beverages such as green tea and red wine is associated with a reduced risk of cardiovascular disease and certain types of cancers (Vainio and Weiderpress 2006). Plant polyphenols are essential components of human diet and the above chemopreventive properties have been attributed to the ingestion of these secondary metabolites. Plant polyphenols are both capable of generating as well as scavenging

S. Hadi, Ph.D. (✉) • M. Farhan
Department of Biochemistry, AMU, Aligarh, Uttar Pradesh 202001, India
e-mail: smhadi@vsnl.com

M.F. Ullah, A. Ahmad (eds.), *Critical Dietary Factors in Cancer Chemoprevention*,
DOI 10.1007/978-3-319-21461-0_3

reactive oxygen species (ROS) and therefore can act both as pro-oxidants and antioxidants. Since ROS can promote cancer by generating mutations and activating biochemical pathways that promote cell proliferation, they were earlier considered as dietary mutagens (Bjeldanes and Chang 1977). However, in the last decade there has been increasing realization that the anticancer property of polyphenols is related to their pro-oxidant action (Hadi et al. 2007, 2010). In this context, it is important to note that most clinically used anticancer agents are themselves capable of inducing cancer under appropriate conditions (Lavie et al. 2008). Most interestingly, there are several studies to suggest that plant polyphenols are cytotoxic to cancer cells whereas normal cells are refractory to such an action (Inoue et al. 1994; Khan et al. 2014).

2 Evidence of Pro-oxidant Action as Anticancer Mechanism

In the last decade or so, we in our lab have been working in elucidating a putative anticancer mechanism of plant polyphenols that involves mobilization of endogenous copper ions and consequent pro-oxidant action leading to cellular DNA breakage (Hadi et al. 2000). This property is related to the number and position of hydroxyl groups in the polycyclic structure of polyphenols (Jain et al. 1999). For example, the parent compound of stilbenes (trans-stilbene) (Azmi et al. 2006) which does not possess any hydroxyl group is ineffective in cellular DNA degradation. It must be noted that copper is a major metal ion present in the nucleus and its level is considerably elevated in almost all malignancies (Hadi et al. 2010; Gupte and Mumper 2008). The elevated copper level in malignant cells facilitates electron transfer between polyphenols and copper leading to formation of Cu(I) whose reoxidation in the presence of molecular oxygen leads to ROS formation (Rahman et al. 1989). This would account for the preferential cytotoxicity of plant polyphenols for cancer cells. In addition to the evidence we have deduced, there is considerable supporting data in the literature which suggests that pro-oxidant action of plant polyphenols rather than their antioxidant property is important for their anticancer properties. These include the relatively low reduction potential of copper versus other metal ions in cells such as iron and the fact that the hydroxyl radical whose diffusion radius is very small has the possibility of being generated close to the cellular DNA as copper ions are bound to GC base pairs (Govindaraju et al. 2013). Inspite of compelling epidemiological and experimental evidence in favor of anticancer property of plant polyphenols, these compounds have failed to reduce incidence of cancer in human clinical trials (Elizabeth et al. 2014). The reason is possibly the fact that plant polyphenols are rapidly metabolized and eliminated before sufficiently cytotoxic intracellular concentrations are achieved for the required length of time (Asensi et al. 2002). Thus, there is considerable skepticism about the benefits of plant polyphenols as anticancer or cancer preventive agents. Indeed, the antioxidants *n*-acetyl cysteine and vitamin E were recently shown to actually increase cancer mortality in a mouse model (Sayin et al. 2014). However, given the chemical structure of *n*-acetyl cysteine and vitamin E, they do not appear to be efficient copper chelators and this possibly explains their non-effect in a tumor model.

Ascorbic acid is the other endogenous antioxidant and it is well established that it possesses both antioxidant as well pro-oxidant properties (Ullah et al. 2011; Yen et al. 2002). Levine and coworkers (Chen et al. 2008) have demonstrated that pharmacological ascorbic acid concentrations achievable through intravenous administration were cytotoxic to many types of cancer cells in vivo and significantly impeded tumor progression without toxicity to normal tissues. Although an interesting mechanism of action was suggested that involved ascorbic acid-induced formation of H_2O_2 in the extracellular fluid leading to the observed cytotoxic effects, the authors were not clear about the molecular basis for the relative resistance of normal cells. Moreover, it is well known that H_2O_2 is freely permeable to both normal and cancer cells (Halliwell 2003; Clement et al. 2002; Shamim et al. 2008). In one of our papers (Ullah et al. 2011), we have explained the relative resistance of normal cells by showing that ascorbic acid is a good reducer of copper and is capable of mobilizing copper from chromatin in a mechanism similar to that of plant polyphenols. Thus, the structural differences between various antioxidants are important in determining whether a given antioxidant could also serve as a pro-oxidant and be effective against cancer cells.

Ascorbic acid is already used by many clinicians as an adjunct to chemotherapy in cancer patients (Vollbracht et al. 2011). Similarly plant polyphenols have been shown to potentiate the efficacy of radiotherapy in various tumors (Garg et al. 2005). Clearly the usefulness of antioxidants for cancer prevention and therapeutic action particularly those that are capable of mobilizing chromatin-bound copper cannot be discounted. The answer possibly lies in using plant polyphenols as lead compounds to synthesize novel molecules that are capable of binding and reducing copper but have greater bioavailability. It is now recognized that a vast majority of agents used to directly kill cancer cells such as ionizing radiation and chemotherapeutic agents work through generating reactive oxygen species that block key steps in the cell cycle (Watson 2013).

3 Conclusion

Thus, the current interest in anticancer research has moved to curing of cancer on the biochemistry of cancer cells. In this context, our studies assume considerable significance as they provide a basis for designing novel anticancer compounds based on targeting elevated copper levels in cancer cells.

References

Asensi M, Medina I, Ortega A, Corretera J, Carmen-Bano M, Obrador E, Estrela MJ (2002) Inhibition of cancer growth by resveratrol is related to its low bioavailability. Free Radic Biol Med 33:387–398

Azmi AS, Bhat SH, Hanif S, Hadi SM (2006) Plant polyphenols mobilize endogenous copper in human peripheral lymphocytes leading to oxidative DNA breakage: a putative mechanism for anticancer properties. FEBS Lett 580:533–538

Bjeldanes LF, Chang GW (1977) Mutagenic activity of quercetin and related compounds. Science 197:577–578

Chen Q, Espey MG, Sun AY, Pooput C, Kirk KL, Krishna MC, Khosh DB, Drisko J, Levine M (2008) Pharmacologic doses of ascorbate act as a prooxidant and decrease growth aggressive tumor xenografts in mice. Proc Natl Acad Sci U S A 105:11105–11109

Clement MV, Long LH, Ramalingam J, Halliwell B (2002) The cytotoxicity of dopamine may be an artifact of cell culture. J Neurochem 81:414–421

Elizabeth GP, Navdeep SC, David AT (2014) The promise and perils of antioxidants for cancer patients. N Engl J Med 371:177

Garg AK, Buchholz TA, Aggarwal BB (2005) Chemosensitization and radiosensitization of tumors by plant polyphenols. Antioxid Redox Signal 7:1630–1647

Govindaraju M, Shekar HS, Sateesha SB, Vasudeva P, Raju KR, Rao S, Rao KSJ, Rajamma AJ (2013) Copper interactions with DNA of chromatin and its role in neurodegenerative disorders. J Pharm Anal 3:354–359

Gupte A, Mumper RG (2008) Elevated copper and oxidative stress in cancer cells as a target for cancer treatment. Cancer Treat Rev 35:32–46

Hadi SM, Asad SF, Singh S, Ahmad A (2000) Putative mechanism for anticancer and apoptosis inducing properties of plant derived polyphenolic compounds. IUBMB Life 50:167–171

Hadi SM, Bhat SH, Azmi AS, Hanif S, Shamim U, Ullah MF (2007) Oxidative breakage of cellular DNA by plant polyphenols: a putative mechanism for anticancer properties. Semin Cancer Biol 17:370–376

Hadi SM, Ullah MF, Azmi AS, Ahmad A, Shamim U, Zubair H, Khan HY (2010) Resveratrol mobilizes endogenous copper in human peripheral lymphocytes leading to oxidative DNA breakage: a putative mechanism for chemoprevention of cancer. Pharm Res 27:979–988

Halliwell B (2003) Oxidative stress in cell culture: an under appreciated problem? FEBS Lett 540:3–6

Inoue M, Suzuki R, Koide T, Sakaguchi N, Ogihara Y, Yabu Y (1994) Antioxidant, gallic acid, induces apoptosis in HL60RG cells. Biochem Biophys Res Commun 204:898–904

Jain A, Martin MC, Parveen N, Khan NU, Parish JH, Hadi SM (1999) Reactivities of flavonoids with different hydroxyl substituents for the cleavage of DNA in the presence of Cu(II). Phytother Res 13:1–4

Khan HY, Zubair H, Faisal M, Ullah MF, Farhan M, Sarkar FH, Ahmad A, Hadi SM (2014) Plant polyphenol induced cell death in human cancer cells involves mobilization of intracellular copper ions and reactive oxygen species generation: a mechanism for cancer chemopreventive action. Mol Nutr Food Res 58:437–446

Lavie O, Barnett-Griness O, Narod SA, Rennert G (2008) The risk of developing uterine sarcoma after tamoxifen use. Int J Gynecol Cancer 18:352–356

Rahman A, Shahabuddin A, Hadi SM, Parish JH, Ainley K (1989) Strand scission in DNA induced by quercetin and Cu(II): role of Cu(I) and oxygen free radicals. Carcinogenesis 10:1833–1839

Sayin VI, Ibrahim MX, Larsson E, Nilsson JA, Lindahl P, Bergo MO (2014) Antioxidants accelerate lung cancer progression in mice. Sci Transl Med 6:221ra15

Shamim U, Hanif S, Ullah MF, Azmi AS, Hadi SM (2008) Plant polyphenols mobilize nuclear copper in human peripheral lymphocytes leading to oxidatively generated DNA breakage: implications for an anticancer mechanism. Free Radic Res 42:764–772

Ullah MF, Khan HY, Zubair H, Shamim U, Hadi SM (2011) The antioxidant ascorbic acid mobilizes nuclear copper leading to a prooxidant breakage of cellular DNA: implications for chemotherapeutic action against cancer. Cancer Chemother Pharmacol 67:103–110

Vainio H, Weiderpress E (2006) Fruit and vegetables in cancer prevention. Nutr Cancer 54:111–142

Vollbracht C, Schneider B, Leendert V, Weiss G, Auerbach L, Beuth J (2011) Intravenous vitamin C administration improves quality of life in breast cancer patients during chemo-/radiotherapy and aftercare: results of a retrospective, multicentre, epidemiological cohort study in Germany. In Vivo 25:983–990

Watson J (2013) Oxidants, antioxidants and the current incurability of metastatic cancers. Open Biol 3:120144

Yen GC, Duh PD, Tsai HL (2002) Antioxidant and pro-oxidant properties of ascorbic acid and gallic acid. Food Chem 79:307–313

Part II
Elements of Dietary Approaches to Cancer Chemoprevention

Phytocomplexity: The Key to Rational Chemoprevention

Sushma R. Gundala, M. Hope Robinson, and Ritu Aneja

Abstract Current chemotherapies have been derived from and inspired by the varied natural repository of phytochemicals and have been the linchpin of cancer treatment for years. However, isolation of individual active ingredients has proven to be expensive while offering narrow therapeutic windows and associated toxicities. In contrast, whole foods are endowed with an intricate natural balance among their constituent phytochemicals and have proven to impart optimal health benefits, leading to an enhanced interest in dietary interventions to treat as well as prevent cancer. Several dietary agents including fruits, vegetables, and spices have been investigated for their therapeutic and preventive efficacies. However, their incorporation in therapeutic regimens has been unsuccessful due to inadequate research emphasis on *phytocomplexity*, the intricate and dynamic interactions among pharmacologically active plant chemicals, and their inactive counterparts within their natural milieu, which affect the absorption, distribution, metabolism, and excretion of the constituent phytochemicals, conferring bioactivity on the plant-derived foods. This chapter illustrates the need to acknowledge the role of phytocomplexity and the possibility of synergistic activity in the current approach pertaining to dietary agents.

1 Role of Dietary Phytochemicals in Chemotherapy and Chemoprevention

Cancer is arguably the deadliest modern illness with its high incidence, puzzling questions surrounding its causes, and the challenges of its prevention and treatment modalities. As devastating as the effects of the disease can be, the treatments can be equally debilitating and frequently ineffective and often result in long-term morbidity for patients. Cancer can occur due to internal factors like inherited mutations and environmental factors such as lifestyle choices, exposure to carcinogens, or infectious organisms (Anand et al. 2008). Although some of the environmental factors leading to cancer are unavoidable, epidemiological studies have shown that

S.R. Gundala • M.H. Robinson • R. Aneja (✉)
Department of Biology, Georgia State University, Atlanta, GA 30303, USA
e-mail: raneja@gsu.edu

M.F. Ullah, A. Ahmad (eds.), *Critical Dietary Factors in Cancer Chemoprevention*,
DOI 10.1007/978-3-319-21461-0_4

lifestyle choices regarding tobacco use, sun exposure, diet, and exercise could affect the onset of this deadly disease. One-third of the estimated cancer cases in the United States have been linked to obesity, lack of physical activity, and improper diet and nutrition (Hanahan and Weinberg 2000, 2011). Though several treatment modalities are in place including surgery, radiation, chemotherapy, immunotherapy, laser therapy, etc., they have all met with limited success. Currently, chemotherapy is the most prominent treatment for cancer, which employs the use of a single molecule or multidrug combinatory therapy that targets multiple aspects of the disease. A vast majority of the drugs thus employed have been individual components identified and purified from the unlimited archive of plant chemicals.

Nature abounds in fruits, vegetables, and other plants in a myriad of colors, flavors, aromas, and textures. Plants have evolved under the same conditions as humans and were subject to similar environmental stressors, resulting in the survival and propagation of only those capable of producing protective defensive chemicals, known as phytochemicals (Liu 2004). These compounds are often associated with a reduced risk of major chronic diseases in humans as well and recently have been the object of an explosive increase in research, resulting in the discovery and promotion of these plant chemicals as highly effective medications such as aspirin from willow, vinblastine from vinca, taxol from pacific yew, catechins from green tea, resveratrol from grapes, proanthocyanidins from grape seed extracts, isothiocyanates from cruciferous vegetables, and curcuminoids from turmeric (Surh 2003; Surh et al. 2001; Quideau et al. 2011). Extensive research of the chemopreventive mechanisms inherent in bioactive phytochemicals has provided crucial clues as to how to modulate the physiological cascades within cancer cells in an effort to fight against this malicious disease. Several such classes of phytochemicals including phenolic compounds, anthocyanins, terpenoids, aromatic acids, vitamins, carotenoids, alkaloids, and glucosinolates have been shown to be selective and nontoxic in nature, and effective in one or more of the three phases of carcinogenesis, suggesting a role for these compounds in both prevention and treatment of cancer (Liu 2004; Mehta et al. 2010).

However, the beneficial effects of fruits, vegetables, and other plants may also be appreciated when ingested as part of the human diet, and in fact may confer superior health benefits as a whole food rather than individual constituents. Several initiatives including Five-a-Day and Savor the Spectrum have been issued by the National Cancer Institute (NCI) to emphasize the importance of including fruits and vegetables in the daily diet as a part of chemopreventive measures (Colli and Amling 2009; Steinkellner et al. 2001; Traka et al. 2008). In 2012, the American Cancer Society published "Guidelines on Nutrition and Physical Activity for Cancer Prevention" which recommends a healthy diet emphasizing plant foods as opposed to nutritional supplements, even suggesting that synergistic effects are possible upon consumption of whole foods (Kushi et al. 2012). Substantial evidence has revealed that a wholesome diet comprised of fruits, vegetables, and whole grains, including the accompanying dietary fibers, has protective and preventive effects against various cancers. With an intricate network of phytochemicals and a preserved natural balance among their constituents as bestowed by Mother Nature, whole foods have thus been drawing attention to dietary interventions for treatment and prevention of cancer.

2 Phytocomplexity Among Whole Food Extracts: The Art of Simplicity in a Puzzle of Complexity

There is a great deal of research regarding plant-based foods and the potential to exploit the natural compounds contained therein for therapeutic benefit, but this research also casts doubt on the prevailing reductionist focus on individual constituents as opposed to the whole food. Although this approach of disassembly has provided many promising leads, it has thus far failed to yield an individual component acting alone that definitively suppresses carcinogenesis significantly in humans without inflicting serious toxicity to the patient. There have been several trials in the past employing individual phytochemicals like β-carotene, α-tocopherol, etc., but with no evidence of health benefits (Greenberg et al. 1994; Liu 2004; Tsao et al. 2004). Vitamins and minerals like B6, folic acid, iron, magnesium, zinc, and copper were also found to have therapeutic properties (Surh 2003). However, it has been revealed that these phytochemicals must be consumed in large quantities to achieve the physiologically relevant doses capable of delivering optimal health benefits (Potter 2014). Such high doses of bioactive phytochemicals often result in cellular and organ toxicity. Similarly, current plant-based chemotherapeutic drugs exert undesirable side effects, despite their lower effective doses, thus categorizing them as toxic drugs. Clinical trials of several individual constituents also led to startling observations indicating that they may increase the risk of lung and colorectal cancer (1994; Albanes et al. 2000; Greenwald et al. 2007; Klein et al. 2001). The idea of purifying a single agent from a complex natural material has led us to mistakenly assume that only one or a few components of a plant are responsible for the efficacy.

Researchers and drug industries have invested in designing and producing purified drugs directed toward specific ligands acting on disease targets, but the recent years have witnessed an increasing failure of such "targeted" agents. These outcomes were mainly due to the fact that cancer has a multifactorial pathogenesis and aiming at a single target in a specific pathway cannot be completely effective in eradicating cancer, as metastasis and relapse are prominent during these therapies. Additionally, such a selective approach has been found to result in unexpected biochemical effects, leading to toxicity (Liu 2004). To address these failures, scientists have focused on multitargeted therapies employing combination chemotherapy, where a concoction of two or more chemotherapeutic drugs is administered, but the toxicity issues persisted.

The solution to this baffling issue rests with Mother Nature, particularly in the form of whole foods. The current approach does not consider the prospects of natural phytochemical cocktails that can deliver maximum health benefits due to phytocomplexity, the intricate and dynamic interactions among pharmacologically active plant chemicals and their inactive counterparts within their natural milieu, which affect the absorption, distribution, metabolism, and excretion of the constituent phytochemicals,conferring bioactivity on the plant-derived foods. Clearly overlooked in the existing paradigm, the natural balance among various constituent phytochemicals in whole foods may not only solve the toxicity issues resulting from high doses of single components, but would also allow the multiple target approach using a single dose. In contrast to individual components, the additive and synergistic interactions among these phytochemicals support multiple roles as diverse as preventing DNA mutations, impeding cell cycle, inhibiting cell proliferation, inducing apoptosis, and even modifying immune responses. These outcomes may be due to their physiological functions, i.e., modulations in the solubility, absorption, biotransformation, and even elimination of these active ingredients. The complexity of phytochemical interactions in whole foods thus delivers desired beneficial effects while possibly eliminating the harmful effects associated with individual components (Liu 2004). Several mechanistic factors such as bioavailability, cellular transport mechanisms, prodrug activation and deactivation of active drug entities, biotransformation, and elimination, all driven by phytocomplexity, are known to govern the efficacy of whole foods.

Every fruit and vegetable is made up of a defined ratio of phytochemicals targeting multiple sites in the body upon ingestion. To accurately access effectiveness, it is crucial to maintain the bioactivity and ratio of the constituent phytochemicals found in whole foods. Critical factors of the scientific research process including possible degradation of active constituents or the quality of plant material processing and fractionation processes could result in loss of or poor activity of isolated entities from whole extracts. Furthermore, lack of understanding pertaining to interactions among constituent phytochemicals, in vivo physiological interplay, and the possibility of biotransformation and absorption at the target sites may have led to ignoring whole foods as effective chemotherapeutic and chemopreventive agents despite their infinite advantages. Hence, acknowledging and preserving the phytocomplexity of whole foods while evaluating their therapeutic efficacies is critical to this research.

In all these noble efforts, we have overlooked that the complex mixture of constituents in plants is like a puzzle; each piece separately can only hint at the potential beauty of the whole image, but when fit together in the right ratios and combinations while acknowledging phytocomplexity, an astounding work of art may be revealed.

This chapter attempts to emphasize the role of phytocomplexity while discussing several phytochemical-rich fruits and vegetables common to the American diet. Among the various phytochemical groups including vitamins, carotenoids, phenolics, alkaloids, nitrogen-containing compounds, and organosulfur compounds, phenolics are likely the most researched and are believed to be responsible for many of the observed anticancer properties of fruits and vegetables (Huang et al. 2010; Wang et al. 2011). For example, Broccoli, a cruciferous vegetable, has the highest phenolic content among vegetables routinely consumed in the USA (Liu 2004), while apples are at the top of the list of fruits, second only to cranberries for phenolic content (USDA 2011). Tomatoes are known for containing the carotenoid lycopene, which has been the subject of extensive research, particularly in regard to prostate cancer, the second leading cause of cancer-related deaths in the USA (Tanaka et al. 2012). While previously less prominent in the American diet, both pomegranates and ginger produce abundant phytochemicals and have been gaining attention in recent years for their valuable benefits to human health (Baliga et al. 2011; Butt and Sultan 2011; Karna et al. 2012; Reuben et al. 2012). A careful analysis and evaluation of the research on apples, pomegranates, tomatoes, cruciferous vegetables, and ginger illustrates the phytocomplexity involved in the exploration of phytochemicals and the possibility of chemopreventive and chemotherapeutic benefits to human health.

2.1 The Appeal of the Apple: Its Countless Core Values

Apples are a ubiquitous fruit, available worldwide in many cultivars, each containing an assortment of phytochemicals represented mainly by polyphenolics. Several investigations have illustrated an inverse relationship between apple intake and a number of cancers, notably lung and colorectal cancers (Boyer and Liu 2004; Feskanich et al. 2000). Other studies have linked a lower risk of lung cancer with intake of dietary flavonoids including quercetin and catechin, key phytochemicals found in apples (Boyer and Liu 2004; Arts et al. 2001; Knekt et al. 1997; Le Marchand et al. 2000). Numerous studies lend support to the idea that apple products benefit human health by many possible mechanisms, acting individually and in concert with each other. Some of the health benefits of apples include antimutagenic, anti-inflammatory, antioxidant, antiproliferative, and apoptosis-inducing activities in addition to modulation of carcinogen metabolism (Gerhauser 2008). Chemical analysis has provided a wealth of information about the constituents found in apples. Aside from water, fiber, carbohydrates, and minerals, apples contain antioxidants such as vitamin C and a number of polyphenols including chlorogenic acid, epicatechin, phloretin glycosides, procyanidin, and quercetin glycosides (Lee et al. 2003). The quantity and assortment of phytochemicals in apples varies widely, dependent on cultivar, growing conditions, and the timing of fruit harvest.

The distribution of phytochemicals in apples also has important implications when assessing its potential health benefits. Apple peels have been found to contain 3–6 times the polyphenolic content, 2–6 times more antioxidant activity, and have exhibited more potent inhibition of cancer cell growth when compared to the flesh, highlighting the importance of consuming the whole apple in order to achieve optimum benefits (Wolfe et al. 2003). The antioxidant capacity of apple phytochemicals has been well established, with quercetin, catechin, epicatechin, and procyanadin demonstrating the most efficacy, even greater than the well-known antioxidant vitamin C (ascorbic acid) (Eberhardt et al. 2000; Lee et al. 2003). In comparison, greater antiproliferative activity was ascribed to phloridzin, procyanidins, and epicatechin (Serra et al. 2010). While not completely unexpected, the lack of correlation suggests that the observed bioactivities of apples may not be a result of antioxidant activity, but may involve additional targets and mechanisms and could indicate the presence of synergistic interactions between constituents.

2.1.1 Quercetin: The Lone Fighter

Among the polyphenols in apples, quercetin, a dietary flavonoid primarily ingested in onions and apples, has been extensively researched, with quercetin glucosides and their metabolites proving to have powerful antiproliferative and pro-apoptotic activity as well as antioxidative function (Gibellini et al. 2011; Russo et al. 2012). In addition, quercetin displays activity in all phases of carcinogenesis by acting on multiple attributes and processes of cancer initiation, promotion, and progression (Russo et al. 2012). In vitro studies have shown that quercetin inhibits cellular proliferation in several cancer cell lines including cervical, breast, prostate, pancreatic, brain, liver, and colon cancers at a wide range of doses between 17.1 and 178 μM as shown in Table **1** (Chou et al. 2010; Senthilkumar et al. 2011; Vidya Priyadarsini et al. 2010; Harris et al. 2012; He and Liu 2008; Michaud-Levesque et al. 2012; Zhang et al. 2012).

Animal studies have further confirmed the chemopreventive and chemotherapeutic properties of quercetin. Administration of quercetin to rats provided protection from sodium fluoride-induced oxidative stress in *N*-Nitrosodiethylamine (NDEA)-induced hepatocarcinoma (Nabavi et al. 2012; Seufi et al. 2009). Chemopreventive effect was observed with a significant reduction in the incidence and

Table 1 Antiproliferative activity of quercetin

Cell line	Reported IC_{50} (μM)	Concentration (in μg/mL)	Citations
Cervical HeLa	80	24.18	Priyadarsini et al. (2011)
Breast MCF-7	92.4	27.93	Chou et al. (2010)
Prostate PC-3	100	30.22	Senthilkumar et al. (2011)
Pancreatic MIA PaCa-2	178	53.80	Harris et al. (2012)
Glioblastoma U87	17.1	5.17	Michaud-levesque et al. (2012)
Glioblastoma T98G	24.3	7.34	Michaud-levesque et al. (2012)
Colon LoVo	40.2	12.15	Zhang et al. (2012)
Breast MCF-7	30.8	9.31	Zhang et al. (2012)
Liver HepG2	40.9	12.36	He and Liu (2008)
Breast MCF-7	137.5	41.56	He and Liu (2008)

tumor burden of 7,12-dimethylbenz[a] anthracene (DMBA)-induced hamster buccal pouch carcinomas when simultaneously treated by intragastric administration of quercetin, while hamsters treated after DMBA was discontinued benefitted from a significant delay in tumor growth (Priyadarsini et al. 2011). Quercetin provided a reduction of tumor burden in lung and mammary carcinomas as well as decreased incidence of aberrant crypt foci and pre-neoplastic lesions of the colon (Gibellini et al. 2011). Taken together, these results demonstrate the potential of quercetin in prevention and treatment of cancer, but also serve to illustrate the need for further mechanistic in vitro and in vivo research of this apple flavonoid.

While the data on quercetin are compelling, the role of other components in quercetin containing foods has become a subject of debate. In apples, there is preliminary evidence that procyanidins may exert stronger antioxidant and antiproliferative activity than quercetin (Gerhauser 2008). An apple juice procyanidin fraction inhibited proliferation of colon cancer cells more effectively than another fraction with catechin, epicatechin, and quercetin, even at double the dose (Gosse et al. 2005). Further inquiry in a rat model concurred by exhibiting a 50 % reduction in the number of pre-neoplastic colonic lesions in rats fed with 0.01 % procyanidin fraction added to drinking water when compared to control rats (Gosse et al. 2005). Apple procyanidins exhibited 2.5× higher antiproliferative activity than apple polyphenols in mouse melanoma cells and 5× higher in mouse mammary cells, results that were also supported by follow-up in vivo research (Miura et al. 2008). A comparison of the antiproliferative activity of apple waste fractions of extractable polyphenols (EPP) and non-extractable polyphenols (NEPP) in cervical, hepatic, and colon cancer cell lines suggested that the NEPP fraction, containing mostly anthocyanidins, exerted higher inhibitory activity in all cell lines (Tow et al. 2011). In addition to cyanidins, several triterpenoids isolated from apple peels have exhibited significant antiproliferative activity in liver, breast, and colon cancer cells at doses ranging from 4.7 μM to 136 μM (He and Liu 2007). Although continued research on these individual apple phytochemicals is vital to discover molecular drug targets and mechanisms, a comprehensive understanding of the interactions between these varied and plentiful constituents of apples warrants serious consideration.

2.1.2 A Whole Apple a Day Fights the Disease Away

While numerous studies have focused on the bioactivity of single phytochemicals, there is considerable data on whole apples, apple juices, and apple extracts, which supply ample evidence of synergistic effects between apple components. Apple extracts have shown in vitro efficacy in a broad array of cancer cell lines, and significant inhibition of mammary carcinogenesis, skin papillomas, solid tumors, and metastasis of lung and lymph nodes has been reported in several in vivo investigations.

Whole apple extracts from nine cultivars native to Portugal were evaluated in colon and gastric cancer cells, reporting significant antiproliferative activity from all cultivars with effective doses (ED_{50}s) from 9.0 to 49.0 mg/mL (Serra et al. 2010). Intriguingly, the cultivar with the most antiproliferative activity did not have the highest quercetin content. In fact, an extract containing nearly four times the quercetin was a less potent inhibitor of cell growth, suggesting that while quercetin does have anticancer activity, it is not working alone and the observed bioactivity can be attributed to other compounds or synergy between the complex blend of phytochemicals in apples. Inhibition of breast cancer cell proliferation was accomplished by apple extracts in both MCF-7 estrogen receptor (ER)-positive cells and with twice the efficacy in ER-negative MDA-MB-231 cells (Sun and Liu 2008; Yoon and Liu 2007). Separately, apple peel extracts significantly suppressed cell growth in breast cancer cells overexpressing ErbB2 as well as those with normal levels of ErbB2 (Reagan-Shaw et al. 2010). Additionally, both androgen-dependent and androgen-independent prostate cancer cell proliferation was inhibited by these apple peel extracts, which could prove advantageous in some chemo-resistant cancers (Reagan-Shaw et al. 2010).

Oral administration of whole apple extracts equivalent to human consumption of 1, 3, and 6 apples per day demonstrated dose-dependent reduction of mammary tumor incidence and tumor burden in rats (Liu et al. 2005, 2009). A comparison of clear and cloudy apple juice ingestion in a rat colon cancer model revealed considerably increased preventive potential of cloudy apple juice despite comparable polyphenolic content of the two juices with the exception of 30 % more procyanidins and a fourfold increase of pectin in the cloudy juice (Barth et al. 2005). While clear apple juice provided modest reductions in genetic damage and proliferation, rats given cloudy apple juice were observed to develop 50 % fewer large aberrant crypt foci (ACF) as well as a significant decrease in the total number of these pre-neoplastic lesions (Barth et al. 2005). Subsequent research compared cloudy apple juice to polyphenolic and cloudy fractions as well as a combination of the two fractions in an effort to ascertain the fraction of the juice with the most potent anticancer properties (Barth et al. 2007). While all preparations reduced hyperproliferation of epithelial cells in the colon as evidenced by the percentage of BrdU-positive cells, cloudy apple juice outperformed the juice fractions and even the combination fraction in reducing DNA damage and provided a 35 % decrease in the development of large ACF. One of the prevailing theories for the effectiveness of natural products holds that the polyphenols are the active "ingredient." These studies illustrate that it is the sum of the components, not just the polyphenols that impart the anticancer benefits seen with apple products (Barth et al. 2007).

There are only a few reports of direct comparisons between whole extracts and individual apple compounds including an in vitro investigation with colon cancer cells comparing an apple flavonoid extract, individual phytochemicals, and a synthetic extract mimicking the original (Veeriah et al. 2006). The natural apple extract was five times more effective than quercetin alone with an EC_{50} of 31.0 μM (phloridzin-equivalents, Ph.E) compared to 148.4 μM for quercetin. The synthetic extract, with an EC_{50} of 59.9 μM Ph.E, was more effective than quercetin but still not as effective as the natural extract (Veeriah et al. 2006), suggesting that there are other components in the natural extract that were not quantified and included in the synthetic extract, lending further support to the idea of superior benefits from whole foods.

An interesting comparison of a whole apple extract, quercetin 3-β-D-glucoside (Q3G), and a combination of the two showed that while both Q3G and apple extracts efficiently inhibited proliferation in MCF-7 breast cancer cells, the combination of the two was considerably more effective, resulting in an EC_{50} which was twofold lower than apple extracts and fourfold lower than Q3G (Yang and Liu 2009). These results suggest that improving on existing combinations from nature may yield more effective treatments than reducing these foods down to their most active ingredient.

Explorations of the anticancer properties of quercetin and whole apple extract have yielded convincing evidence to demonstrate synergy in apples. As shown in Table **1**, in most studies, the doses of quercetin required to inhibit cancer cell proliferation were between 17.1 and 178 μM (5.17 and 53.8 μg/mL), but as a portion of the whole apple extract, quercetin comprises just 0.0000193–0.0072 % meaning its contribution to the observed anticancer effects of whole apple extract amounts to only 0.001737–11.1816 μg/mL, a 2–5-fold difference (Table 2). Clearly, quercetin is only one piece of a complex puzzle (Fig. 1) when it comes to chemoprevention with apples. It is reasonable to suggest that no single component in apples can produce the benefits summarized in this review.

Extensive in vitro and in vivo studies have demonstrated the potential health benefits of apples with the majority of literature supporting both the health benefits from apples and the concept of synergy in apples, implying that this fruit should be consumed frequently and in forms utilizing the whole apple. Future research of mechanisms, molecular targets, and the interactions between apple components may provide direction on how best to capitalize on apple's benefits.

2.2 Pomegranate: Pomtastic Truths About a Time-Honored Healing Fruit

Pomegranates have been consumed as food, used as medicine, and featured prominently in a number of ancient religious traditions. Despite its long history of human applications, scientific research of this fruit is still relatively new, having started in

Table 2 Antiproliferative activity of whole apple extracts with Quercetin contribution to the effect of the whole

Material tested	Cell line	IC_{50} (in mg/mL)	Contribution range of quercetin to IC_{50} (μg/mL) of Whole apple extract		Citations
			Low	High	
Bravo de Esmolfe	Colon HT29	37	0.007141	2.664	Serra (2010)
Malapio Fino		24.8	0.0047864	1.7856	
Malapio de Serra		37	0.007141	2.664	
Pero Pipo		49	0.009457	3.528	
Golden		42.2	0.0081446	3.0384	
Starking		24.1	0.0046513	1.7352	
Fuji		25.8	0.0049794	1.8576	
Gala Galaxy		48	0.009264	3.456	
Reineta Parda		21.1	0.0040723	1.5192	
Bravo de Esmolfe	Gastric MKN45	15	0.002895	1.08	Serra (2010)
Malapio Fino		11.9	0.0022967	0.8568	
Malapio de Serra		19.8	0.0038214	1.4256	
Pero Pipo		13.2	0.0025476	0.9504	
Golden		26.3	0.0050759	1.8936	
Starking		15	0.002895	1.08	
Fuji		17.2	0.0033196	1.2384	
Gala Galaxy		23.8	0.0045934	1.7136	
Reineta Parda		9	0.001737	0.648	
Red Delicious (whole extract)	Breast MCF-7	65.1	0.0125643	4.6872	Yoon and Liu (2007)
Red Delicious (whole extract)		70.7	0.0136451	5.0904	Yang and Liu (2009)
Red Delicious (phenolic extract)		69.9	0.0134907	5.0328	Sun and Liu (2008)
Red Delicious (phenolic extract)	Breast MDA-MB-231	35.2	0.0067936	2.5344	Sun and Liu (2008)
Apple juice extract	Colon HT-29	31 μM	0.005983	2.232	Veeriah et al. (2006)
Synthetic apple extract		59.9 μM	0.0115607	4.3128	
Rome Beauty (flesh + peel)	Liver HepG2	26.5	0.0051145	1.908	Wolfe et al. (2003)
Rome Beauty (peel)		12.4	0.0023932	0.8928	
Idared (flesh + peel)		125.1	0.0241443	9.0072	
Idared (peel)		13.6	0.0026248	0.9792	
Cortland (flesh)		103.9	0.0200527	7.4808	
Cortland (flesh + peel)		74.1	0.0143013	5.3352	
Cortland (peel)		15.7	0.0030301	1.1304	
Golden Delicious (flesh)		155.3	0.0299729	11.1816	
Golden Delicious (flesh + peel)		107.7	0.0207861	7.7544	
Golden Delicious (peel)		20.2	0.0038986	1.4544	

Quercetin content of apples is in the range 0.0000193–0.0072 %

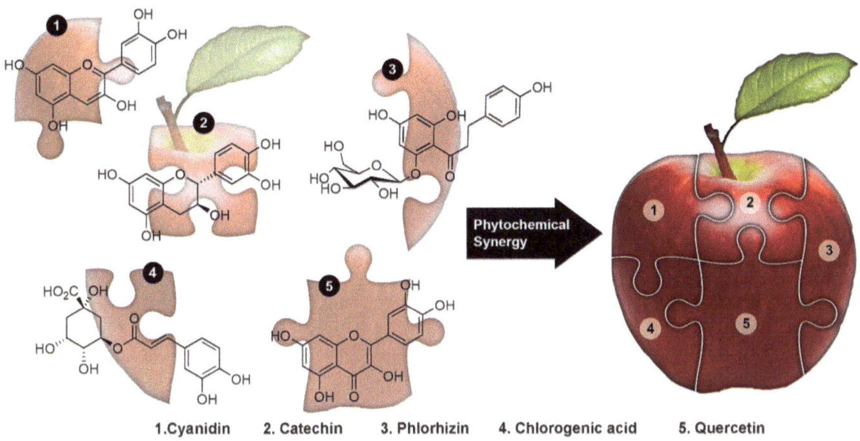

Fig. 1 *The in'cider truth about apples*: The apple phytochemicals including cyanidins, catechins, phlorhizin, chlorogenic acid, quercetin, etc., are nothing but the mystifying puzzle pieces of whole apples, which were brought together into a phytocomplex by Mother Nature to confer synergized health benefits

earnest approximately 20 years ago. Investigations of pomegranate fruit extracts (PFE), fractions, or purified compounds indicate that pomegranate has antioxidant, antiproliferative, anti-invasion, anti-angiogenic, and pro-apoptotic activity in a wide range of cancer cell lines (Adhami et al. 2009; Lansky and Newman 2007; Syed et al. 2007; Faria and Calhau 2011). In addition to data from in vitro evaluations, animal studies have confirmed the efficacy of pomegranate, even leading to human clinical research (Adhami et al. 2009). The phytocomplexity in pomegranates is driven by at least 124 different phytochemicals (Fig. 2), comprised primarily of ellagitannins specific to pomegranate, punicalagins, which can be hydrolyzed to ellagic acid, in addition to anthocyanins and flavonols (Faria and Calhau 2011; Heber 2011; Banerjee et al. 2012). The quantity of any of these polyphenols in pomegranate products is dependent on the preparation methods, with considerably greater amounts of polyphenols in extracts made from whole fruit juices as opposed to extracts from the juice of the arils only (Faria and Calhau 2011; Lansky et al. 2005).

2.2.1 Ellagic Acid: The Hydrolyzed Antioxidant Tannin

Of these compounds, ellagic acid (EA) quickly became the phytochemical of research focus, demonstrating potent antioxidant and anticarcinogenic capabilities (Jurenka 2008). In vitro studies suggest an antiproliferative role for EA in a wide range of cancer cell lines. Neuroblastoma cell growth was inhibited by EA in

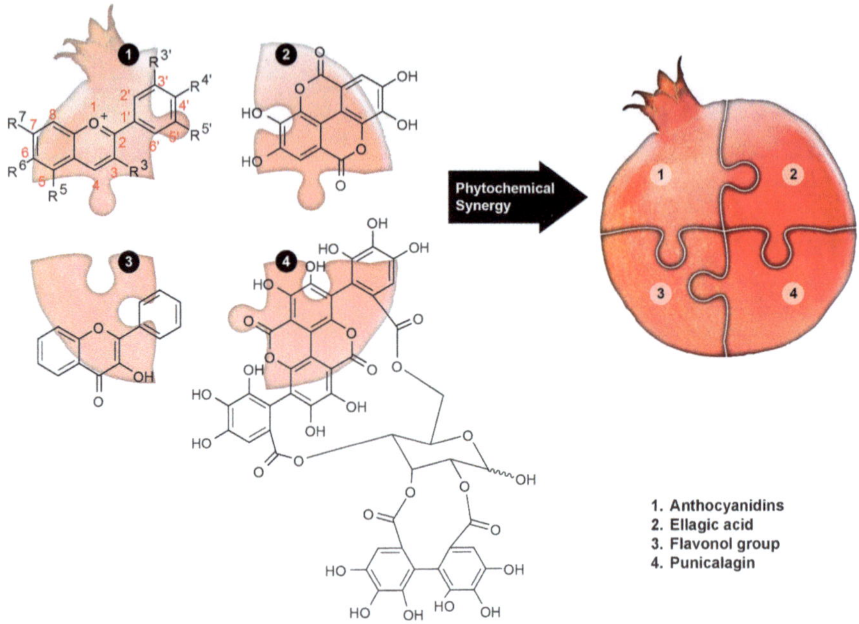

Fig. 2 *Poms pack the punch in their paunch*: Like there are no extra pieces in the universe, anthocyanidins, ellagic acid, flavonols, punicalgins, etc., make up the complex pomegranate jigsaw puzzle to exercise synergy, thus providing optimal health benefits

concentrations between 10 and 30 μM (Fjaeraa and Nanberg 2009). As shown in Table 3, treatment with EA was also observed to significantly reduce cell growth in breast, prostate, colon, skin, ovarian, oral cavity, and bone cancer cells with IC_{50} doses between 21.5 and 462 μM (6.5–139.6 μg/mL) (Han et al. 2006; Kasimsetty et al. 2010; Malik et al. 2011; Seeram et al. 2007).

In vivo research has demonstrated that a diet supplemented with EA in an estrogen-induced mammary tumor rat model significantly reduced the incidence of tumors by 19 %, tumor volume by 65 %, and tumor multiplicity by 41 % when compared to rats given a control diet (Aiyer and Gupta 2010). A mouse skin cancer model resulted in significant inhibition of DMBA-induced epidermal hyperplasia with topical application of EA while the incidence of aberrant crypt foci was significantly reduced in a DMH-induced colon cancer rat model (Kowalczyk et al. 2009; Umesalma and Sudhandiran 2010). Hamster buccal pouch carcinoma also induced by DMBA was nonexistent in hamsters with EA-supplemented diet, although hyperplasia was evident upon histopathological evaluation (Vidya Priyadarsini et al. 2012).

Table 3 Antiproliferative activity of ellagic acid

Cell line	Reported IC_{50} (μM)	Concentration (in μg/mL)	Citations
Prostate PC-3	80	24.18	Malik et al. (2011)
Human osteogenic sarcoma	21.5	6.50	Han et al. (2006)
Prostate LNCaP	62.4	18.86	Seeram et al. (2007)
Prostate LNCaP-AR	78.7	23.87	Seeram et al. (2007)
Prostate DU145	74.3	22.45	Seeram et al. (2007)
Prostate 22RV1	108.7	32.85	Seeram et al. (2007)
Breast BT-549	198	59.84	Kasimsetty et al. (2010)
Colon HT-29	462	139.60	Kasimsetty et al. (2010)
Oral KB	300	90.66	Kasimsetty et al. (2010)
Melanoma SK-MEL	132	39.89	Kasimsetty et al. (2010)
Ovarian SK-OV-3	222	67.09	Kasimsetty et al. (2010)

Cellular and animal investigations have thus presented strong evidence that EA is a promising phytochemical for the prevention and treatment of cancer. However, the doses required to provide these beneficial effects are considerably higher than the physiologically attainable blood plasma level of 0.018–0.033 μM (Mertens-Talcott et al. 2006; Seeram et al. 2004, 2006). Since inquiries into the anticancer properties of pomegranate phytochemicals other than EA have also shown potential for chemoprevention and treatment, the spotlight has turned to focus on properties of the whole pomegranate.

2.2.2 Whole Pomegranate Extract: The Highly Effective Antioxidant Concoction

Confirmation of the anticancer benefits of whole pomegranate has been provided by a number of animal studies of prostate, skin, and lung cancer. Inhibition of proliferation by pomegranate extracts has been explored in several in vitro studies of prostate, lung, oral, and colon cell lines with 30–100 % inhibition of proliferation observed with doses from 10 to 150 μg/mL (Khan et al. 2007b; Malik et al. 2005; Seeram et al. 2005). Intriguingly, one of these studies determined that greater antiproliferative activity was provided by whole pomegranate juice when compared to a total pomegranate tannin extract, punicalagin, and ellagic acid at normalized concentrations of punicalagin (Seeram et al. 2005). Pomegranate juice metabolites, including ellagic acid and urolithin A, were found to be synergistically interacting among themselves, thus emphasizing the idea of phytocomplexity, to inhibit growth of PC-3 and DU145 cells, even causing death by affecting the cell cycle kinetics and induction of apoptosis (Vicinanza et al. 2013). Pomegranate extract was also found to inhibit proliferation of breast cancer cells while inducing apoptosis (Shirode et al. 2014). The authors attribute the antiproliferative effects to reduced DNA repair gene expression and induction of double-stranded DNA damage (Shirode et al. 2014). Pancreatic cancer cell growth was decreased with anIC_{50}value of 50 μg/mL while higher doses of 100 and 125 μg/mL were required for two oral cancer lines (Nair et al. 2011; Weisburg et al. 2010). In contrast, prostate cancer cells were inhibited by a whole pomegranate fruit extract (PFE) with an observed IC_{50} value of only 5.7 μg/mL (Sartippour et al. 2008). In addition to antiproliferative activity, a protective role for PFE was suggested when UVA- and UVB-induced damage in normal human epithelial keratinocytes (NHEK) was inhibited by treatment with PFE (Afaq et al. 2005a; Syed et al. 2006). Follow-up studies in mice further illustrated the photochemopreventive potential of pomegranate with oral administration of PFE demonstrating inhibition of UVB-induced damage and early carcinogenesis (Afaq et al. 2010). A summary of these studies is found in Table **4**.

Prostate cancer was significantly inhibited in mouse xenograft models upon oral ingestion of PFE resulting in 35–60 % reduction in tumor volumes, delays in tumor incidence, and significantly increased survival times (Seeram et al. 2007; Malik et al. 2005; Adhami et al. 2012; Sartippour et al. 2008). Efficacy of PFE against lung cancer was explored in a xenograft model and a Benzo(a)pyrene [B(a)P] and *N*-nitroso-*tris*-chloroethylurea (NTCU)-induced model, both of which involved oral administration of PFE to mice which produced delayed progression of tumors, significantly increased survival time, and over 50 % reduction in tumor volume (Khan et al. 2007a, b). A 33 % tumor growth inhibition of tobacco smoke-induced lung adenomas was observed upon daily oral administration of pomegranate fruit

Table 4 Antiproliferative activity of whole pomegranate extract

Cell line	Reported IC_{50} (μg/mL) of whole pomegranate extract	Contribution of ellagic acid to IC_{50} (μg/mL) of whole pomegranate extract	Citations
Pancreas PANC-1	50	1.35	Nair et al. (2011)
Oral HSC-2	100	2.70	Weisburg et al. (2010)
Tongue CAL-27	125	3.38	Weisburg et al. (2010)
Prostate LNCaP	5.7	0.15	Sartippour et al. (2008)
Endothelial HUVEC	6.7	0.18	Sartippour et al. (2008)

Ellagic acid is present at an abundance of 2.7 % in whole pomegranate extract

extract (Naghma Khan et al. 2013). Skin tumors induced by 12-*O*-tetradecanoylphorbol-13-acetate (TPA) developed later, were fewer in number, and weighed less in mice treated with topical applications of PFE as opposed to control mice (Afaq et al. 2005b).

An initial human trial treating 46 men with rising prostate-specific antigen (PSA) values after primary treatment indicated a significant increase in the average PSA doubling time (PSADT) with daily oral ingestion of 8 oz of pomegranate juice. Untreated PSADT averaged 15 months while PSADT for treated patients averaged 54 months. As this was an open-label, single-arm, small clinical trial, future investigations are planned that will include more patients and placebo controls (Pantuck et al. 2006). More recently,a similar result of lengthened PSADT was observed in a randomized, double-blind phase II clinical trial, where PSA levels even declined in about 13 % of patients in the test group treated with pomegranate extract (POMx) (Paller et al. 2013). However, in direct contrast another placebo-controlled clinical trial in Switzerland re-reported that daily pomegranate intake does not influence the PSA levels when compared to the placebo group (Stenner-Liewen et al. 2013). It is important to note that these studies involved different populations, with the Swiss study treating advanced prostate cancer patients. Additionally, the studies used different preparations of pomegranate, a critical factor in this kind of research. The initial trial by Pantuck et al. used a juice made from crushing the whole fruit while the other studies used pomegranate extract capsules or a juice product that included 27 % pomegranate extract. As the quantity and composition of phytochemicals can vary widely based on preparation methods, the use of different study populations and products could be responsible for these contradictory results.

Several studies providing comparisons between whole products and fractions or constituents of pomegranate have suggested an additive or synergistic effect with treatment by whole pomegranate products. In pancreatic cancer cells, PFE treatment was observed to induce cell cycle arrest and inhibited cell proliferation at an IC_{50} of 50 μg/mL, while a dose of 25–30 μM (7.55–9.07 μg/mL) produced the same results with ellagic acid. Given that ellagic acid comprises only 2.7 % of PFE, its contribution to the effects provided by whole pomegranate extract equates to only 1.35 μg/mL, indicating a minimum fivefold difference in the concentration of EA required when administered as an isolated compound (Nair et al. 2011). Additionally, a comparison between pomegranate extract and paclitaxel determined that PFE inhibited cell proliferation more quickly and more effectively than this standard chemotherapeutic drug (Nair et al. 2011).

Pomegranate juice (PJ) exhibited greater inhibition of proliferation than constituent compounds punicalagin, ellagic acid, and a standardized total pomegranate extract in a variety of cancer cell lines (Seeram et al. 2005). While all treatments demonstrated dose-dependent reductions in cell growth, the inhibition provided by PJ at very low doses was not achievable by other compounds without considerable increases in dosage. Similarly, a comparison of pomegranate juice (PJ), POMx (whole extract), punicalagin, and ellagic acid revealed superior antiproliferative activity of PJ in all three prostate cancer cell lines evaluated (Hong et al. 2008). It is important to note that both PJ and POMx were processed from the whole pomegranate and should therefore provide similar levels of inhibition, but the effects of POMx did not approach those of PJ until higher doses were utilized.

An interesting study evaluating antiproliferative activity of individual pomegranate phytochemicals compared to the whole extract found that while both the extract and the phytochemicals inhibited proliferation and reduced viability of mouse mammary cancer stem cells in a time- and dose-related manner, the doses of phytochemicals were higher than those found in the whole extract. EA inhibited cell growth with an IC_{50} of ~7.5 μM (2.27 μg/mL), but its contribution to the IC_{50} of PE was 1.35 μg/mL, a difference of 41 %, suggesting that the effect of EA is enhanced when administered as part of the whole extract (Dai et al. 2010).

Evaluation of the reported effective doses for whole pomegranate extracts versus ellagic acid provides considerable evidence for synergistic interactions between naturally occurring phytochemicals in pomegranates. Pomegranate extracts proved to be effective in doses between 50 and 200 μg/mL, providing an ellagic acid content between 0.15 and 5.4 μg/mL (Table **4**). In contrast, the IC_{50}s for ellagic acid were reported to be between 22 and 462 μM, correlating to 6.5–139.6 μg/mL (Table 3), which are substantially higher, thus lending support to our idea that greater anticancer activity can be observed with whole foods than with constituents alone.

2.3 What Tomatoes Truly Bring to the Table: Juicy Facts

According to the United States Department of Agriculture, the average American consumes more than seventy pounds of tomato products each year, primarily in the form of sauces and other processed tomato products (Lucier 2011). Numerous epidemiological studies investigating diet and disease have suggested that consumption of tomato products or the carotenoid lycopene from tomatoes is associated with a reduced risk of cancer (Campbell et al. 2004; Chan et al. 2006, 2009; Etminan et al. 2004; Giovannucci et al. 2007). Multiple analyses of the prospective Health Professional's Follow-up Study has uncovered an inverse relationship between tomato product intake and prostate cancer (PC) suggesting a significantly lower risk of PC for subjects who consumed two to four servings of tomato sauce per week (Giovannucci et al. 2007). A more recent report from a prospective hospital-based multicenter case–control study also demonstrated an inverse relationship between tomato/tomato products and PC (Salem et al. 2011). Additionally, tomato was found to significantly reduce the odds ratio of pancreatic cancer (Jansen et al. 2011). While no causality has been proven, the available data collectively support the idea that consumption of tomatoes and tomato products containing lycopene may have anticarcinogenic activity. Mounting evidence from cellular and animal studies in addition to human clinical trials seems to validate the continued research into this commonly consumed food. While variations exist dependent on cultivar, growing conditions, and processing, tomatoes contain carotenoids, flavonoids, and other important phytochemicals like phytoene, phytofluene, beta-carotene, lycopene, quercetin, kaempferol, and vitamins (Capanoglu et al. 2008). As observed with apples and pomegranates, the presence and concentration of compounds can be vastly different in the flesh as opposed to the skin of tomatoes and inclusion of the tomato skin and seeds is important to the phytochemical content, antioxidant potential, and the associated anticancer properties (Capanoglu et al. 2008).

2.3.1 Lycopene: The Red Carotenoid

Much of the early tomato research focused on lycopene, a fat-soluble carotenoid providing the red pigment found in red tomatoes, watermelon, and other fruits (Kelkel et al. 2011). There is agreement that lycopene is a powerful antioxidant, often referred to as the most efficient carotenoid quencher of singlet oxygen (Di Mascio et al. 1989). In addition to antioxidant properties, lycopene displays potent anticancer activity including inhibition of cell growth, anti-inflammatory effects, cell cycle arrest, and alteration of cell signaling pathways (Kelkel et al. 2011). Interestingly, absorption of lycopene is affected by cooking as heat processing results in higher levels of cis-lycopene, the form found in human plasma, as opposed to the trans configuration dominant in fresh tomatoes (Tan et al. 2010). Raw tomatoes have an estimated lycopene concentration of 8.8–42 μg/g, whereas the range for tomato juice and tomato sauce is 86–100 and 63–131 μg/g, respectively (Russo et al. 2010). The bioavailability of lycopene can also be increased with the addition of lipids to the processing or ingestion of tomato products (Tan et al. 2010). However, there seems to be a maximum level of absorption regardless of the dose administered, suggesting the presence of saturable absorptive mechanisms (Diwadkar-Navsariwala et al. 2003). Keeping these factors in mind, cellular, animal, and human studies have provided considerable evidence for chemoprevention by lycopene.

Lycopene has been shown to significantly inhibit the proliferation of prostate, liver, lung, breast, and colon cancer cell lines with inhibition of at least 50 % cell growth for doses between 1.3 and 50 μM, concentrations that are well above the reported serum lycopene concentration of 0.34 and 0.65 μM achievable upon acute lycopene supplementation (Burgess et al. 2008; Diwadkar-Navsariwala et al. 2003; Hwang and Bowen 2005a, b; Hwang and Lee 2006; Koh et al. 2010; Salman et al. 2007; Tang et al. 2008; Palozza et al. 2010; Takeshima et al. 2014; Asmah Rahmat et al. 2002). Lycopene may exert more suppressive activity in androgen-independent prostate cancer cells as demonstrated by IC_{50}s of 26.6 and 40.3 μM compared to 168.5 μM for an androgen-dependent cell line (Tang et al. 2005). These studies are summarized in Table 5. However, several limitations exist in assessing the in vitro efficacy of tomato products containing lycopene as they are particularly sensitive to light, oxygen, and temperature in addition to their incompatibility as hydrophobic molecules in aqueous culture media (Ford et al. 2011; Hwang and Bowen 2005a).

Table 5 Antiproliferative activity of lycopene or tomatine

Tomato phytochemical	Cell line	Reported IC_{50} (μM)	Concentration (in μg/mL)	Citations
Lycopene	Breast MCF-7	42.8	22.9	Takeshima et al. (2014)
Lycopene	Breast SK-BR-3	41	22	Takeshima et al. (2014)
Lycopene	Breast MDA-MB-468	41.7	22.4	Takeshima et al. (2014)
Lycopene	Breast H-Ras MCF10A	1.3	0.698	Koh et al. (2010)
Lycopene	Breast MDA-MB-231	13.4	7.19	Koh et al. (2010)
Lycopene	Colon HT-29	10	5.37	Tang et al. (2008)
Lycopene	Prostate DU-145	26.6	14.28	Tang et al. (2005)
Lycopene	Prostate PC-3	40.3	21.64	Tang et al. (2005)
Lycopene	Prostate LNCaP	168.5	90.46	Tang et al. (2005)
Lycopene	Liver HepG2	42.4	22.8	Rahmat et al. (2002)
Lycopene	Breast MDA-MB-231	21	11.3	Rahmat et al. (2002)
α-Tomatine	Liver HepG2	41.6	43	Friedman et al. (2009)
α-Tomatine	Breast MCF-7	4.9	5.1	Friedman et al. (2009)

Animal experiments have reinforced the link between lycopene and reduced risk of carcinogenesis. Androgen-independent xenograft prostate tumor growth rate in rats was significantly reduced from ~50 to 76 % by oral ingestion of lycopene with a correlating reduction in tumor volume of ~43–81 % for doses between 10 and 300 mg/kg (Tang et al. 2005). Oral consumption of lycopene has also been found to inhibit hepatoma tumor metastasis and reduce colon cancer tumor growth in nude mice models in addition to upregulating antioxidant and immune system activity in a gastric cancer rat model (Huang et al. 2008; Luo and Wu 2011; Tang et al. 2011). Human clinical studies of lycopene are under way and a number of these studies investigating lycopene's purported anticancer benefits will likely provide valuable information regarding absorption, disposition, and any chemopreventive or therapeutic properties of lycopene.

The anticarcinogenic properties of tomatoes have also been attributed to flavonoids, which have individually displayed antiproliferative effects but when combined with other flavonoids the effects were far more striking, strongly suggestive of additive interactions between these phytochemicals (Campbell et al. 2004;

2006). Another line of research investigated the tomato glycoalkaloid referred to as tomatine, found in green tomatoes, with promising initial results (Friedman et al. 2009).

2.3.2 Whole Tomatoes: The Ripened Efficacy

A 2007 review of earlier clinical trials concluded that while lycopene containing tomato products are significantly beneficial, the effects are not the result of lycopene exclusively, but rather the combination of phytochemicals and other components in the whole tomato (Basu and Imrhan 2007). Research on whole tomatoes and the phytocomplexity found naturally in tomatoes has provided support for this conclusion. As observed with other foods reviewed here, the results have suggested that superior benefits may be realized by utilizing the whole tomato (Fig. 3) as opposed to selectively using only one component.

Colon adenocarcinoma cell growth was inhibited and apoptosis induced in a dose-dependent manner by tomato digestate from in vitro simulated digestion of a tomato genetically engineered to be β-carotene rich (Palozza et al. 2009). A dose of 100 mL/L of tomato digestate inhibited cell growth by 55 %. This dose corresponds to a β-carotene concentration of 0.08 μM, but when purified β-carotene was compared in an identical assay, doses as high as 10 μM did not inhibit cell growth as effectively as tomato digestate, suggesting the involvement of other compounds or processes (Palozza et al. 2009). LycoC, a lycopene phytocomplex with 6 % purified lycopene, inhibited HL60 leukemia cells at concentrations between 10 and 25 μM which corresponds to a lycopene concentration of 0.6–1.5 μM (Ettorre et al. 2010). Explorations of extraction methods and cytotoxity in HT29 colon cancer cells determined the IC_{50}s of 62.5 μg/mL for the petroleum ether extract and 87.0 μg/mL for an in vitro digested tomato extract (Guil-Guerrero et al. 2011). In another study, Bhaumik et al. have performed cell growth inhibition studies employing a variety of tomato extracts prepared in various solvents including methanol, ethanol, acetone, and chloroform against HeLa cells. Results from this study revealed that these tomato extracts exhibited moderate efficacy with IC_{50} values ranging from 57 to 69 μg/mL (Bhaumik 2014).

A comparison of the effects on human sera of ingestion of lycopene-rich red tomatoes (RTS), lycopene-free yellow tomatoes (YTS), and purified lycopene (LYS) confirmed similar lycopene concentrations in RTS and LYS sera, but produced some surprising results in terms of anticarcinogenic gene expression (Talvas et al. 2010). While increases in beneficial gene expression were observed in RTS and YTS, decreases of anticarcinogenic and increases of pro-carcinogenic gene expression were revealed with evaluation of LYS sera samples, suggesting that the food matrix in whole tomatoes may provide positive benefits and modulate negative effects. While cell proliferation was unaffected by any of the samples at physiological levels, it may be important to note that cells in this experiment were exposed to the human subject sera for only 24 h while a number of other studies have utilized 48 h or longer exposures (Talvas et al. 2010).

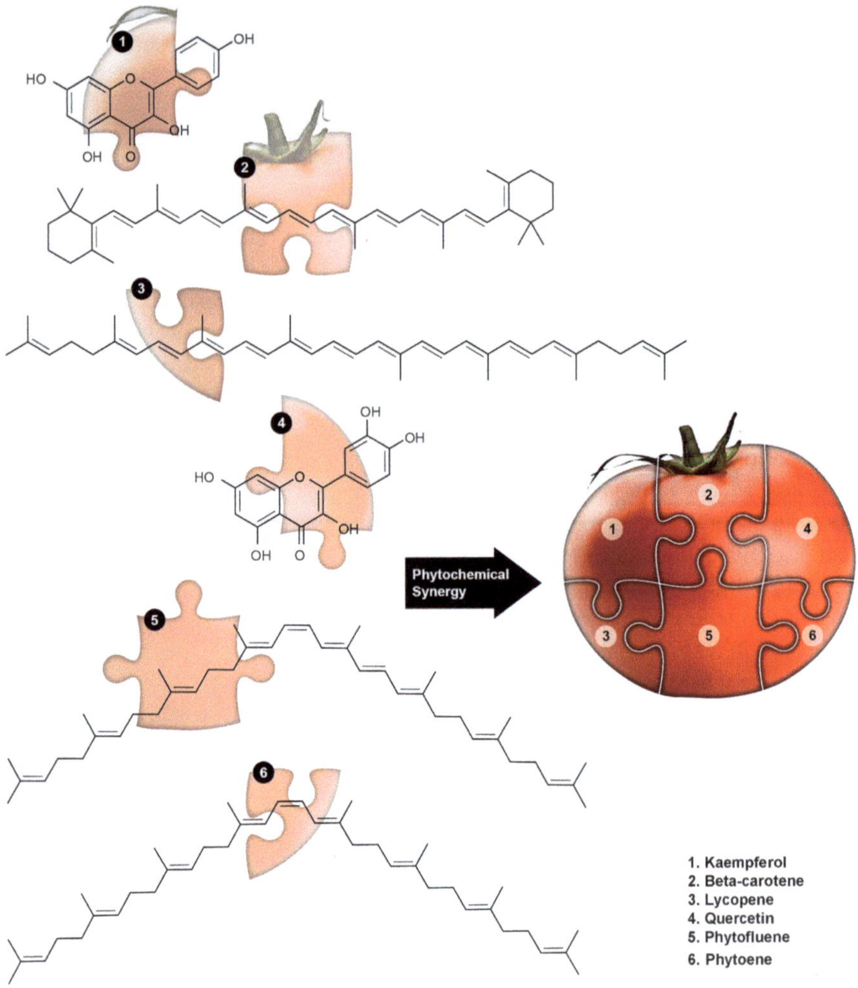

Fig. 3 *Tomato is to salsa as phytocomplexity is to well-being*: The excellent chemotherapeutic and chemopreventive benefits offered by a whole tomato are the result of phytochemical synergy activated when its constituents including kaempferol, β-carotene, lycopene, quercetin, phytofluenes, phytoenes, etc., fit together as pieces in a puzzle

Not all investigations into the anticancer properties of tomatoes have focused on lycopene. Research of the isolated green tomato glycoalkaloid tomatine revealed growth inhibition of stomach, liver, colon, and breast cancer cell lines when treated with purified α-tomatine. Inhibition was also observed in normal liver cells. When extracts of a variety of green tomatoes were tested, a number of them were also found to inhibit these cell lines. A comparison of the IC_{50}s for purified tomatine and the quantities of tomatine in the green tomato extracts suggests that the blend of glycoalkaloids found in these tomatoes is more effective than the individual

Table 6 Antiproliferative activity of tomato extract

Substance evaluated	Cell line	Reported IC_{50} (μg/mL) of tomato product	Contribution of phytochemical to IC_{50} (μg/mL) of whole tomato extract	Citations
Lycopene				
LycoC (6 % lycopene)	Leukemia HL60	5.37–13.4	0.32–0.8	Ettorre et al. (2010)
Petroleum ether extract of tomato	Colon HT-29	62.5	0.0146	Guil-Guerrero et al. (2011)
Tomato digestate	Colon HT-29	87	0.0204	Guil-Guerrero et al. (2011)
Ethanolic extract of tomato	Cervical HeLa	68.2	3.75	Bhaumik et al. (2014)
α-Tomatine				
Sancheri, small green	Liver HepG2	12.3	0.00386	Friedman et al. (2009)
Sancheri, medium green	Liver HepG2	3.2	0.0003456	Friedman et al. (2009)
Sancheri, large green	Liver HepG2	1	0.0000575	Friedman et al. (2009)
Yoyo, green tomato	Liver HepG2	0.8	0.0000664	Friedman et al. (2009)
Chobok Power, small green	Liver HepG2	0.2	0.0000231	Friedman et al. (2009)
Rokusanmaru, small green	Liver HepG2	0.9	0.0000842	Friedman et al. (2009)
Sancheri, small green	Breast MCF-7	377	0.118	Friedman et al. (2009)
Sancheri, medium green	Breast MCF-7	0.33	0.0000356	Friedman et al. (2009)
Sancheri, large green	Breast MCF-7	241	0.0139	Friedman et al. (2009)
Yoyo, green tomato	Breast MCF-7	<0.1	0	Friedman et al. (2009)
Chobok Power, small green	Breast MCF-7	18.7	0.00216	Friedman et al. (2009)
Rokusanmaru, small green	Breast MCF-7	9	0.000842	Friedman et al. (2009)

Lycopene is present at an abundance of 0.88–5.5 % in whole tomato extract
Tomatine abundance in these extracts varied and is listed in Table 2 of Friedman 2009

component. Results for HepG2 liver cancer cells and MCF-7 breast cancer cells are shown in Tables 5 and 6.

Animal studies have also provided evidence of an additive effect in whole tomato products as opposed to single components. Rats fed with whole tomato powder experienced longer prostate cancer-free survival when compared to those fed with lycopene beadlets, even though the concentration of lycopene was nearly twelve times higher in the beadlets (Boileau et al. 2003). Intriguingly, comparison of lycopene concentrations in plasma showed higher levels in rats fed with lycopene, but the levels were not twelve times higher, suggesting better uptake from the tomato powder and possible synergy from the combination of phytochemicals in tomatoes (Boileau et al. 2003). In direct contradiction to these findings, a similar study reported in 2010 failed to replicate this result, indicating instead that mice fed with the lycopene beadlets experienced a lower incidence of prostate cancer. A plausible explanation of the discrepancy may be provided by the composition of the tomato products as this experiment used a tomato paste product produced without the skin and seeds while the earlier investigation used a tomato powder comprised of the whole tomato (Konijeti et al. 2010).

To gain further insights into synergy between phytochemicals in tomatoes, several studies have been performed using modified tomato products. FruHis, a carbohydrate derivative found in dehydrated tomato products, was found to display robust synergy with lycopene both in vitro and in vivo (Mossine et al. 2008). Although tumor incidence was reduced in rats fed with tomato paste or tomato powder, longer survival was seen in rats fed with tomato paste supplemented with FruHis (Mossine et al. 2008). A dietary supplement of tomato powder processed to provide ketosamine and maximize flavonoids and carotenoids showed significant chemopreventive efficacy in transgenic adenocarcinoma of the mouse prostate (TRAMP) mice (Pannellini et al. 2010). Control diet enhanced with 10 % tomato powder displayed lower incidence of poorly differentiated carcinoma, delayed progression to adenocarcinoma, and significantly increased survival time. This study indicates that a tomato-rich diet is effective in preventing prostate cancer in TRAMP mice, which suggests prevention with tomato products may also be possible in humans (Pannellini et al. 2010). Significantly reduced numbers of altered hepatic foci were observed in rats fed with diets containing equal amounts of lycopene in either a pure compound or tomato extract, although gene expression indicated different mechanism may have been involved (Wang et al. 2010).

A frequently reported human trial of 32 diagnosed prostate cancer patients involving increased tomato sauce intake for 3 weeks prior to prostatectomy resulted in decreased prostate-specific antigen levels and increased serum and prostate tissue levels of lycopene (Bowen et al. 2002; Chen et al. 2001; Kim et al. 2003; Stacewicz-Sapuntzakis and Bowen 2005). Another small clinical trial asking newly diagnosed prostate cancer patients to consume lycopene capsules for 3 weeks prior to surgery concurred, demonstrating decreased PSA levels and less tumor growth than control patients. This study is particularly relevant because these capsules were comprised of lycopene in the tomato matrix including other bioactive compounds (Kucuk et al. 2001, 2002). While these results are intriguing, these studies were very small and conducted in patients with known disease providing no information regarding prevention of primary cancer.

A 2010 review by Tan et al. confirms the need for more research, but contrary to the common reductionist approach of extracting the most effective single compound, it was proposed that the development of a tomato-based food product with a consistent phytochemical profile should be the goal of cancer prevention efforts (Tan et al. 2010). Additionally, they believe this can best be accomplished by an interdisciplinary approach utilizing horticulturalists, food scientists, cancer biologists, and clinical investigators (Tan et al. 2010).

2.4 *Many Heads Are Better Than One: Phytochemicals in Broccoli florets Synergize to Energize*

Cruciferous vegetables (CV), named for the cross-shaped appearance of their flowers, are a rich source of organosulfur compounds that give these vegetables their signature aroma and taste and are believed to be the phytochemicals responsible for the observed anticancer properties (Higdon et al. 2007). Cabbage, Brussels sprouts, watercress, radish, and broccoli are some examples of these vegetables that are common to human diets over most of the world. The relationship between the intake of cruciferous vegetables and various cancers generally indicates an inverse association, particularly when comparisons are made between the highest and lowest intake groups (Lam et al. 2009). While a number of epidemiological studies have reported a lower incidence of cancers for those people who eat the most cruciferous vegetables, many studies have been inconclusive. Given the inherent difficulties of prospective and case–control studies, this is not surprising and serves to highlight the need for better methods of evaluation. Analysis of CV can be problematic due to several known genetic polymorphisms of the glutathione S-transferase (GST) family of enzymes that are key in isothiocyanate processing (Herr and Buchler 2010; Kim and Park 2009; Latte et al. 2011). It is likely that this is not an isolated problem and may factor into the assessment of many fruits and vegetables (Lampe 2009a).

Epidemiological evidence seems to support the refrain of mothers to "eat your broccoli" and has been followed up with considerable research seeking to find the individual molecule with the most health benefits. Cruciferous vegetables provide a bountiful supply of bioactive phytochemicals working together to provide synergistic health benefits (Fig. 4). In addition to organosulfur compounds from glucosinolates (GS), carotenoids and polyphenolic flavonoids kaempferol and quercetin are also represented (Moreno et al. 2006). The concentrations of these compounds differ widely between the different types of CV and different cultivars, with even more variability for growing conditions and harvest times (Bjorkman et al. 2011). Found primarily in crucifers, GS are biologically inactive until hydrolyzed by myrosinase, a heat-inactivated enzyme segregated from GS in the

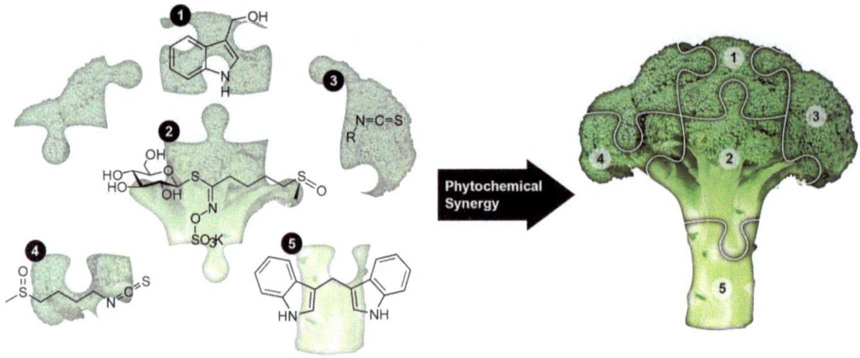

Fig. 4 *Broccoli: What's not to like?* Every puzzle has a solution and one of Nature's cleverest solutions is Broccoli. The isothiocyanates, sulforaphane, indole-3-carbinol, glucoraphanin, 3,3′-diindolylmethane, and broccoli constituents are assembled together in defined ratios making broccoli the "superfood" with utmost therapeutic benefits

plant that is released upon mechanical disruption of cells (Vasanthi et al. 2009; Herr and Buchler 2010). The resulting indole isothiocyanates and isothiocyanates (ITC) include idole-3-carbinol (I3C), 3,3′-diindolylmethane (DIM), benzyl isothiocyanate (BITC), phenethyl isothiocyanate (PEITC), and sulforaphane (SF) (Moreno et al. 2006).

Studies investigating these individual phytochemicals have provided a wealth of information. Proliferation of cancer cell lines representing breast, colon, liver, and androgen-dependent prostate was inhibited by I3C at a wide range of IC_{50}s between 5 and 300 μM (Mossine et al. 2008; Wang et al. 2012; Pappa et al. 2006; Saw et al. 2011). DIM inhibition of cell proliferation was achieved with IC50s between 8 and 60 μM for breast, prostate, colon, and liver cancer cell lines (Jin 2011; Wang et al. 2012; Cho et al. 2011; Pappa et al. 2006; Saw et al. 2011). In vitro research of BITC and PEITC has been less common but colon cancer cell growth was suppressed by 50 % with doses of 5.1 and 2.4 μM, respectively, and also in a separate experiment by PEITC in a range of doses between 7.1 and 10.0 μM (Pappa et al. 2006; Visanji et al. 2004). PEITC was also effective against liver cancer cells at anIC_{50} of ~51 μM (Saw et al. 2011). Flavonoids have known anticancer properties and the flavonoid extract of broccoli leaf inhibited colon, liver, ovarian, and lung cancer cell lines with IC_{50}s between 79.77 and 104.43 mg/ml (Wang and Zhang 2012).

Animal studies have added to the evidence for cancer prevention and treatment with broccoli constituent phytochemicals. In a tobacco smoke carcinogen-induced lung adenocarcinoma mouse model, I3C administered in the diet either post-initiation or during progression demonstrated phase-dependent anticancer properties with early administration of I3C resulting in reduced multiplicity of microscopic lesions and tumors, while administration during progression decreased the number of large tumors, inhibiting the development of lung adenocarcinoma while seemingly increasing the number of small tumors (Qian et al. 2011). Prostate cancer progression in TRAMP mice was delayed by adding either DIM or PEITC to the feed (Cho et al. 2011; Powolny et al. 2011). Intraperitoneal sulforaphane treatment of breast cancer xenograft tumors in mice resulted in tumors half the size of untreated mice (Li et al. 2010). Subsequent reimplantation of cells from these treated tumors failed to generate tumors while untreated cells rapidly developed tumors suggesting possible targeting of stem cells by sulforaphane. Breast cancer xenografts were also inhibited by oral ingestion of DIM, resulting in a 60 % decrease in tumor volume for treated mice (Jin 2011).

2.4.1 Sulforaphane: The Organosulfur Antioxidant

Sulforaphane (SF) has been the most extensively researched of all CV phytochemicals with data in a broad range of cancers (Lampe 2009b). It has been shown to suppress the proliferation of cancer cells of various tissue origins including breast, ovarian, cervical, glioma, oral, etc. (Chaudhuri et al. 2007; Huang et al. 2012; Jee et al. 2011; Jin 2011; Sharma et al. 2011; Pawlik et al. 2013). In vitro evaluation of CV phytochemicals against colon cancer cells revealed potential selectivity by SF with an IC_{50} in non-tumorigenic cells approximately double the IC_{50} for a tumorigenic cell line (Zeng et al. 2011). Normal prostate cell proliferation was largely unaffected by doses up to 15 μM, a dose that induced 2.5 times the caspase activity in prostate cancer cells. Additional evidence of selectivity was provided in normal lymphocytes as doses of sulforaphane as high as 100 μM failed to decrease the viability of these cells (Sharma et al. 2011). Two studies exploring SF antiproliferative efficacy in bladder cancer determined IC_{50}s from 6.6 to 26.9 μM depending on cell line and time of treatment (Shan et al. 2006; Tang et al. 2006). These results are summarized in Table 7.

Research of a combination treatment using sulforaphane and DIM provided some contrasting results with dose-dependent antagonism or synergy. At physiologically relevant low doses, the combination proved to be antagonistic while high doses appeared to be additive or weakly synergistic (Pappa et al. 2007). Higher concentrations of CV components were required to reduce liver cancer cell growth as SF and PEITC had IC_{50}s ~20 μM, while doses of ~51 and ~135 μM were needed for DIM and I3C (Saw et al. 2011). Interestingly, synergistic induction of antioxidant response elements (ARE) was observed in some, but not all, combinations of indoles and isothiocyanates. Further investigations, including comparisons with whole extracts, may provide insight into the results of these studies.

Clearly, the individual phytochemicals present in cruciferous vegetables have potential as chemopreventive and therapeutic compounds. The narrow focus and contradictory results provided by these studies leave many questions, some of which may be answered by evaluating whole extracts for anticancer activity.

Table 7 Antiproliferative activity of sulforaphane

Cell line	Reported IC_{50} (μM)	Concentration (in μg/mL)	Citations
Bladder UM-UC-3	6.6	1.170	Tang et al. (2006)
Bladder T24	15.9	2.819	Shan et al. (2006)
Glioma GBM 8401	35.52	6.297	Huang et al. (2012)
Colon 40-16 (HCT116 derived)	6.6	1.170	Pappa et al. (2006)
Colon 379.2 (HCT116 derived)	6.8	1.206	Pappa et al. (2006)
Liver HepG2-C8	20	3.546	Saw et al. (2011)
Oral tongue carcinoma YD10B	3	5.319	Jee et al. (2011)
Ovarian SKOV3	40	7.092	Chaudhuri et al. (2007)
Breast SUM159	10	1.773	Li et al. (2010)
Breast MCF-7	16	2.837	Li et al. (2010)
Breast MDA MB 231	21	3.72	Pawlik et al. (2013)
Breast MCF-7	19	3.369	Pawlik et al. (2013)
Breast MDA MB 468	20	3.546	Pawlik et al. (2013)
Breast SKBR-3	25	4.432	Pawlik et al. (2013)

2.4.2 Eat Your Whole Broccoli

A screening of 34 common vegetables indicated that cruciferous vegetables demonstrated some degree of selective inhibition in all tumor cell lines tested (Boivin et al. 2009). Tissue-specific differences in sensitivity were apparent with prostate and stomach cancer cells being most sensitive followed by kidney, pancreatic, and lung cancer cells. Interestingly, the antiproliferative activity seemed to be disconnected from the antioxidant capacity, which led the authors to conclude that multiple mechanisms, essentially driven by phytocomplexity, were at work to confer optimal efficacy to whole broccoli extract. Colon cancer cell proliferation was inhibited by raw extracts of Brussels sprouts and broccoli while a raw extract of watercress provided significant DNA damage protection and invasion inhibition (Boyd et al. 2006; Ferrarini et al. 2012; Smith et al. 2005). A broccoli sprout extract (BSE) prepared to maximize isothiocyanate content was observed to inhibit proliferation of human bladder cancer cells with an IC_{50} of 6.8 μM while purified sulforaphane exhibited similar inhibition with an IC_{50} of 6.6 μM, leading the authors to conclude that the antiproliferative effects of BSE were due solely to isothiocyanates (Tang et al. 2006). However, other phytochemicals such as flavonoids could play a part in anticancer effects and a full analysis of the extract could provide critical information regarding the phytocomplexity of these compounds after being subjected to the heat processing involved in creating this extract. Prostate cancer cell proliferation was inhibited by broccoli sprout extracts with IC_{50}s equivalent to SF concentrations of 3.3–4.4 μg/mL. Selenium-enriched

Table 8 Antiproliferative activity of broccoli extract

Material tested	Cell line	Reported IC_{50} (µg/mL)	Contribution of sulforaphane to IC_{50} of whole extract (in µg/mL)	Citations
Broccoli sprout extract	Lung A549	81.94	15.73	Yang and Zhang (2011)
	Ovarian OVCAR-3	78.6	15.09	Yang and Zhang (2011)
Broccoli sprout extract	Prostate LNCaP	19× dilution	3.51	Abdulah et al. (2009)
Selenium-enriched extract		32× dilution	1.75	Abdulah et al. (2009)
Broccoli sprout extract	Prostate PC-3	20× dilution	3.33	Abdulah et al. (2009)
Selenium-enriched extract		28× dilution	2.00	Abdulah et al. (2009)
Broccoli sprout extract	Prostate DU-145	15× dilution	4.43	Abdulah et al. (2009)
Selenium-enriched extract		30× dilution	1.86	Abdulah et al. (2009)

Sulforaphane is present at an abundance of 1.15 % in whole broccoli sprout extract

broccoli sprout extracts exhibited IC_{50}s at even lower concentrations between 1.75 and 2 µg/mL (Abdulah et al. 2009). These findings are shown in Table 8.

While a comparison between sulforaphane-induced inhibition and inhibition produced by whole CV extracts may indicate that SF is largely responsible for the antiproliferative effects, more research is needed as there are few studies investigating the anticancer properties of whole extracts of cruciferous vegetables. However, compelling evidence for the benefits of eating the whole plant can be found in a number of in vivo studies.

Broccoli has shown benefits in skin cancer prevention with topical application of broccoli sprout extract to mice skin increasing the induction of phase 2 protective enzymes (Dinkova-Kostova et al. 2007). In an experimental model intended to represent human childhood sun exposure, mice chronically exposed to UV radiation were fed either a control diet or a diet supplemented with broccoli sprout extracts resulting in significantly fewer and smaller non-melanoma skin tumors in supplement fed mice than mice fed with the control diet (Dinkova Kostova et al. 2010). Detoxification enzymes were increased to a similar degree in rats fed with a diet supplemented either with freeze-dried broccoli containing intact glucosinolates (GS) or purified sulforaphane (SF) despite a concentration of SF more than double the concentration of GS (Keck et al. 2003). Additional evidence was provided by analysis of urinary metabolites, which were threefold greater in rats ingesting purified SF, thus confirming that induction of antioxidant enzymes was not due solely to SF and is likely a result of the inherent phytocomplexity. Rats fed with a freeze-dried aqueous extract of broccoli sprouts prior to initiation and then throughout the study experienced significant dose-dependent inhibition of bladder cancer when compared to the rats ingesting the control diet, making the case for cancer prevention with cruciferous vegetables (Munday et al. 2008). A crossover experiment of the effects of steamed broccoli consumption in young healthy smokers indicated a 41 % reduction in DNA damage, while an earlier study comparing smokers and nonsmokers demonstrated a significant decrease in DNA strand breaks in broccoli consuming subjects, regardless of smoking status (Riso et al. 2009, 2010). This effect was temporary as levels returned to normal when tested ten days after discontinuing ingestion of broccoli, emphasizing the need for regular consumption to achieve the observed protective benefits.

Further evidence of the importance of eating whole foods as opposed to supplements of individual compounds is provided by another study, where human subjects ingesting fresh broccoli sprouts excreted five times more sulforaphane metabolites and eight times more erucin metabolites when compared to subjects consuming a broccoli supplement (Clarke et al. 2011). Components in the food matrix, for example, myrosinase, are critical for absorption and are often not found in supplements. Glucosinolate derivatives crambene, PEITC, and I3C demonstrated some degree of efficacy on the induction of detoxification enzymes, but they were considerably more potent when administered in various combinations (Nho and Jeffery 2001; Staack et al. 1998; Wallig et al. 1998). Additional research to determine if the induction of these enzymes resulted in chemoprevention concluded that high doses of a crambene and I3C combination were protective, while relevant low dietary doses were not effective (Wallig et al. 2005). Such data from combination experiments highlight the need for additional research with regard to phytocomplexity.

2.5 *Ginger, The Intricate Spice: Spike Your Health with a Zing*

The rhizome of *Zingiber officinale*, commonly known as ginger, is widely consumed as a spice worldwide and commonly employed as medicine, but is not a substantive part of most human diets. Ginger is believed to have been cultivated and used in food and medicine for over 5000 years by humans living in India and China and has now become common over most of the world (Bode and Dong 2011). It has diverse uses, from aphrodisiac to anti-arthritic food spice to anti-inflammatory agent with most applications related to gastrointestinal issues like nausea (Baliga et al. 2011). More recently, the anticancer properties of ginger have been reported through in vitro and in vivo studies and extensive efforts have been made to discover the individual phytochemicals with the most activity against cancer including investigations of gingerols, shogaols, paradols, and zingerones (Baliga et al. 2011; Peng et al. 2012). Further efforts have been made to elucidate the mechanisms by which ginger induces phase 2 enzymes and apoptosis in addition to inhibiting angiogenesis, metastasis, cell cycle progression, and posttranslational modification (Butt and Sultan 2011).

2.5.1 Ginger Phenolics: Bullets With Multiple Targets

The majority of in vitro studies investigating the anticancer efficacy of one or more of the individual ginger phytochemicals reveal that gingerols and shogaols are the most effective ginger phenolics. Of all the ginger phenolics, 6-gingerol (6G), 8-gingerol (8G), 10-gingerol (10G), and 6-shogaol (6S) have been extensively studied so far. Among the gingerols, 6G is the most abundant in fresh ginger and seems to possess potent anticancer activity including antioxidant, anti-inflammatory, and antiproliferative actions (Baliga et al. 2011; Oyagbemi et al. 2010). While present in fresh ginger in smaller amounts, 6S is plentiful in dried and heat-treated ginger and has proven to be equally if not more effective than 6G as an anticancer agent in many studies (Baliga et al. 2011; Peng et al. 2012; Rhode et al. 2007; Sang et al. 2009; Weng et al. 2010). Both 6G and 6S have been shown to inhibit invasion, cell adhesion, and migration and 6G also has efficacy against metastasis and angiogenesis (Peng et al. 2012; Rhode et al. 2007; Weng et al. 2010; Weng and Yen 2012). Inhibition of cell proliferation by 6G has been demonstrated in cervical, liver, skin, colon, pancreatic, and lung cancer cell lines with IC_{50}s between 50 μM and 400 μM (Cheng et al. 2011; Kim et al. 2008; Nigam et al. 2009; Park et al. 2006; Sang et al. 2009; Yang et al. 2010). Greater efficacy has been reported with 6S in cervical, liver, colon, and lung cancer cells as well as in prostate, nasopharyngeal, neuroblastoma, and oral cancer cell lines with a much lower range of IC_{50} values from 3.7 to 100 μM (Table 9) (Chen et al. 2010; Cheng et al. 2011; Gan et al. 2011; Hung et al. 2009; Peng et al. 2012; Sang et al. 2009).

In vivo investigations of the individual ginger phytochemicals have revealed anticancer activity against skin, lung, liver, breast, cervical, bladder, and colorectal cancers (Baliga et al. 2011; Butt and Sultan 2011). Skin cancer development was delayed and the incidence, multiplicity, and volume of tumors were reduced by topical application of 6G, although the anticancer effects of GS were more pronounced when compared to 6G (Nigam et al. 2010; Park et al. 1998; Wu et al. 2010). Lung cancer metastasis was considerably suppressed by 6-gingerol as evidenced by a significant reduction in the number of metastatic colonies (Kim et al. 2005). Treatment with 6G resulted in reduced colon tumor volume and significantly longer survival of the treated mice (Jeong et al. 2009).

2.5.2 Ginger Extract: Whole Is Greater Than the Sum of Its Parts

As observed with other foods reviewed here, very little research has been conducted that directly compares individual phytochemicals to the whole plant. However,

Table 9 Antiproliferative activity of ginger phenolics

Cell line	Reported IC_{50} (in μM)	Concentration (in μg/mL)	Citations
6-Gingerol			
Pancreas BxPC-3	405.3	119.3	Park et al. (2006)
Pancreas HPAC	387.4	114	Park et al. (2006)
Cervical HeLa	>50		Cheng et al. (2011)
Colon HCT15	30.05	30.05	Kim et al. (2008)
Liver HepG2	304.27	89.6	Yang et al. (2010)
Lung A549	17.43	17.43	Kim et al. (2008)
Lung H-1299	150	44.2	Sang et al. (2009)
Oral OC2	74.2	21.8	Chen et al. (2010)
Ovarian SK-OV-3	15.72	15.72	Kim et al. (2008)
Skin A431	300	88.3	Nigam et al. (2009)
Skin SK-MEL-2	20.94	20.94	Kim et al. (2008)
6-Shogaol			
Colon HCT116	4.3	1.19	Gan et al. (2011)
Colon HCT15	1.76	1.76	Kim et al. (2008)
Liver BEL 7404	11.8	3.26	Peng et al. (2012)
Lung A549	1.47	1.47	Kim et al. (2008)
Lung A549	22.9	6.33	Peng et al. (2012)
Lung A549	55.4	1.53	Hung et al. (2009)
Lung H-1299	8	2.21	Sang et al. (2009)
Neuroblastoma SH-SY5Y	3.7	1.02	Gan et al. (2011)
Oral OC2	15.6	4.31	Chen et al. (2010)
Ovarian SK-OV-3	1.05	1.05	Kim et al. (2008)
Prostate PC-3	100	27.64	Peng et al. (2012)
Respiratory CNE	43.8	12.11	Peng et al. (2012)
Respiratory KB	7.4	2.05	Peng et al. (2012)
Skin SK-MEL-2	1.13	1.13	Kim et al. (2008)

evaluations of whole ginger extracts have provided valuable information regarding the potent anticancer activity of the whole food. Ginger extract was found to induce dose-dependent inhibition of cell proliferation and apoptosis in HEp-2 (HeLa derived) cells at an IC_{50} dose of 900 μg/mL by means of increased superoxide production (Vijaya Padma et al. 2007). Three ovarian cancer cell lines (SKOV3, A2780, and ES-2) and a line of untransformed human ovarian surface epithelium (HOSE) cells were treated with whole ginger extract resulting in significant growth inhibition of the cancer cells at doses under 50 μg/mL, while the HOSE cells were relatively unaffected even at double the dose (Rhode et al. 2007). Interestingly, aqueous extract of ginger (GAE), devoid of gingerols and shogaols, decreased in vitro cell viability and induced apoptosis with IC_{50}s of 239.4 and 253.4 μg/mL in human lung and cervical cancer cells respectively, emphasizing the anticancer potential of other less-abundant components in whole ginger (Choudhury et al. 2010). Antiproliferative studies against breast cancer cell lines involving different ginger varieties revealed that the ginger variety (rhizomes) grown under elevated CO2 concentration exhibited the highest anticancer and antioxidant activities against MCF-7 and MDA-MB-231 cells (Rahman et al. 2011). These findings are represented in Table 10.

Animal studies with whole ginger have contributed to the case for whole foods rather than components. Significant inhibition of the expression of skin tumor promotion markers, considerably lower incidence of skin papillomas, and a dose-dependent decrease in tumor multiplicity and burden were demonstrated in mice treated with whole ginger extract (Katiyar et al. 1996). Ginger extract fed ad libitum in the water of SHN virgin mice delayed mammary tumorigenesis and reduced the incidence of tumors (Nagasawa et al. 2002). An exploration of the efficacy of oral administration of GE against colon cancer initiation and progression in rats resulted in no tumors in the group representing the initiation phase and only one rat in ten developed a tumor in the post-initiation group suggesting a possible role for GE in the prevention and treatment of colon cancer (Manju and Nalini 2005; Manju et al. 2006). Ginger extract ingestion was also shown to significantly decrease early indicators of hepatocarcinogenesis, providing protection from liver cancer in male Wistar rats (Habib et al. 2008; Mansour et al. 2010; Yusof et al. 2008).

Recently, we have conducted a comprehensive evaluation of ginger extract for the prevention and treatment of prostate cancer in our laboratory (Brahmbhatt et al. 2013; Gundala et al. 2014; Karna et al. 2012; Mukkavilli et al. 2014). Treating five cancer cell lines and two normal cell lines revealed selective inhibition of proliferation, cell cycle arrest, and apoptosis induction. The reported effective range for 6G is 300–400μM (88–177 μg/ml), but in this study using whole ginger, the amount of 6G in the IC_{50} dose is only 5.38 μg/ml (18 μM), suggesting that 6G is likely not the only active ingredient and that there may be synergistic reactions between constituent phytochemicals (Karna et al. 2012). In further investigations of this concept, individual phytochemicals from ginger were compared, including 6G, 8G, 10G, and 6S, separately and in a variety of combinations with each other and with whole ginger extract. Significant antiproliferative synergy was observed in a number of these combinations, suggesting that a focus on optimal combinations of phytochemicals may provide greater anticancer benefits than the current reductionist thinking of isolating the most active phytochemical (Brahmbhatt et al. 2013). An analysis of available data for in vitro proliferation studies provides a striking contrast between the IC_{50} doses of 6G and 6S and their estimated equivalent dose as part of a whole ginger extract. When cells were treated with 6G alone, the average required dose was 37.3 μg/mL, but as a percentage of the IC_{50} dose of whole ginger, only 2.5 μg/mL are present in the extract, a 15-fold difference. As a more effective inhibitor of cell growth the results for 6S are not as dramatic, but the average IC_{50} of 4.53 μg/mL is threefold higher than the 1.39 μg/mL concentration available in whole ginger (Brahmbhatt et al. 2013). This study revealed that not

Table 10 Antiproliferative activity of whole ginger extract

Material tested	Cell line	Reported IC_{50} (in μg/mL)	Contribution towards efficacy of whole ginger extract (in μg/mL)		Citations
			6G	6S	
Aqueous whole extract (lacks G & S)	Cervical HeLa	253.4	3.73	2.06	Choudhury et al. (2010)
Whole	Liver Hep-2	900	13.24	7.33	Vijaya Padma et al. (2007)
Aqueous whole extract (lacks G and S)	Lung A549	239.4	3.52	1.95	Choudhury et al. (2010)
Whole (Fulbaria)	Breast MCF-7	52	0.77	0.42	Rahman et al. (2011)
Whole (Syedpuri)	Breast MCF-7	47	0.69	0.38	Rahman et al. (2011)
Whole-high CO_2 (Fulbaria)	Breast MCF-7	34.8	0.51	0.28	Rahman et al. (2011)
Whole-high CO_2 (Syedpuri)	Breast MCF-7	25.7	0.38	0.21	Rahman et al. (2011)
Whole (Fulbaria)	Breast MDA-MB-231	62.8	0.92	0.51	Rahman et al. (2011)
Whole (Syedpuri)	Breast MDA-MB-231	38.8	0.57	0.32	Rahman et al. (2011)
Whole-high CO2 (Fulbaria)	Breast MDA-MB-231	32.53	0.48	0.26	Rahman et al. (2011)
Whole-high CO2 (Syedpuri)	Breast MDA-MB-231	30.2	0.44	0.25	Rahman et al. (2011)
Whole	Prostate C4-2	523	7.69	4.26	Karna et al. (2012)
Whole	Prostate C4-2B	240	3.53	1.95	Karna et al. (2012)
Whole	Prostate LNCaP	95	1.40	0.77	Karna et al. (2012)
Whole	Prostate PC-3	250	3.68	2.04	Karna et al. (2012)

G gingerols, *S* shogaols
6-gingerol and 6-shogaol are present at an abundance of 1.47 % and 0.84 % in whole ginger extract, respectively

only do these phenolics exhibit synergistic and additive interactions among themselves, but also show similar effects when GE was further enriched with each of them.

This observation further led to our investigation of in vivo synergy among ginger biophenolics (Gundala et al. 2014). It was clearly evident that 6G, 8G, 10G, and 6S were not the only ones contributing toward GE's efficacy, but the remaining partners also exhibit synergistic and/or additive interactions to impart remarkable efficacy to GE. Our data demonstrated the existence of in vivo interactions among GE phytochemicals as evidenced by the tumor growth-inhibiting efficacy of GE (~68 %) compared to that of an artificial mixture, Mix (~28 %), comprised 6G, 8G, 10G, and 6S in the same ratios as they exist in their natural form (Gundala et al. 2014). The superior efficacy of GE by 40 % unmasked other partners that contribute toward GE's remarkable activity in addition to 6G, 8G, 10G, and 6S. Further confirmation of this hypothesis was observed upon testing the sub-fraction of ginger extract called GE-Mix that lacked the four bioactive components, for its in vivo anticancer efficacy (Gundala et al. 2014). Surprisingly, GE-Mix showed ~35 % inhibition of tumor growth indicating that the less known partners other than 6G, 8G, 10G, and 6S also possess significant anticancer potential. Furthermore, pharmacokinetic (PK) profiling of the four GE components upon oral administration of 250 mg/kg of GE or Mix revealed that there were multiple $C_{\max}$ peaks observed in the evaluation of GE (Gundala et al. 2014). This multiple peaking phenomenon, often associated with recirculation of compounds from intestine to systemic circulation after getting eliminated through bile, was not observed when GE phytochemicals were administered as a Mix. Further, the plasma concentrations of the four GE components were only transiently observed when consumed in the Mix form. β-glucuronidase hydrolysis of both plasma and feces samples obtained post-intravenous administration of pure ginger biophenolics confirmed that the gingerols reenter the liver via the hepatic portal vein from the intestine for reabsorption into the systemic circulation, a phenomenon known as enterohepatic recirculation (EHR). Gingerols when fed as GE mimicked this phenomenon and thus may aid in the enhanced availability of ginger phenolics at the target sites in their natural setting (Gundala et al. 2014). This study further emphasizes the existence of phytocomplexity, where collaborative interplay among GE phytochemicals (Fig. 5) confers maximum therapeutic benefits due to favorable absorption kinetics and bioavailability. Enzyme inhibition assays revealed that GE is not a potent inhibitor of the phase I drug metabolizing cytochrome P450 enzymes (Mukkavilli et al. 2014). Also, GE was found to have no potential herb–drug interactions, thus rendering it safe for consumption along with other clinical drugs (Mukkavilli et al. 2014). The observations pertaining possible EHR of gingerols when delivered in their natural matrix are compelling and provide impetus to investigate and design novel combinations/dietary supplements for prostate cancer management.

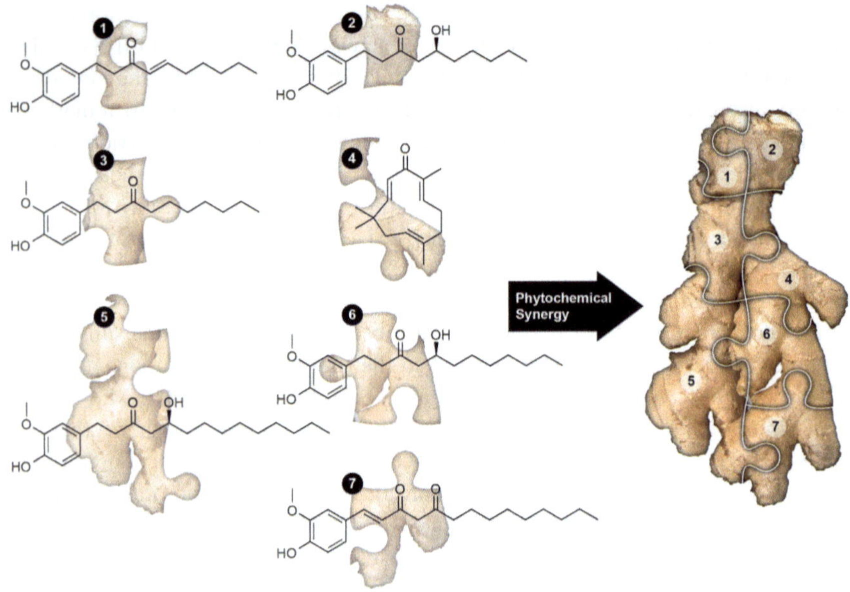

1. 6-shogaol 2. 6-gingerol 3. Paradol 4. Zerumbone 5. 10-gingerol 6. 8-gingerol 7. 1-dehydro-10-gingerdione

Fig. 5 *Whole Ginger's manifold contributions to the cuisine of health*: The optimal therapeutic potential lies in ginger, with its phenolics, including the gingerols, shogaols, paradols, zerumbone, gingerdiones, and many others, collaborate to puzzle and confound the fatal adversary, i.e., cancer

3 The Whole Truth and Nothing But the Truth: Significance of Synergy Among Dietary Phytochemicals

It is now understood that a detailed evaluation of the fate of the constituent phytochemicals and in vivo mechanisms of action upon consumption of whole foods is required in order to employ whole foods as therapeutic and preventive agents. Decades of research has indicated that several constituent phytochemicals of whole foods compete with each other or interact among themselves to attack specific sites of metabolically active tumors to impart improved efficacy. The phytocomplexity inherent in whole plant foods and spices requires a shift in the current paradigm of isolating the individual phytochemicals for their activity. Additionally, there could be several mechanisms through which these phytochemicals act in parallel at the target sites. The existence of synergistic interactions among phytochemicals has long been known and is intrinsic to the activity of whole foods. Such synergistic mixtures of phytochemicals naturally present in plant foods at low concentrations may even prevent DNA mutations, impede cell cycle, inhibit cell proliferation, and induce apoptosis in cancer cells as well as modify immune responses more effectively than individual components that comprise the plant food.

Whole foods have been evaluated for their capacity to deliver "pharmacodynamic synergy," where the effect due to combination of phytochemicals is greater than the additive sum of effects of individual phytochemicals (Fig. 6), to enhance the overall therapeutic index (Danielsson et al. 2011). For example, as stated earlier, the highest antioxidant activity was observed in case of the combination of polyphenols in pomegranate juice in contrast to the constituent polyphenols alone. Recent observations pertaining to ginger phenolics also suggest the significance of pharmacodynamic synergy in whole foods, which may cause a great decrease in the concentration of effective doses while preserving efficacy. Furthermore, apart from the pharmacodynamic synergy, phytocomplexity also offers compelling supplementary in vivo benefits in terms of "pharmacokinetic synergy," where the less active or non-active constituents of whole foods assist the most-active constituent phytochemicals to target specific sites of action either by improving bioavailability or by decreasing metabolism and excretion (Yang et al. 2014). Recent reports on ginger biophenolics revealed that upon oral administration of whole ginger extract, such pharmacokinetic synergy is exhibited to enhance the bioavailability of individual ginger phenols. Along with improving the bioavailability, pharmacokinetic synergy (Fig. 6) might also induce resistance-reversal mechanisms and other complementary mechanisms like immunomodulation. Thus, all the abovementioned data related to whole food phytochemicals not only emphasize the complexity of natural matrices but also signify the role of the "unsung heroes," the other silently partnering constituents, which might actually be responsible for the improved efficacy of the active ingredients when delivered in their natural forms.

Information pertaining to the extent of absorption of active phytochemicals as measured by the plasma, urine, and/or feces concentrations upon oral administration of whole foods is required to understand the in vivo fate of phytochemicals. Further, bioavailability parameters including maximum plasma concentration (C_{max}), time taken to reach C_{max} (T_{max}), area under the plasma concentration–time curve (AUC), and elimination half-life need to be evaluated in order to determine the right dosage of whole foods to achieve maximum anticancer benefits. Though the efficacy of several whole food extracts has been determined, this level of detailed pharmacokinetic evaluation is limited. Thus, it is important to investigate the untapped arena, i.e., pharmacodynamic and pharmacokinetic synergies of whole foods, in order to exploit their therapeutic efficacies to further design and interpret the intervention studies employing fruits and vegetables.

4 Conclusion

Like the age-old adage "prevention is better than cure," it is becoming increasingly clear that chemoprevention is the best way to fight cancer rather than attempting to cure it with toxic chemotherapeutics once it manifests. Lifestyle aspects such as diet and exercise have become the objects of intense focus in developing novel

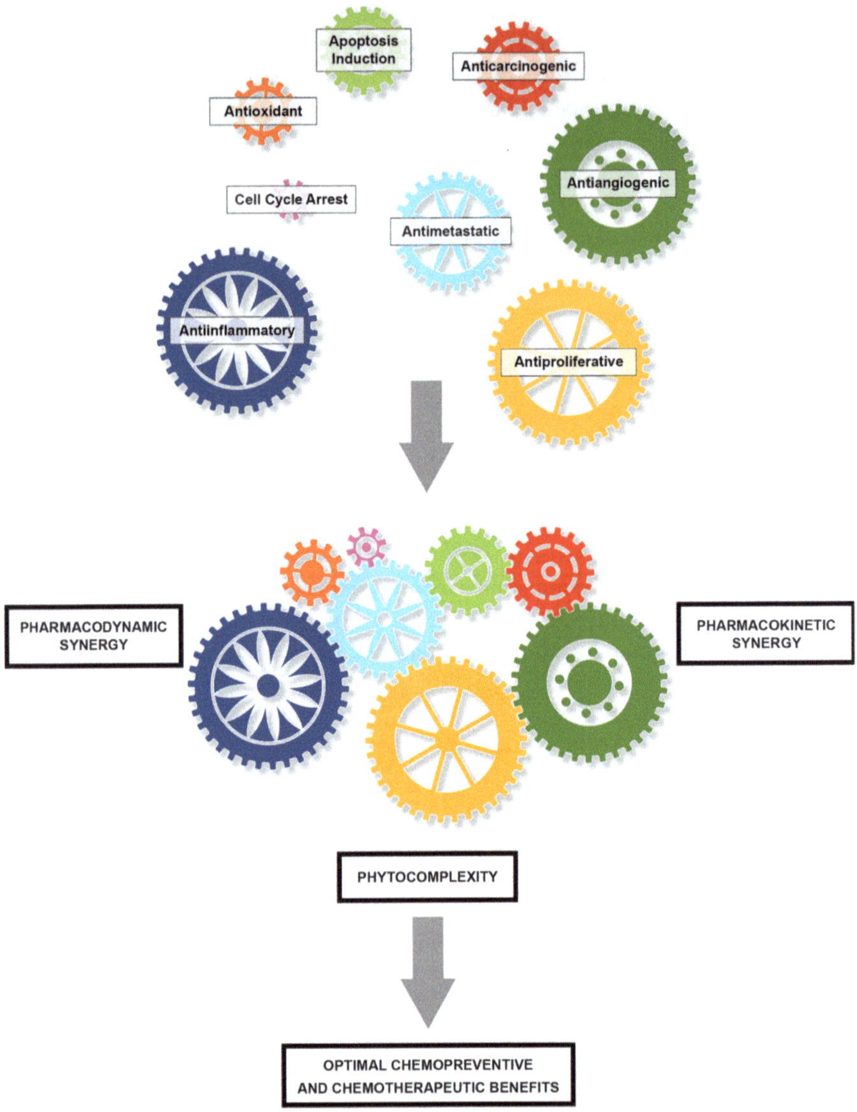

Fig. 6 *The untiring machines with immense outputs!* Unique chemotherapeutic and chemopreventive benefits conferred, via inhibition of cell proliferation, angiogenesis, metastasis, carcinogenesis, induction of cell cycle arrest, apoptosis, and/or antioxidant and anti-inflammatory properties, by constituent phytochemicals of whole foods are fueled by the infinite capabilities, including pharmacokinetic and pharmacodynamic synergies of the nature's own phytocomplexity, like the limitless output of a well-oiled machine

chemoprevention modalities. Dietary interventions could prove to be cost-effective and nontoxic options in treating cancer as the constituent phytochemicals of whole food agents can deliver maximum therapeutic benefits via pharmacodynamic and pharmacokinetic synergies. While increased consumption of fruits and vegetables is often associated with reduced risk of cancer, dietary agents have not been exploited to their fullest potential in developing safer and inexpensive chemopreventive approaches. Various factors including choice of test population, age and lifestyle of the subjects in test groups, and most importantly, the phytocomplexity of the enigmatic whole foods have not been focused upon in earlier attempts. Additionally, there have not been ideal preclinical models to study chemoprevention in vivo before human trials, thus restricting the choice of potential agents. Essentially, the pharmacokinetic and pharmacodynamics synergies associated with whole foods along with the prospects of improved bioavailability, biotransformation, and absorption of the constituent active entities at the target sites possibly due to the interactions of the "silent" partners are crucial aspects that cannot be ignored as they may provide the rationale for innovative chemopreventive strategies.

Although this chapter focuses on the evidence for synergy in whole plant foods, contradictory results do exist and should be considered when embarking on an exploration of plants and their effects on human health. In addition to the five plant foods that are our main focus here, research has discovered many other plants and plant compounds with beneficial functions such as EGCG from tea and curcumin from the spice turmeric, which have been extensively investigated for human health benefits. While much of the research into plant-based cancer prevention and treatment has concentrated on individual compounds existing in plants, a growing body of evidence holds that the complex blend of phytochemicals found in whole foods presents an additive or synergistic effect that is superior to the individual components, suggesting that Mother Nature may be the best combinatorial chemist and future research should be geared toward identification of optimal phytochemical combinations rather than exclusively on single constituents.

References

(1994) The effect of Vitamin E and beta carotene on the incidence of lung cancer and other cancers in male smokers. N Engl J Med 330:1029–1035

Abdulah R, Faried A, Kobayashi K, Yamazaki C, Suradji EW, Ito K, Suzuki K, Murakami M, Kuwano H, Koyama H (2009) Selenium enrichment of broccoli sprout extract increases chemosensitivity and apoptosis of LNCaP prostate cancer cells. BMC Cancer 9:414

Adhami VM, Khan N, Mukhtar H (2009) Cancer chemoprevention by pomegranate: laboratory and clinical evidence. Nutr Cancer 61:811–815

Adhami VM, Siddiqui IA, Syed DN, Lall RK, Mukhtar H (2012) Oral infusion of pomegranate fruit extract inhibits prostate carcinogenesis in the TRAMP model. Carcinogenesis 33:644–651

Afaq F, Malik A, Syed D, Maes D, Matsui MS, Mukhtar H (2005a) Pomegranate fruit extract modulates UV-B-mediated phosphorylation of mitogen-activated protein kinases and activation of nuclear factor kappa B in normal human epidermal keratinocytes paragraph sign. Photochem Photobiol 81:38–45

Afaq F, Saleem M, Krueger CG, Reed JD, Mukhtar H (2005b) Anthocyanin- and hydrolyzable tannin-rich pomegranate fruit extract modulates MAPK and NF-kappaB pathways and inhibits skin tumorigenesis in CD-1 mice. Int J Cancer 113:423–433

Afaq F, Khan N, Syed DN, Mukhtar H (2010) Oral feeding of pomegranate fruit extract inhibits early biomarkers of UVB radiation-induced carcinogenesis in SKH-1 hairless mouse epidermis. Photochem Photobiol 86:1318–1326

Aiyer HS, Gupta RC (2010) Berries and ellagic acid prevent estrogen-induced mammary tumorigenesis by modulating enzymes of estrogen metabolism. Cancer Prev Res (Phila) 3:727–737

Albanes D, Malila N, Taylor PR, Huttunen JK, Virtamo J, Edwards BK, Rautalahti M, Hartman AM, Barrett MJ, Pietinen P, Hartman TJ, Sipponen P, Lewin K, Teerenhovi L, Hietanen P, Tangrea JA, Virtanen M, Heinonen OP (2000) Effects of supplemental alpha-tocopherol and beta-carotene on colorectal cancer: results from a controlled trial (Finland). Cancer Causes Control 11:197–205

Anand P, Kunnumakkara AB, Sundaram C, Harikumar KB, Tharakan ST, Lai OS, Sung B, Aggarwal BB (2008) Cancer is a preventable disease that requires major lifestyle changes. Pharm Res 25:2097–2116

Arts IC, Hollman PC, Bueno de Mesquita HB, Feskens EJ, Kromhout D (2001) Dietary catechins and epithelial cancer incidence: the Zutphen elderly study. Int J Cancer 92:298–302

Baliga MS, Haniadka R, Pereira MM, D'Souza JJ, Pallaty PL, Bhat HP, Popuri S (2011) Update on the chemopreventive effects of ginger and its phytochemicals. Crit Rev Food Sci Nutr 51:499–523

Banerjee N, Talcott S, Safe S, Mertens-Talcott SU (2012) Cytotoxicity of pomegranate polyphenolics in breast cancer cells in vitro and vivo: potential role of miRNA-27a and miRNA-155 in cell survival and inflammation. Breast Cancer Res Treat 136:21–34

Barth SW, Fahndrich C, Bub A, Dietrich H, Watzl B, Will F, Briviba K, Rechkemmer G (2005) Cloudy apple juice decreases DNA damage, hyperproliferation and aberrant crypt foci development in the distal colon of DMH-initiated rats. Carcinogenesis 26:1414–1421

Barth SW, Faehndrich C, Bub A, Watzl B, Will F, Dietrich H, Rechkemmer G, Briviba K (2007) Cloudy apple juice is more effective than apple polyphenols and an apple juice derived cloud fraction in a rat model of colon carcinogenesis. J Agric Food Chem 55:1181–1187

Basu A, Imrhan V (2007) Tomatoes versus lycopene in oxidative stress and carcinogenesis: conclusions from clinical trials. Eur J Clin Nutr 61:295–303

Bhaumik A, Upender Kumar M, Sravan Kumar P, Khan KA, Srinivas CH (2014) The bioactive compounds obtained from the tomatoes (Solanum lycopersicum L.) act as potential anticancer agents against the human cervicle adenocarcinoma. Asian Journal of Medical and Pharmaceutical Sciences 2:169–173

Bjorkman M, Klingen I, Birch AN, Bones AM, Bruce TJ, Johansen TJ, Meadow R, Molmann J, Seljasen R, Smart LE, Stewart D (2011) Phytochemicals of Brassicaceae in plant protection and human health--influences of climate, environment and agronomic practice. Phytochemistry 72:538–556

Bode AM, Dong Z (2011) The amazing and mighty ginger. In: Benzie IFF, Wachtel-Galor S (eds) Herbal medicine: biomolecular and clinical aspects, 2nd edn. CRC Press, Boca Raton, FL

Boileau TW, Liao Z, Kim S, Lemeshow S, Erdman JW Jr, Clinton SK (2003) Prostate carcinogenesis in N-methyl-N-nitrosourea (NMU)-testosterone-treated rats fed tomato powder, lycopene, or energy-restricted diets. J Natl Cancer Inst 95:1578–1586

Boivin D, Lamy S, Lord-Dufour S, Jackson J, Beaulieu E, Cote M, Moghrabi A, Barrette S, Gingras D, Beliveau R (2009) Antiproliferative and antioxidant activities of common vegetables: A comparitive study. Food Chem 112:374–380

Bowen P, Chen L, Stacewicz-Sapuntzakis M, Duncan C, Sharifi R, Ghosh L, Kim HS, Christov-Tzelkov K, van Breemen R (2002) Tomato sauce supplementation and prostate cancer: lycopene accumulation and modulation of biomarkers of carcinogenesis. Exp Biol Med (Maywood) 227:886–893

Boyd LA, Mccann MJ, Hashim Y, Bennett RN, Gill CI, Rowland IR (2006) Assessment of the anti-genotoxic, anti-proliferative, and anti-metastatic potential of crude watercress extract in human colon cancer cells. Nutr Cancer 55:232–241

Boyer J, Liu RH (2004) Apple phytochemicals and their health benefits. Nutr J 3:5

Brahmbhatt M, Gundala SR, Asif G, Shamsi SA, Aneja R (2013) Ginger phytochemicals exhibit synergy to inhibit prostate cancer cell proliferation. Nutr Cancer 65:263–272

Burgess LC, Rice E, Fischer T, Seekins JR, Burgess TP, Sticka SJ, Klatt K (2008) Lycopene has limited effect on cell proliferation in only two of seven human cell lines (both cancerous and noncancerous) in an in vitro system with doses across the physiological range. Toxicol In Vitro 22:1297–1300

Butt MS, Sultan MT (2011) Ginger and its health claims: molecular aspects. Crit Rev Food Sci Nutr 51:383–393

Campbell JK, Canene-Adams K, Lindshield BL, Boileau TW, Clinton SK, Erdman JW Jr (2004) Tomato phytochemicals and prostate cancer risk. J Nutr 134:3486S–3492S

Campbell JK, King JL, Harmston M, Lila MA, Erdman JW Jr (2006) Synergistic effects of flavonoids on cell proliferation in Hepa-1c1c7 and LNCaP cancer cell lines. J Food Sci 71: S358–S363

Capanoglu E, Beekwilder J, Boyacioglu D, Hall R, de Vos R (2008) Changes in antioxidant and metabolite profiles during production of tomato paste. J Agric Food Chem 56:964–973

Chan JM, Holick CN, Leitzmann MF, Rimm EB, Willett WC, Stampfer MJ, Giovannucci EL (2006) Diet after diagnosis and the risk of prostate cancer progression, recurrence, and death (United States). Cancer Causes Control 17:199–208

Chan R, Lok K, Woo J (2009) Prostate cancer and vegetable consumption. Mol Nutr Food Res 53:201–216

Chaudhuri D, Orsulic S, Ashok BT (2007) Antiproliferative activity of sulforaphane in Akt-overexpressing ovarian cancer cells. Mol Cancer Ther 6:334–345

Chen L, Stacewicz-Sapuntzakis M, Duncan C, Sharifi R, Ghosh L, van Breemen R, Ashton D, Bowen PE (2001) Oxidative DNA damage in prostate cancer patients consuming tomato sauce-based entrees as a whole-food intervention. J Natl Cancer Inst 93:1872–1879

Chen CY, Yang YH, Kuo SY (2010) Effect of [6]-shogaol on cytosolic Ca2+ levels and proliferation in human oral cancer cells (OC2). J Nat Prod 73:1370–1374

Cheng X-L, Liu Q, Peng Y-B, Qi L-W, Li P (2011) Steamed ginger (Zingiber officinale): Changed chemical profile and increased anticancer potential. Food Chem 129:1785–1792

Cho HJ, Park SY, Kim EJ, Kim JK, Park JH (2011) 3,3'-Diindolylmethane inhibits prostate cancer development in the transgenic adenocarcinoma mouse prostate model. Mol Carcinog 50:100–112

Chou CC, Yang JS, Lu HF, Ip SW, Lo C, Wu CC, Lin JP, Tang NY, Chung JG, Chou MJ, Teng YH, Chen DR (2010) Quercetin-mediated cell cycle arrest and apoptosis involving activation of a caspase cascade through the mitochondrial pathway in human breast cancer MCF-7 cells. Arch Pharm Res 33:1181–1191

Choudhury D, Das A, Bhattacharya A, Chakrabarti G (2010) Aqueous extract of ginger shows antiproliferative activity through disruption of microtubule network of cancer cells. Food Chem Toxicol 48:2872–2880

Clarke JD, Riedl K, Bella D, Schwartz SJ, Stevens JF, Ho E (2011) Comparison of isothiocyanate metabolite levels and histone deacetylase activity in human subjects consuming broccoli sprouts or broccoli supplement. J Agric Food Chem 59:10955–10963

Colli JL, Amling CL (2009) Chemoprevention of prostate cancer: what can be recommended to patients? Curr Urol Rep 10:165–171

Dai Z, Nair V, Khan M, Ciolino HP (2010) Pomegranate extract inhibits the proliferation and viability of MMTV-Wnt-1 mouse mammary cancer stem cells in vitro. Oncol Rep 24:1087–1091

Danielsson M, Rosenthal-Aizman K, Bergsson G, Unden A (2011) Pharmacodynamic synergy strictly dependent on the co-operative aggregation of enantiomers of cyclic peptides in the bacterial cell membrane. Bioorg Med Chem Lett 21:5262–5265

di Mascio P, Kaiser S, Sies H (1989) Lycopene as the most efficient biological carotenoid singlet oxygen quencher. Arch Biochem Biophys 274:532–538

Dinkova-Kostova AT, Fahey JW, Wade KL, Jenkins SN, Shapiro TA, Fuchs EJ, Kerns ML, Talalay P (2007) Induction of the phase 2 response in mouse and human skin by sulforaphane-containing broccoli sprout extracts. Cancer Epidemiol Biomarkers Prev 16:847–851

Dinkova-Kostova AT, Fahey JW, Benedict AL, Jenkins SN, Ye L, Wehage SL, Talalay P (2010) Dietary glucoraphanin-rich broccoli sprout extracts protect against UV radiation-induced skin carcinogenesis in SKH-1 hairless mice. Photochem Photobiol Sci 9:597–600

Diwadkar-Navsariwala V, Novotny JA, Gustin DM, Sosman JA, Rodvold KA, Crowell JA, Stacewicz-Sapuntzakis M, Bowen PE (2003) A physiological pharmacokinetic model describing the disposition of lycopene in healthy men. J Lipid Res 44:1927–1939

Eberhardt MV, Lee CY, Liu RH (2000) Antioxidant activity of fresh apples. Nature 405:903–904

Etminan M, Takkouche B, Caamano-Isorna F (2004) The role of tomato products and lycopene in the prevention of prostate cancer: a meta-analysis of observational studies. Cancer Epidemiol Biomarkers Prev 13:340–345

Ettorre A, Frosali S, Andreassi M, di Stefano A (2010) Lycopene phytocomplex, but not pure lycopene, is able to trigger apoptosis and improve the efficacy of photodynamic therapy in HL60 human leukemia cells. Exp Biol Med (Maywood) 235:1114–1125

Faria A, Calhau C (2011) The bioactivity of pomegranate: impact on health and disease. Crit Rev Food Sci Nutr 51:626–634

Ferrarini L, Pellegrini N, Mazzeo T, Miglio C, Galati S, Milano F, Rossi C, Buschini A (2012) Anti-proliferative activity and chemoprotective effects towards DNA oxidative damage of fresh and cooked Brassicaceae. Br J Nutr 107:1324–1332

Feskanich D, Ziegler RG, Michaud DS, Giovannucci EL, Speizer FE, Willett WC, Colditz GA (2000) Prospective study of fruit and vegetable consumption and risk of lung cancer among men and women. J Natl Cancer Inst 92:1812–1823

Fjaeraa C, Nanberg E (2009) Effect of ellagic acid on proliferation, cell adhesion and apoptosis in SH-SY5Y human neuroblastoma cells. Biomed Pharmacother 63:254–261

Ford NA, Elsen AC, Zuniga K, Lindshield BL, Erdman JW Jr (2011) Lycopene and apo-12'-lycopenal reduce cell proliferation and alter cell cycle progression in human prostate cancer cells. Nutr Cancer 63:256–263

Friedman M, Levin CE, Lee SU, Kim HJ, Lee IS, Byun JO, Kozukue N (2009) Tomatine-containing green tomato extracts inhibit growth of human breast, colon, liver, and stomach cancer cells. J Agric Food Chem 57:5727–5733

Gan FF, Nagle AA, Ang X, Ho OH, Tan SH, Yang H, Chui WK, Chew EH (2011) Shogaols at proapoptotic concentrations induce G (2)/M arrest and aberrant mitotic cell death associated with tubulin aggregation. Apoptosis 16:856–867

Gerhauser C (2008) Cancer chemopreventive potential of apples, apple juice, and apple components. Planta Med 74:1608–1624

Gibellini L, Pinti M, Nasi M, Montagna JP, de Biasi S, Roat E, Bertoncelli L, Cooper EL, Cossarizza A (2011) Quercetin and cancer chemoprevention. Evid Based Complement Alternat Med 2011:591356

Giovannucci E, Liu Y, Platz EA, Stampfer MJ, Willett WC (2007) Risk factors for prostate cancer incidence and progression in the health professionals follow-up study. Int J Cancer 121:1571–1578

Gosse F, Guyot S, Roussi S, Lobstein A, Fischer B, Seiler N, Raul F (2005) Chemopreventive properties of apple procyanidins on human colon cancer-derived metastatic SW620 cells and in a rat model of colon carcinogenesis. Carcinogenesis 26:1291–1295

Greenberg ER, Baron JA, Tosteson TD, Freeman DH Jr, Beck GJ, Bond JH, Colacchio TA, Coller JA, Frankl HD, Haile RW et al (1994) A clinical trial of antioxidant vitamins to prevent colorectal adenoma. Polyp Prevention Study Group. N Engl J Med 331:141–147

Greenwald P, Anderson D, Nelson SA, Taylor PR (2007) Clinical trials of vitamin and mineral supplements for cancer prevention. Am J Clin Nutr 85:314S–317S

Guil-Guerrero JL, Ramos-Bueno R, Rodriguez-Garcia I, Lopez-Sanchez C (2011) Cytotoxicity screening of several tomato extracts. J Med Food 14:40–45

Gundala SR, Mukkavilli R, Yang C, Yadav P, Tandon V, Vangala S, Prakash S, Aneja R (2014) Enterohepatic recirculation of bioactive ginger phytochemicals is associated with enhanced tumor growth-inhibitory activity of ginger extract. Carcinogenesis 35:1320–1329
Habib SH, Makpol S, Abdul Hamid NA, Das S, Ngah WZ, Yusof YA (2008) Ginger extract (Zingiber officinale) has anti-cancer and anti-inflammatory effects on ethionine-induced hepatoma rats. Clinics (Sao Paulo) 63:807–813
Han DH, Lee MJ, Kim JH (2006) Antioxidant and apoptosis-inducing activities of ellagic acid. Anticancer Res 26:3601–3606
Hanahan D, Weinberg RA (2000) The hallmarks of cancer. Cell 100:57–70
Hanahan D, Weinberg RA (2011) Hallmarks of cancer: the next generation. Cell 144:646–674
Harris DM, Li L, Chen M, Lagunero FT, Go VL, Boros LG (2012) Diverse mechanisms of growth inhibition by luteolin, resveratrol, and quercetin in MIA PaCa-2 cells: a comparative glucose tracer study with the fatty acid synthase inhibitor C75. Metabolomics 8:201–210
He X, Liu RH (2007) Triterpenoids isolated from apple peels have potent antiproliferative activity and may be partially responsible for apple's anticancer activity. J Agric Food Chem 55:4366–4370
He X, Liu RH (2008) Phytochemicals of apple peels: isolation, structure elucidation, and their antiproliferative and antioxidant activities. J Agric Food Chem 56:9905–9910
Heber D (2011) Pomegranate Ellagitannins. In: Benzie IFF, Wachtel-Galor S (eds) Herbal medicine: biomolecular and clinical aspects, 2nd edn. CRC Press, Boca Raton, FL
Herr I, Buchler MW (2010) Dietary constituents of broccoli and other cruciferous vegetables: implications for prevention and therapy of cancer. Cancer Treat Rev 36:377–383
Higdon JV, Delage B, Williams DE, Dashwood RH (2007) Cruciferous vegetables and human cancer risk: epidemiologic evidence and mechanistic basis. Pharmacol Res 55:224–236
Hong MY, Seeram NP, Heber D (2008) Pomegranate polyphenols down-regulate expression of androgen-synthesizing genes in human prostate cancer cells overexpressing the androgen receptor. J Nutr Biochem 19:848–855
Huang CS, Liao JW, Hu ML (2008) Lycopene inhibits experimental metastasis of human hepatoma SK-Hep-1 cells in athymic nude mice. J Nutr 138:538–543
Huang WY, Cai YZ, Zhang Y (2010) Natural phenolic compounds from medicinal herbs and dietary plants: potential use for cancer prevention. Nutr Cancer 62:1–20
Huang TY, Chang WC, Wang MY, Yang YR, Hsu YC (2012) Effect of sulforaphane on growth inhibition in human brain malignant glioma GBM 8401 cells by means of mitochondrial- and MEK/ERK-mediated apoptosis pathway. Cell Biochem Biophys 63:247–259
Hung JY, Hsu YL, Li CT, Ko YC, Ni WC, Huang MS, Kuo PL (2009) 6-Shogaol, an active constituent of dietary ginger, induces autophagy by inhibiting the AKT/mTOR pathway in human non-small cell lung cancer A549 cells. J Agric Food Chem 57:9809–9816
Hwang ES, Bowen PE (2005a) Effects of lycopene and tomato paste extracts on DNA and lipid oxidation in LNCaP human prostate cancer cells. Biofactors 23:97–105
Hwang ES, Bowen PE (2005b) Effects of tomato paste extracts on cell proliferation, cell-cycle arrest and apoptosis in LNCaP human prostate cancer cells. Biofactors 23:75–84
Hwang ES, Lee HJ (2006) Inhibitory effects of lycopene on the adhesion, invasion, and migration of SK-Hep1 human hepatoma cells. Exp Biol Med (Maywood) 231:322–327
Jansen RJ, Robinson DP, Stolzenberg-Solomon RZ, Bamlet WR, de Andrade M, Oberg AL, Hammer TJ, Rabe KG, Anderson KE, Olson JE, Sinha R, Petersen GM (2011) Fruit and vegetable consumption is inversely associated with having pancreatic cancer. Cancer Causes Control 22:1613–1625
Jee HG, Lee KE, Kim JB, Shin HK, Youn YK (2011) Sulforaphane inhibits oral carcinoma cell migration and invasion in vitro. Phytother Res 25:1623–1628
Jeong CH, Bode AM, Pugliese A, Cho YY, Kim HG, Shim JH, Jeon YJ, Li H, Jiang H, Dong Z (2009) [6]-Gingerol suppresses colon cancer growth by targeting leukotriene A4 hydrolase. Cancer Res 69:5584–5591

Jin Y (2011) 3,3'-Diindolylmethane inhibits breast cancer cell growth via miR-21-mediated Cdc25A degradation. Mol Cell Biochem 358:345–354
Jurenka JS (2008) Therapeutic applications of pomegranate (Punica granatum L.): a review. Altern Med Rev 13:128–144
Karna P, Chagani S, Gundala SR, Rida PC, Asif G, Sharma V, Gupta MV, Aneja R (2012) Benefits of whole ginger extract in prostate cancer. Br J Nutr 107:473–484
Kasimsetty SG, Bialonska D, Reddy MK, Ma G, Khan SI, Ferreira D (2010) Colon cancer chemopreventive activities of pomegranate ellagitannins and urolithins. J Agric Food Chem 58:2180–2187
Katiyar SK, Agarwal R, Mukhtar H (1996) Inhibition of tumor promotion in SENCAR mouse skin by ethanol extract of Zingiber officinale rhizome. Cancer Res 56:1023–1030
Keck AS, Qiao Q, Jeffery EH (2003) Food matrix effects on bioactivity of broccoli-derived sulforaphane in liver and colon of F344 rats. J Agric Food Chem 51:3320–3327
Kelkel M, Schumacher M, Dicato M, Diederich M (2011) Antioxidant and anti-proliferative properties of lycopene. Free Radic Res 45:925–940
Khan N, Afaq F, Kweon MH, Kim K, Mukhtar H (2007a) Oral consumption of pomegranate fruit extract inhibits growth and progression of primary lung tumors in mice. Cancer Res 67:3475–3482
Khan N, Hadi N, Afaq F, Syed DN, Kweon MH, Mukhtar H (2007b) Pomegranate fruit extract inhibits prosurvival pathways in human A549 lung carcinoma cells and tumor growth in athymic nude mice. Carcinogenesis 28:163–173
Khan N, Sullivan R, Hoang T, Dittakavi T, Mukhtar H (2013) In: Abstract 194: delay in the progression of lung adenoma to adenocarcinoma in mice by oral consumption of pomegranate fruit extract. Cancer Research, Proceedings: AACR 104th Annual Meeting 2013
Kim MK, Park JH (2009) Conference on "Multidisciplinary approaches to nutritional problems". Symposium on "Nutrition and health". Cruciferous vegetable intake and the risk of human cancer: epidemiological evidence. Proc Nutr Soc 68:103–110
Kim HS, Bowen P, Chen L, Duncan C, Ghosh L, Sharifi R, Christov K (2003) Effects of tomato sauce consumption on apoptotic cell death in prostate benign hyperplasia and carcinoma. Nutr Cancer 47:40–47
Kim EC, Min JK, Kim TY, Lee SJ, Yang HO, Han S, Kim YM, Kwon YG (2005) [6]-Gingerol, a pungent ingredient of ginger, inhibits angiogenesis in vitro and in vivo. Biochem Biophys Res Commun 335:300–308
Kim JS, Lee SI, Park HW, Yang JH, Shin TY, Kim YC, Baek NI, Kim SH, Choi SU, Kwon BM, Leem KH, Jung MY, Kim DK (2008) Cytotoxic components from the dried rhizomes of Zingiber officinale Roscoe. Arch Pharm Res 31:415–418
Klein EA, Thompson IM, Lippman SM, Goodman PJ, Albanes D, Taylor PR, Coltman C (2001) SELECT: the next prostate cancer prevention trial. Selenum and Vitamin E Cancer Prevention Trial. J Urol 166:1311–1315
Knekt P, Jarvinen R, Seppanen R, Hellovaara M, Teppo L, Pukkala E, Aromaa A (1997) Dietary flavonoids and the risk of lung cancer and other malignant neoplasms. Am J Epidemiol 146:223–230
Koh MS, Hwang JS, Moon A (2010) Lycopnene Inhibits Proliferation, Invasion and Migration of Human Breast Cancer Cells. Biomol Therap 18:92–98
Konijeti R, Henning S, Moro A, Sheikh A, Elashoff D, Shapiro A, Ku M, Said JW, Heber D, Cohen P, Aronson WJ (2010) Chemoprevention of prostate cancer with lycopene in the TRAMP model. Prostate 70:1547–1554
Kowalczyk MC, Walaszek Z, Kowalczyk P, Kinjo T, Hanausek M, Slaga TJ (2009) Differential effects of several phytochemicals and their derivatives on murine keratinocytes in vitro and in vivo: implications for skin cancer prevention. Carcinogenesis 30:1008–1015
Kucuk O, Sarkar FH, Sakr W, Djuric Z, Pollak MN, Khachik F, Li YW, Banerjee M, Grignon D, Bertram JS, Crissman JD, Pontes EJ, Wood DP Jr (2001) Phase II randomized clinical trial of

lycopene supplementation before radical prostatectomy. Cancer Epidemiol Biomarkers Prev 10:861–868
Kucuk O, Sarkar FH, Djuric Z, Sakr W, Pollak MN, Khachik F, Banerjee M, Bertram JS, Wood DP Jr (2002) Effects of lycopene supplementation in patients with localized prostate cancer. Exp Biol Med (Maywood) 227:881–885
Kushi LH, Doyle C, McCullough M, Rock CL, Demark-Wahnefried W, Bandera EV, Gapstur S, Patel AV, Andrews K, Gansler T, American Cancer Society Nutrition & Physical Activity Guidelines Advisory Commitee (2012) American Cancer Society Guidelines on nutrition and physical activity for cancer prevention: reducing the risk of cancer with healthy food choices and physical activity. CA Cancer J Clin 62:30–67
Lam TK, Gallicchio L, Lindsley K, Shiels M, Hammond E, Tao XG, Chen L, Robinson KA, Caulfield LE, Herman JG, Guallar E, Alberg AJ (2009) Cruciferous vegetable consumption and lung cancer risk: a systematic review. Cancer Epidemiol Biomarkers Prev 18:184–195
Lampe JW (2009a) Interindividual differences in response to plant-based diets: implications for cancer risk. Am J Clin Nutr 89:1553S–1557S
Lampe JW (2009b) Sulforaphane: from chemoprevention to pancreatic cancer treatment? Gut 58:900–902
Lansky EP, Newman RA (2007) Punica granatum (pomegranate) and its potential for prevention and treatment of inflammation and cancer. J Ethnopharmacol 109:177–206
Lansky EP, Jiang W, Mo H, Bravo L, Froom P, Yu W, Harris NM, Neeman I, Campbell MJ (2005) Possible synergistic prostate cancer suppression by anatomically discrete pomegranate fractions. Invest New Drugs 23:11–20
Latte KP, Appel KE, Lampen A (2011) Health benefits and possible risks of broccoli—an overview. Food Chem Toxicol 49:3287–3309
le Marchand L, Murphy SP, Hankin JH, Wilkens LR, Kolonel LN (2000) Intake of flavonoids and lung cancer. J Natl Cancer Inst 92:154–160
Lee KW, Kim YJ, Kim DO, Lee HJ, Lee CY (2003) Major phenolics in apple and their contribution to the total antioxidant capacity. J Agric Food Chem 51:6516–6520
Li Y, Zhang T, Korkaya H, Liu S, Lee HF, Newman B, Yu Y, Clouthier SG, Schwartz SJ, Wicha MS, Sun D (2010) Sulforaphane, a dietary component of broccoli/broccoli sprouts, inhibits breast cancer stem cells. Clin Cancer Res 16:2580–2590
Liu RH (2004) Potential synergy of phytochemicals in cancer prevention: mechanism of action. J Nutr 134:3479S–3485S
Liu RH, Liu J, Chen B (2005) Apples prevent mammary tumors in rats. J Agric Food Chem 53:2341–2343
Liu JR, Dong HW, Chen BQ, Zhao P, Liu RH (2009) Fresh apples suppress mammary carcinogenesis and proliferative activity and induce apoptosis in mammary tumors of the Sprague–Dawley rat. J Agric Food Chem 57:297–304
Lucier G, Glaser L (2011) Vegetables and melons outlook. Economic Research Service, USDA
Luo C, Wu XG (2011) Lycopene enhances antioxidant enzyme activities and immunity function in N-methyl-N'-nitro-N-nitrosoguanidine-enduced gastric cancer rats. Int J Mol Sci 12:3340–3351
Malik A, Afaq F, Sarfaraz S, Adhami VM, Syed DN, Mukhtar H (2005) Pomegranate fruit juice for chemoprevention and chemotherapy of prostate cancer. Proc Natl Acad Sci U S A 102:14813–14818
Malik A, Afaq S, Shahid M, Akhtar K, Assiri A (2011) Influence of ellagic acid on prostate cancer cell proliferation: a caspase-dependent pathway. Asian Pac J Trop Med 4:550 555
Manju V, Nalini N (2005) Chemopreventive efficacy of ginger, a naturally occurring anticarcinogen during the initiation, post-initiation stages of 1,2 dimethylhydrazine-induced colon cancer. Clin Chim Acta 358:60–67
Manju V, Viswanathan P, Nalini N (2006) Hypolipidemic effect of ginger in 1,2-dimethyl hydrazine-induced experimental colon carcinogenesis. Toxicol Mech Methods 16:461–472

Mansour MA, Bekheet SA, Al-Rejaie SS, Al-Shabanah OA, Al-Howiriny TA, Al-Rikabi AC, Abdo AA (2010) Ginger ingredients inhibit the development of diethylnitrosoamine induced premalignant phenotype in rat chemical hepatocarcinogenesis model. Biofactors 36:483–490

Mehta RG, Murillo G, Naithani R, Peng X (2010) Cancer chemoprevention by natural products: how far have we come? Pharm Res 27:950–961

Mertens-Talcott SU, Jilma-Stohlawetz P, Rios J, Hingorani L, Derendorf H (2006) Absorption, metabolism, and antioxidant effects of pomegranate (Punica granatum l.) polyphenols after ingestion of a standardized extract in healthy human volunteers. J Agric Food Chem 54:8956–8961

Michaud-Levesque J, Bousquet-Gagnon N, Beliveau R (2012) Quercetin abrogates IL-6/STAT3 signaling and inhibits glioblastoma cell line growth and migration. Exp Cell Res 318:925–935

Miura T, Chiba M, Kasai K, Nozaka H, Nakamura T, Shoji T, Kanda T, Ohtake Y, Sato T (2008) Apple procyanidins induce tumor cell apoptosis through mitochondrial pathway activation of caspase-3. Carcinogenesis 29:585–593

Moreno DA, Carvajal M, Lopez-Berenguer C, Garcia-Viguera C (2006) Chemical and biological characterisation of nutraceutical compounds of broccoli. J Pharm Biomed Anal 41:1508–1522

Mossine VV, Chopra P, Mawhinney TP (2008) Interaction of tomato lycopene and ketosamine against rat prostate tumorigenesis. Cancer Res 68:4384–4391

Mukkavilli R, Gundala SR, Yang C, Donthamsetty S, Cantuaria G, Jadhav GR, Vangala S, Reid MD, Aneja R (2014) Modulation of cytochrome P450 metabolism and transport across intestinal epithelial barrier by ginger biophenolics. PLoS One 9, e108386

Munday R, Mhawech-Fauceglia P, Munday CM, Paonessa JD, Tang L, Munday JS, Lister C, Wilson P, Fahey JW, Davis W, Zhang Y (2008) Inhibition of urinary bladder carcinogenesis by broccoli sprouts. Cancer Res 68:1593–1600

Nabavi SM, Nabavi SF, Eslami S, Moghaddam AH (2012) In vivo protective effects of quercetin against sodium fluoride-induced oxidative stress in the hepatic tissue. Food Chem 132:931–935

Nagasawa H, Watanabe K, Inatomi H (2002) Effects of bitter melon (Momordica charantia l.) or ginger rhizome (Zingiber offifinale rosc) on spontaneous mammary tumorigenesis in SHN mice. Am J Chin Med 30:195–205

Nair V, Dai Z, Khan M, Ciolino HP (2011) Pomegranate extract induces cell cycle arrest and alters cellular phenotype of human pancreatic cancer cells. Anticancer Res 31:2699–2704

Nho CW, Jeffery E (2001) The synergistic upregulation of phase II detoxification enzymes by glucosinolate breakdown products in cruciferous vegetables. Toxicol Appl Pharmacol 174:146–152

Nigam N, Bhui K, Prasad S, George J, Shukla Y (2009) [6]-Gingerol induces reactive oxygen species regulated mitochondrial cell death pathway in human epidermoid carcinoma A431 cells. Chem Biol Interact 181:77–84

Nigam N, George J, Srivastava S, Roy P, Bhui K, Singh M, Shukla Y (2010) Induction of apoptosis by [6]-gingerol associated with the modulation of p53 and involvement of mitochondrial signaling pathway in B[a]P-induced mouse skin tumorigenesis. Cancer Chemother Pharmacol 65:687–696

Oyagbemi AA, Saba AB, Azeez OI (2010) Molecular targets of [6]-gingerol: Its potential roles in cancer chemoprevention. Biofactors 36:169–178

Paller CJ, Ye X, Wozniak PJ, Gillespie BK, Sieber PR, Greengold RH, Stockton BR, Hertzman BL, Efros MD, Roper RP, Liker HR, Carducci MA (2013) A randomized phase II study of pomegranate extract for men with rising PSA following initial therapy for localized prostate cancer. Prostate Cancer Prostatic Dis 16:50–55

Palozza P, Bellovino D, Simone R, Boninsegna A, Cellini F, Monastra G, Gaetani S (2009) Effect of beta-carotene-rich tomato lycopene beta-cyclase (tlcy-b) on cell growth inhibition in HT-29 colon adenocarcinoma cells. Br J Nutr 102:207–214

Palozza P, Colangelo M, Simone R, Catalano A, Boninsegna A, Lanza P, Monego G, Ranelletti FO (2010) Lycopene induces cell growth inhibition by altering mevalonate pathway and Ras signaling in cancer cell lines. Carcinogenesis 31:1813–1821

Pannellini T, Iezzi M, Liberatore M, Sabatini F, Iacobelli S, Rossi C, Alberti S, di ILIO C, Vitaglione P, Fogliano V, Piantelli M (2010) A dietary tomato supplement prevents prostate cancer in TRAMP mice. Cancer Prev Res (Phila) 3:1284–1291

Pantuck AJ, Leppert JT, Zomorodian N, Aronson W, Hong J, Barnard RJ, Seeram N, Liker H, Wang H, Elashoff R, Heber D, Aviram M, Ignarro L, Belldegrun A (2006) Phase II study of pomegranate juice for men with rising prostate-specific antigen following surgery or radiation for prostate cancer. Clin Cancer Res 12:4018–4026

Pappa G, Lichtenberg M, Iori R, Barillari J, Bartsch H, Gerhauser C (2006) Comparison of growth inhibition profiles and mechanisms of apoptosis induction in human colon cancer cell lines by isothiocyanates and indoles from Brassicaceae. Mutat Res 599:76–87

Pappa G, Strathmann J, Lowinger M, Bartsch H, Gerhauser C (2007) Quantitative combination effects between sulforaphane and 3,3'-diindolylmethane on proliferation of human colon cancer cells in vitro. Carcinogenesis 28:1471–1477

Park KK, Chun KS, Lee JM, Lee SS, Surh YJ (1998) Inhibitory effects of [6]-gingerol, a major pungent principle of ginger, on phorbol ester-induced inflammation, epidermal ornithine decarboxylase activity and skin tumor promotion in ICR mice. Cancer Lett 129:139–144

Park YJ, Wen J, Bang S, Park SW, Song SY (2006) [6]-Gingerol induces cell cycle arrest and cell death of mutant p53-expressing pancreatic cancer cells. Yonsei Med J 47:688–697

Pawlik A, Wiczk A, Kaczynska A, Antosiewicz J, Herman-Antosiewicz A (2013) Sulforaphane inhibits growth of phenotypically different breast cancer cells. Eur J Nutr 52:1949–1958

Peng F, Tao Q, Wu X, Dou H, Spencer S, Mang C, Xu L, Sun L, Zhao Y, Li H, Zeng S, Liu G, Hao X (2012) Cytotoxic, cytoprotective and antioxidant effects of isolated phenolic compounds from fresh ginger. Fitoterapia 83:568–585

Potter JD (2014) The failure of cancer chemoprevention. Carcinogenesis 35:974–982

Powolny AA, Bommareddy A, Hahm ER, Normolle DP, Beumer JH, Nelson JB, Singh SV (2011) Chemopreventative potential of the cruciferous vegetable constituent phenethyl isothiocyanate in a mouse model of prostate cancer. J Natl Cancer Inst 103:571–584

Priyadarsini RV, Vinothini G, Murugan RS, Manikandan P, Nagini S (2011) The flavonoid quercetin modulates the hallmark capabilities of hamster buccal pouch tumors. Nutr Cancer 63:218–226

Qian X, Melkamu T, Upadhyaya P, Kassie F (2011) Indole-3-carbinol inhibited tobacco smoke carcinogen-induced lung adenocarcinoma in A/J mice when administered during the post-initiation or progression phase of lung tumorigenesis. Cancer Lett 311:57–65

Quideau S, Deffieux D, Douat-Casassus C, Pouysegu L (2011) Plant polyphenols: chemical properties, biological activities, and synthesis. Angew Chem Int Ed Engl 50:586–621

Rahman S, Salehin F, Iqbal A (2011) In vitro antioxidant and anticancer activity of young Zingiber officinale against human breast carcinoma cell lines. BMC Complement Altern Med 11:76

Rahmat A, Rosli R, Wan Mohd Zain WN, Susi E, Huzaimah AS (2002) Antiproliferative activity of pure lycopene compared to both extracted lycopene and juices from watermelon. J Med Sci 2:55–58

Reagan-Shaw S, Eggert D, Mukhtar H, Ahmad N (2010) Antiproliferative effects of apple peel extract against cancer cells. Nutr Cancer 62:517–524

Reuben SC, Gopalan A, Petit DM, Bishayee A (2012) Modulation of angiogenesis by dietary phytoconstituents in the prevention and intervention of breast cancer. Mol Nutr Food Res 56:14–29

Rhode J, Fogoros S, Zick S, Wahl H, Griffith KA, Huang J, Liu JR (2007) Ginger inhibits cell growth and modulates angiogenic factors in ovarian cancer cells. BMC Complement Altern Med 7:44

Riso P, Martini D, Visioli F, Martinetti A, Porrini M (2009) Effect of broccoli intake on markers related to oxidative stress and cancer risk in healthy smokers and nonsmokers. Nutr Cancer 61:232–237

Riso P, Martini D, Moller P, Loft S, Bonacina G, Moro M, Porrini M (2010) DNA damage and repair activity after broccoli intake in young healthy smokers. Mutagenesis 25:595–602

Russo M, Spagnuolo C, Tedesco I, Russo GL (2010) Phytochemicals in cancer prevention and therapy: truth or dare? Toxins (Basel) 2:517–551

Russo M, Spagnuolo C, Tedesco I, Bilotto S, Russo GL (2012) The flavonoid quercetin in disease prevention and therapy: facts and fancies. Biochem Pharmacol 83:6–15

Salem S, Salahi M, Mohseni M, Ahmadi H, Mehrsai A, Jahani Y, Pourmand G (2011) Major dietary factors and prostate cancer risk: a prospective multicenter case–control study. Nutr Cancer 63:21–27

Salman H, Bergman M, Djaldetti M, Bessler H (2007) Lycopene affects proliferation and apoptosis of four malignant cell lines. Biomed Pharmacother 61:366–369

Sang S, Hong J, Wu H, Liu J, Yang CS, Pan MH, Badmaev V, Ho CT (2009) Increased growth inhibitory effects on human cancer cells and anti-inflammatory potency of shogaols from Zingiber officinale relative to gingerols. J Agric Food Chem 57:10645–10650

Sartippour MR, Seeram NP, Rao JY, Moro A, Harris DM, Henning SM, Firouzi A, Rettig MB, Aronson WJ, Pantuck AJ, Heber D (2008) Ellagitannin-rich pomegranate extract inhibits angiogenesis in prostate cancer in vitro and in vivo. Int J Oncol 32:475–480

Saw CL, Cintron M, Wu TY, Guo Y, Huang Y, Jeong WS, Kong AN (2011) Pharmacodynamics of dietary phytochemical indoles I3C and DIM: Induction of Nrf2-mediated phase II drug metabolizing and antioxidant genes and synergism with isothiocyanates. Biopharm Drug Dispos 32:289–300

Seeram NP, Lee R, Heber D (2004) Bioavailability of ellagic acid in human plasma after consumption of ellagitannins from pomegranate (Punica granatum L.) juice. Clin Chim Acta 348:63–68

Seeram NP, Adams LS, Henning SM, Niu Y, Zhang Y, Nair MG, Heber D (2005) In vitro antiproliferative, apoptotic and antioxidant activities of punicalagin, ellagic acid and a total pomegranate tannin extract are enhanced in combination with other polyphenols as found in pomegranate juice. J Nutr Biochem 16:360–367

Seeram NP, Henning SM, Zhang Y, Suchard M, Li Z, Heber D (2006) Pomegranate juice ellagitannin metabolites are present in human plasma and some persist in urine for up to 48 hours. J Nutr 136:2481–2485

Seeram NP, Aronson WJ, Zhang Y, Henning SM, Moro A, Lee RP, Sartippour M, Harris DM, Rettig M, Suchard MA, Pantuck AJ, Belldegrun A, Heber D (2007) Pomegranate ellagitannin-derived metabolites inhibit prostate cancer growth and localize to the mouse prostate gland. J Agric Food Chem 55:7732–7737

Senthilkumar K, Arunkumar R, Elumalai P, Sharmila G, Gunadharini DN, Banudevi S, Krishnamoorthy G, Benson CS, Arunakaran J (2011) Quercetin inhibits invasion, migration and signalling molecules involved in cell survival and proliferation of prostate cancer cell line (PC-3). Cell Biochem Funct 29:87–95

Serra AT, Matias AA, Frade RFM, Duarte RO, Feliciano RP, Bronze MR, Figueira ME, Carvalho A, Duarte CMM (2010) Characterization of traditional and exotic apple varieties from Portugal. Part 2—Antioxidant and antiproliferative activities. J Funct Foods 2:46–53

Seufi AM, Ibrahim SS, Elmaghraby TK, Hafez EE (2009) Preventive effect of the flavonoid, quercetin, on hepatic cancer in rats via oxidant/antioxidant activity: molecular and histological evidences. J Exp Clin Cancer Res 28:80

Shan Y, Sun C, Zhao X, Wu K, Cassidy A, Bao Y (2006) Effect of sulforaphane on cell growth, G (0)/G(1) phase cell progression and apoptosis in human bladder cancer T24 cells. Int J Oncol 29:883–888

Sharma C, Sadrieh L, Priyani A, Ahmed M, Hassan AH, Hussain A (2011) Anti-carcinogenic effects of sulforaphane in association with its apoptosis-inducing and anti-inflammatory properties in human cervical cancer cells. Cancer Epidemiol 35:272–278

Shirode AB, Kovvuru P, Chittur SV, Henning SM, Heber D, Reliene R (2014) Antiproliferative effects of pomegranate extract in MCF-7 breast cancer cells are associated with reduced DNA repair gene expression and induction of double strand breaks. Mol Carcinog 53:458–470

Smith TK, Lund EK, Clarke RG, Bennett RN, Johnson IT (2005) Effects of Brussels sprout juice on the cell cycle and adhesion of human colorectal carcinoma cells (HT29) in vitro. J Agric Food Chem 53:3895–3901

Staack R, Kingston S, Wallig MA, Jeffery EH (1998) A comparison of the individual and collective effects of four glucosinolate breakdown products from brussels sprouts on induction of detoxification enzymes. Toxicol Appl Pharmacol 149:17–23

Stacewicz-Sapuntzakis M, Bowen PE (2005) Role of lycopene and tomato products in prostate health. Biochim Biophys Acta 1740:202–205

Steinkellner H, Rabot S, Kassie F, Knasmuller S (2001) Dietary induction of phase II enzymes: a promising strategy for protection against DNA-reactive intermediates in man? Adv Exp Med Biol 500:629–633

Stenner-Liewen F, Liewen H, Cathomas R, Renner C, Petrausch U, Sulser T, Spanaus K, Seifert HH, Strebel RT, Knuth A, Samaras P, Muntener M (2013) Daily pomegranate intake has no impact on PSA levels in patients with advanced prostate cancer—results of a Phase IIb. Randomized Controlled Trial. J Cancer 4:597–605

Sun J, Liu RH (2008) Apple phytochemical extracts inhibit proliferation of estrogen-dependent and estrogen-independent human breast cancer cells through cell cycle modulation. J Agric Food Chem 56:11661–11667

Surh YJ (2003) Cancer chemoprevention with dietary phytochemicals. Nat Rev Cancer 3:768–780

Surh YJ, Chun KS, Cha HH, Han SS, Keum YS, Park KK, Lee SS (2001) Molecular mechanisms underlying chemopreventive activities of anti-inflammatory phytochemicals: down-regulation of COX-2 and iNOS through suppression of NF-kappa B activation. Mutat Res 480–481:243–268

Syed DN, Malik A, Hadi N, Sarfaraz S, Afaq F, Mukhtar H (2006) Photochemopreventive effect of pomegranate fruit extract on UVA-mediated activation of cellular pathways in normal human epidermal keratinocytes. Photochem Photobiol 82:398–405

Syed DN, Afaq F, Mukhtar H (2007) Pomegranate derived products for cancer chemoprevention. Semin Cancer Biol 17:377–385

Takeshima M, Ono M, Higuchi T, Chen C, Hara T, Nakano S (2014) Anti-proliferative and apoptosis-inducing activity of lycopene against three subtypes of human breast cancer cell lines. Cancer Sci 105:252–257

Talvas J, Caris-Veyrat C, Guy L, Rambeau M, Lyan B, Minet-Quinard R, Lobaccaro JM, Vasson MP, George S, Mazur A, Rock E (2010) Differential effects of lycopene consumed in tomato paste and lycopene in the form of a purified extract on target genes of cancer prostatic cells. Am J Clin Nutr 91:1716–1724

Tan HL, Thomas-Ahner JM, Grainger EM, Wan L, Francis DM, Schwartz SJ, Erdman JW Jr, Clinton SK (2010) Tomato-based food products for prostate cancer prevention: what have we learned? Cancer Metastasis Rev 29:553–568

Tanaka T, Shnimizu M, Moriwaki H (2012) Cancer chemoprevention by carotenoids. Molecules 17:3202–3242

Tang L, Jin T, Zeng X, Wang JS (2005) Lycopene inhibits the growth of human androgen-independent prostate cancer cells in vitro and in BALB/c nude mice. J Nutr 135:287–290

Tang L, Zhang Y, Jobson HE, Li J, Stephenson KK, Wade KL, Fahey JW (2006) Potent activation of mitochondria-mediated apoptosis and arrest in S and M phases of cancer cells by a broccoli sprout extract. Mol Cancer Ther 5:935–944

Tang FY, Shih CJ, Cheng LH, Ho HJ, Chen HJ (2008) Lycopene inhibits growth of human colon cancer cells via suppression of the Akt signaling pathway. Mol Nutr Food Res 52:646–654

Tang FY, Pai MH, Wang XD (2011) Consumption of lycopene inhibits the growth and progression of colon cancer in a mouse xenograft model. J Agric Food Chem 59:9011–9021
Tow WW, Premier R, Jing H, Ajlouni S (2011) Antioxidant and antiproliferation effects of extractable and nonextractable polyphenols isolated from apple waste using different extraction methods. J Food Sci 76:T163–T172
Traka M, Gasper AV, Melchini A, Bacon JR, Needs PW, Frost V, Chantry A, Jones AM, Ortori CA, Barrett DA, Ball RY, Mills RD, Mithen RF (2008) Broccoli consumption interacts with GSTM1 to perturb oncogenic signalling pathways in the prostate. PLoS One 3, e2568
Tsao AS, Kim ES, Hong WK (2004) Chemoprevention of cancer. CA Cancer J Clin 54:150–180
Umesalma S, Sudhandiran G (2010) Chemomodulation of the antioxidative enzymes and peroxidative damage in the colon of 1,2-dimethyl hydrazine-induced rats by ellagicacid. Phytother Res 24(Suppl 1):S114–S119
USDA (2011) Food availability (per capita) fruit. USDA
Vasanthi HR, Mukherjee S, Das DK (2009) Potential health benefits of broccoli- a chemico-biological overview. Mini Rev Med Chem 9:749–759
Veeriah S, Kautenburger T, Habermann N, Sauer J, Dietrich H, Will F, Pool-Zobel BL (2006) Apple flavonoids inhibit growth of HT29 human colon cancer cells and modulate expression of genes involved in the biotransformation of xenobiotics. Mol Carcinog 45:164–174
Vicinanza R, Zhang Y, Henning SM, Heber D (2013) Pomegranate Juice Metabolites, Ellagic Acid and Urolithin A, Synergistically Inhibit Androgen-Independent Prostate Cancer Cell Growth via Distinct Effects on Cell Cycle Control and Apoptosis. Evid Based Complement Alternat Med 2013:247504
Vidya Priyadarsini R, Senthil Murugan R, Maitreyi S, Ramalingam K, Karunagaran D, Nagini S (2010) The flavonoid quercetin induces cell cycle arrest and mitochondria-mediated apoptosis in human cervical cancer (HeLa) cells through p53 induction and NF-kappaB inhibition. Eur J Pharmacol 649:84–91
Vidya Priyadarsini R, Kumar N, Khan I, Thiyagarajan P, Kondaiah P, Nagini S (2012) Gene expression signature of DMBA-induced hamster buccal pouch carcinomas: modulation by chlorophyllin and ellagic acid. PLoS One 7, e34628
Vijaya Padma V, Arul Diana Christie S, Ramkuma KM (2007) Induction of apoptosis by ginger in HEp-2 cell line is mediated by reactive oxygen species. Basic Clin Pharmacol Toxicol 100:302–307
Visanji JM, Duthie SJ, Pirie L, Thompson DG, Padfield PJ (2004) Dietary isothiocyanates inhibit Caco-2 cell proliferation and induce G2/M phase cell cycle arrest, DNA damage, and G2/M checkpoint activation. J Nutr 134:3121–3126
Wallig MA, Kingston S, Staack R, Jefferey EH (1998) Induction of rat pancreatic glutathione S-transferase and quinone reductase activities by a mixture of glucosinolate breakdown derivatives found in Brussels sprouts. Food Chem Toxicol 36:365–373
Wallig MA, Heinz-Taheny KM, Epps DL, Gossman T (2005) Synergy among phytochemicals within crucifers: does it translate into chemoprotection? J Nutr 135:2972S–2977S
Wang B, Zhang X (2012) Inhibitory effects of Broccolini leaf flavonoids on human cancer cells. Scanning 34:1–5
Wang Y, Ausman LM, Greenberg AS, Russell RM, Wang XD (2010) Dietary lycopene and tomato extract supplementations inhibit nonalcoholic steatohepatitis-promoted hepatocarcinogenesis in rats. Int J Cancer 126:1788–1796
Wang S, Meckling KA, Marcone MF, Kakuda Y, Tsao R (2011) Synergistic, additive, and antagonistic effects of food mixtures on total antioxidant capacities. J Agric Food Chem 59:960–968
Wang TT, Schoene NW, Milner JA, Kim YS (2012) Broccoli-derived phytochemicals indole-3-carbinol and 3,3'-diindolylmethane exerts concentration-dependent pleiotropic effects on prostate cancer cells: comparison with other cancer preventive phytochemicals. Mol Carcinog 51:244–256

Weisburg JH, Schuck AG, Silverman MS, Ovits-Levy CG, Solodokin LJ, Zuckerbraun HL, Babich H (2010) Pomegranate extract, a prooxidant with antiproliferative and proapoptotic activities preferentially towards carcinoma cells. Anticancer Agents Med Chem 10:634–644

Weng CJ, Yen GC (2012) Chemopreventive effects of dietary phytochemicals against cancer invasion and metastasis: phenolic acids, monophenol, polyphenol, and their derivatives. Cancer Treat Rev 38:76–87

Weng CJ, Wu CF, Huang HW, Ho CT, Yen GC (2010) Anti-invasion effects of 6-shogaol and 6-gingerol, two active components in ginger, on human hepatocarcinoma cells. Mol Nutr Food Res 54:1618–1627

Wolfe K, Wu X, Liu RH (2003) Antioxidant activity of apple peels. J Agric Food Chem 51:609–614

Wu H, Hsieh MC, Lo CY, Liu CB, Sang S, Ho CT, Pan MH (2010) 6-Shogaol is more effective than 6-gingerol and curcumin in inhibiting 12-O-tetradecanoylphorbol 13-acetate-induced tumor promotion in mice. Mol Nutr Food Res 54:1296–1306

Yang J, Liu RH (2009) Synergistic effect of apple extracts and quercetin 3-beta-D-glucoside combination on antiproliferative activity in MCF-7 human breast cancer cells in vitro. J Agric Food Chem 57:8581–8586

Yang Y, Zhang X (2011) In vitro antitumor activity of broccolini seeds extracts. Scanning 33:402–404

Yang G, Zhong L, Jiang L, Geng C, Cao J, Sun X, Ma Y (2010) Genotoxic effect of 6-gingerol on human hepatoma G2 cells. Chem Biol Interact 185:12–17

Yang Y, Zhang Z, Li S, Ye X, Li X, He K (2014) Synergy effects of herb extracts: pharmacokinetics and pharmacodynamic basis. Fitoterapia 92:133–147

Yoon H, Liu RH (2007) Effect of selected phytochemicals and apple extracts on NF-kappaB activation in human breast cancer MCF-7 cells. J Agric Food Chem 55:3167–3173

Yusof YA, Ahmad N, Das S, Sulaiman S, Murad NA (2008) Chemopreventive efficacy of ginger (Zingiber officinale) in ethionine induced rat hepatocarcinogenesis. Afr J Tradit Complement Altern Med 6:87–93

Zeng H, Trujillo ON, Moyer MP, Botnen JH (2011) Prolonged sulforaphane treatment activates survival signaling in nontumorigenic NCM460 colon cells but apoptotic signaling in tumorigenic HCT116 colon cells. Nutr Cancer 63:248–255

Zhang H, Zhang M, Yu L, Zhao Y, He N, Yang X (2012) Antitumor activities of quercetin and quercetin-5',8-disulfonate in human colon and breast cancer cell lines. Food Chem Toxicol 50:1589–1599

The Ketogenic Diet as an Adjuvant Therapy for Brain Tumors and Other Cancers

Kenneth S. Brooks, Eric C. Woolf, and Adrienne C. Scheck

Abstract Altered metabolism was first identified in cancer cells by Otto Warburg, who identified a higher reliance on anaerobic glycolysis rather than cellular respiration even in the presence of sufficient oxygen levels, a phenomenon called the Warburg Effect. Deregulated metabolism is now considered a driving hallmark of cancer and an attractive therapeutic target. While a great deal of work is being done to find genetic therapeutic targets that can be used for personalized medicine, current targeted approaches are typically ineffective because tumors are heterogeneous and contain multiple genetic subpopulations. This often precludes a particular targeted molecule from being found on all cells. In contrast to many genetic alterations, dysregulation of metabolism resulting in the need for high amounts of glucose is found in virtually all cancer cells. Targeting metabolism by reducing blood glucose may be a way to inhibit tumor growth since this, to a large extent, should circumvent the inherent problems associated with tumor heterogeneity. Methods that also provide an energy source for normal tissues such as ketones should reduce side effects associated with an overall reduction in blood glucose. The high-fat, low carbohydrate, and protein ketogenic diet (KD) results in reduced blood glucose and increased blood ketones, as does caloric restriction and fasting. In preclinical mouse models of malignant brain tumors, animals fed a KD had increased survival, particularly when used in combination with radiation or chemotherapy. Metabolic modulation through the use of a KD, caloric restriction, or fasting has been found to change the expression of a number of genes and pathways thought to inhibit tumor growth. Metabolic therapy has also recently been explored in other cancer types. In this chapter, we will examine the mechanisms underlying the KD which suggests its potential as an adjuvant therapy for cancer treatment.

K.S. Brooks • E.C. Woolf • A.C. Scheck (✉)
Neuro-Oncology Research, Barrow Neurological Institute, 350 W Thomas Rd., Phoenix, AZ 85013, USA
e-mail: Adrienne.scheck@dignityhealth.org

M.F. Ullah, A. Ahmad (eds.), *Critical Dietary Factors in Cancer Chemoprevention*,
DOI 10.1007/978-3-319-21461-0_5

1 Introduction

Every year, ~14,000 new cases of malignant glioma are diagnosed in the United States. Brain tumors are also the second leading cause of cancer deaths among children and young adults. Glioblastoma (GBM) or grade IV astrocytoma is the most aggressive grade of this disease. The standard of care is surgery followed by radiation and chemotherapy. Like many cancers, brain tumor cells tend to infiltrate adjoining tissue; however, unlike other cancers, complete surgical resection is hampered by the eloquent nature of the brain. While radiation and chemotherapy with alkylating agents such as temozolomide are somewhat effective, again the location can reduce the efficacy of these therapies. Radiation is typically targeted to the tumor to reduce toxicity to normal brain tissue, and the blood–brain barrier limits the number of chemotherapies that are effective. Thus, once a tumor recurs following chemotherapy with temozolomide, there are few additional chemotherapeutic agents with demonstrated efficacy for the treatment of brain tumors. Cells that survive initial therapies typically regrow, and these tumors often recur rapidly. Recurrent tumor is typically resistant to additional chemotherapy and the use of additional radiation can be hazardous due to toxicity to normal brain (Weller et al. 2012). For these reasons, median survival of patients diagnosed with a GBM is 12–18 months and there is less than a 10 % 5-year survival rate (Anton et al. 2012; Bloch et al. 2012). This underscores the need for new therapies for the treatment of malignant brain tumors.

The human genome project has spawned a virtual explosion of tools for the study of the molecular underpinnings of human disease. In-depth molecular analysis of malignant gliomas has been done by The Cancer Genome Atlas consortium (The Cancer Genome Atlas Research Group 2008) and other groups (Brennan et al. 2009; Brennan 2011; Lee et al. 2008; Verhaak et al. 2010). This data has shown that not all GBMs have the same molecular basis. This has fueled the idea that therapies can be tailored to the molecular traits of an individual person's disease, so-called "personalized medicine." The ultimate goal of these studies is the identification of therapeutic targets and a better understanding of how to determine the best patients for these specific targeted agents (Masui et al. 2012). While studies such as these may ultimately prove useful, to date they have met with limited success. This is likely due to the heterogeneity seen in most solid tumors. In fact, biopsies taken from different regions of the same tumor can sometimes suggest that the tumor has components of more than one GBM subtype (Gill et al. 2014; Patel et al. 2014). Advances in survival and quality of life rely on new therapeutic strategies, especially those that can enhance the efficacy of current treatment options without damaging the normal brain.

2 Tumor Metabolism

Alterations in the metabolism of cancer cells, what we now call the "Warburg effect" or aerobic glycolysis, were first described by Otto Warburg in 1927 (Warburg et al. 1927). Cancer cells use glycolysis to provide energy and biomolecules regardless of the availability of oxygen. This results in the production of fewer ATP molecules per molecule of glucose, and thus tumor cells require large amounts of glucose. This shift toward increased glycolytic flux in the cytosol and away from the tricarboxylic acid cycle and oxidative phosphorylation in the mitochondria occurs very early in tumorigenesis. This allows for rapid cell proliferation even under conditions of hypoxia and in the presence of dysfunctional mitochondria. Since Warburg's discovery, metabolism has been of interest in the cancer field, but it often seemed overshadowed by discoveries of oncogenes, tumor suppressor genes, growth factor pathways, molecular subtypes of cancers, etc. There is a resurgence of interest in metabolism as a central theme in cancer, and we continue to find that metabolic pathways intersect and often regulate key components of tumor initiation, progression, and therapy response (Nijsten and van Dam 2009; Wolf et al. 2010). In fact, altered metabolism has been referred to as a hallmark of cancer (Cantor and Sabatini 2012; Ward and Thompson 2012).

The term "metabolic remodeling" has been used to describe some of the metabolic changes that can occur in cancer cells, and a wide variety of oncogenes have been found to be involved in metabolism (Obre and Rossignol 2015). For example, the tumor suppressor protein p53 which plays a pivotal role in the cellular responses to hypoxia, DNA damage, and oncogene activation has recently been found to regulate glycolysis and assist in maintaining mitochondrial integrity (Puzio-Kuter 2011). MYC has been found to activate glutaminolysis and lipid synthesis from citrate (Obre and Rossignol 2015). The overactivation of the stress-responsive PI3K/AKT signaling pathway, typical in many cancers, has also been closely linked to metabolism and under low glucose conditions results in rapid tumor cell death (Marie and Shinjo 2011; Robey and Hay 2009; Yang et al. 2009). Furthermore, Hypoxia-inducible factor 1 (HIF-1) may, at least in part, provide the molecular basis for the Warburg effect. HIF-1 can "reprogram" cellular metabolism in response to oxygen availability. In doing so, it contributes to the cancer cell phenotype in a number of ways. HIF-1 expression is activated by hypoxia, which subsequently activates the transcription of genes involved in angiogenesis (VEGF and other cytokines) in an attempt to improve tissue perfusion. This often results in the formation of abnormal blood vessels that contribute to metastasis in some cancers, and can increase inflammation and edema in brain tumors. Loss of function of phosphatase and tensin homologue (PTEN) or mutation of p53 also increases HIF-1, as does the accumulation of reactive oxygen species (ROS). We now know that cancer cell metabolism is far more complex than originally thought and a number of cancer-associated mutations affect metabolism, and there are numerous reviews on the subject (Cantor and Sabatini 2012; Gatenby and Gillies 2004; Semenza 2013; Vander Heiden et al. 2009; Ward and Thompson 2012). The fact that metabolic dysregulation is seen in virtually all tumor cells has led to suggestions that a promising therapeutic strategy may be to exploit this feature. One potential way to achieve this goal is through the use of the therapeutic ketogenic diet (KD) or physiologically similar methods, such as caloric restriction or intermittent fasting.

3 The Ketogenic Diet

The ketogenic diet (KD) is more correctly referred to as "metabolic therapy" rather than a "diet." This high-fat low protein/carbohydrate diet is used to treat refractory epilepsy (Cross 2013; Kim and Rho 2008) in children, and more recently in some adults. The diet is not without side effects; however, these are typically readily managed when the patient has appropriate supervision by a registered dietitian skilled in its use. The KD has been shown to have neuroprotective effects and there are now studies to determine its efficacy for a number of neurological disorders, including Alzheimer's disease, traumatic brain injury, and amyotrophic lateral sclerosis (Maalouf et al. 2009; Stafstrom and Rho 2012). The KD increases blood ketones and decreases blood glucose by simulating the physiological response to fasting, thus leading to high rates of fatty acid oxidation and an increase in the production of acetyl coenzyme A (acetyl-CoA). When the amount of acetyl-CoA exceeds the capacity of the tricarboxylic acid cycle to utilize it, there is an increase in the production of the ketone bodies β-hydroxybutyrate (βHB) and acetoacetate (ACA), which can be used as an energy source in the brain (Cahill and Veech 2003; Morris 2005; Vanitallie and Nufert 2003; Veech et al. 2001). The metabolic alterations found in cancer cells are generally thought to reduce their ability to be "flexible" regarding their primary energy source, and thus they require glucose and are unable to use ketones like normal cells (Fredericks and Ramsey 1978; Maurer et al. 2011; Seyfried et al. 2011; Seyfried 2012; Seyfried and Mukherjee 2005; Tisdale and Brennan 1983; Zhou et al. 2007). Normal cells readily use ketones as an alternate energy source and are thus unaffected by the ketogenic diet. In contrast, the reduction in glucose inhibits the growth of tumor cells. Thus, when used as a therapy, the KD can take advantage of the Warburg effect. In addition, work in the epilepsy field and more recent work in cancer research have shown that the effects of the ketogenic diet extend far beyond the simple growth inhibitory effects of reduced glucose. We used a cell line derived from a recurrent human glioblastoma to demonstrate the in vitro effect of adding ketones to media containing glucose (Scheck et al. 2012). The AO2V4 cell line was derived from a recurrent human glioblastoma and grown in Waymouth's MAB 87/3 media supplemented with 20 % fetal calf serum. When 10 mM βHB plus ACA was added to complete media, cell growth was significantly inhibited. There was additional growth inhibition when 1,3-*bis*(2-chloroethyl)-1 nitrosourea (BCNU, carmustine), one of the chemotherapeutic agents given to this patient prior to tumor recurrence, compared to either ketones or BCNU alone. More recent work has shown that the ketones themselves exert antitumor effects separate from the effects of reduced blood glucose (Magee et al. 1979; Scheck et al. 2012; Skinner et al. 2009). This chapter addresses the utility of increasing blood ketones and reducing blood glucose for the treatment of brain tumors.

4 Gene Expression

Studies done in our laboratory using a GL261/C57BL/6 mouse model of malignant glioma demonstrated that the KD exerts a global effect on the aberrant genetic landscape found in tumors (Scheck et al. 2012). We compared gene expression in tumor tissue and tissue from the contralateral non-tumor containing side of the brain using cDNA array technology. This work showed that overall gene expression in tumor from animals fed the KD was shifted more toward the gene expression found in non-tumor containing tissue from animals fed either the KD or standard diet (Stafford et al. 2010) (Fig. 1). Furthermore, the changes in gene expression were different in tumor tissue compared to that seen in the contralateral non-tumor containing side of the brain (Stafford et al. 2010), a finding similar to that of Maurer (Maurer et al. 2011) who demonstrated differential effects of 3-hydroxybutyrate (in vitro) and a non-calorie-restricted ketogenic diet (in vivo) on normal glia versus glioma cells and tumors. Differences in the response of normal cells versus tumor cells are likely to be due to the alterations in metabolism that are a hallmark of cancer. However, the global nature of these differences has been somewhat surprising, and while the underlying mechanism(s) of these pluripotent effects has not been elucidated, it may be based at least in part on epigenetic changes. Epigenetic changes are heritable alterations in gene activity that are not due to DNA sequence changes (Baylin and Jones 2011). These changes include chromatin remodeling, histone modifications, DNA methylation, and alterations in microRNA pathways, all of which have now been linked to gene expression changes and metabolism in many cancers, including brain tumors (Venneti and Thompson 2013; Yun et al. 2012). In fact, the epigenetic changes found in some cancers are now being looked at as potential therapeutic targets. New therapies such as histone deacetylase (HDAC) inhibitors are actively being tested for their ability to reverse the abnormal gene expression patterns inherent to the cancer epigenome and for their ability to enhance other antitumor therapies (Azad et al. 2013; Qureshi and Mehler 2013). Support for the idea that the effects of the ketogenic diet may be due, at least in part, to changes in the genome comes from a recent study demonstrating that β-hydroxybutyrate (βHB), the major ketone elevated in the blood as a result of the ketogenic diet, can also inhibit HDAC, thus altering the epigenetic landscape in much the same way as the HDAC inhibitors currently being tested (Shimazu et al. 2013). While direct effects of the KD on epigenetic changes in brain tumors have not yet been shown, it has been shown to reverse the major epigenetic modifications seen in the brains of epileptic rats (Kobow et al. 2013), thus

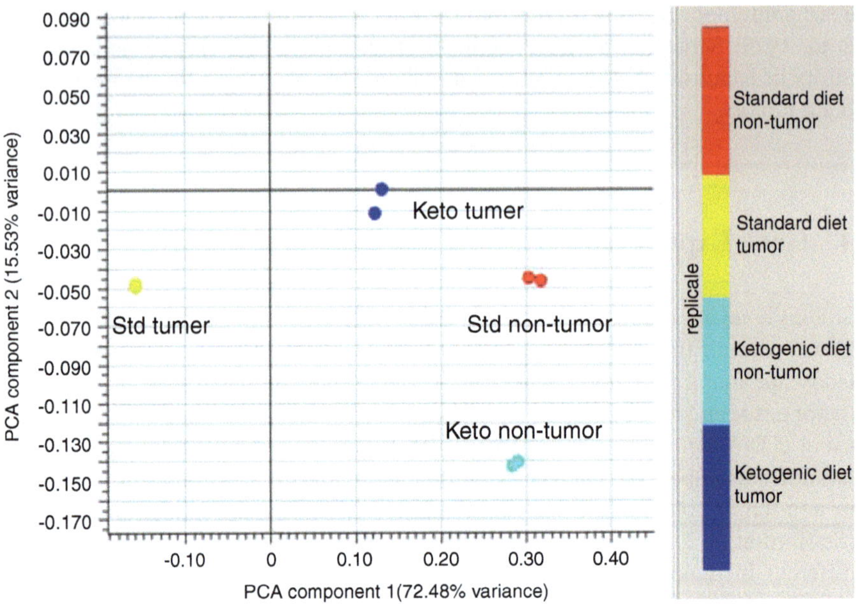

Fig. 1 *The KD alters overall gene expression to more closely resemble that seen in normal brain.* Total cellular RNA was isolated from the tumor and the non-tumor containing contralateral side of the brain. Gene expression was analyzed using Affymetrix GeneChip® Mouse Genome 430 2.0 arrays (Affymetrix, Santa Clara, CA). A two-way ANOVA for interaction showed that the data from the tumor sample obtained from mice fed a SD are clearly separate from the data obtained from the other three conditions. This analysis implies that the KD is driving the overall gene expression in the tumor to be more normal, that is, to be more like gene expression seen in the non-tumor containing tissue. Reprinted from (Stafford et al. 2010)

suggesting that this may indeed be one mechanism through which ketogenic diet exerts its antitumor effect.

5 Growth Factor Signaling

A number of growth factor signaling pathways are critical to the formation and progression of malignant brain tumors. Insulin-like growth factor 1 (IGF-I) is one such growth factor that supports the growth of the number of cancers including brain tumors (Arcaro 2013; Haisa 2013; Hummel et al. 2013; Negi et al. 2013; Singh et al. 2014; Weroha and Haluska 2012). We have shown that IGF1 expression is markedly reduced in tumors from mice fed a KD compared to those fed a standard diet (Fig. 2). Similar results have been found by others using caloric restriction in a variety of mouse models of malignant brain tumors (Marsh et al. 2008; Seyfried et al. 2003; Shelton et al. 2010). cDNA array analysis also showed a reduction in the expression of RAS p21 protein activator 1 and mitogen-

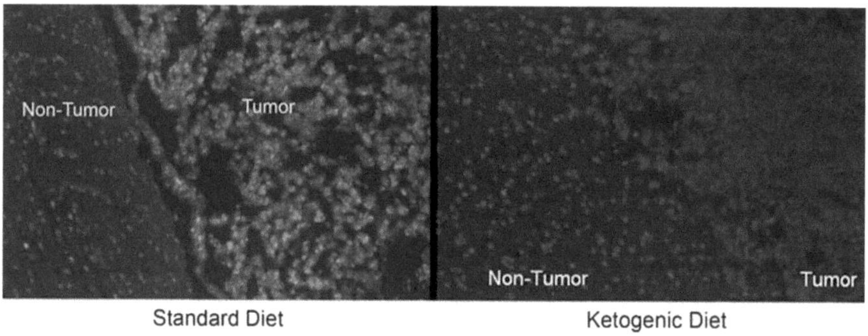

Fig. 2 *Immunohistochemical analysis of Insulin Growth Factor 1 (IGF1)*. There is an increase in the expression of IGF1 in tumor tissue relative to non-tumor in animals fed a standard diet. In animals fed a ketogenic diet, the IGF1 expression in tumor tissue is reduced to the level of the adjacent non-tumor tissue. Reprinted from (Scheck et al. 2012)

activated protein kinase 8 (c-Jun N-terminal kinase, JNK) in tumors from animals fed a KD (Scheck et al. 2012). These proteins participate in the platelet-derived growth factor and epidermal growth factor receptor tyrosine kinase signaling pathways, suggesting that the KD may act as a "pan-growth factor inhibitor."

Growth factor pathways also intersect with metabolism through the PI3K/Akt pathway which can be activated by a number of receptor tyrosine kinase growth factor pathways or activated Ras (Cantor and Sabatini 2012). The PI3K/Akt pathway is also closely linked to glucose metabolism and has been called the "Warburg kinase" (Robey and Hay 2009). Recent studies have shown that the action of Akt is fairly complex and may have different effects on tumor cell survival and growth depending on the genetic background of the cell (such as EGFR amplification, etc.), glucose and oxygen availability, therapy, and other environmental stimuli (Chautard et al. 2010; Elstrom et al. 2004; Eyler et al. 2008; Fan and Weiss 2010; Gallia et al. 2009; Li et al. 2009; Los et al. 2009; Marsh et al. 2008; Rao et al. 2005; Robey and Hay 2009; Vadlakonda et al. 2013). A complete discussion of the role of Akt, HIF-1, and other genes in tumor growth and metabolism is outside the scope of this chapter, but readers are referred to the cited review papers.

6 Reactive Oxygen Species

While the mechanisms underlying the anticancer effects of the KD are not completely understood, the literature regarding the KD in epilepsy has provided some insight. A number of these studies have involved the putative role of changes in the level of reactive oxygen species (ROS) and seizure control. ROS are involved in a variety of cellular processes including autophagic/apoptotic responses to genotoxic stress, pathways involved in the regulation of inflammation, response to hypoxia, and nutrient deprivation—to name a few. Rho and colleagues have shown that ROS production in the brain is reduced in animals fed a ketogenic diet (Kim and Rho 2008; Maalouf et al. 2007). Cancer cells often have increased levels of ROS resulting from a variety of intrinsic and external sources including mitochondrial alterations (Liang and Grootveld 2011), aberrant expression of components of cellular antioxidant systems, chronic inflammation, tobacco, viruses, and environmental pollutants to name just a few (Gupta et al. 2012; Weinberg and Chandel 2009; Fruehauf and Meyskens 2007). They regulate vascular endothelial growth factor (VEGF) and HIF-1 (Weinberg and Chandel 2009) and thus have been implicated in angiogenesis and tumor growth. We have demonstrated a reduction in ROS in tumors from mice fed a KD and changes in the expression of genes involved in oxidative stress pathways (Stafford et al. 2010). Amigo and Kowaltowski (2014) described a similar effect using CR. While the specific downstream effects of this have not yet been fully elucidated, alterations in tumor ROS levels are sure to have profound effects on tumor growth.

7 Anti-angiogenic Effects

One major hallmark of brain tumors is the rapid stimulation of blood vessels that supply the nutrients needed to sustain rapid cellular growth. This vessel growth is favored by the uncontrolled production of angiogenic stimulators and the absence of inhibitors. Vascular endothelial growth factor (VEGF) is considered a driving factor in angiogenesis and has thus become a prime target for anti-angiogenic therapy (El-Kenawi and El-Remessy 2013). To this end, the FDA approved bevacizumab, a monoclonal antibody targeting VEGF, for use in GBMs. While this drug may help to reduce edema, especially following radiation, it often results in adverse effects and it affords little if any improvement in overall survival (Field et al. 2014; Patel et al. 2012).

Studies as far back as 1914 have suggested that restricted food intake can target tumor blood supply and reduce tumor growth (Rous 1914). More recently, it has been suggested that caloric restriction (CR), which also reduces blood glucose and raises blood ketones, reduces growth and angiogenic biomarker expression in prostate cancer and breast cancer (De Lorenzo et al. 2011; Mukherjee et al. 1999; Phoenix et al. 2010; Thompson et al. 2004). Seyfried and colleagues recently showed that CR promoted vessel maturation by preventing vascular VEGF signaling in the CT-2A mouse astrocytoma model (Urits et al. 2012), and they have demonstrated reduced angiogenesis in a number of other mouse glioma models using caloric restriction (Mukherjee et al. 2002, 2004; Seyfried et al. 2011; Shelton et al. 2010; Zhou et al. 2007). Further, CR was shown to normalize a number of factors involved in tumor vessel instability and weakness (including VEGF) as well as reducing peritumoral edema in a mouse model using human U87 glioma cells (Jiang and Wang 2013). In the GL261 mouse glioma model, we found that when fed ad libitum the KD decreased tumor vasculature, reduced peritumoral edema, and altered the expression of genes involved in angiogenesis (Woolf et al. 2015), despite the fact that the expression of VEGF was unchanged (Scheck et al. 2012). Taken together, these results suggest that another effect of metabolic therapy may be to target angiogenesis activity, thus mimicking the beneficial effects of bevacizumab.

8 Anti-inflammatory Effects

The blood vessels formed by rapid angiogenesis in gliomas are often leaky, leading to peritumoral inflammation and edema. Inflammation can also be increased by treatment such as radiation therapy. Inflammation and edema can promote tumor growth, and reduce patient quality of life due to increased pressure-related symptoms and side effects of the high-dose steroids often used for treatment. We have shown that increasing blood ketones affects a number of tumor-related gene networks and alters the expression of genes involved in the cellular response to oxidative stress in tumor tissue, notably cyclooxygenase 2 (COX-2), an important mediator of inflammation (Stafford et al. 2010). A separate study using the KD in combination with radiation therapy in the same mouse model demonstrated reduced expression of both COX-2 and Nf-κB while reducing the production of ROS (Woolf et al. 2013). Similar results have demonstrated reduced expression of pro-inflammatory markers, cyclooxygenase-2 (COX-2), nuclear factor kappa B (NF-κB), and macrophage inflammatory protein (MIP-2) using caloric restriction in mouse models of astrocytoma (Mulrooney et al. 2011) and colon cancer (Harvey et al. 2013).

9 KD as an Adjuvant Therapy

Although evidence suggests that the KD provides antitumor benefits on its own, perhaps the most effective use of the KD is in combination with standard cancer therapies such as radiation and chemotherapy. The KD greatly enhanced survival in a mouse model of malignant glioma when combined with TMZ when compared to either treatment alone (Scheck et al. 2011). In addition, a separate study showed that 9 out of 11 animals maintained on the KD and treated with radiation had complete and sustained remission of their implanted tumors, even after being switched back to a standard rodent diet (Fig. 3) (Abdelwahab et al. 2012). Allen et al. reported similar results when the KD is combined with radiation and chemotherapy in a lung cancer xenograft model (Allen et al. 2013). That is, they found decreased tumor growth rate and increased survival. CR and short-term fasting have also been found to be synergistic with radiation and other anticancer therapeutics in both preclinical and clinical studies (Champ et al. 2013, 2014; Klement and Champ

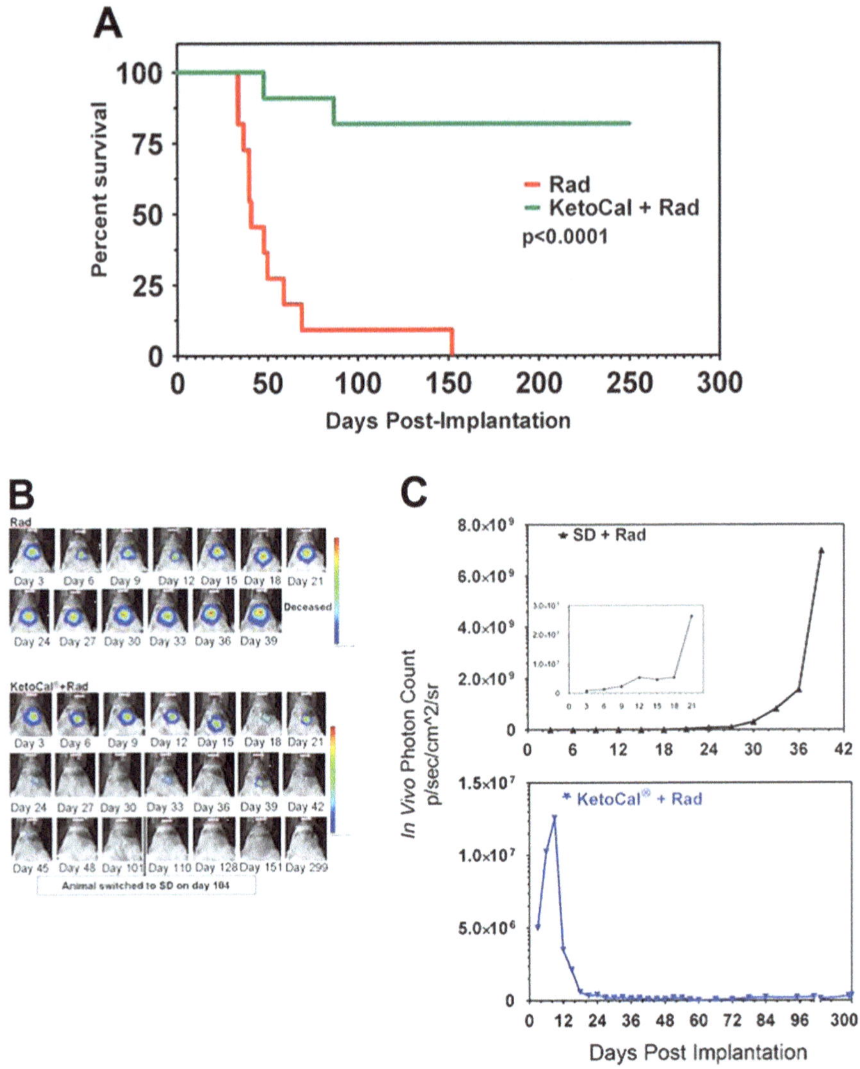

Fig. 3 *Radiation in combination with the ketogenic diet causes tumor regression.* On days 3 and 5 postimplantation animals received 4 Gy of radiation. The tumor completely regressed in 9 of the 11 animals fed a ketogenic diet. Animals were switched back to standard diet on day 101 and maintained for an additional 200 days and no tumor regrowth was detected. (**a**) Kaplan–Meier survival plot; (**b**) bioluminescence in representative animals treated with radiation and fed a standard diet vs. radiation plus the ketogenic diet; (**c**) bioluminescent signal plotted as in vivo photon count versus days postimplantation. Reprinted from (Abdelwahab et al. 2012)

2014; Lee et al. 2010, 2012; Poff et al. 2013; Raffaghello et al. 2008, 2010; Safdie et al. 2012; Saleh et al. 2013; Seyfried et al. 2012).

The effectiveness of radiation therapy is due to a number of factors including relative damage done to tumor cells versus normal tissue and the ability of normal cells and tumor cells to repair the damage (Klement and Champ 2014). Radiation works, in part, by creating ROS through the radiolysis of water. The ROS damage the DNA and other macromolecules, causing sublethal damage that can become lethal if not repaired. The potentiation of radiation therapy by the KD or caloric restriction seems paradoxical in light of our data demonstrating a reduction in ROS in tumors from animals maintained on a KD (Stafford et al. 2010). However, radiation effects do not only occur through ROS, and radiation can directly damage DNA and other cellular macromolecules. Furthermore, in addition to reactive oxygen species, radiation causes the production of reactive nitrogen species (RNS), a potential source of macromolecular damage following radiation (Saenko et al. 2013). Whether the KD and/or caloric restriction reduces the formation of RNS is as yet unknown. In fact, the main effect of the KD or CR may not be in altering the amount of radiation-induced damage, but may in fact be in modulating the ability of tumor and normal cells to repair radiation-induced damage (Klement and Champ 2014; Santivasi and Xia 2014). Studies have shown that caloric restriction can enhance DNA repair in normal cells (Heydari et al. 2007); however, this may not be the case in tumor cells, and the differential response of tumor cells and normal cells to genotoxic stress may be mediated by reduced IGF1 and glucose in the tumor cells. In fact, a number of studies have shown that reduction of activation of the PI3K/Akt pathway, activation of the adenosine monophosphate-activated protein kinase (AMPK) signaling pathway, and reduction of receptor tyrosine kinase growth factor pathways can all reduce radioresistance in tumor cells (Choi et al. 2014; Danhier et al. 2013; Gil Del Alcazar et al. 2014; Li et al. 2014; Medova et al. 2013; Munshi and Ramesh 2013; Sanli et al. 2014; Wang et al. 2013; Zhang et al. 2014). These reports provide additional support for the use of the KD or caloric restriction as an adjuvant therapy for the treatment of gliomas.

10 Neuroprotection

There is a resurgence of interest in the use of the KD for the treatment of medically refractory epilepsy and increasing interest in the use of this therapy for the treatment of malignant brain tumors. While the majority of the research in this field focuses on slowing tumor growth and enhancing the efficacy of current therapeutic modalities, the KD may have additional benefits for cancer patients. Evidence suggests that the ketogenic diet may also protect normal brain tissue from the genotoxic stress that is a typical "side effect" of radiation and chemotherapy. We have demonstrated that gene expression changes in the tumor tissue from animals fed the KD were not the same as those in the non-tumor containing contralateral side of the brain (Scheck et al. 2012; Stafford et al. 2010). This allows for the hypothesis that while the neuroprotective activity of the KD does not protect the *tumor* from the therapeutic benefits of radiation and chemotherapy, it may reduce the deleterious side effects of cranial radiation on normal brain. A recent publication showed that fasting, which elevates blood ketones, not only sensitizes many types of cancer cells to standard therapies but may promote the protection of normal tissue from the toxicity associated with radiation and chemotherapy (Lee et al. 2012). Additional studies are needed to support this hypothesis; however, the potential benefit of protecting the normal brain from decreased cognitive function due to radiation toxicity would be of great importance, particularly for the treatment of pediatric brain tumors.

11 KD in Other Cancers

Although much of the research regarding the anticancer benefits of the KD has focused on brain tumors, this type of metabolic therapy has also recently been explored in other cancer types. For example, Gluschnaider et al. used the MMTV-PyMT oncomouse model to demonstrate that a KD suppressed breast tumor growth (Gluschnaider et al. 2014). Likewise, Allen et al. showed that the KD enhanced radiation and chemotherapy responses in a mouse lung xenograft model by increasing oxidative stress in both NCI-H292 and A549 lung xenograft models (Allen et al. 2013). The use of a no carbohydrate ketogenic diet (NCKD) in prostate cancer models has also been examined. A recent study demonstrated that an NCKD significantly slowed tumor growth and prolonged survival in a prostate cancer xenograft model (Freedland et al. 2008). Studies in prostate cancer xenograft models demonstrated that the NCKD significantly reduces tumor volume (Kim et al. 2012) and alters pathways linked to apoptosis, inflammation, and insulin resistance (Mavropoulos et al. 2009). A KD supplemented with omega-3 fatty acids and medium chain triglycerides was shown to delay tumor growth in a mouse xenograft model of gastric cancer. The use of the KD in models of cancer-associated cachexia has also been studied. Shukla et al. showed that a KD reduced glycolytic flux and glutamine uptake in a number of pancreatic cell lines. They identified decreased pancreatic cancer cell growth as well as a dose-dependent induction of apoptosis in the presence of ketone bodies in vitro. Likewise, in the presence of ketones, pancreatic cancer cells had a reduced expression and activity of the oncogene c-Myc and reduced cachexic markers. They also showed a reduction of tumor growth and cachexia in an animal model of pancreatic cancer (Shukla et al. 2014).

Although the mechanisms behind the KD have not been completely identified and extend beyond the reduction in blood glucose and increase in blood ketones, recent studies in cancer research suggest that the KD may provide therapeutic benefits in a variety of cancer types. This demonstrates that more research is warranted to better understand the mechanisms behind the KD as well as the different physiological responses which occur based upon cancer type and location.

12 KD in Humans

Studies of glucose utilization in cancer go back prior to the 1980s, including studies of metabolism and cancer cachexia (Fearon et al. 1988; Tisdale et al. 1987). These and other studies suggested that the ketogenic diet consisting of a high percentage of medium chain triglycerides (MCT) along with various supplements resulted in weight gain and improved nitrogen balance in both animals and humans. In 1995, Nebeling and colleagues published a case report in which they used a similar ketogenic diet based on MCT oil to treat 2 female pediatric patients with advanced stage malignant brain tumors (Nebeling et al. 1995; Nebeling and Lerner 1995). They demonstrated that dietary-induced ketosis decreased the availability of glucose to the tumor without causing a decrease in patient weight for overall nutritional status. Furthermore, both children had long-term tumor management (Nebeling et al. 1995). The 2nd case report was published in 2010 by Zuccoli and coworkers (2010). This patient was a 65-year-old female with multicentric glioblastoma. She was put on a 4:1 (ratio of fats:carbohydrate plus protein) calorie restricted (600 kcal/day) ketogenic diet during radiation and chemotherapy. During this time her body weight dropped by 20 %, she had reduced blood glucose, increased urinary ketones, and, most importantly, no observable brain tumor by either fluorodeoxyglucose Positron Emission Tomography (FDG-PET) or magnetic resonance imaging (MRI). The tumor recurred 10 weeks after the patient resumed her normal eating habits and she succumbed to her disease less than 2 years after diagnosis. While this patient did not experience long-term tumor control after cessation of the diet, this report demonstrated that the diet could be tolerated, even when used in a calorie-restricted setting. Results of a phase 1 clinical trial were reported in 2011 by a German group. Tolerability of a restricted calorie ketogenic diet was tested in 16 patients with a variety of advanced (end-stage) cancers. There were no severe side effects and 5 of the 16 patients were able to complete the 3-month treatment. These 5 patients had stable disease while on the diet. Two of the 11 remaining patients died early following the beginning of the trial, one was unable to tolerate the diet and dropped out immediately, 2 patients dropped out for personal reasons, one was unable to continue the diet for more than a month, and 3 had disease progression within less than 2 months of starting the diet and one dropped out to resume chemotherapy. While this trail demonstrated tolerability and favorable side-effect profile, the antitumor efficacy could not be assessed due to the variety and severity of disease in the patients. More recently, a number of prospective clinical trials have been initiated. A study in Germany is evaluating the efficacy of a calorie-restricted ketogenic diet and transient fasting during re-irradiation for patients with recurrent GBM (ClinicalTrials.gov NCT01754350). Michigan State University is directing a similar trial evaluating a calorie-restricted KD for recurrent GBM (ClinicalTrials.gov NCT01535911). A third clinical trial is evaluating the KD as adjunctive treatment in refractory/end-stage GBM (ClinicalTrials.gov NCT01865162). The goals for all of these studies are to obtain data on the safety, efficacy, and tolerability of the KD as an adjunctive therapy for patients with GBM. The only study using the KD as an up-front, concurrent therapy has recently been approved and is now open for enrollment at St. Joseph's Hospital and Medical Center and Barrow Neurological Institute in Phoenix, Arizona (ClinicalTrials.gov NCT02046187). This trial for patients with primary GBM will evaluate the classic 4:1 ketogenic diet therapy during radiation treatment and concurrent temozolomide followed by the modified Atkins Diet (1:1 fat:carbohydrate plus protein) during temozolomide treatment.

The case reports described above along with numerous anecdotal reports suggest that the KD may be a promising anticancer therapy; however, more work is needed to determine how to best utilize this and other metabolic therapies for the treatment of tumors. Most of the information regarding the best way to use the ketogenic diet comes from the epilepsy literature. Further research is needed to determine optimum blood ketone and glucose levels for anticancer effects. In addition, a variety of ketogenic diets are used for seizure control and it is not clear if one or more of the different formulations will provide the best results for cancer patients. Finally, while the KD has a long record of safety in the epilepsy community, side effects that occur when used in combination with cancer therapies may differ in type or severity. This data will come from carefully controlled clinical trials that include input from registered dietitians well-versed in the use of the KD. Patient enrollment into clinical trials requires "buy-in" from the medical community. Physicians must be educated on the therapeutic value of metabolic alteration as an adjuvant therapy, even if it results in a small amount of healthy weight loss, since the current dogma is to avoid weight loss in patients undergoing chemotherapy for fear of increased fatigue and further decline in overall patient health. As with any decision regarding therapy, the patient's overall condition, including nutritional status, must be taken into account.

Concern about patients' quality of life is sometimes given as a reason not to employ KD. Compliance can be made more difficult by the use of steroids (prescribed for peritumoral edema) that often increase hunger and raise blood glucose levels. To address this, our clinical trial includes an analysis of both patient and caregiver quality of life. Quality of life measurements are being added to more clinical trials, as the importance of this has become recognized at the national level (Boele et al. 2013; Dirven et al. 2014; van den Bent et al. 2011). While some clinicians are concerned that compliance will reduce quality of life, the patients that do remain on the KD often comment that this allows them to participate in their own therapy. Despite these caveats, the existing preclinical data suggesting antitumor efficacy and a synergistic effect with standard therapies provide a strong impetus to conduct controlled clinical trials, particularly those that will shed light on the interactions between the KD and other therapies.

13 Conclusion

Improvements in the survival and quality of life for patients with malignant brain tumors require the implementation of new therapeutic modalities, especially those that increase the efficacy of current therapies without increasing toxic side effects. While the rapid accumulation of data defining the molecular and genetic aberrations present in these tumors has suggested a host of targets for the development of new therapies, targeted therapies tried to date have met with limited success. This is at least in part due to the molecular heterogeneity of these tumors that prevents any one target from being present on all cells. In contrast, metabolic dysregulation is present in virtually all tumor cells and there is increased interest in using metabolic therapies such as the ketogenic diet for the treatment of various cancers, especially brain tumors. Preclinical data have demonstrated that the antitumor effects of the KD and caloric restriction are multifaceted, and alterations in energy metabolism can inhibit cancer cell growth and increase the tumor's response to therapy. This provides a strong impetus to continue work designed to elucidate the mechanisms through which the KD exerts its anticancer effects, as well as suggesting the need for the design of controlled clinical trials that will shed light on the most effective way to implement metabolic therapies in combination with standard therapies for the treatment of malignant disease. This is a novel therapeutic paradigm, and we have only begun to scratch the surface of its potential.

References

Abdelwahab MG, Fenton KE, Preul MC, Rho JM, Lynch A, Stafford P, Scheck AC (2012) The ketogenic diet is an effective adjuvant to radiation therapy for the treatment of malignant glioma. PLoS One 7(5), e36197

Allen BG, Bhatia SK, Buatti JM, Brandt KE, Lindholm KE, Button AM, Szweda LI, Smith B, Spitz DR, Fath MA (2013) Ketogenic diets enhance oxidative stress and radio-chemo-therapy responses in lung cancer xenografts. Clin Cancer Res 19(14):3905–3913

Amigo I, Kowaltowski AJ (2014) Dietary restriction in cerebral bioenergetics and redox state. Redox Biol 2:296–304

Anton K, Baehring JM, Mayer T (2012) Glioblastoma multiforme: overview of current treatment and future perspectives. Hematol Oncol Clin North Am 26(4):825–853

Arcaro A (2013) Targeting the insulin-like growth factor-1 receptor in human cancer. Front Pharmacol 4:30

Azad N, Zahnow CA, Rudin CM, Baylin SB (2013) The future of epigenetic therapy in solid tumours--lessons from the past. Nat Rev Clin Oncol 10(5):256–266

Baylin SB, Jones PA (2011) A decade of exploring the cancer epigenome—biological and translational implications. Nat Rev Cancer 11(10):726–734

Bloch O, Han SJ, Cha S, Sun MZ, Aghi MK, McDermott MW, Berger MS, Parsa AT (2012) Impact of extent of resection for recurrent glioblastoma on overall survival: clinical article. J Neurosurg 117(6):1032–1038

Boele FW, Heimans JJ, Aaronson NK, Taphoorn MJ, Postma TJ, Reijneveld JC, Klein M (2013) Health-related quality of life of significant others of patients with malignant CNS versus non-CNS tumors: a comparative study. J Neurooncol 115(1):87–94

Brennan C (2011) Genomic profiles of glioma. Curr Neurol Neurosci Rep 11(3):291–297
Brennan C, Momota H, Hambardzumyan D, Ozawa T, Tandon A, Pedraza A, Holland E (2009) Glioblastoma subclasses can be defined by activity among signal transduction pathways and associated genomic alterations. PLoS One 4(11), e7752
Cahill GF Jr, Veech RL (2003) Ketoacids? Good medicine? Trans Am Clin Climatol Assoc 114:149–161
Cantor JR, Sabatini DM (2012) Cancer cell metabolism: one hallmark, many faces. Cancer Discov 2(10):881–898
Champ CE, Baserga R, Mishra MV, Jin L, Sotgia F, Lisanti MP, Pestell RG, Dicker AP, Simone NL (2013) Nutrient restriction and radiation therapy for cancer treatment: when less is more. Oncologist 18(1):97–103
Champ CE, Palmer JD, Volek JS, Werner-Wasik M, Andrews DW, Evans JJ, Glass J, Kim L, Shi W (2014) Targeting metabolism with a ketogenic diet during the treatment of glioblastoma multiforme. J Neurooncol 117(1):125–131
Chautard E, Loubeau G, Tchirkov A, Chassagne J, Vermot-Desroches C, Morel L, Verrelle P (2010) Akt signaling pathway: a target for radiosensitizing human malignant glioma. Neuro Oncol 12(5):434–443
Choi EJ, Cho BJ, Lee DJ, Hwang YH, Chun SH, Kim HH, Kim IA (2014) Enhanced cytotoxic effect of radiation and temozolomide in malignant glioma cells: targeting PI3K-AKT-mTOR signaling, HSP90 and histone deacetylases. BMC Cancer 14:17
Cross JH (2013) New research with diets and epilepsy. J Child Neurol 28(8):970–974
Danhier P, De Saedeleer CJ, Karroum O, De PG, Porporato PE, Jordan BF, Gallez B, Sonveaux P (2013) Optimization of tumor radiotherapy with modulators of cell metabolism: toward clinical applications. Semin Radiat Oncol 23(4):262–272
De Lorenzo MS, Baljinnyam E, Vatner DE, Abarzua P, Vatner SF, Rabson AB (2011) Caloric restriction reduces growth of mammary tumors and metastases. Carcinogenesis 32 (9):1381–1387
Dirven L, Taphoorn MJ, Reijneveld JC, Blazeby J, Jacobs M, Pusic A, La SE, Stupp R, Fayers P, Efficace F (2014) The level of patient-reported outcome reporting in randomised controlled trials of brain tumour patients: a systematic review. Eur J Cancer 50(14):2432–2448
El-Kenawi AE, El-Remessy AB (2013) Angiogenesis Inhibitors in Cancer Therapy: Mechanistic perspective on classification and treatment rationales. Br. J, Pharmacol
Elstrom RL, Bauer DE, Buzzai M, Karnauskas R, Harris MH, Plas DR, Zhuang H, Cinalli RM, Alavi A, Rudin CM, Thompson CB (2004) Akt stimulates aerobic glycolysis in cancer cells. Cancer Res 64(11):3892–3899
Eyler CE, Foo WC, LaFiura KM, McLendon RE, Hjelmeland AB, Rich JN (2008) Brain cancer stem cells display preferential sensitivity to Akt inhibition. Stem Cells 26(12):3027–3036
Fan QW, Weiss WA (2010) Targeting the RTK-PI3K-mTOR axis in malignant glioma: overcoming resistance. Curr Top Microbiol Immunol 347(279-96):279–296
Fearon KC, Borland W, Preston T, Tisdale MJ, Shenkin A, Calman KC (1988) Cancer cachexia: influence of systemic ketosis on substrate levels and nitrogen metabolism. Am J Clin Nutr 47 (1):42–48
Field KM, Jordan JT, Wen PY, Rosenthal MA, Reardon DA (2014) Bevacizumab and glioblastoma: Scientific review, newly reported updates, and ongoing controversies. Cancer 10
Fredericks M, Ramsey RB (1978) 3-Oxo acid coenzyme A transferase activity in brain and tumors of the nervous system. J Neurochem 31(6):1529–1531
Freedland SJ, Mavropoulos J, Wang A, Darshan M, Demark-Wahnefried W, Aronson WJ, Cohen P, Hwang D, Peterson B, Fields T, Pizzo SV, Isaacs WB (2008) Carbohydrate restriction, prostate cancer growth, and the insulin-like growth factor axis. Prostate 68(1):11–19
Fruehauf JP, Meyskens FL Jr (2007) Reactive oxygen species: a breath of life or death? Clin Cancer Res 13(3):789–794

Gallia GL, Tyler BM, Hann CL, Siu IM, Giranda VL, Vescovi AL, Brem H, Riggins GJ (2009) Inhibition of Akt inhibits growth of glioblastoma and glioblastoma stem-like cells. Mol Cancer Ther 8(2):386–393

Gatenby RA, Gillies RJ (2004) Why do cancers have high aerobic glycolysis? Nat Rev Cancer 4:891–899

Gil Del Alcazar CR, Hardebeck MC, Mukherjee B, Tomimatsu N, Gao X, Yan J, Xie XJ, Bachoo R, Li L, Habib AA, Burma S (2014) Inhibition of DNA Double-Strand Break Repair by the Dual PI3K/mTOR Inhibitor NVP-BEZ235 as a Strategy for Radiosensitization of Glioblastoma. Clin, Cancer Res

Gill BJ, Pisapia DJ, Malone HR, Goldstein H, Lei L, Sonabend A, Yun J, Samanamud J, Sims JS, Banu M, Dovas A, Teich AF, Sheth SA, McKhann GM, Sisti MB, Bruce JN, Sims PA, Canoll P (2014) MRI-localized biopsies reveal subtype-specific differences in molecular and cellular composition at the margins of glioblastoma. Proc Natl Acad Sci U S A 111(34):12550–12555

Gluschnaider U, Hertz R, Ohayon S, Smeir E, Smets M, Pikarsky E, Bar-Tana J (2014) Long-chain Fatty Acid analogues suppress breast tumorigenesis and progression. Cancer Res 74 (23):6991–7002

Group TCGAR (2008) Comprehensive genomic characterization defines human glioblastoma genes and core pathways. Nature 455(7216):1061–1068

Gupta SC, Hevia D, Patchva S, Park B, Koh W, Aggarwal BB (2012) Upsides and downsides of reactive oxygen species for cancer: The roles of reactive oxygen species in tumorigenesis, prevention and therapy. Antioxid Redox Signal 16(11):1295–1322

Haisa M (2013) The type 1 insulin-like growth factor receptor signalling system and targeted tyrosine kinase inhibition in cancer. J Int Med Res 41(2):253–264

Harvey AE, Lashinger LM, Otto G, Nunez NP, Hursting SD (2013) Decreased systemic IGF-1 in response to calorie restriction modulates murine tumor cell growth, nuclear factor-kappaB activation, and inflammation-related gene expression. Mol Carcinog 52(12):997–1006

Heydari AR, Unnikrishnan A, Lucente LV, Richardson A (2007) Caloric restriction and genomic stability. Nucleic Acids Res 35(22):7485–7496

Hummel TR, Chow LM, Fouladi M, Franz D (2013) Pharmacotherapeutic management of pediatric gliomas : current and upcoming strategies. Paediatr Drugs 15(1):29–42

Jiang YS, Wang FR (2013) Caloric restriction reduces edema and prolongs survival in a mouse glioma model. J Neurooncol 114(1):25–32

Kim DY, Rho JM (2008) The ketogenic diet and epilepsy. Curr Opin Clin Nutr Metab Care 11 (2):113–120

Kim HS, Masko EM, Poulton SL, Kennedy KM, Pizzo SV, Dewhirst MW, Freedland SJ (2012) Carbohydrate restriction and lactate transporter inhibition in a mouse xenograft model of human prostate cancer. BJU Int 110(7):1062–1069

Klement RJ, Champ CE (2014) Calories, carbohydrates, and cancer therapy with radiation: exploiting the five R's through dietary manipulation. Cancer Metastasis Rev 33(1):217–29

Kobow K, Kaspi A, Harikrishnan KN, Kiese K, Ziemann M, Khurana I, Fritzsche I, Hauke J, Hahnen E, Coras R, Muhlebner A, El-Osta A, Blumcke I (2013) Deep sequencing reveals increased DNA methylation in chronic rat epilepsy. Acta Neuropathol 126(5):741–756

Lee Y, Scheck AC, Cloughesy TF, Lai A, Dong J, Farooqi HK, Liau LM, Horvath S, Mischel PS, Nelson SF (2008) Gene expression analysis of glioblastomas identifies the major molecular basis for the prognostic benefit of younger age. BMC Med Genomics 1:52

Lee C, Safdie FM, Raffaghello L, Wei M, Madia F, Parrella E, Hwang D, Cohen P, Bianchi G, Longo VD (2010) Reduced levels of IGF-1 mediate differential protection of normal and cancer cells in response to fasting and improve chemotherapeutic index. Cancer Res 70 (4):1564–1572

Lee C, Raffaghello L, Brandhorst S, Safdie FM, Bianchi G, Martin-Montalvo A, Pistoia V, Wei M, Hwang S, Merlino A, Emionite L, de Cabo R, Longo VD (2012) Fasting cycles retard growth of tumors and sensitize a range of cancer cell types to chemotherapy. Sci Transl Med 4 (124):124ra27

Li HF, Kim JS, Waldman T (2009) Radiation-induced Akt activation modulates radioresistance in human glioblastoma cells. Radiat Oncol 4:43

Li W, Guo F, Wang P, Hong S, Zhang C (2014) miR-221/222 confers radioresistance in glioblastoma cells through activating Akt independent of PTEN status. Curr Mol Med 14 (1):185–195

Liang BC, Grootveld M (2011) The importance of mitochondria in the tumourigenic phenotype: gliomas as the paradigm (review). Int J Mol Med 27(2):159–171

Los M, Maddika S, Erb B, Schulze-Osthoff K (2009) Switching Akt: from survival signaling to deadly response. Bioessays 31(5):492–495

Maalouf M, Sullivan PG, Davis L, Kim DY, Rho JM (2007) Ketones inhibit mitochondrial production of reactive oxygen species production following glutamate excitotoxicity by increasing NADH oxidation. Neuroscience 145(1):256–264

Maalouf M, Rho JM, Mattson MP (2009) The neuroprotective properties of calorie restriction, the ketogenic diet, and ketone bodies. Brain Res Rev 59(2):293–315

Magee BA, Potezny N, Rofe AM, Conyers RA (1979) The inhibition of malignant cell growth by ketone bodies. Aust J Exp Biol Med Sci 57(5):529–539

Marie SK, Shinjo SM (2011) Metabolism and brain cancer. Clinics (SaoPaulo) 66(Suppl 1):33–43

Marsh J, Mukherjee P, Seyfried TN (2008) Akt-dependent proapoptotic effects of dietary restriction on late-stage management of a phosphatase and tensin homologue/tuberous sclerosis complex 2-deficient mouse astrocytoma. Clin Cancer Res 14(23):7751–7762

Masui K, Cloughesy TF, Mischel PS (2012) Review: molecular pathology in adult high-grade gliomas: from molecular diagnostics to target therapies. Neuropathol Appl Neurobiol 38 (3):271–291

Maurer GD, Brucker DP, Bahr O, Harter PN, Hattingen E, Walenta S, Mueller-Klieser W, Steinbach JP, Rieger J (2011) Differential utilization of ketone bodies by neurons and glioma cell lines: a rationale for ketogenic diet as experimental glioma therapy. BMC Cancer 11 (315):315

Mavropoulos JC, Buschemeyer WC III, Tewari AK, Rokhfeld D, Pollak M, Zhao Y, Febbo PG, Cohen P, Hwang D, Devi G, Demark-Wahnefried W, Westman EC, Peterson BL, Pizzo SV, Freedland SJ (2009) The effects of varying dietary carbohydrate and fat content on survival in a murine LNCaP prostate cancer xenograft model. Cancer Prev Res (Phila) 2(6):557–565

Medova M, Aebersold DM, Zimmer Y (2013) The molecular crosstalk between the MET receptor tyrosine kinase and the DNA damage response-biological and clinical aspects. Cancers(Basel) 6(1):1–27

Morris AAM (2005) Cerebral ketone body metabolism. J Inherit Metab Dis 28:109–121

Mukherjee P, Sotnikov AV, Mangian HJ, Zhou JR, Visek WJ, Clinton SK (1999) Energy intake and prostate tumor growth, angiogenesis, and vascular endothelial growth factor expression. J Natl Cancer Inst 91(6):512–523

Mukherjee P, El-Abbadi MM, Kasperzyk JL, Ranes MK, Seyfried TN (2002) Dietary restriction reduces angiogenesis and growth in an orthotopic mouse brain tumour model. Br J Cancer 86 (10):1615–1621

Mukherjee P, Abate LE, Seyfried TN (2004) Antiangiogenic and proapoptotic effects of dietary restriction on experimental mouse and human brain tumors. Clin Cancer Res 10 (16):5622–5629

Mulrooney TJ, Marsh J, Urits I, Seyfried TN, Mukherjee P (2011) Influence of caloric restriction on constitutive expression of NF-kappaB in an experimental mouse astrocytoma. PLoS One 6 (3), e18085

Munshi A, Ramesh R (2013) Mitogen-Activated Protein Kinases and Their Role in Radiation Response. Genes Cancer 4(9-10):401–408

Nebeling LC, Lerner E (1995) Implementing a ketogenic diet based on medium-chain triglyceride oil in pediatric patients with cancer. J Am Diet Assoc 95(6):693–697

Nebeling LC, Miraldi F, Shurin SB, Lerner E (1995) Effects of a ketogenic diet on tumor metabolism and nutritional status in pediatric oncology patients: two case reports. J Am Coll Nutr 14(2):202–208
Negi A, Ramarao P, Kumar R (2013) Recent advancements in small molecule inhibitors of insulin-like growth factor-1 receptor (IGF-1R) tyrosine kinase as anticancer agents. Mini Rev Med Chem 13(5):653–681
Nijsten MW, van Dam GM (2009) Hypothesis: using the Warburg effect against cancer by reducing glucose and providing lactate. Med Hypotheses 73(1):48–51
Obre E, Rossignol R (2015) Emerging concepts in bioenergetics and cancer research: Metabolic flexibility, coupling, symbiosis, switch, oxidative tumors, metabolic remodeling, signaling and bioenergetic therapy. Int J Biochem Cell Biol 59C:167–181. doi:10.1016/j.biocel.2014.12.008
Patel M, Vogelbaum MA, Barnett GH, Jalali R, Ahluwalia MS (2012) Molecular targeted therapy in recurrent glioblastoma: current challenges and future directions. Expert. Opin. Investig, Drugs
Patel AP, Tirosh I, Trombetta JJ, Shalek AK, Gillespie SM, Wakimoto H, Cahill DP, Nahed BV, Curry WT, Martuza RL, Louis DN, Rozenblatt-Rosen O, Suva ML, Regev A, Bernstein BE (2014) Single-cell RNA-seq highlights intratumoral heterogeneity in primary glioblastoma. Science 344(6190):1396–1401
Phoenix KN, Vumbaca F, Fox MM, Evans R, Claffey KP (2010) Dietary energy availability affects primary and metastatic breast cancer and metformin efficacy. Breast Cancer Res Treat 123(2):333–344
Poff AM, Ari C, Seyfried TN, D'Agostino DP (2013) The ketogenic diet and hyperbaric oxygen therapy prolong survival in mice with systemic metastatic cancer. PLoS One 8(6), e65522
Puzio-Kuter AM (2011) The role of p53 in metabolic regulation. Genes Cancer 2(4):385–391
Qureshi IA, Mehler MF (2013) Developing epigenetic diagnostics and therapeutics for brain disorders. Trends Mol Med 19(12):732–741
Raffaghello L, Lee C, Safdie FM, Wei M, Madia F, Bianchi G, Longo VD (2008) Starvation-dependent differential stress resistance protects normal but not cancer cells against high-dose chemotherapy. Proc Natl Acad Sci U S A 105(24):8215–8220
Raffaghello L, Safdie F, Bianchi G, Dorff T, Fontana L, Longo VD (2010) Fasting and differential chemotherapy protection in patients. Cell Cycle 9(22):4474–4476
Rao RD, Mladek AC, Lamont JD, Goble JM, Erlichman C, James CD, Sarkaria JN (2005) Disruption of parallel and converging signaling pathways contributes to the synergistic antitumor effects of simultaneous mTOR and EGFR inhibition in GBM cells. Neoplasia 7 (10):921–929
Robey RB, Hay N (2009) Is Akt the "Warburg kinase"?-Akt-energy metabolism interactions and oncogenesis. Semin Cancer Biol 19(1):25–31
Rous P (1914) The influence of diet on transplanted and spontaneous mouse tumors. J Exp Med 20 (5):433–451
Saenko Y, Cieslar-Pobuda A, Skonieczna M, Rzeszowska-Wolny J (2013) Changes of reactive oxygen and nitrogen species and mitochondrial functioning in human K562 and HL60 cells exposed to ionizing radiation. Radiat Res 180(4):360–366
Safdie F, Brandhorst S, Wei M, Wang W, Lee C, Hwang S, Conti PS, Chen TC, Longo VD (2012) Fasting enhances the response of glioma to chemo- and radiotherapy. PLoS One 7(9), e44603
Saleh AD, Simone BA, Palazzo J, Savage JE, Sano Y, Dan T, Jin L, Champ CE, Zhao S, Lim M, Sotgia F, Camphausen K, Pestell RG, Mitchell JB, Lisanti MP, Simone NL (2013) Caloric restriction augments radiation efficacy in breast cancer. Cell Cycle 12(12):1955–1963
Sanli T, Steinberg GR, Singh G, Tsakiridis T (2014) AMP-activated protein kinase (AMPK) beyond metabolism: a novel genomic stress sensor participating in the DNA damage response pathway. Cancer Biol Ther 15(2):156–169
Santivasi WL, Xia F (2014) 2014. Ionizing radiation-induced DNA damage, response, and repair. Antioxid Redox Signal 21(2):251–9

Scheck AC, Abdelwahab MG, Stafford P, Kim DY, Iwai S, Preul MC, Rho JM (2011) Mechanistic studies of the ketogenic diet as an adjuvant therapy for malignant gliomas. Cancer Res 70 (8 Suppl):638, Ref Type: Abstract

Scheck AC, Abdelwahab MG, Fenton K, Stafford P (2012) The ketogenic diet for the treatment of glioma: Insights from genetic profiling. Epilepsy Res 100:327–337

Semenza GL (2013) HIF-1 mediates metabolic responses to intratumoral hypoxia and oncogenic mutations. J Clin Invest 123(9):3664–3671

Seyfried TN (2012) Cancer as a metabolic disease: on the origin, management and prevention of cancer. John Wiley and Sons Inc, Hoboken, NJ

Seyfried TN, Mukherjee P (2005) Targeting energy metabolism in brain cancer: review and hypothesis. Nutr Metab 2:30–38

Seyfried TN, Sanderson TM, El-Abbadi MM, McGowan R, Mukherjee P (2003) Role of glucose and ketone bodies in the metabolic control of experimental brain cancer. Br J Cancer 89 (7):1375–1382

Seyfried TN, Kiebish MA, Marsh J, Shelton LM, Huysentruyt LC, Mukherjee P (2011) Metabolic management of brain cancer. Biochim Biophys Acta 1807(6):577–594

Seyfried TN, Marsh J, Shelton LM, Huysentruyt LC, Mukherjee P (2012) Is the restricted ketogenic diet a viable alternative to the standard of care for managing malignant brain cancer? Epilepsy Res 100(3):310–326

Shelton LM, Huysentruyt LC, Mukherjee P, Seyfried TN (2010) Calorie restriction as an anti-invasive therapy for malignant brain cancer in the VM mouse. ASN Neuro 2(3), e00038

Shimazu T, Hirschey MD, Newman J, He W, Shirakawa K, Le MN, Grueter CA, Lim H, Saunders LR, Stevens RD, Newgard CB, Farese RV Jr, de Cabo R, Ulrich S, Akassoglou K, Verdin E (2013) Suppression of oxidative stress by beta-hydroxybutyrate, an endogenous histone deacetylase inhibitor. Science 339(6116):211–214

Shukla SK, Gebregiworgis T, Purohit V, Chaika NV, Gunda V, Radhakrishnan P, Mehla K, Pipinos II, Powers R, Yu F, Singh PK (2014) Metabolic reprogramming induced by ketone bodies diminishes pancreatic cancer cachexia. Cancer Metab 2:18

Singh P, Alex JM, Bast F (2014) Insulin receptor (IR) and insulin-like growth factor receptor 1 (IGF-1R) signaling systems: novel treatment strategies for cancer. Med Oncol 31(1):805

Skinner R, Trujillo A, Ma X, Beierle EA (2009) Ketone bodies inhibit the viability of human neuroblastoma cells. J Pediatr Surg 44(1):212–216

Stafford P, Abdelwahab MG, Kim DY, Preul MC, Rho JM, Scheck AC (2010) The ketogenic diet reverses gene expression patterns and reduces reactive oxygen species levels when used as an adjuvant therapy for glioma. Nutr Metab (Lond) 7:74

Stafstrom CE, Rho JM (2012) The ketogenic diet as a treatment paradigm for diverse neurological disorders. Front Pharmacol 3:59

Thompson HJ, McGinley JN, Spoelstra NS, Jiang W, Zhu Z, Wolfe P (2004) Effect of dietary energy restriction on vascular density during mammary carcinogenesis. Cancer Res 64 (16):5643–5650

Tisdale MJ, Brennan RA (1983) Loss of acetoacetate coenzyme A transferase activity in tumours of peripheral tissues. Br J Cancer 47(2):293–297

Tisdale MJ, Brennan RA, Fearon KC (1987) Reduction of weight loss and tumour size in a cachexia model by a high fat diet. Br J Cancer 56(1):39–43

Urits I, Mukherjee P, Meidenbauer J, Seyfried TN (2012) Dietary restriction promotes vessel maturation in a mouse astrocytoma. J Oncol 2012:264039

Vadlakonda L, Dash A, Pasupuleti M, Anil KK, Reddanna P (2013) The Paradox of Akt-mTOR Interactions. Front Oncol 3:165

van den Bent MJ, Wefel JS, Schiff D, Taphoorn MJ, Jaeckle K, Junck L, Armstrong T, Choucair A, Waldman AD, Gorlia T, Chamberlain M, Baumert BG, Vogelbaum MA, MacDonald DR, Reardon DA, Wen PY, Chang SM, Jacobs AH (2011) Response assessment in neuro-oncology (a report of the RANO group): assessment of outcome in trials of diffuse low-grade gliomas. Lancet Oncol 12(6):583–593

Vander Heiden MG, Cantley LC, Thompson CB (2009) Understanding the Warburg effect: the metabolic requirements of cell proliferation. Science 1029–1033

Vanitallie TB, Nufert TH (2003) Ketones: metabolism's ugly duckling. Nutr Rev 61(10):327–341

Veech RL, Chance B, Kashiwaya Y, Lardy HA, Cahill GF Jr (2001) Ketone bodies, potential therapeutic uses. IUBMB Life 51(4):241–247

Venneti S, Thompson CB (2013) Metabolic modulation of epigenetics in gliomas. Brain Pathol 23 (2):217–221

Verhaak RG, Hoadley KA, Purdom E, Wang V, Qi Y, Wilkerson MD, Miller CR, Ding L, Golub T, Mesirov JP, Alexe G, Lawrence M, O'Kelly M, Tamayo P, Weir BA, Gabriel S, Winckler W, Gupta S, Jakkula L, Feiler HS, Hodgson JG, James CD, Sarkaria JN, Brennan C, Kahn A, Spellman PT, Wilson RK, Speed TP, Gray JW, Meyerson M, Getz G, Perou CM, Hayes DN (2010) Integrated genomic analysis identifies clinically relevant subtypes of glioblastoma characterized by abnormalities in PDGFRA, IDH1, EGFR, and NF1. Cancer Cell 17 (1):98–110

Wang Y, Yuan JL, Zhang YT, Ma JJ, Xu P, Shi CH, Zhang W, Li YM, Fu Q, Zhu GF, Xue W, Lei YH, Gao JY, Wang JY, Shao C, Yi CG, Wang H (2013) Inhibition of both EGFR and IGF1R sensitized prostate cancer cells to radiation by synergistic suppression of DNA homologous recombination repair. PLoS One 8(8), e68784

Warburg O, Wind F, Negelein E (1927) The metabolism of tumors in the body. J Gen Physiol 8 (6):519–530

Ward PS, Thompson CB (2012) Metabolic reprogramming: A cancer hallmark even Warburg did not anticipate. Cancer Cell 21:297–308

Weinberg F, Chandel NS (2009) Reactive oxygen species-dependent signaling regulates cancer. Cell Mol Life Sci 66(23):3663–3673

Weller M, Stupp R, Hegi M, Wick W (2012) Individualized targeted therapy for glioblastoma: fact or fiction? Cancer J 18(1):40–44

Weroha SJ, Haluska P (2012) The insulin-like growth factor system in cancer. Endocrinol Metab Clin North Am 41(2):335–50, vi

Wolf A, Agnihotri S, Guha A (2010) Targeting metabolic remodeling in glioblastoma multiforme. Oncotarget 1(7):552–562

Woolf EC, Curley KL, Liu Q, Turner GH, Charlton JA, Preul MC, Scheck AC (2015) The ketogenic diet alters the hypoxic response and affects expression of proteins associated with angiogenesis, invasive potential and vascular permeability in a mouse glioma model. PLoS One 10(6):e0130357

Woolf EC, Stafford P, Abdelwahab MG, Fenton KE, Preul MC, Scheck AC (2013) The ketogenic diet potentiates radiation therapy in a mouse model of glioma: effects on inflammatory pathways and reactive oxygen species. Cancer Res 73:4441

Yang C, Sudderth J, Dang T, Bachoo RG, McDonald JG, DeBerardinis RJ (2009) Glioblastoma cells require glutamate dehydrogenase to survive impairments of glucose metabolism or Akt signaling. Cancer Res 69(20):7986–7993

Yun J, Johnson JL, Hanigan CL, Locasale JW (2012) Interactions between epigenetics and metabolism in cancers. Front Oncol 2:163

Zhang H, Gu C, Yu J, Wang Z, Yuan X, Yang L, Wang J, Jia Y, Liu J, Liu F (2014) Radiosensitization of glioma cells by TP53-induced glycolysis and apoptosis regulator knockdown is dependent on thioredoxin-1 nuclear translocation. Free Radic Biol Med 69C:239–248

Zhou W, Mukherjee P, Kiebish MA, Markis WT, Mantis JG, Seyfried TN (2007) The calorically restricted ketogenic diet, an effective alternative therapy for malignant brain cancer. Nutr Metab (Lond) 4:5

Zuccoli G, Marcello N, Pisanello A, Servadei F, Vaccaro S, Mukherjee P, Seyfried TN (2010) Metabolic management of glioblastoma multiforme using standard therapy together with a restricted ketogenic diet: case report. Nutr Metab 7:33–53

The Role of Organosulfur Compounds Derived From *Allium* Vegetables in Cancer Prevention and Therapy

Ajay Bommareddy, Adam L. VanWert, Dan F. McCune, Sarah L. Brozena, Zbigniew Witczak, and Shivendra V. Singh

Abstract Organosulfur compounds (OSCs) are a group of small molecules commonly present in *Allium* vegetables, such as garlic, onions chives, and shallots that have garnered scientific interest for their noted health benefits. OSCs have been evaluated for their potential to prevent or treat major diseases including cancer. Epidemiological evidence of inverse association between increased intake of *Allium* vegetables and cancer risk is now substantiated by animal studies wherein true causal relationships between OSCs and cancer prevention have been found. This chapter summarizes the chemistry, metabolism, and bioavailability of commonly studied OSCs and the latest developments regarding their anticarcinogenic effects in cell culture and animal models. Data pertinent to clinical trials assessing safety and anticancer efficacy of OSCs are also discussed.

Abbreviations

5-FU	5-Fluorouracil
AA	Aristolochic acid
ALT	Alanine aminotransferase
AST	Aspartate aminotransferase
B[a]P	Benzo[a]pyrene
CA	Cancer
CCl4	Carbon tetrachloride
COX-2	Cyclooxygenase 2
CYP 2E1	Cytochrome P450 isoenzyme 2E1
DADS	Diallyl disulfide

A. Bommareddy (✉) • A.L. VanWert • D.F. McCune • S.L. Brozena • Z. Witczak
Department of Pharmaceutical Sciences, Nesbitt School of Pharmacy, Wilkes University, 84 W South St, Wilkes-Barre, PA 18766, USA
e-mail: ajay.bommareddy@wilkes.edu

S.V. Singh
Department of Pharmacology and Chemical Biology, University of Pittsburgh Cancer Institute, University of Pittsburgh School of Medicine, Pittsburgh, PA, USA

M.F. Ullah, A. Ahmad (eds.), *Critical Dietary Factors in Cancer Chemoprevention*,
DOI 10.1007/978-3-319-21461-0_6

DAS	Diallyl sulfide
DATS	Diallyl trisulfide
DMBA	7,12-Dimethylbenz[a]anthracene
DMH	Dimethylhydrazine
DR4 and DR5	Death receptor
ERK	Extracellular signal-regulated kinase
GST	Glutathione-*S*-transferase
HDACs	Histone deacetylases
HMG-CoA	3-Hydroxy-3-methyl-glutaryl-Coenzyme A
HUVEC	Human umbilical vein endothelial cells
i.p.	Intraperitoneal
JNK	c-Jun N-terminal kinases
MNNG	Methylnitronitrosoguanidine
MMP	Matrix metalloprotease
NAC	*N*-acetyl-L-cysteine
NDEA	*N*-nitrosodiethylamine
NDMA	*N*-nitrosodimethylamine
NDN	*N*-diethylnitrosamine
NMBA	*N*-nitrosomethylbenzylamine
NF-κB	Nuclear factor-κB
NKK	(methylnitrosamino)1-(3-pyridyl)-1-butanone
NMU	*N*-methylnitrosourea
OSCs	Organosulfur compounds
PAH	Polycyclic aromatic hydrocarbon
PBS	Phosphate-buffered saline
PCNA	Proliferating cell nuclear antigen
PFE	Pomegranate fruit extract
PK	Pharmacokinetic
ppm	Parts per million
PSA	Prostate-specific antigen
pSTAT3	Phosphorylated signal transducer and activator of transcription 3
q3d	Every 3 days
q4d	Every 4 days
qod	Every other day
qd	Every day
ROS	Reactive Oxygen Species
s.c.	Subcutaneous
SAC	*S*-allylcysteine
SAMC	*S*-allylmercaptocysteine
S-NaCl	Saturated sodium chloride
TPA	12-*O*-tetradecanoylphorbol 13-acetate
TRAIL	Tumor necrosis factor-related apoptosis-inducing ligand
TRAMP	Transgenic adenoma of a mouse prostate
VC	Vinyl carbamate
XIAP	X-linked inhibitor of apoptosis protein
Z-ajoene	Z isomer of ajoene

1 Introduction

Beneficial properties of *Allium* vegetables, especially garlic, have been recognized for thousands of years. It has been suggested that garlic can enhance stamina, physical strength, and increase longevity, in addition to functioning as an analgesic, antimicrobial, and antiseptic (Bianchini and Vainio 2001). Together with other types of *Allium* vegetables such as onions, shallots, leeks, and chives, garlic is one of the most commonly consumed foods. Each garlic clove weighs roughly 2–4 g and the average intake varies considerably from individual to individual. In the United States, the average intake of garlic has been estimated to be 0.6 g per week or less, while in other countries, e.g., China, the intake may be close to 20 g or more (reviewed by Milner 2004).

Published data provides undeniable evidence for health-promoting effects of *Allium* vegetables and their constituents. It has been well documented that *Allium* vegetables and their constituents can reduce the risk of major chronic diseases, including cardiovascular diseases, diabetes, and cancer, in addition to their immunomodulatory benefits, protection against infections, and anti-aging effects (Agarwal 1996; Milner 2001; Rahman 2001; Powolny et al. 2011). Studies focusing on garlic and its OSCs in the past three decades have provided a substantial body of evidence demonstrating their ability to prevent or treat various diseases. Several investigations focusing on pharmacological effects of *Allium* vegetables and related OSCs have documented an inverse association with disease development. The anticancer properties of *Allium* vegetables are well supported by epidemiological studies (Shukla and Kalra 2007). Even though the mechanistic details associated with health benefits of OSCs remain partially unknown, the usage of garlic and its products continues to grow. This chapter first introduces the constituents of garlic, including metabolites produced after disruption of its cellular integrity, their molecular mechanisms of anticancer action, and preclinical and clinical evidence for their safety and efficacy. The chapter then concludes with summary and future directions.

2 Chemistry and Metabolism

The primary sulfur-containing compounds in intact garlic are γ-glutamyl-*S*-alk(en)yl-L-cysteines that are hydrolyzed or oxidized to *S*-allylcysteine (SAC) and *S*-alk(en)yl-L-cysteine sulfoxide(alliin) (Fig. 1a). When garlic is processed by crushing or chewing, compounds in the intact garlic are converted into several volatile OSCs within a short period of time. Allinase, a key vacuolar enzyme, is responsible for the conversion of alliin into allicin. The transiently formed and highly unstable

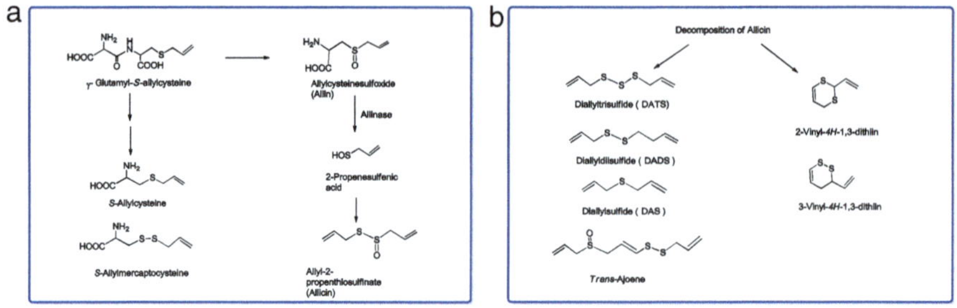

Fig. 1 (**a**) Formation of OSCs upon chewing/crushing of whole garlic cloves. (**b**) Chemical structures of commonly studied OSCs that are produced from allicin

compound, allicin (Fig. 1b) is converted into various OSCs including diallyl sulfide (DAS), diallyl disulfide (DADS), diallyl trisulfide (DATS), ajoene, and dithiins (Higdon 2007; Block et al. 1984; Block 1992; Amagase et al. (review) 2001).

3 Pharmacological Attributes of OSCs in Relation to Anticancer Effects

3.1 Induction of Apoptosis

The process of apoptosis is highly dysregulated in cancer cells contributing to abnormal cell growth, thus leading to increased tumor burden. OSCs have the potential of inducing apoptosis and contributing to the growth suppression of cancer cells. Sundaram and Milner (1996a, b) showed induction of apoptosis by DADS in colon cancer cells. Further studies focused on elucidation of the mechanistic details of apoptosis induction by OSCs have revealed the involvement of Bcl-2 class proteins. For example, apoptosis induction by DATS was more pronounced in prostate cancer cells PC-3 and DU-145 compared to DAS and DADS and that the induction of apoptosis was correlated with a decrease in Bcl-2 levels and reduced Bcl2:Bax interaction activating the mitochondria-mediated intrinsic pathway (Xiao et al. 2004). In the same study, it was also identified that DATS-induced hyperphosphorylation of Bcl-2 was mediated in part by c-Jun N-terminal kinases (JNK) and ERK1/2. Subsequent studies from the same group showed that DATS induces apoptosis in LNCaP prostate cancer cells by increasing Bak protein levels and decreasing Bcl-2 and Bcl-xL protein levels (Kim et al. 2007). However, ectopic expression of Bcl-2 conferred protection against DATS-induced apoptosis only in PC-3 cells and not LNCaP cells (Xiao et al. 2004; Kim et al. 2007). It was reasoned that the genotypic differences between these cells, including their p53 status and androgen responsiveness, were responsible for the observed differential effect. Similarly, in other cancer models such as lung cancer, neuroblastoma, breast cancer, and skin cancer, OSCs were shown to increase the ratio of Bax/Bcl-2, upregulating Bax protein levels and decreasing the levels of Bcl-2 and Bcl-xL proteins (Hong et al. 2000; Karmakar et al. 2007; Nakagawa et al. 2001; Li et al. 2002a, b; Wang et al. 2010, 2012a, b).

It is interesting to point out that OSCs have little or no effect on normal cells, although the mechanism underlying their selectivity for cancer cells is not completely understood. For example, the PrEC normal prostate epithelial cells were more resistant to DATS-induced apoptosis than prostate cancer cells (Kim et al. 2007). Similarly, DAS or DADS administration induced apoptosis in SH-SY5Y neuroblastoma cells and did not impact the viability of primary neurons (Karmakar et al. 2007). In a different study, ajoene caused apoptotic cell death in human leukemia cells but had no effect on normal peripheral mononuclear blood cells (Dirsch et al. 1998).

3.2 Modulation of Carcinogen Metabolism

Multiple studies indicate that chemopreventive effect of OSCs is at least in part due to their ability to inhibit the activation of carcinogens and/or increase detoxification of the activated metabolites. *N*-nitrosodimethylamine (NDMA) is a by-product of industrial processes, while 4-(methylnitrosamino)1-(3-pyridyl)-1-butanone (NKK) is a carcinogen found in tobacco smoke. Their toxicity and carcinogenicity is dependent upon activation by the Phase 1 drug-metabolizing enzyme, CYP 2E1. Early studies utilizing in vitro cell culture and in vivo animal models revealed that OSC treatment prevented cytotoxicity and tumor formation induced by NDMA and NKK (Hong et al. 1992). Furthermore, it was suggested that OSCs inhibit P450 2E1 by both competitive inhibition and suicide inactivation (Brady et al. 1991). OSCs may also protect against acetaminophen toxicity in mice via inhibition of CYP2E1 (Wang et al. 1996). More recent evidence confirmed that oral OSC treatment at 100–400 mg/kg depressed CYP2E1 activity in male Sprague–Dawley rats in a dose-dependent manner. This correlated with statistically significant reductions in serum alanine aminotransferase (ALT) and aspartate aminotransferase (AST) activity following treatment with the hepatotoxicant thioacetamide (Kim et al. 2014), indicating a reduction in liver damage.

Experimental evidence suggests that OSCs may also enhance the detoxification of carcinogens via induction of Phase 2 drug-metabolizing enzymes. One recent study confirmed that oil-soluble garlic compounds activate metabolizing enzymes that detoxify carcinogens. This resulted in a reduction of the development of mammary cancer in animals and suppression of growth of human breast cancer cells in culture (Tsubura et al. 2011). Earlier studies demonstrated the ability of OSCs to prevent benzo(a)pyrene (BP)-induced for stomach tumorigenesis in mice. The authors attributed this to increased expression of NAD(P)H:quinone oxidoreductase (NQO), an enzyme implicated in the detoxification of activated quinone metabolites of BP (Singh et al. 1998). Munday and Munday (2001) documented increases in the activity of the Phase II enzymes NQO and glutathione-*S*-transferase

(GST) in rat tissues following oral doses of both DADS and DATS. OSCs enhanced glutathione content of intestinal mucosa and liver in irradiated Swiss albino mice (Chittezhath and Kuttan 2006). Oil-soluble OSCs induced GST phosphorylation via activation of c-Jun NH_2-terminal kinase (JNK) in neuroblastoma cells (Filomeni et al. 2003). Studies have confirmed activation of GST by JNK in normal rat liver cells (Tsai et al. 2011).

In summary, OSCs act as a double-edged sword in chemoprevention by inhibiting carcinogen activation by Phase 1 enzymes while simultaneously enhancing detoxification of activated carcinogenic intermediates via induction of Phase 2 enzymes (Herman-Antosiewicz et al. 2007).

3.3 *Inhibition of Cell Cycle Progression*

Numerous studies have demonstrated the antiproliferative effects of DATS in a variety of cancer cell types, including liver, gastric, colon, prostate, lung, bladder, and skin cancer cells. The DATS appear to induce cell cycle arrest in the G2/M phase; however, the mechanism by which this occurs may be cell-type specific (for review see Antony and Singh 2011; Yi and Su 2013). In colon cancer cells, DADS-induced G2/M phase arrest was associated with hyperphosphorylation and decreased expression of cell division cycle 25C phosphatase (Cdc25C), inhibition of cdc2 kinase activation, and decreased formation of cdc2/cyclin B1 complex formation (Knowles and Milner 2000). Similarly, Xiao et al. (2005) demonstrated destruction and hyperphosphorylation of Cdc25C and inhibition of cdc2/cyclin B1 kinase activity in prostate cancer cells upon treatment with DATS. This effect was dependent upon generation of reactive oxygen species (ROS). Wang et al. (2010) demonstrated increased ROS generation in DATS-treated skin cancer cells. ROS production associated with G2/M arrest was also seen in neuroblastoma (Filomeni et al. 2003), colon (Song et al. 2009), and lung (Wu et al. 2009) cancer cells.

A role for checkpoint 1 kinase (Chk1) in OSC-mediated cell cycle arrest was also proposed. Chk1 is normally activated in response to DNA damage and results in cell cycle arrest prior to DNA repair or apoptosis. It has been found that SATS-induced mitotic arrest is dependent upon activation of Chk1 in prostate cancer cells and gastric cancer cells (Herman-Antosiewicz and Singh 2005; Ling et al. 2010).

Cell cycle arrest in liver tumor cells was associated with decreased cyclin-dependent kinase 7 protein levels and increased cyclin B1 protein levels (Wu et al. 2004). OSC-induced mitotic arrest in human leukemic cells was attributed to activation and nuclear translocation of nuclear factor-κB (NF-κB) followed by NF-κB binding to the promoter region of cyclin-dependent kinase inhibitor 1 (p21) (Dasgupta and Bandyopadhyay 2013). OSC induced upregulation of p21 was also demonstrated in a study utilizing colon cancer cells (Liao et al. 2009). Multiple studies have associated mitogen-activated protein kinase (MAPK) activation with G2/M arrest. DADS have been shown to trigger cell cycle arrest in both colon cancer (Knowles and Milner 2003) and lung carcinoma cells (Hui et al. 2008). In both studies, this was associated with increased activity of extra-cellular signal-regulated kinase (ERK). In contrast, DADS-mediated arrest in gastric tumor cells was associated with upregulation of p38 MAPK (Yuan et al. 2004). Finally, several studies have identified OSC binding sites on components of tumor cell cytoskeleton and correlated morphological changes to the cytoskeleton with G2/M arrest (Hosono et al. 2005; Xiao et al. 2005; Aquilano et al. 2010).

Cell cycle arrest, if sustained, provides a powerful preventative mechanism to the growth of tumors both in vitro and in vivo. In some of the studies cited above, cell cycle arrest was transient, but was then followed by apoptosis (Xiao et al. 2005; Song et al. 2009; Aquilano et al. 2010; Dasgupta and Bandyopadhyay 2013). Regardless of the mechanism by which it occurs, cell cycle arrest appears to be a common pharmacological effect of OSCs in cancer cells.

3.4 Induction of Reactive Oxygen Species

Accumulating evidence suggests a role for reactive oxygen species (ROS) in cancer cell apoptosis by OSCs. DADS-induced apoptosis in SH-SY5Y neuroblastoma cells was associated with ROS generation (Karmakar et al. 2007). Likewise, ajoene-induced apoptosis in human promyelocleukemic cells was linked to ROS and activation of NF-κB (Dirsch et al. 1998). Studies involving prostate cancer cells (Kim et al. 2007), basal cell carcinoma (Wang et al. 2012a, b), MCF-7 breast cancer cells (Na et al. 2012), and leukemia cells (Choi and Park 2012) also reported that DATS-induced apoptosis was mediated through ROS generation.

The precise mechanism by which DATS causes ROS generation is not fully understood, but some advances in this context are worthy of discussion. For example, apoptosis induction and cell cycle arrest by DADS and DATS were shown to be mediated through increased intracellular calcium (Park et al. 2002; Wang et al. 2010). Cell cycle arrest and apoptosis induction by DATS in prostate cancer cells was shown to be mediated by ROS, generated through increase in labile iron due to proteasomal degradation of ferritin (Antosiewicz et al. 2006). Wang et al. (2010) showed that DATS-dependent calcium increase in basal cell carcinoma (BCC) cells was accompanied by intracellular ROS generation. The ROS generation by OSCs was also linked with the generation of hydrogen sulfide (H_2S) where it was shown that OSCs can be converted to H_2S in human red blood cells (Benavides et al. 2007). More recently, it was shown that DATS-induced H_2S is associated with the generation of ROS and activation of mitochondria-mediated apoptosis pathway in human breast cancer MCF-7 cells (Na et al. 2012). Based on these studies, it is evident that OSC-dependent ROS generation is crucial for their anticancer effects.

3.5 Inhibition of Angiogenesis and Cell Invasion

Inhibition of angiogenesis, which is required for tumor growth, is another major effect of some OSCs. Mousa and colleagues demonstrated the anti-angiogenic potential of alliin as it inhibited the tube formation, dependent on fibroblast growth factor-2 and vascular endothelial growth factor (VEGF) both in human endothelial cells and in a chick chorioallantoic membrane assay (Mousa and Mousa 2005). In the same study, the authors also showed that the anti-angiogenic potential of alliin, which was in part mediated by increase in cellular nitric oxide and p53 protein expression, increased in the presence of vitamin C and vitamin E. The DATS-associated anti-angiogenic properties were examined in human umbilical vein endothelial cells (HUVEC). DATS was shown to inhibit formation of capillary-like tube structure and migration by HUVECs. Mechanistic details revealed suppression of VEGF secretion, downregulation of VEGF receptor-2 protein level, and inactivation of Akt upon treatment with DATS (Xiao et al. 2006a, b).

The effect of OSCs on migration and invasion of cancer cells has also been studied. Ajoene administration inhibited B16/BL6 melanoma cell adhesion to LEC1 cells in vitro and also significantly inhibited lung metastasis in C57BL/6 mice injected with B16/Bl6 melanoma cells (Taylor et al. 2006). Similarly, DADS treatment resulted in the inhibition of HUVEC cell proliferation and activity of matrix metalloprotease-2 (MMP-2) and MMP-9 (Meyer et al. 2004). The DATS administration in a transgenic mouse model of prostate cancer (Transgenic Adenocarcinoma of Mouse Prostate; TRAMP) not only prevented the development of poorly differentiated prostate cancer but also inhibited pulmonary metastasis multiplicity (Singh et al. 2008). In a study using osteosarcoma cells, DATS was shown to exhibit antitumor activity by targeting Notch1 signaling and inhibiting cell invasion and angiogenesis partly through downregulation of VEGF, MMP-2, and MMP-9 (Li et al. 2013). DAS, DADS, and DATS were shown to inhibit migration, invasion, and angiogenesis. For example, exposure of human colon cancer Colo 205 cells to all three OSCs resulted in inhibition of PI3K, Ras, MEKK3, MKK7, ERK1/2, JNK1/2, and p38 which correlated with the inhibition of MMP-2, -7, and -9, essential for cell migration and invasion (Lai et al. 2013). DATS was also shown to inhibit mRNA and protein levels of VEGF and MMP-2, -7, and -9 in human colon cancer HT29 cells (Lai et al. 2015). In addition to reducing MMP levels, inhibitory effects of DADS in Colo 205 cells and LNCaP cells were also found to be associated with reduced levels of proteins associated with tight junctions functionality [Lai et al. (2013), Shin et al. (2010), for review see Yi and Su (2013)].

3.6 Immunomodulation

Immunomodulatory effects of garlic and its OSCs have been reported (for a review, see Schafer and Kaschula 2014). Studies have identified that garlic and its constituents can effectively strengthen the host immune system within the tumor against the immunosuppressive activity of an emerging tumor (Schafer and Kaschula 2014). Aged garlic extract along with an anticancer agent suppressed tumor growth of sarcoma-180 and Lewis Lung carcinoma LL/2 cells injected in mice by inducing cellular immune response through the activation of NK cells and cytotoxic T cells (Kyo et al. 1998). In addition, aged garlic extract was also found to stimulate lymphocyte proliferation, macrophages phagocytosis, and lymphocyte infiltration into tumors and enhanced NK cell number and activity (Schafer and Kaschula 2014). A recent study showed that intra-tumor inoculation of a protein fraction of fresh garlic bulbs was more efficient than garlic extract in infiltrating the tumor with CD8+ T cells (Ebrahimi et al. 2013). DADS downregulated the levels of CCL-2 (an important chemokine which favors tumor cell migration and expansion) induced by TNF-α in MDA-MB 231 breast cancer cells (Bauer et al. 2014). It was reasoned that CCL-2 release by breast cancer cells may be regulated by pro-inflammatory cytokines through NF-κB or ERK.

Even though studies have identified conflicting evidence (for a review, see Schafer and Kaschula 2014) with the immunomodulation properties of OSCs, it is noteworthy to mention that immunomodulatory effects of OSCs may contribute to their overall anticancer activity.

3.7 *Modulation of Histone Acetylation*

Balance between histone acetylation and deacetylation is crucial for regulation of gene expression essential for normal cellular processes. However, this balance is often lost in cancer cells, favoring their uncontrolled growth and progression. Discovery of agents that can either block the activity of histone deacetylases (HDACs) or promote the histone acetylation activity is crucial in combating cancer development. There are examples of clinical success of this approach (vorinostat). Studies have shown that garlic and its compounds have the potential of both increasing histone acetylation and inhibiting HDAC activity (for reviews, see Druense-Pecollo and Latino-Martel 2011; Yi and Su 2013). For example, DADS caused an increase in the acetylation of histones H3 and H4 in DS19 and K562 human leukemic cells. Acetylation was also induced in rat hepatoma and human breast cancer cells by DADS and its metabolite, allylmercaptan. Moreover, in the same study it was shown that allylmercaptan was more potent in inhibiting HDAC compared to DADS (Lea et al. 1999). The induction of histone acetylation by *S*-allylmercaptocysteine (SAMC), allicin, and DADS in various cancer models was also shown (Lea and Randolph 2001; Lea et al. 2001). DADS was also shown to promote cellular accumulation in G2/M phase by decreasing HDAC activity and increasing histone H3 and H4 acetylation, thus causing an increase in p21 mRNA and protein levels in colon cancer CaCo-2 and HT29 cells (Druesne et al. 2004). A recent study showed that DATS-induced acetylation of histones H3 and H4 and inhibition of HDAC activity contributed to the inhibition of glioblastoma xenograft growth (Wallace et al. 2013).

4 Preclinical In Vivo Evidence for Chemopreventive Effects of OSCs

A wealth of literature exists characterizing effects of *Allium*-derived OSCs on prevention of cancer initiation and promotion. The primary compounds investigated include the oil-soluble DATS, DADS, DAS, and ajoene, and the major water-soluble component SAC. With the exception of ajoene, these compounds have received roughly equal attention in the literature.

4.1 DATS

Although other OSCs have received significant attention for their chemopreventive ability against carcinogens, the majority of preclinical studies with DATS used rodents that either received a cancerous cell implant or were genetically susceptible to cancer. The major cancers investigated with DATS include lung, colon, liver, prostate, skin, and breast, with a predominance of prostate cancer studies. These studies were initiated in 2005 (Table 1).

Female BALB/c nude mice with human lung adenocarcinoma cell (A549) xenografts showed significantly retarded tumor growth with no apparent side effects when given a DATS oral gavage of 0.6 nmol every other day for 30 days (Li et al. 2012). Singh et al. (2008) studied the ability of oral DATS (1 and 2 mg/day, thrice weekly for 13 weeks) to inhibit lung metastasis from prostate cancer in TRAMP mice. DATS administration did not reduce the incidence of metastasis, but multiplicity was lower in the treatment group compared with control.

Female nude mice subcutaneously implanted with human colon cancer cells (HCT-15) exhibited a marked reduction in tumor volume relative to control after 25 days of DATS treatment at 6 mg/kg IV every 3 days initiated 7 days after xenograft implantation (Hosono et al. 2005). Statistical significance was not reported, but average tumor volume was less in the treatment group versus control mice. Wu et al. (2011) found that female BALB/c mice with mouse colon carcinoma cell (CT-26) allografts had significantly reduced tumor volumes and weights when administered DATS at 50 mg/kg by oral gavage every 4 days starting 4 weeks prior to cell inoculation.

In a unique study by Zhang et al. (2007), polybutylcyanoacrylate nanoparticles containing DATS were tested for 2 weeks of treatment against orthotopically transplanted HepG2 liver cancer cells. The subcutaneously grown tumors were subsequently implanted under the envelope of the liver in BALB/c nude mice. IV

Table 1 Preclinical studies on DATS

Lead author	Year	Animal	Cancer	Carcinogen	Treatment	Results
Hosono	2005	Mice (female nude)	Colon: HCT-15 xenograft s.c.	No	6 mg/kg via tail vein q3d from day 7 to 25	Prevented colon tumors (*P* value not reported but tumor volume was on average < 1/3 of control after 25 days)
Xiao	2006	Mice (male athymic)	Prostate:PC-3 cell s.c. xenograft	No	Oral gavage 6 μmol, 3×/week	Tumor growth was slowed without causing weight loss (3-fold smaller in 20 days). DATS caused more apoptotic bodies and more Bax and Bak expression (pro-apoptotic proteins), but did not inhibit angiogenesis
Zhang	2007	Mice (BALB/c nude) orthotopic transplantation	Liver: HCC HepG2 xenografts into liver	No	Liver-targeted intravenous polybutylcyanoacrylate nanoparticles of DATS (1.5 mg/kg qod, 2 weeks)	DATS-nano. distributed differently than DATS alone (highly liver targeted, while DATS alone showed renal predominant targeting. Both targeted spleen similarly and substantially). DATS-nano retarded growth of hepatoma compared to DATS, nano., or saline, with no weight loss. PCNA and Bcl-2 proteins were downregulated in DATS-nano

(continued)

Table 1 (continued)

Lead author	Year	Animal	Cancer	Carcinogen	Treatment	Results
Singh	2008	Mice (TRAMP)	Prostate and Lung	No	Oral gavage 1 and 2 mg/day, 3×/week, 13 weeks	Inhibited progression to poorly differentiated prostate CA and pulmonary metastasis multiplicity (not incidence of metastasis) w/out side effects. Dorsolateral prostate showed decreased cell proliferation from DATS and induction of cyclinB1 and securin protein. DATS did not increase apoptosis or affect angiogenesis or natural killer or dendritic cell function
Shankar	2008	Mice (BALB/c nude)	Prostate: orthotopic PC-3 cell implant into prostate	No	Oral DATS (daily 5days/week 40 mg/kg)	Inhibited growth of prostate CA without causing weight loss. Co-treatment w/DATS and TRAIL was more effective at growth inhibition, DR4 and DR5 protein induction, caspase-8-activation, and apoptosis induction than either agent alone. DATS inhibited angiogenesis and metastasis-related protein expression and Akt and NF-kB activation. This effect was stronger when combined with TRAIL
Stan	2009	Mice (TRAMP)	Prostate	No	Oral gavage of DATS (2 mg/day, 3×/week, 13 weeks)	Suppressed androgen receptor protein expression in poorly differentiated prostate cancer

Chandra-Kuntal	2010	Mice (TRAMP)	Prostate	No	The 2 mg-treated mice from (Singh et al. 2008)	The reduction in poorly differentiated prostate tissue correlated with a decrease in the oncogenic protein pSTAT3. When STAT3 was made constitutively active in cells, the response to DATS was not attenuated. Thus, inhibition of STAT3 activation alone is not required for DATS's pro-apoptotic effect
Shrotriya	2010	Mice	Skin	DMBA and TPA	Pretreatment of skin (25 μmol topical) 30 min before TPA	DATS more effective than other allyl sulfides (DATS > DADS > DAS) in suppressing TPA-induced COX-2 expression. DATS reduced DNA binding of activator protein 1 (AP-1), a transcription factor for COX-2. DATS also reduced JNK and Akt activation. DATS significantly reduced incidence and multiplicity of papillomas
Wu	2011	Mice (female BALB/c)	Colon: i.p. CT-26 cell allograft	No	DATS (10 or 50 mg/kg) i.p. q4d 4 weeks prior to cell inoculation	50 mg/kg reduced tumor volume and weight significantly
Kim	2011	Mice (TRAMP)	Prostate	No	2 mg/day/mouse, 3×/week for 13 weeks beginning at 8 weeks of age	Dorsolateral prostates from treated mice showed significant downregulation of XIAP and induction of Survivin protein vs. control mice. Ectopic expression of XIAP partially reversed the DATS-induced apoptosis

(continued)

Table 1 (continued)

Lead author	Year	Animal	Cancer	Carcinogen	Treatment	Results
Li	2012	Mice (female BALB/c nude)	Lung: A549 cell s.c. xenografts	No	Oral gavage, 6 μM in 100 μl PBS qod (0.6 nmol total mass) for 30 days	Slowed growth of xenografts with no apparent side effects (no weight loss)
Na	2012	Mice (BALB/c female)	Breast: thoracic implant w/human MCF-7 Breast CA cells	17-β-estradiol implanted device	Oral (5 μmol/kg, 2×/week for 1 month)	Inhibited growth of xenografts. In cells, DATS induced apoptosis that was dependent on JNK. DATS-induced cell apoptosis and JNK activation was reduced by *N*-acetyl-L-cysteine (NAC). DATS increased DNA binding of AP-1, which was blocked by NAC or JNK inhibitor

Treatment was DATS unless otherwise noted. Results are statistically significant unless otherwise indicated

Abbreviations: 5-FU, 5-fluorouracil; AA, aristolochic acid; B[a]P, benzo[a]pyrene; CA, cancer; CCl4, carbon tetrachloride; COX-2, cyclooxygenase 2; CYP 2E1, cytochrome P450 isoenzyme 2E1; DADS, diallyl disulfide; DAS, diallyl sulfide; DATS, diallyl trisulfide; DMBA, 7,12-dimethylbenz[a]anthracene; DMH, Dimethylhydrazine; DR4 and DR5, death receptor 4 and 5; GST, glutathione-*S*-transferase; HMG-CoA, 3-hydroxy-3-methyl-glutaryl-Coenzyme A; i. p., intraperitoneal; MNNG, methylnitronitrosoguanidine; NAC, *N*-acetyl-L-cysteine; NDEA, *N*-nitrosodiethylamine; NDMA, *N*-nitrosodimethylamine; NDN, *N*-diethylnitrosamine; NMBA, *N*-nitrosomethylbenzylamine; NMU, *N*-methylnitrosourea; PAH, polycyclic aromatic hydrocarbon; PBS, phosphate buffered saline; PCNA, proliferating cell nuclear antigen; PFE, pomegranate fruit extract; PK, pharmacokinetic; ppm, parts per million; PSA, prostate specific antigen; pSTAT3, phosphorylated signal transducer and activator of transcription 3; q3d, every 3 days; q4d, every 4 days; qod, every other day; s.c., subcutaneous; SAC, S-allylcysteine; S-NaCl, saturated sodium chloride; TPA, 12-*O*-tetradecanoylphorbol 13-acetate; TRAIL, tumor necrosis factor-related apoptosis-inducing ligand; VC, vinyl carbamate; XIAP, X-linked inhibitor of apoptosis protein; Z-ajoene, Z isomer of ajoene; qd, every day

DATS or DATS-filled nanoparticles were injected every other day for 14 days at 1.5 mg/kg. The DATS nanoparticles were markedly more liver targeted than DATS alone, which showed predominantly renal localization. Both formulations showed significant spleen distribution. Moreover, DATS nanoparticles retarded growth of liver tumors more than DATS with no weight loss. To determine a molecular basis for the result, PCNA and Bcl-2 proteins were assessed. Both were downregulated in the tumors from DATS nanoparticle-treated mice compared with control tumors.

In preclinical prostate cancer studies on DATS, investigators mostly employed the TRAMP model or grown xenografts with PC-3 cell implantation. Studies with TRAMP mice focused on changes in protein expression of cell growth and apoptosis related proteins, while the follow-up ones directly assessed effectiveness against tumor growth. Kim et al. (2011) found that DATS given at 2 mg/day thrice weekly for 13 weeks caused significant downregulation of XIAP while inducing survivin protein in TRAMP mice. Ectopic expression of XIAP partially reversed DATS-induced apoptosis in prostate cancer cells, strengthening the contention that DATS-induced XIAP downregulation is important for induction of apoptosis. Stan and Singh (2009) demonstrated that the same dose and schedule of DATS suppressed androgen receptor (AR) protein expression in poorly differentiated prostate cancer in TRAMP mice. Therefore, there is evidence indicating that DATS can both trigger apoptosis and attenuate prostate cancer-promoting receptor expression.

Oral gavage of DATS in TRAMP mice at either 1 or 2 mg/day, three times a week for 13 weeks, significantly inhibited progression to poorly differentiated prostate cancer, and showed a trend toward a reduction in prostate weight, albeit not significant (Singh et al. 2008). Dorsolateral prostate showed reduced cell proliferation from DATS treatment and induction of cyclinB1 and securin protein. DATS did not increase apoptosis or affect angiogenesis. In Chandra-Kuntal and Singh (2010), mice from the same study were further assessed. The reduction in poorly differentiated prostate cancer cells from the 2 mg DATS treatment group in Singh et al. (2008) correlated with a decrease in phosphorylated STAT3, an oncogenic protein. However, forced expression of STAT3 in prostate cancer cells did not attenuate the response to DATS, indicating that inhibition of STAT3 activation is not required for the preventive effect of DATS.

Xiao et al. 2006a, b found that oral DATS at 6 μmol thrice weekly significantly slowed tumor growth in male nude mice subcutaneously implanted with PC-3 cells. Tumors were 2/3 smaller in treated mice in 20 days vs. untreated mice. DATS caused more apoptotic bodies and increased expression of Bax and Bak (pro-apoptotic proteins). However, DATS did not inhibit angiogenesis, and was apparently not toxic, as demonstrated by lack of weight loss. Shankar et al. (2008) approached PC-3 cell implantation differently by implanting directly into the prostate rather than studying the cells' subcutaneous growth. They found that oral DATS given every day 5 days a week at 40 mg/kg inhibited growth of the prostate cancer implant vs. control. When DATS was combined with TRAIL (tumor necrosis factor-related apoptosis-inducing ligand), the combination was even more effective at growth inhibition than DATS. TRAIL-R1/DR4 and TRAIL-R2/DR5 protein induction, caspase-8 activation, and apoptosis induction were also greater with the combination than either agent alone. DATS also inhibited angiogenesis and metastasis-related protein expression and Akt and NF-κB activation, but again did so more strongly when combined with TRAIL (Shankar et al. 2008).

The two-stage murine model of skin cancer with DMBA (dimethylbenz[a] anthracene) as the initiator and TPA (tetradecanoylphorbol-13-acetate) as the promoter was employed to test the cancer protective effect of DATS (Shrotriya et al. 2010). Topical DATS at 25 μmol 30 min before TPA application was effective in suppressing TPA-induced COX-2 expression. COX-2 suppression appeared to have been caused by a DATS-triggered reduction in DNA binding of activator protein 1 (AP-1), a transcription factor for COX-2. DATS also reduced JNK and Akt activation, and moreover, reduced the incidence and multiplicity of skin papillomas. COX-2 has been linked with skin cancer through its inflammatory role in the body, thus providing a mechanistic explanation for the reduced papilloma formation.

Na et al. (2012) employed BALB/c mice implanted with human breast cancer cells (MCF-7) directly into the thoracic area and promoted with estradiol-releasing implanted devices. Oral DATS at 5 μmol/kg twice weekly for 1 month inhibited xenograft growth.

Cell studies indicated that DATS induced apoptosis that was dependent on JNK. DATS increased DNA binding of AP-1. This may appear to be in contrast to the skin cancer study by Shrotriya et al. (2010) with respect to AP-1 effects; however, in Shrotriya et al. (2010), DATS's effects on AP-1 DNA binding were assessed in the context of TPA-promoted skin cancer, whereas in Na et al. (2012) DATS's effects on AP-1 DNA binding were assessed in the presence of estradiol-promoted breast cancer. Thus, DATS effects on AP-1 are likely context/environment dependent.

4.2 DADS

DADS have been assessed in treatment or prevention of cancers of the skin, mammary tissue, liver, colon, kidney, and stomach, in addition to leukemia. Earlier studies generally employed cancer initiators and promoters (two-stage model), whereas later studies relied heavily on xenografts of various cancer cell types (Table 2).

Dwivedi et al. (1992) employed the SENCAR mice, which are sensitive to two-stage skin cancer induction. Topical DADS (1 mg) 30 min prior to DMBA initiation and 30 min before each recurrent TPA administration inhibited skin papilloma formation from the 9th week of promotion. Survival of mice was also increased after DADS treatment. The mechanism of chemoprevention by DADS in this study is unclear, but authors postulated the modulation of bioactivation of DMBA by DADS.

Table 2 Preclinical studies on DADS

Lead author	Year	Animal	Cancer	Carcinogen	Treatment	Results
Dwivedi	1992	SENCAR (two-stage model-sensitive) Mice	Skin	DMBA and TPA	Topical DADS and DAS (1 mg/100 μl) administered 30 min before DMBA and 30 min before TPA	Inhibited skin papilloma formation from the 9th week of promotion and increased survival
Ip	1992	Rats	Mammary	DMBA	Gavage 1.8 mmol/kg at 96, 48, and 24 h before 10 mg intragastric DMBA, single dose	Protected in the initiation phase (61 % reduction in tumor incidence and 56 % reduction in total tumor number), somewhat more so than DAS
Takahashi	1992	Rats (male F344)	Liver, colon, kidney: two-step cancer models	*N*-diethylnitrosamine i.p. (200 mg/kg) and other carcinogens sequentially	DADS (50 mg/kg) or DAS (200 mg/kg) gavage, 3×/week for 6 weeks after NDN, or for 24 weeks after admin. of other carcinogens	DADS inhibited colon and renal CA. DAS increased levels of a liver cancer-associated protein, but an increased risk for liver cancer was not confirmed
Sundaram	1996	Mice (female)	Colon: human colon tumor cell line s.c. xenograft, HCT-15	No	1 mg 3×/week by gavage or i.p.	I.p. Reduced tumor volume by 69 % without apparent toxicity. Gavage was also effective, but less than i.p.. DADS was as efficacious as 5-FU. DADS and 5-FU combined was no more effective than either alone. DADS also reduced 5-FU toxicity by unknown mechanism

(continued)

Table 2 (continued)

Lead author	Year	Animal	Cancer	Carcinogen	Treatment	Results
Singh	1996	Mice (BALB/c nude)	Subcutaneous implant of H-ras oncogene-transformed NIH 3T3 (fibroblast) cell xenograft	No	Oral administration (33 μmol thrice weekly)	Delayed and inhibited tumor growth. Inhibition of tumor growth correlated with inhibition of $p21^{H\text{-}ras}$ membrane association. DADS also inhibited hepatic and tumoral HMG-CoA reductase. Suggested that inhibition of prenylation may be the therapeutic mechanism
Suzui	1997	Rats (SD, female)	Mammary	2-amino-1-methyl-6-phenylimidazo[4,5-b] pyridine	200 ppm in diet	Reduced the number of mammary tumors per rat
Xiang	2005	Mice (BALB/c nude)	Gastric: s.c.human gastric CA MGC803 cell xenograft	No	50, 100, and 200 mg/kg i.p. 3×/week	Reduced xenograft tumor weight compared to control by 27.8 %, 66.1 %, and 73 %. PCNA expression was inhibited
Yang	2006	Mice (BALB/c w	Leukemia: mouse WEHI-3 leukemia cell injection	No	25 μM/100 μL (2.5 nmol total) oral qd	Decreased percentage of MAC-3 marker. DADS decreased the weights of liver and spleen. WEHI-3 cells normally enlarge the spleen

Liao	2007	Mice (BALB/c nude)	Colon:s.c.SW480 cell implanted	No	i.p.30 mg/kg qod	Inhibition of tumor growth was seen from 16 days after implantation to termination of the experiment at 32 days. PCNA was reduced
Tang	2013	Mice (BALB/c nude)	Gastric: cells s.c. implantMGC-803 gastric cells	No	i.p. 100 mg/kg (frequency not reported) and intratumoral miRNAs	DADS alone reduced tumor growth with a more noticeable effect as the study progressed to termination at 28 days. Micro RNAs that were shown to be upregulated in response to DADS treatment in MGC-803 cells (i.e., miR-200b and miR-22) enhanced the effects of DADS

Treatment was DADS unless otherwise noted. Results are statistically significant unless otherwise indicated
Abbreviations listed under Table 1

Ip et al. (1992) assessed effects of DADS against DMBA-induced mammary tumors in rats. Oral DADS at 1.8 mmol/kg given 96, 48, and 24 h before intragastric DMBA (10 mg) reduced mammary tumor incidence by 61 % and total tumor yield by 56 %. DAS also significantly reduced both incidence and yield, but was weaker than DADS. Suzui et al. (1997) tested DADS against 2-amino-1-methyl-6-phenylimidazo[4,5-b]pyridine-induced mammary tumors in rats. DADS at 200 ppm in the diet significantly reduced the total number of mammary tumors per rat by 63 % and trended toward a reduction in tumor incidence.

Sundaram and Milner (1996a, b) used a human colon tumor cell line, HCT-15, to study anticancer effects of DADS. Intraperitoneal or intragastric DADS treatment (1 mg thrice weekly) reduced tumor volume without apparent toxicity. The intraperitoneal route was more effective (69 % reduction in volume) than the later. DADS was as effective as 5-fluorouracil (5-FU), a well-established antineoplastic drug. Interestingly, concomitant DADS and 5-FU was no more effective than either agent alone, but DADS reduced 5-FU toxicity. This finding indicated that DADS might inhibit the pharmacological action of 5-FU or perhaps affect its bioavailability. Liao et al. (2007) tested efficacy against SW480 colon cancer cells implanted subcutaneously in BALB/C nude mice and found that intraperitoneal DADS (30 mg/kg) inhibited tumor growth and reduced proliferating cell nuclear antigen (PCNA) expression.

Xiang et al. (2005) implanted human gastric cancer cells, MGC803, subcutaneously into nude BALB/c mice. Three different doses of DADS, 50, 100, and 200 mg/kg intraperitoneally thrice weekly reduced tumor weight compared to control by 27.8 %, 66.1 %, and 73 %, respectively. This dose–response profile may indicate that a ceiling effect will be exhibited by DADS at least with respect to this tumor type. Subsequently, Tang et al. (2013) used coadministration of DADS and a microRNA (miR-200b and miR-22) that is upregulated in response to DADS treatment in MGC803 cells. The combination treatment enhanced the effects of DADS against the subcutaneously implanted cancer cells in nude BALB/c mice.

Takahashi et al. (1992) aimed for a comprehensive approach by sequentially introducing carcinogens to male F344 rats that targeted different organs. *N*-diethylnitrosamine was one of the primary carcinogens used in the study. DADS were administered, after initiation, at a dose of 200 mg/kg thrice weekly for 6–24 weeks depending on the organ under investigation. DADS significantly inhibited colon adenoma and renal nephroblastoma; however, although the related garlic constituent, DAS, trended toward inhibiting colon adenoma, significance was not achieved. Moreover, DAS did not appear to exhibit any effect on renal cancer. Perhaps as important as determining therapeutic targets for DADS is the identification of cancers that do not respond to DADS. In this study, 100 % of animals acquired alveolar hyperplasia, but neither DADS nor DAS exhibited any chemopreventive ability in lung. In addition, urinary bladder cell hyperplasia was not significantly inhibited by DADS or DAS. It is possible that the statistical power of the study was a limiting factor, particularly because only 35 % of animals exhibited bladder hyperplasia. This would require highly consistent results to recognize a true difference between treatment groups. Other cancers were relatively rare in the study, precluding any assessment of DADS or DAS efficacy. It is worth noting that DAS-treated animals exhibited induction of placental glutathione-*S*-transferase (GST-P), an enzyme considered to be indicative of a pre-neoplastic state. Thus, this study suggests that DAS may promote liver cancer. Unfortunately, later studies were not designed to assess and confirm this hepatic finding, as they focused on different organs.

The majority of studies with DADS are aimed at specific organs or tissues; however, Singh et al. (1996) took a different approach. They used an H-ras oncogene-transformed fibroblast cell line (NIH 3T3) in xenografts in nude BALB/c mice. When cells were implanted subcutaneously, oral administration of DADS delayed and inhibited tumor growth, which correlated with a reduction in membrane association of $p21^{H\text{-}ras}$. Interestingly, DADS also inhibited hepatic and tumoral 3-hydroxy-3-methyl-glutaryl-CoA (HMG-CoA) reductase, an enzyme important in prenylation, and thus anchoring of proteins, e.g., Ras, in the plasma membrane. Therefore, the investigation indicates that DADS may reduce extracellular growth signal sensitivity in cancer cells.

4.3 DAS

Studies on DAS in relation to cancer began in the late 1980s. It has commonly been studied for its effects on skin cancer, but has also been assessed for neoplasms of the esophagus, stomach, mammary tissue, liver, colon, and kidney (Table 3). One of the first studies on DAS, by Wargovich et al. (1988), focused on esophageal cancer initiated by *N*-nitrosomethylbenzylamine (NMBA) in rats. DAS, when given at 200 mg/kg orally 3 h prior to NMBA (3 and 5 mg/kg), inhibited DNA damage by up to 64 % and inhibited tumor formation completely with high statistical significance. DAS inhibited gastric and hepatic metabolism of NMBA, thus indicating that DAS could prevent the formation of DNA-alkylating metabolites. However, whether DAS inhibited esophageal cancer by inhibiting metabolism of NMBA is unknown, as this mechanism would suggest that the carcinogenic metabolite(s) of NMBA can target esophageal cells via the basolateral aspect after reaching the systemic circulation. In a later study by Wargovich et al. (1992), DAS again showed a significant ability to suppress initiation of esophageal cancer by NMBA; however, a dose dependence was clearly observed. That is, 10 mg/kg DAS gavage weekly for 5 weeks (3 h prior to NMBA) failed to inhibit esophageal cancer or papillomas, while 100 mg/kg weekly reduced tumor incidence by 34 %, tumor multiplicity by 53 %, papilloma multiplicity by 42 %, and squamous cell carcinoma by 88 %, all statistically significantly. A very important distinction was made in this study, as when DAS, 200 mg/kg weekly, was given after NMBA treatment it was completely ineffective at preventing tumors or papillomas.

As described in the previous section, Dwivedi et al. (1992) employed the SENCAR mouse model to test DAS in parallel with DADS. When given topically, either DAS or DADS, 1 mg, 30 min prior to DMBA and 30 min before each TPA

Table 3 Preclinical studies on DAS

Lead Author	Year	Animal	Cancer	Carcinogen	Treatment	Results
Wargovich	1988	Rats	Esophageal	NMBA, 3 and 5 mg/kg	200 mg/kg, oral) 3 h prior to NMBA	Inhibited DNA damage (56-64 %). DAS totally inhibited tumor formation and reduced hepatic metabolism of NMBA. Thus, DAS inhibits monoalkylating carcinogens in the GI tract
Dwivedi	1992	SENCAR Mice	Skin	DMBA and TPA	Topical DADS and DAS (1 mg/100 μl) administered 30 min before DMBA and 30 min before TPA	Inhibited skin papilloma formation from the 9th week of promotion and increased survival
Wargovich	1992	Rats (Sprague Dawley)	Esophagus	NMBA (3 mg/kg 1×/week for 5 weeks	– 10 mg/kg or 100 mg/kg gavage 1x/week, 5 weeks, 3 h prior to NMBA (initiation) – 200 mg/kg 1×/week after NMBA treatments were completed (post-initiation	Strongly inhibited during initiation, reducing tumor incidence (34 % red), papillomas (43 % red), and squamous cell carcinoma (88 % red), but was completely ineffective if given post-initiation until the end of the study (15 weeks total)
Ip	1992	Rats	Mammary	DMBA (10 mg intragastric single dose)	Gavage 1.8 mmol/kg at 96, 48, and 24 h before DMBA	Protected in the initiation phase (61 % reduction in tumor incidence and 56 % reduction in total tumor number), somewhat more so than DAS
Takahashi	1992	Rats (male F344)	Liver, Colon, Kidney	NDN (i.p. 200 mg/kg) and other carcinogens (two-step liver and organ CA models)	Intragastric DADS (50 mg/kg) or DAS (200 mg/kg) 3×/week for 6 weeks after NDN, or for 24 weeks after second carcinogens	DADS inhibited colon and renal CA. DAS increased levels of a liver cancer-associated protein, but an increased risk for liver cancer was not confirmed

Hadjiolov	1993	Rats (male BD-6)	Gastric	AA (oral, 2 × 10 mg/kg/week, 3 months)	150 mg/kg intragastric 24 and 4 h prior to AA	AA induced stomach, bladder, and thymus tumors after 12 weeks. DAS reduced the incidence of stomach carcinoma/sarcoma from 45 % to 10 % (DAS once 4 h before AA) or 0 % (DAS 24 and 4 h before AA), but did not reduce the incidence of the preceding papillomas (a strong trend in this direction was seen). DAS also decreased DNA damage in stomach. AA caused a hyperplastic urothelium, but was poor at causing bladder cancer. DAS did not prevent this hyperplasia. Total tumor burden reduction in the bodies was from 60 % to 10 % w/single admin. DAS and to 0 % w/double admin. DAS
Surh	1995	ICR Mice	Skin	VC (topical) and NDMA	Gavage, 8 μmol 10 min prior to VC	Reduced papilloma incidence apparently by reducing the CYP 2E1-mediated metabolism of NDMA (reduced N-demethylation)
Singh	1998a	Mice (Swiss albino)	Skin	Topical DMBA and TPA	Topical, 250 μg 3×/week for 3 weeks for anti-initiation and 1 h prior to each promotion treatment	Delayed onset of tumors, reduced number of tumors. Several mice remained tumor free until termination of the study

(continued)

Table 3 (continued)

Lead Author	Year	Animal	Cancer	Carcinogen	Treatment	Results
Singh	1998b	Mice (female Swiss albino)	Skin	DMBA or Benzo[a]pyrene	Topical 1 h before, or 1 h after DMBA or BaP	Protected against skin CA. Administration of DAS 1 h prior was more effective at reducing the average tumor number per mouse (28 week period). B[a]P-induced tumors were better prevented when DAS was given after, rather than before, contrasting with DMBA. DAS was much more effective in all respects against B[a]P-induced cancer vs. DMBA. DAS is therefore effective against PAH-induced mouse skin cancer
George	2011	Mice (male BALB/c)	Skin	DMBA and TPA	Topical 3×/week, 250 μg, or topical 125 μg combined with PFE in drink	Delayed onset and tumor incidence by 55 % and 45 %. When combined with PFE, the prevention was synergistic (84 %). PFE alone worked slightly better than DAS alone, but both were effective. Combination was more effective in decreasing expression of phosphoERK1/2, phosphoJNK1, and reducing activity of NF-κB, IKK-α, and decreasing phosphorylated IκB-α

Treatment was DAS unless otherwise noted. Results are statistically significant unless otherwise indicated
Abbreviations listed under Table 1

administration, inhibited skin papilloma formation from the 9th week of promotion and increased survival. As described previously, the authors suggested the possibility of modified bioactivation of DMBA by DAS and DADS as the mechanism of chemoprevention. Several later studies continued with the assessment of DAS against chemically induced skin cancer. Singh and Shukla (1998a) also used the two-stage model of skin cancer (DMBA then TPA). In the study, topical DAS (250 μg thrice weekly for 3 weeks) given prior to the topical initiator, DMBA, but not prior to each promoter application, significantly delayed the onset of tumors and reduced the total number of tumors by 81 % compared to vehicle control. When 250 μg of DAS was given topically 1 h prior to each topical promoter treatment, but not prior to initiation with DMBA, the total number of tumors was reduced by 76 %. Singh and Shukla (1998b) tested DAS against skin cancer induced by DMBA or benzo[a]pyrene (BaP) without the use of a promotion phase. Topical DAS given 1 h *prior* to topical DMBA 3 times per week for 28 weeks significantly reduced the multiplicity of skin tumors in female Swiss albino mice. When DAS was given 1 h *after* DMBA, the chemopreventive effect remained, but was somewhat attenuated. DAS also inhibited BaP-induced skin tumors, but in contrast to DMBA experiments, it trended toward a stronger chemopreventive potential when applied after BaP. The reason for this contrast with respect to timing-dependent efficacy of DAS against these two different carcinogens remains unknown. Some plausible factors to consider are potential differences in the transdermal permeation rates of the carcinogens or in the time delay before toxicodynamic effects are exhibited. In a more recent study, George et al. (2011) found that topical DAS (250 μg thrice weekly) delayed onset and incidence of skin tumors in male BALB/c mice by 55 % and 45 %, respectively, when started in parallel with a standard two-stage skin cancer carcinogen treatment (DMBA and TPA). Efficacy was increased (84 % tumor reduction) when DAS was combined with pomegranate fruit extract (PFE) in drinking water. PFE, incidentally, showed significant efficacy by itself. From the molecular aspect, DAS reduced expression of phospho-ERK1/2, phospho-JNK1, and phospho-IκB-α, and reduced activity of NF-κB and IKK-α. Again, when DAS was combined with PFE, the effect on all of these molecular indicators was stronger. Thus, this report demonstrated that DAS and DAS + PFE (DAS < DAS + PFE) may work to inhibit a common cell proliferation pathway in skin cancer.

In a study described in the previous section, Ip et al. (1992) assessed DAS and DADS against DMBA-induced mammary tumors in rats. Gastric gavage of DAS at 1.8 mmol/kg given 96, 48, and 24 h before intragastric DMBA (10 mg) significantly reduced mammary tumor incidence by 39 % and total tumor yield by 41 %. DADS showed superior efficacy to DAS in both measures.

The details of a study by Takahashi ct al. (1992) comparing DAS and DADS in liver, colon, and renal cancer, induced by various carcinogens, have also been described above. Briefly, DAS had a tendency to inhibit colon adenoma, but failed to reach significance. Further, DAS failed to reduce renal cancer, alveolar hyperplasia, or bladder cell hyperplasia, and induced a marker of pre-neoplasia, namely GST-P, in liver. In a different study, Surh et al. (1995) showed that 250 μM DAS inhibited N-demethylation of NDMA in rat liver extract by 27 %, indicating that at least some metabolic activity was affected by DAS. Thus, whether DAS is hepatoprotective or detrimental in the presence of a carcinogen very likely depends on the metabolic fate of the specific carcinogen in question, and how DAS influences that fate. Further, whether DAS alone increases the risk of liver cancer remains an important unanswered question.

Hadjiolov et al. (1993) deviated to some extent from the commonly studied carcinogens when assessing DAS against aristolochic acid (AA)-induced gastric cancer. AA is a potent carcinogen found in some herbal preparations that is capable of inducing a variety of tumors in several organs. AA induced stomach, bladder, and thymus tumors after 12 weeks of exposure in male BD-6 rats. Intragastric DAS (150 mg/kg) reduced the incidence of stomach carcinomas and sarcomas from 45 % to 10 % when given 4 h before AA, and from 45 % to 0 % when given twice, 24 and 4 h, before AA. DAS decreased gastric DNA damage, but did not appear to reduce bladder cell hyperplasia. The total tumor burden was reduced from 60 % to 10 % with single administration of DAS, and from 60 % to 0 % with double administration of DAS prior to AA.

4.4 *Ajoene*

Of all major OSCs in garlic, ajoene has received the least attention in animal studies. To date, such studies have involved skin cancer, melanoma, hepatocarcinoma, and an ascites-derived sarcoma (Table 4). Li et al. (Li et al. 2002a, b) studied one stereoisomer, Z-ajoene, against subcutaneously implanted sarcoma 180 (an ascites/peritoneal-derived mouse cancer) and mouse hepatocarcinoma 22. Z-Ajoene, 8 mg/kg IP daily, significantly reduced sarcoma growth by 32 %, and 4 mg/kg IP daily significantly reduced hepatocarcinoma growth by 42 %. Nishikawa et al. (2002) employed the two-stage model of skin cancer with DMBA and TPA in ICR mice wherein they demonstrated that 250 μg topical ajoene, given 1 h before each TPA treatment, reduced the multiplicity of skin cancer to 4.9 % of that observed in ajoene-naïve mice at 18 weeks. Taylor et al. (2006) used the C57BL/6 B16/BL6 mouse melanoma model to show that 25 mg/kg of IP ajoene given every other day reduced primary tumor growth and lung metastases.

4.5 *SAC*

As one of the major water-soluble constituents of garlic, SAC has been studied quite extensively in animal models for its chemopreventive properties (Table 5). In animal models, it has extensive oral bioavailability and is excreted variably depending on the species. Although in rats it is significantly renally eliminated as the *N*-acetyl-*S*-allylcysteine (NSAC) metabolite, mice show less of this metabolite,

Table 4 Preclinical studies on ajoene

Lead author	Year	Animal	Cancer	Carcinogen	Treatment	Results
Li	2002	Mice (Kunming Swiss)	Sarcoma 180, Hepatocarcinoma 22 s.c.inj	No	– 8 mg/kg i.p. qd – 4 mg/kg i.p. qd (Pure Z-ajoene was used)	Inhibited tumor growth by 32 % (sarcoma, 8 mg/kg dose) and 42 % (hepatocarcinoma,4 mg/kg dose) when initiated after tumor implantation
Nishikawa	2002	Mice (ICR)	Skin	DMBA and TPA	250 μg topically 1 h before each TPA admin	Suppressed skin cancer (4.9 % the number of tumors compared with control group at 18 weeks)
Taylor	2006	Mice (C57BL/6 B16/BL6 mouse melanoma cell tumor model)	Melanoma: s.c. implant	No	5, 15, 25 μg/g i.p qod from day 1 to day 28 (sacrifice day)	Highest dose inhibited primary tumor growth and lung metastasis. Endothelial cell adhesion by the tumor was also inhibited

Treatment was ajoene unless otherwise noted. Results are statistically significant unless otherwise indicated
Abbreviations listed under Table 1

Table 5 Preclinical studies on SAC

Lead author	Year	Animal	Cancer	Carcinogen	Treatment	Results
Nagae	1993	Rats, Mice, Dogs	N/A, PK study	N/A	12.5, 25, or 50 mg/kg orally	87–100 % bioavailability. Partial renal excretion in rats, 50 % in *N*-acetyl form, 1 % as SAC. Partial renal excretion in mice as SAC (16.5 % of dose) and *N*-acetyl-SAC (7.2 % of dose). <1 % renal excretion of SAC or *N*-acetyl-SAC in dogs
Hatono	1996	Rats (male Fischer-344)	Colon	DMH	0.125 or 0.25 g/kg of diet (~9 or ~18 mg/kg body weight)	Decreased aberrant crypt foci (precursors of colon CA) by 33 and 54 % in groups given 40 or 80 % of the maximum tolerated dose during initiation. Treatment in the promotion period had no effect on crypt foci. GST activity was increased 41 % by SAC 12 h after as single oral dose (3.5 mmol/kg) and was maintained for 72 h. GST was upregulated in the small bowel and liver. Concluded that SAC is chemopreventive likely by bolstering detoxification systems
Cohen	1999	Rats	Mammary	NMU	666 or 2000 ppm in diet (~167 mg/kg/day higher dose)	Was ineffective at preventing tumors when given beginning 7 days before initiation of NMU and thereafter 18 weeks post-NMU. SAC blood concentration was below the limit of detection of the HPLC system. Nonlinear dose effects were proposed for discrepancy with other studies

Velmurugan	2003	Rats (Wistar)	Gastric	MNNG (200 mg/kg on days 0 and 14) then by S-NaCl (1 ml 3 days during weeks 0–3)	Intragastric, 200 mg/kg, 3×/week, starting on the day following 1st exposure to MNNG, then thereafter	Suppressed the incidence of gastric tumors and increased the antioxidant status in the stomach, blood, and liver
Sundaresan	2003	Rats (Wistar)	Liver	NDEA then CCl_4 i.p.	200 mg/kg gavage on alternate days vs. carcinogen	Inhibited tumor incidence and elevated antioxidants while decreasing lipid peroxidation
Velmurugan	2005	Wistar Rats	Gastric	MNNG (200 mg/kg on days 0 and 14) then by S-NaCl (1 ml 3 days during weeks 0–3)	Intragastric 100 mg/kg, 3×/week, starting on the day following 1st exposure to MNNG, then thereafter	Suppressed gastric cancer, but was enhanced with lycopene (1.25 mg/kg thrice weekly), which also inhibited gastric cancer alone. Apoptosis appeared to be the mechanism
Chu	2006	Mice (nude)	Prostate: CWR22R s.c. xenograft (androgen-independent)	No	1000 mg/kg i.p. qd, 7 weeks	Inhibited xenograft growth with no apparent toxicity. Serum PSA declined, and E-cadherin and gamma-catenin expression was restored, indicating inhibition of invasion. Apoptosis increased with a reduction in Bcl-2 and increase in active caspase-3
Sundaresan et al.	2008	Rats (Wistar)	Liver	NDEA (i.p.), then s.c. CCl_4.	200 mg/kg gavage initiated day 1 (frequency of admin. not reported)	Inhibited tumor incidence and increased reduced glutathione levels, superoxide dismutase, and catalase in NDEA-induced hepatocarcinogenesis

(continued)

Table 5 (continued)

Lead author	Year	Animal	Cancer	Carcinogen	Treatment	Results
Ng	2012	Mice (male BALB/c nude)	Liver: xenograft of MHCC97L (human liver CA cells) s.c., then implanted in liver	No	1 mg/kg/day (route of admin. not reported) starting 1 week after xenograft	Did not reduce incidence of established tumors, but reduced tumor volume (by 74 %). Trended toward reducing lung metastasis (87.5 % w/out SAC, 37.5 % w/SAC), but did not reach significance unless combined with cisplatin (1 mg/kg/day). In vitro, SAC caused apoptosis and necrosis (caspase-3 and caspase-9 upregulation, Bcl-2 and Bcl-xL and PCNA suppression). Migration was inhibited in vitro, associated with upregulated E-cadherin
Pai	2012	Mice (BALB/c nude)	Oral: s.c.xenograft w/ CAL-27 (human oral cancer) cells	No	– Low dose (5 mg/kg oral qd) – High dose (40 mg/kg oral qd)l	Dose dependently inhibited xenograft growth and suppressed phosphorylation of Akt, mTOR, inhibitor of kappa-B-alpha, and ERK1/2 in tumor tissue. Also suppressed cyclin D1 protein expression and increased expression of cell cycle inhibitor p16^{Ink4}. Inhibited expression of COX-2, vimentin, and NF-kB p65 (RelA)

Treatment was SAC unless otherwise noted. Results are statistically significant unless otherwise indicated
Abbreviations listed under Table 1

and more of the parent compound, in the urine (Nagae et al. 1994). In contrast, dogs show very little renal elimination of both compounds (Nagae et al. 1994). SAC and NSAC, of course, bear some resemblance to *N*-acetylcysteine (NAC), the antidote for acetaminophen (paracetamol) toxicity. It is therefore worth noting that NAC has also received some attention for its potential as a more general hepatoprotective compound, as it is able to bolster the glutathione-based detoxification/conjugation system. NAC is thus likely useful also in instances without acetaminophen exposure. This information may be helpful to consider when interpreting studies on SAC.

Studies with SAC have involved cancers of the GI tract, including the oral cavity, stomach, liver, and colon, and mammary and prostate tumors. One of the first studies on SAC in cancer was reported by Hatono et al. (1996). In the study they used dimethylhydrazine (DMH) as both an initiator and promoter of colon cancer in male Fischer-344 rats. When SAC was administered via diet at 0.125 or 0.25 g/kg of food starting one week *prior to* initiation with DMH, and continuously thereafter, aberrant crypt foci (precursors of colon cancer) were reduced by 33 % and 54 %, respectively. In contrast, when SAC was initiated 2 weeks *after* starting DMH it had no effect on aberrant crypt foci. When SAC was given at 1.8 mmol/kg/day to the rats, a significant increase in glutathione-*S*-transferase (GST) activity was seen in the liver, early and middle small intestine, and colon. Further investigation revealed an increase in GST protein expression. Thus, it is probable that SAC is chemopreventive via bolstering detoxification systems in the GI tract and liver. Whether SAC can also act like NAC to increase glutathione stores is unknown, but being devoid of a protonated sulfur may preclude it from having this role.

Velmurugan et al. (2003) assessed SAC against gastric cancer in rats induced by serial administration of *N*-methyl-*N′*-nitro-*N*-nitrosoguanidine (MNNG) and saturated sodium chloride (S-NaCl). Intragastric SAC at 200 mg/kg thrice weekly, starting the day after initiating MNNG, suppressed the incidence of gastric tumors and increased the antioxidant status in the stomach, blood, and liver. When the gastric glutathione/GST system was assessed, it was found that SAC alone or MNNG + S-NaCl alone increased GSH levels and GST activity; however, MNNG + S-NaCl did so to a significantly greater extent. Moreover, MNNG + S-NaCl given concomitantly with SAC yielded the highest increase in GSH concentration and GST activity in the stomach. Therefore, the earlier study by P et al. demonstrating that SAC can induce GST in the liver substantiates these results in stomach. That MNNG + S-NaCl alone increased gastric GST activity likely reflects an "attempt" to protect gastric tissue by fortifying its antioxidant capacity. Again, exactly how SAC triggers GST upregulation is unknown. A subsequent study by Velmurugan et al. (2005) again used intragastric SAC against MNNG + S-NaCl, both given in the same frequency and sequence as in the prior study; however, the dose of SAC was 100 mg/kg thrice weekly instead of 200 mg/kg. This study also found SAC to be chemopreventive against gastric tumors, but efficacy was significantly greater when SAC was combined with thrice-weekly lycopene (1.25 mg/kg), the primary chromophore-bearing molecule in red tomatoes. From a mechanistic aspect, SAC appeared to have reversed the anti-apoptotic effect of

MNNG + S-NaCl in gastric tissue. For example, Bcl-2 overexpression was attenuated by SAC to an extent that approached control levels. There was also a trend for SAC to increase caspase 3 activity that had been reduced by MNNG + S-NaCl, but this was not significant until SAC was combined with lycopene. The expression and functional changes were demonstrated in gastric tissue; however, whether the tissue originated from tumors or unaltered stomach is unclear.

Sundaresan and Subramanian (2003) studied liver cancer in rats induced by a combination of *N*-nitrosodiethylamine (NDEA) and carbon tetrachloride (CCl_4). The carcinogens produced tumors in 6 of 6 rats, but oral gavage of SAC (200 mg/kg given on alternate days than carcinogens) prevented tumors completely (0 of 6) and elevated the antioxidant status. Although circulating levels of reduced glutathione (GSH) were depleted by the carcinogen mix by approximately 50 %, SAC significantly reversed this effect, with GSH returning to 87 % of normal. Moreover, when SAC was given in the absence of carcinogens, the GSH level rose above the control concentration to 116 %. Interestingly, when the same group later assessed changes in liver GSH in response to the same carcinogen (NDEA), their results contrasted somewhat with blood GSH (Sundaresan and Subramanian 2008). That is, whereas NDEA depleted blood GSH, it increased hepatic GSH. However, in both blood and liver, SAC alone increased GSH, and, in addition, GSH was greater in NDEA + SAC vs. NDEA alone in both studies. Sundaresan and Subramanian (2008) also found that hepatic GST activity differed in treatment groups. Specifically, NDEA increased GST activity, which was further increased by adding SAC. SAC alone also significantly increased GST activity vs. control, but to a lesser extent than NDEA or NDEA + SAC. Finally, when Sundaresan and Subramanian (2008) evaluated two additional major detoxification enzymes in the liver, namely superoxide dismutase (SOD) and catalase (CAT), they found that they differed somewhat in response to NDEA and SAC compared to GST. In particular, SOD and CAT activities were reduced by NDEA, an effect that was partially reversed by SAC. Further, SAC alone was able to increase SOD and CAT activities, thus exhibiting some consistency with its effects on GST. In a more recent study, Ng et al. (2012) used male BALB/c nude mice with an orthotopic xenograft of a human metastatic hepatocellular carcinoma cell line (MHCC97L-luc). The cells were grown subcutaneously and then implanted into the liver where they were monitored with an in vivo imaging system. SAC, given at 1 mg/kg/day, did not reduce incidence of established tumors, but significantly reduced tumor volume (74 % reduction). SAC trended toward reducing lung metastases (i.e., 87.5 % without SAC, 37.5 % with SAC), but did not reach statistical significance unless combined with the anticancer/DNA-binding drug cisplatin. In vitro, albeit at very high concentrations (i.e., 5 to 40 mM), SAC dose dependently induced apoptosis and necrosis with an accompanying stimulation of caspases 3 and 9 and suppression of Bcl-2, Bcl-xL, and PCNA. E-cadherin expression was also increased, which corresponded to impaired migration in vitro. Therefore, perhaps surprisingly, SAC showed in vivo efficacy against liver cancer at blood concentrations that were likely at least 100 times lower than those shown to trigger cell death in vitro. Without knowing the hepatic concentration of SAC, or the potency of its metabolite(s), these in vivo results are somewhat difficult to compare and contrast with the in vitro results.

Pai et al. (2012) assessed SAC against a human oral cancer cell line subcutaneous xenograft, CAL-27, in BALB/c nude mice. SAC dose dependently inhibited subcutaneous tumor growth and suppressed phosphorylation of Akt, mTOR, inhibitor of κ-B-α, and ERK1/2. SAC reduced expression of cyclin D1 protein, cyclooxygenase-2 (COX-2), vimentin, and NF-κB-65 (RelA), and increased expression of cell cycle inhibitor $p16^{Ink4}$. Thus, SAC exhibited a broad scope of antiproliferative activity at the molecular level.

Cohen et al. (1999) assessed SAC against *N*-methylnitrosourea (NMU)-induced mammary tumors in rats. Dietary SAC (2,000 ppm or approximately 167 mg/kg/day) initiated 7 days before NMU and continued for 18 weeks after NMU was ineffective at preventing tumors. The authors reported that the blood SAC concentration was below the limit of detection of the HPLC method used, but analysis of metabolites was not performed. The authors suggested that the lack of efficacy, which contrasted with other studies on SAC, may be due to nonlinear dose effects. However, this is the only study assessing SAC against NMU-induced mammary tumors. Therefore, given the considerably high dose, and the fact that the majority of other SAC studies were on the GI tract (prior to complete metabolism), the results may indeed be accurate in this unique study.

Although prostate cancer has been studied quite extensively with some organosulfur compounds, e.g., DATS, SAC has received little attention. Chu et al. (2006) used nude mice implanted subcutaneously with a human androgen-independent prostate cancer cell line, CWR22R. SAC, 1000 mg/kg intraperitoneally daily for 7 weeks, inhibited tumor growth significantly by 62.4 % with no apparent toxicity. Serum PSA declined significantly by about 50 % compared to untreated xenograft-bearing mice. E-cadherin and γ-catenin expression wes restored, indicating an inhibition of invasiveness by SAC. Apoptosis increased with a significant reduction in Bcl-2 and an increase in cleaved caspase-3 in response to SAC.

5 Clinical Trials with *Allium* Vegetables as a Source of OSCs

Clinical validation of the positive results from cell culture and animal models was undertaken in a few population-based studies which investigated the protective benefits of *Allium* vegetables and their constituents. To date, most of the clinical trials looked into the chemopreventive properties of *Allium* vegetables on various cancers particularly those of the digestive tract. In the Prostate, Lung, Colorectal, and Ovarian Screening (PLCO) Trial from 1993 to 2001, men and women were screened for colorectal cancer where 29,413 control subjects were compared to 3057 cases with at least one adenoma of the distal large bowel to investigate the association of fruit and vegetable intake and the risk of colorectal adenoma development. The study concluded that diets high in fruits and dark-green vegetables, deep yellow vegetables, and garlic and onions are associated with decreased risk of colorectal adenomas (Millen et al. 2007). In a small double-blind randomized clinical trial which studied the use of high-dose aged garlic extracts (AGE) to reduce the number of colorectal adenomas, 37 patients were randomly assigned to receive either high (2.4 mL/day) or low (0.16 mL/day) dose of AGE after adenomas larger than 5 mm were removed by polypectomy. It was identified that the number of colorectal adenomas in the control group increased steadily, but patients who received high dose had significant reductions in size and number after one year of treatment (Tanaka et al. 2006). Association of aged garlic extract or oil and gastric cancer was studied in a factorial double-blind, placebo-controlled trial, the Shandong Intervention Trial (Ma et al. 2012). 3365 participants with *Helicobacter pylori*, associated with increased gastric lesions and cancer, were either treated with two weeks of antibiotics or long-term administration (7.3 years) of aged garlic extract and oil, or a vitamin supplement. A 14.7 year follow-up showed a non-statistically significant reduction in gastric cancer incidence and mortality with garlic and vitamin treatment groups (Ma et al. 2012). Data from the European Prospective Investigation into Cancer and Nutrition study were also used to study gastric cancer (GC) and adenocarcinomas of the esophagus (ADO). Baseline data was collected in 521,457 men and women in ten European countries. After an average of 6.5 years follow-up, 330 gastric cancer and 65 adenocarcinoma of the esophagus cases were diagnosed and used as the case subjects. Although there was no reduction in ADO, there was a borderline significant negative association between onion and garlic intake and intestinal gastric cancer risk (Millen et al. 2007).

Clinical trials also looked at the effect of organosulfur compounds in cancers affecting women. Data from the European Prospective Investigation into Cancer and Nutrition study was used to study the effect of fruit and vegetable consumption on the risk of epithelial ovarian cancer. 325,640 female participants with no incidence of cancer were interviewed and reassessed after an average of 6.3 years. There were 581 cases of primary invasive epithelial ovarian cancer after this time period. A high consumption of garlic and onion had a borderline significant reduction of cancer risk (Schulz et al. 2005). Data from the Shanghai Women's Health Study (SWHS) and Shanghai Men's Health Study (SMHS) were used to study the relationship between food groups and liver cancer risk. A total of 132,837 Chinese men and women were surveyed about their lifestyle and nutritional habits. After a follow-up of 10.9 years (SWHS) or 5.5 years (SMHS), 267 liver cancer cases were diagnosed in the two years following study enrollment. High intake of *Allium* vegetables such as garlic was shown to be associated with a significantly decreased liver cancer risk (Zhang et al. 2013).

An Italian case–control study looked at the relationship between onion and garlic intake and endometrial cancer. 454 endometrial cancer cases and 908 controls were interviewed after being admitted to the same hospitals for a wide spectrum of acute, non-neoplastic conditions. The consumption of garlic showed a nonsignificant decrease in risk at low levels and significant decrease in risk of endometrial cancer at high levels of garlic consumption (Galeone et al. 2008). A hospital-based study in Northwest China studied the effects of various foods on the risk of developing multiple myeloma (MM). The study consisted of 220 confirmed MM cases and 220 individually matched patient controls. High shallot and garlic intake was significantly associated with a reduced risk of multiple MM (Wang et al. 2012a, b). A similar hospital-based case–control study which looked at the effect of diet on prostate cancer concluded a borderline risk reduction in those subjects who consumed more than 5.5 g of garlic a week (Salem et al. 2011).

6 Concluding Remarks and Future Perspectives

At this juncture, significant evidence has mounted to support the use of *Allium* vegetables and their constituents in cancer chemoprevention. That is not to say that regular use of *Allium*-derived OSCs will *protect* against all cancers or at all times, but rather that an overall protective influence appears to be observed with regular exposure to these compounds. As can be gleaned from the preceding discussion, compounds in intact garlic exhibit quite a complex series of chemical modifications when sliced, chewed, or pulverized. Mechanistic, preclinical, and clinical studies on these compounds have provided us with a wealth of information. There is significant evidence demonstrating that these compounds can induce apoptosis and inhibit cell cycle progression in neoplastic cells, perhaps selectively over normal cells. The molecular mediators of these actions remain an intense area of investigation and a subject of controversy. For example, it remains unknown whether the MAPK pathway is upregulated or downregulated by OSCs to prevent cancer, as results have been conflicting. Similarly, although production of ROS has gained support as a therapeutic mechanism of action of some OSCs, at least one OSC, namely SAC, appears to induce a systemic antioxidant state. These discrepancies in mechanistic details must be resolved; however, they cannot overshadow the clear evidence of the benefits of OSCs. In contrast to the aforementioned controversy, a quite consistent mechanistic explanation for the protection against carcinogens, by OSCs, is the upregulation of very important detoxification systems within various tissues. For example, in both cell work and animal studies, OSCs from garlic consistently upregulate both GST expression and activity, and increase the abundance of its co-substrate, namely, reduced glutathione (GSH). Furthermore, various OSCs exhibit a complementary effect on Phase I-metabolizing enzymes. That is, they can inhibit formation of toxic carcinogen metabolites via inhibiting CYP 2E1. These beneficial effects can be extrapolated to suggest that garlic-derived OSCs likely provide a general hepatoprotection and reduce the toxicity of noncarcinogenic chemicals (e.g., acetaminophen). Other putative anticancer effects of OSCs, such as immunomodulation and anti-angiogenesis, remain controversial, but evidence continues to accumulate in these areas.

The antineoplastic potential of OSCs is exhibited quite extensively in animal models. A variety of cancers have been significantly suppressed in rodents, either at the initiation stage, the promotion stage, or both. In brief, DATS has shown utility against colon, prostate, liver, skin, and breast neoplasms. DADS exhibited efficacy against gastric and colon cancers in particular, and also some utility against skin and other cancers. DAS has shown particular efficacy against carcinogen-induced skin cancer as well as various gastrointestinal-type cancers. Ajoene has not received much attention, but may be effective against skin and hepatic cancers. As the major water-soluble constituent of garlic, SAC has demonstrated utility against carcinogen-induced and implanted liver tumors, as well as efficacy in the majority of the gastrointestinal tract. Prospective clinical trials and epidemiological studies on garlic and onions have become more common starting in 2005. The summary from these investigations is that garlic is likely beneficial in cancer chemoprevention. Some studies have shown a statistically significant protective action of garlic, while others have shown a promising trend in this direction. It appears that achieving statistical significance can be challenging at times, particularly because the incidence of some of the cancers studied was quite low during the duration of the studies. Achieving greater statistical power in future studies will undoubtedly reveal a more precise therapeutic role for *Allium* vegetables in chemoprevention. Finally, clinical investigations have largely used total garlic, rather than the isolated OSCs assessed in animal studies. This informational gap must be closed to facilitate confident and meaningful decisions in the future.

References

Agarwal KC (1996) Therapeutic actions of garlic constituents. Med Res Rev 16(1):111–124

Amagase H, Petesch BL, Matsuura H et al (2001) Intake of garlic and its bioactive components. J Nutr 131(3s):955S–962S

Antony ML, Singh SV (2011) Molecular mechanisms and targets of cancer chemoprevention by garlic-derived bioactive compound diallyl trisulfide. Indian J Exp Biol 49(11):805–816

Antosiewicz J, Herman-Antosiewicz A, Marynowski SW, Singh SV (2006) c-Jun NH(2)-terminal kinase signaling axis regulates diallyl trisulfide-induced generation of reactive oxygen species and cell cycle arrest in human prostate cancer cells. Cancer Res 66(10):5379–86

Aquilano K, Vigilanza P, Filomeni G et al (2010) Tau dephosphorylation and microfilaments disruption are upstream events of the anti-proliferative effects of DADS in SH-SY5Y cells. J Cell Mol Med 14(3):564–577

Bauer D, Mazzio E, Soliman KF et al (2014) Diallyl disulfide inhibits TNFalpha-induced CCL2 release by MDA-MB-231 cells. Anticancer Res 34(6):2763–2770

Benavides GA, Squadrito GL, Mills RW et al (2007) Hydrogen sulfide mediates the vasoactivity of garlic. Proc Natl Acad Sci U S A 104(46):17977–17982

Bianchini F, Vainio H (2001) *Allium* vegetables and organosulfur compounds: do they help prevent cancer? Environ Health Perspect 109(9):893–902

Block E (1992) The organosulfur chemistry of the Genus *Allium*-Implications for the organochemistry of sulfur. Angew Chemie 31(9):1135–1178

Block E, Ahmad S, Jain MK et al (1984) The chemistry of alkyl thiosulfate esters. 8. (E, Z)-Ajoene: a potent antithrombotic agent from garlic. J Am Chem Soc 106(26):8295–8296

Brady JF, Ishizaki H, Fukuto JM et al (1991) Inhibition of cytochrome P-450 2E1 by diallyl sulfide and its metabolites. Chem Res Toxicol 4(6):642–647

Chandra-Kuntal K, Singh SV (2010) Diallyl trisulfide inhibits activation of signal transducer and activator of transcription 3 in prostate cancer cells in culture and in vivo. Cancer Prev Res (Phila) 3(11):1473–1483

Chittezhath M, Kuttan G (2006) Radioprotective activity of naturally occurring organosulfur compounds. Tumori 92(2):163–169

Choi YH, Park HS (2012) Apoptosis induction of U937 human leukemia cells by diallyl trisulfide induces through generation of reactive oxygen species. J Biomed Sci 19:50

Chu Q, Lee DT, Tsao SW et al (2006) S-allylcysteine, a water-soluble garlic derivative, suppresses the growth of a human androgen-independent prostate cancer xenograft, CWR22R, under in vivo conditions. BJU Int 99(4):925–932

Cohen LA, Zhao Z, Pittman B et al (1999) S-allylcysteine, a garlic constituent, fails to inhibit N-methylnitrosourea-induced rat mammary tumorigenesis. Nutr Cancer 35(1):58–63

Dasgupta P, Bandyopadhyay SS (2013) Role of di-allyl disulfide, a garlic component in NF-kappaB mediated transient G2-M phase arrest and apoptosis in human leukemic cell-lines. Nutr Cancer 65(4):611–622

Dirsch VM, Gerbes AL, Vollmar AM (1998) Ajoene, a compound of garlic, induces apoptosis in human promyeloleukemic cells, accompanied by generation of reactive oxygen species and activation of nuclear factor kappaB. Mol Pharmacol 53(3):402–407

Druesne N, Pagniez A, Mayeur C et al (2004) Diallyl disulfide (DADS) increases histone acetylation and p21(waf1/cip1) expression in human colon tumor cell lines. Carcinogenesis 25(7):1227–1236

Druesne-Pecollo N, Latino-Martel P (2011) Modulation of histone acetylation by garlic sulfur compounds. Anticancer Agents Med Chem 11(3):254–259

Dwivedi C, Rohlfs S, Jarvis D et al (1992) Chemoprevention of chemically induced skin tumor development by diallyl sulfide and diallyl disulfide. Pharm Res 9(12):1668–1670

Ebrahimi M, Mohammad Hassan Z, Mostafaie A et al (2013) Purified protein fraction of garlic extract modulates cellular immune response against breast transplanted tumors in BALB/c mice model. Cell J 15(1):65–75

Filomeni G, Aquilano K, Rotilio G et al (2003) Reactive oxygen species-dependent c-Jun NH2-terminal kinase/c-Jun signaling cascade mediates neuroblastoma cell death induced by diallyl disulfide. Cancer Res 63(18):5940–5949

Galeone C, Pelucchi C, Dal Maso L et al (2008) *Allium* vegetables intake and endometrial cancer risk. Public Health Nutr 12(9):1576–1579

George J, Singh M, Srivastava AK et al (2011) Synergistic growth inhibition of mouse skin tumors by pomegranate fruit extract and diallyl sulfide: evidence for inhibition of activated MAPKs/ NF-kappaB and reduced cell proliferation. Food Chem Toxicol 49(7):1511–1520

Hadjiolov D, Fernando RC, Schmeiser HH et al (1993) Effect of diallyl sulfide on aristolochic acid-induced forestomach carcinogenesis in rats. Carcinogenesis 14(3):407–410

Hatono S, Jimenez A, Wargovich MJ (1996) Chemopreventive effect of S-allylcysteine and its relationship to the detoxification enzyme glutathione S-transferase. Carcinogenesis 17 (5):1041–1044

Herman-Antosiewicz A, Singh SV (2005) Checkpoint kinase 1 regulates diallyl trisulfide-induced mitotic arrest in human prostate cancer cells. J Biol Chem 280(31):28519–28528

Herman-Antosiewicz A, Powolny AA, Singh SV (2007) Molecular targets of cancer chemoprevention by garlic-derived organosulfides. Acta Pharmacol Sin 28(9):1355–1364

Higdon J (2007) An evidence-based approach to dietary phytochemicals, 1st ed. Thieme Publishers

Hong JY, Wang ZY, Smith TJ et al (1992) Inhibitory effects of diallyl sulfide on the metabolism and tumorigenicity of the tobacco-specific carcinogen 4-(methylnitrosamino)-1-(3-pyridyl)-1-butanone (NNK) in A/J mouse lung. Carcinogenesis 13(5):901–904

Hong YS, Ham YA, Choi JH et al (2000) Effects of allyl sulfur compounds and garlic extract on the expression of Bcl-2, Bax, and p53 in non-small cell lung cancer cell lines. Exp Mol Med 32:127–134

Hosono T, Fukao T, Ogihara J et al (2005) Diallyl trisulfide suppresses the proliferation and induces apoptosis of human colon cancer cells through oxidative modification of beta-tubulin. J Biol Chem 280(50):41487–41493

Hui C, Jun W, Ya LN et al (2008) Effect of *Allium* sativum (garlic) diallyl disulfide (DADS) on human non-small cell lung carcinoma H1299 cells. Trop Biomed 25(1):37–45

Ip C, Lisk DJ, Stoewsand GS (1992) Mammary cancer prevention by regular garlic and selenium-enriched garlic. Nutr Cancer 17(3):279–286

Karmakar S, Banik NL, Patel SJ et al (2007) Garlic compounds induced calpain and intrinsic caspase cascade for apoptosis in human malignant neuroblastoma SH-SY5Y cells. Apoptosis 12(4):671–684

Kim YA, Xiao D, Xiao H et al (2007) Mitochondria-mediated apoptosis by diallyl trisulfide in human prostate cancer cells is associated with generation of reactive oxygen species and regulated by Bax/Bak. Mol Cancer Ther 6(5):1599–1609

Kim SH, Bommareddy A, Singh SV (2011) Garlic constituent diallyl trisulfide suppresses x-linked inhibitor of apoptosis protein in prostate cancer cells in culture and in vivo. Cancer Prev Res (Phila) 4(6):897–906

Kim NH, Lee S, Kang MJ et al (2014) Protective effects of diallyl sulfide against Thioacetamide-induced toxicity: a possible role of cytochrome P450 2E1. Biomol Ther (Seoul) 22(2):149–154

Knowles LM, Milner JA (2000) Diallyl disulfide inhibits p34(cdc2) kinase activity through changes in complex formation and phosphorylation. Carcinogenesis 21(6):1129–1134

Knowles LM, Milner JA (2003) Diallyl disulfide induces ERK phosphorylation and alters gene expression profiles in human colon tumor cells. J Nutr 133(9):2901–2906

Kyo E, Uda N, Suzuki A et al (1998) Immunomodulation and antitumor activities of aged garlic extract. Phytomedicine 5(4):259–267

Lai KC, Hsu SC, Kuo CL et al (2013) Diallyl sulfide, diallyl disulfide, and diallyl trisulfide inhibit migration and invasion in human colon cancer colo 205 cells through the inhibition of matrix metalloproteinase-2, -7, and -9 expressions. Environ Toxicol 28(9):479–488

Lai KC, Hsu SC, Yang JS et al (2015) Diallyl trisulfide inhibits migration, invasion and angiogenesis of human colon cancer HT-29 cells and umbilical vein endothelial cells, and suppresses murine xenograft tumour growth. J Cell Mol Med 19(2):474–484

Lea MA, Randolph VM (2001) Induction of histone acetylation in rat liver and hepatoma by organosulfur compounds including diallyl disulfide. Anticancer Res 21(4A):2841–2845

Lea MA, Randolph VM, Patel M (1999) Increased acetylation of histones induced by diallyl disulfide and structurally related molecules. Int J Oncol 15(2):347–352

Lea MA, Randolph VM, Lee JE et al (2001) Induction of histone acetylation in mouse erythroleukemia cells by some organosulfur compounds including allyl isothiocyanate. Int J Cancer 92(6):784–789

Li M, Ciu JR, Ye Y et al (2002a) Antitumor activity of Z-ajoene, a natural compound purified from garlic: antimitotic and microtubule-interaction properties. Carcinogenesis 23(4):573–579

Li M, Min JM, Cui JR et al (2002b) Z-ajoene induces apoptosis of HL-60 cells: involvement of Bcl-2 cleavage. Nutr Cancer 42(2):241–247

Li W, Tian H, Li L et al (2012) Diallyl trisulfide induces apoptosis and inhibits proliferation of A549 cells in vitro and in vivo. Acta Biochim Biophys Sin (Shanghai) 44(7):577–583

Li Y, Zhang J, Zhang L et al (2013) Diallyl trisulfide inhibits proliferation, invasion and angiogenesis of osteosarcoma cells by switching on suppressor microRNAs and inactivating of Notch-1 signaling. Carcinogenesis 34(7):1601–1610

Liao QJ, Su J, Zhou XT et al (2007) Inhibitory effect of diallyl disulfide on proliferation of human colon cancer cell line SW480 in nude mice. Ai Zheng 26(8):828–832

Liao QJ, Su J, He J et al (2009) Effect of diallyl disulfide on cell cycle arrest of human colon cancer SW480 cells. Ai Zheng 28(2):138–141

Ling H, Wen L, Ji XX et al (2010) Growth inhibitory effect and Chk1-dependent signaling involved in G2/M arrest on human gastric cancer cells induced by diallyl disulfide. Braz J Med Biol Res 43(3):271–278

Ma JL, Zhang L, Brown LM et al (2012) Fifteen-year effects of Helicobacter pylori, garlic, and vitamin treatments on gastric cancer incidence and mortality. J Natl Cancer Inst 104 (6):488–492

Meyer K, Ueberham E, Gebhardt R (2004) Influence of organosulphur compounds from garlic on the secretion of matrix metalloproteinases and their inhibitor TIMP-1 by cultured HUVEC cells. Cell Biol Toxicol 20(4):253–260

Millen AE, Subar AF, Graubard BI et al (2007) Fruit and vegetable intake and prevalence of colorectal adenoma in a cancer screening trial. Am J Clin Nutr 86(6):1754–1764

Milner JA (2001) Mechanisms by which garlic and allyl sulfur compounds suppress carcinogen bioactivation. Garlic and carcinogenesis. Adv Exp Med Biol 492:69–81

Milner J (2004) Organosulfur-garlic compounds and cancer prevention. In: Bao Y, Fenwick R (eds) Phytochemicals in health and disease. Dekker, New York, pp 163–186

Mousa AS, Mousa SA (2005) Anti-angiogenesis efficacy of the garlic ingredient alliin and antioxidants: role of nitric oxide and p53. Nutr Cancer 53(1):104–110

Munday R, Munday CM (2001) Relative activities of organosulfur compounds derived from onions and garlic in increasing tissue activities of quinone reductase and glutathione transferase in rat tissues. Nutr Cancer 40(2):205–210

Na HK, Kim EH, Choi MA et al (2012) Diallyl trisulfide induces apoptosis in human breast cancer cells through ROS-mediated activation of JNK and AP-1. Biochem Pharmacol 84 (10):1241–1250

Nagae S, Ushijima M, Hatono S et al (1994) Pharmacokinetics of the garlic compound S-allylcysteine. Planta Med 60(3):214–217

Nakagawa H, Tsuta K, Kiuchi K et al (2001) Growth inhibitory effects of diallyl disulfide on human breast cancer cell lines. Carcinogenesis 22(6):891–897

Ng KT, Guo DY, Cheng Q et al (2012) A garlic derivative, S-allylcysteine (SAC), suppresses proliferation and metastasis of hepatocellular carcinoma. PLoS One 7(2), e31655

Nishikawa T, Yamada N, Hattori A et al (2002) Inhibition by ajoene of skin-tumor promotion in mice. Biosci Biotechnol Biochem 66(10):2221–2223

Pai MH, Kuo YH, Chiang EP et al (2012) S-Allylcysteine inhibits tumour progression and the epithelial-mesenchymal transition in a mouse xenograft model of oral cancer. Br J Nutr 108 (1):28–38

Park EK, Kwon KB, Park KI et al (2002) Role of Ca(2+) in diallyl disulfide-induced apoptotic cell death of HCT-15 cells. Exp Mol Med 34(3):250–257

Powolny AA, Singh SV, Melov S, Hubbard A, Fisher AL (2011) The garlic constituent diallyl trisulfide increases the lifespan of C. elegans via skn-1 activation. Exp Gerontol 46(6):441–52

Rahman K (2001) Historical perspective on garlic and cardiovascular disease. J Nutr 131 (3s):977S–979S

Salem S, Salahi M, Mohseni M et al (2011) Major dietary factors and prostate cancer risk: a prospective multicenter case–control study. Nutr Cancer 63(1):21–27

Schafer G, Kaschula CH (2014) The immunomodulation and anti-inflammatory effects of garlic organosulfur compounds in cancer chemoprevention. Anticancer Agents Med Chem 14 (2):233–240

Schulz M, Lahmann PH, Boeing H et al (2005) Fruit and vegetable consumption and risk of epithelial ovarian cancer: the European Prospective Investigation into Cancer and Nutrition. Cancer Epidemiol Biomarkers Prev 14(11 Pt 1):2531–2535

Shankar S, Chen Q, Ganapathy S et al (2008) Diallyl trisulfide increases the effectiveness of TRAIL and inhibits prostate cancer growth in an orthotopic model: molecular mechanisms. Mol Cancer Ther 7(8):2328–2338

Shin DY, Kim GY, Kim JI et al (2010) Anti-invasive activity of diallyl disulfide through tightening of tight junctions and inhibition of matrix metalloproteinase activities in LNCaP prostate cancer cells. Toxicol In Vitro 24:1569–1576

Shrotriya S, Kundu JK, Na HK et al (2010) Diallyl trisulfide inhibits phorbol ester-induced tumor promotion, activation of AP-1, and expression of COX-2 in mouse skin by blocking JNK and Akt signaling. Cancer Res 70(5):1932–1940

Shukla Y, Kalra N (2007) Cancer chemoprevention with garlic and its constituents. Cancer Lett 247(2):167–181

Singh A, Shukla Y (1998a) Antitumor activity of diallyl sulfide in two-stage mouse skin model of carcinogenesis. Biomed Environ Sci 11(3):258–263

Singh A, Shukla Y (1998b) Antitumour activity of diallyl sulfide on polycyclic aromatic hydrocarbon-induced mouse skin carcinogenesis. Cancer Lett 131(2):209–214

Singh SV, Mohan RR, Agarwal R et al (1996) Novel anti-carcinogenic activity of an organosulfide from garlic: inhibition of H-RAS oncogene transformed tumor growth in vivo by diallyl disulfide is associated with inhibition of p21H-ras processing. Biochem Biophys Res Commun 225(2):660–665

Singh SV, Pan SS, Srivastava SK et al (1998) Differential induction of NAD(P)H:quinone oxidoreductase by anti-carcinogenic organosulfides from garlic. Biochem Biophys Res Commun 244(3):917–920

Singh SV, Powolny AA, Stan SD et al (2008) Garlic constituent diallyl trisulfide prevents development of poorly differentiated prostate cancer and pulmonary metastasis multiplicity in TRAMP mice. Cancer Res 68(22):9503–9511

Song JD, Lee SK, Kim KM et al (2009) Molecular mechanism of diallyl disulfide in cell cycle arrest and apoptosis in HCT-116 colon cancer cells. J Biochem Mol Toxicol 23(1):71–79

Stan SD, Singh SV (2009) Transcriptional repression and inhibition of nuclear translocation of androgen receptor by diallyl trisulfide in human prostate cancer cells. Clin Cancer Res 15 (15):4895–4903

Sundaram SG, Milner JA (1996a) Diallyl disulfide induces apoptosis of human colon tumor cells. Carcinogenesis 17(4):669–673

Sundaram SG, Milner JA (1996b) Diallyl disulfide suppresses the growth of human colon tumor cell xenografts in athymic nude mice. J Nutr 126(5):1355–1361

Sundaresan S, Subramanian P (2003) S-allylcysteine inhibits circulatory lipid peroxidation and promotes antioxidants in N-nitrosodiethylamine-induced carcinogenesis. Pol J Pharmacol 55 (1):37–42

Sundaresan S, Subramanian P (2008) Prevention of N-nitrosodiethylamine-induced hepatocarcinogenesis by S-allylcysteine. Mol Cell Biochem 310(1-2):209–214

Surh YJ, Lee RC, Park KK et al (1995) Chemoprotective effects of capsaicin and diallyl sulfide against mutagenesis or tumorigenesis by vinyl carbamate and N-nitrosodimethylamine. Carcinogenesis 16(10):2467–2471

Suzui N, Sugie S, Rahman KM et al (1997) Inhibitory effects of diallyl disulfide or aspirin on 2-amino-1-methyl-6-phenylimidazo[4,5-b]pyridine-induced mammary carcinogenesis in rats. Jpn J Cancer Res 88(8):705–711

Takahashi S, Hakoi K, Yada H et al (1992) Enhancing effects of diallyl sulfide on hepatocarcinogenesis and inhibitory actions of the related diallyl disulfide on colon and renal carcinogen esis in rats. Carcinogenesis 13(9):1513–1518

Tanaka S, Haruma K, Yoshihara M et al (2006) Aged garlic extract has potential suppressive effect on colorectal adenomas in humans. J Nutr 136(3 Suppl):821S–826S

Tang H, Kong Y, Guo J et al (2013) Diallyl disulfide suppresses proliferation and induces apoptosis in human gastric cancer through Wnt-1 signaling pathway by up-regulation of miR-200b and miR-22. Cancer Lett 340(1):72–81

Taylor P, Noriega R, Farah C et al (2006) Ajoene inhibits both primary tumor growth and metastasis of B16/BL6 melanoma cells in C57BL/6 mice. Cancer Lett 239(2):298–304

Tsai CW, Liu KL, Lin CY et al (2011) Structure and function relationship study of *Allium* organosulfur compounds on upregulating the pi class of glutathione S-transferase expression. J Agric Food Chem 59(7):3398–3405

Tsubura A, Lai YC, Kuwata M et al (2011) Anticancer effects of garlic and garlic-derived compounds for breast cancer control. Anticancer Agents Med Chem 11(3):249–253

Velmurugan B, Bhuvaneswari V, Nagini S (2003) Effect of S-allylcysteine on oxidant-antioxidant status during N-methyl-N'-nitro-N-nitrosoguanidine and saturated sodium chloride-induced gastric carcinogenesis in Wistar rats. Asia Pac J Clin Nutr 12(4):488–494

Velmurugan B, Mani A, Nagini S (2005) Combination of S-allylcysteine and lycopene induces apoptosis by modulating Bcl-2, Bax, Bim and caspases during experimental gastric carcinogenesis. Eur J Cancer Prev 14(4):387–393

Wallace GC, Haar CP, Vandergrift WA 3rd et al (2013) Multi-targeted DATS prevents tumor progression and promotes apoptosis in ectopic glioblastoma xenografts in SCID mice via HDAC inhibition. J Neurooncol 114(1):43–50

Wang EJ, Li Y, Lin M et al (1996) Protective effects of garlic and related organosulfur compounds on acetaminophen-induced hepatotoxicity in mice. Toxicol Appl Pharmacol 136(1):146–154

Wang HC, Yang JH, Hsieh SC et al (2010) Allyl sulfides inhibit cell growth of skin cancer cells through induction of DNA damage mediated G2/M arrest and apoptosis. J Agric Food Chem 58 (11):7096–7103

Wang HC, Hsieh SC, Yang JH et al (2012a) Diallyl trisulfide induces apoptosis of human basal cell carcinoma cells via endoplasmic reticulum stress and the mitochondrial pathway. Nutr Cancer 64(5):770–780

Wang Q, Wang Y, Ji Z et al (2012b) Risk factors for multiple myeloma: a hospital-based case–control study in Northwest China. Cancer Epidemiol 36(5):439–444

Wargovich MJ, Woods C, Eng VW et al (1988) Chemoprevention of N-nitrosomethylbenzylamine-induced esophageal cancer in rats by the naturally occurring thioether, diallyl sulfide. Cancer Res 48(23):6872–6875

Wargovich MJ, Imada O, Stephens LC (1992) Initiation and post-initiation chemopreventive effects of diallyl sulfide in esophageal carcinogenesis. Cancer Lett 64(1):39–42

Wu CC, Chung JG, Tsai SJ et al (2004) Differential effects of allyl sulfides from garlic essential oil on cell cycle regulation in human liver tumor cells. Food Chem Toxicol 42:1937–1947

Wu XJ, Hu Y, Lamy E, Mersch-Sundermann V (2009) Apoptosis induction in human lung adenocarcinoma cells by oil-soluble allyl sulfides: triggers, pathways, and modulators. Environ Mol Mutagen 50(3):266–275

Wu PP, Liu KC, Huang WW et al (2011) Diallyl trisulfide (DATS) inhibits mouse colon tumor in mouse CT-26 cells allograft model in vivo. Phytomedicine 18(8-9):672–676

Xiang SL, Xiao XL, Ling H et al (2005) Antitumor effect of diallyl disulfide on human gastric cancer MGC803 cells xenograft in nude mice. Ai Zheng 24(8):940–944

Xiao D, Choi S, Johnson DE et al (2004) Diallyl trisulfide-induced apoptosis in human prostate cancer cells involves c-Jun N-terminal kinase and extracellular-signal regulated kinase-mediated phosphorylation of Bcl-2. Oncogene 23(33):5594–5606

Xiao D, Herman-Antosiewicz A, Antosiewicz J et al (2005) Diallyl trisulfide-induced G(2)-M phase cell cycle arrest in human prostate cancer cells is caused by reactive oxygen species-dependent destruction and hyperphosphorylation of Cdc 25 C. Oncogene 24(41):6256–6268

Xiao D, Lew KL, Kim YA et al (2006a) Diallyl trisulfide suppresses growth of PC-3 human prostate cancer xenograft in vivo in association with Bax and Bak induction. Clin Cancer Res 12(22):6836–6843

Xiao D, Li M, Herman-Antosiewicz A et al (2006b) Diallyl trisulfide inhibits angiogenic features of human umbilical vein endothelial cells by causing Akt inactivation and down-regulation of VEGF and VEGF-R2. Nutr Cancer 55(1):94–107

Yang JS, Kok LF, Lin YH et al (2006) Diallyl disulfide inhibits WEHI-3 leukemia cells in vivo. Anticancer Res 26(1A):219–225

Zhang ZM, Yang XY, Deng SH et al (2007) Anti-tumor effects of polybutylcyanoacrylate nanoparticles of diallyl trisulfide on orthotopic transplantation tumor model of hepatocellular carcinoma in BALB/c nude mice. Chin Med J (Engl) 120(15):1336–1342

Zhang W, Xiang YB, Li HL et al (2013) Vegetable-based dietary pattern and liver cancer risk: results from the Shanghai women's and men's health studies. Cancer Sci 104(10):1353–1361

Yi L, Su Q (2013) Molecular mechanisms for the anti-cancer effects of diallyl disulfide. Food Chem Toxicol 57:362–370

Yuan JP, Wang GH, Ling H et al (2004) Diallyl disulfide-induced G2/M arrest of human gastric cancer MGC803 cells involves activation of p38 MAP kinase pathways. World J Gastroenterol 10(18):2731–2734

Epigenetic Impact of Bioactive Dietary Compounds in Cancer Chemoprevention

Gordana Supic, Darja Wagner, and Zvonko Magic

Abstract Epigenetic changes refer to modifications caused by heritable but potentially reversible changes in gene expression not coded in the DNA sequence. Evidence has been provided that various environmental factors and dietary bioactive compounds contribute to cancer development through epigenetic mechanisms. The main mechanisms of epigenetic control in mammals are DNA methylation, histone modifications, and RNA silencing through noncoding RNAs. The inhibition of DNA methyltransferases (DNMTs) involved in DNA methylation of CpG-rich regions of gene promoters and various enzymes involved in the chromatin condensation such as histone deacetylases (HDACs) have been recognized as potent strategies for cancer therapy and chemoprevention. Treatments using natural compounds such as green tea polyphenols, soy isoflavones, curcumin, resveratrol, isothiocyanates, and butyrate (an intestinal product from dietary fiber) modulate DNMT or HDAC gene expression and/or protein levels and activities, indicating that natural compounds could have strong potential to reverse epigenetic changes, without the adverse toxic effects associated with synthetic epigenetic inhibitors used in chemotherapy. Further characterization of the chemopreventive properties of various dietary bioactive compounds is warranted to potentially establish the clinical utility of dietary factors as anticancer compounds either alone or in combination with other dietary factors or clinically relevant therapeutics. Moreover, these characterizations are useful for personalized dietary recommendations and chemopreventive strategies for reducing cancer incidence.

G. Supic (✉) • Z. Magic
Medical Faculty of Military Medical Academy, University of Defense, Belgrade, Serbia

Institute for Medical Research, Military Medical Academy, Crnotravska 17, 11002 Belgrade, Serbia
e-mail: gogasupic@sezampro.rs; zvonkomag@yahoo.co.uk

D. Wagner
Freie Universität Berlin, Kaiserswerther Str. 16-18, 14195 Berlin, Germany
e-mail: darjawagner@gmail.com

M.F. Ullah, A. Ahmad (eds.), *Critical Dietary Factors in Cancer Chemoprevention*,
DOI 10.1007/978-3-319-21461-0_7

1 Introduction

Despite advances in cancer prevention through early detection and modern treatment modalities, cancer remains a major health problem worldwide. A number of recent studies provide strong evidence that various environmental factors and dietary bioactive compounds contribute to cancer development through epigenetic mechanisms. Waddington established the term "epigenetics" to describe developmental processes and the adaptation of an organism to an environment. Nowadays, this term has been modified and refers to mitotically heritable changes in gene expression that are not coded in the DNA sequence (Herman and Baylin 2003; Szyf 2005). The main mechanisms of epigenetic control in mammals are DNA methylation, histone modifications, and RNA interference (RNA silencing) (Fig. 1). Unlike genetic changes, epigenetic changes are potentially reversible, which suggests that they could be influenced by nutrition, environmental factors, or the joint effects of gene–environment interactions. Thus, epigenetic modifications could be a link between cancer, susceptibility genes, and nutrition (Supic et al. 2013). Due to the reversible nature of epigenetic changes, there is growing interest in epigenetic therapies for cancer. Several synthetic epigenetic inhibitors such as DNA methyltransferase (DNMT) and histone deacetylase (HDAC) inhibitors are either approved or undergoing clinical trials for the treatment of various cancers (Magic et al. 2009). However, most synthetic epigenetic inhibitors have shown adverse side effects. Hence, bioactive phytochemicals which are widely available with lesser toxic effects have been tested for their potential role in epigenetic modulation of gene expression in cancer prevention and therapy. A number of bioactive phytochemicals have been identified that potentially alter the expression of key tumor

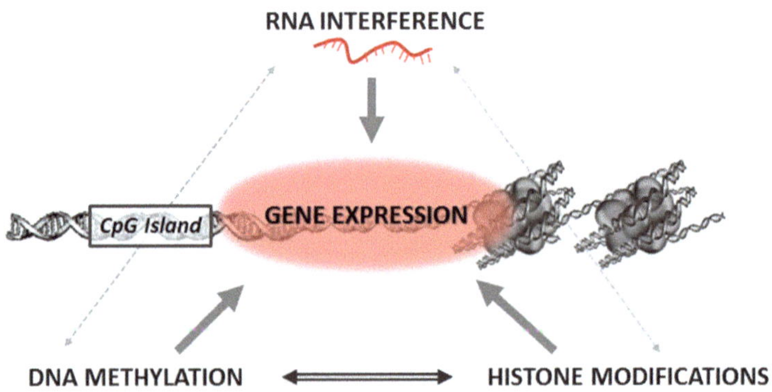

Fig. 1 Cross talk of the epigenetic alterations in cancer. The three classes of epigenetic modifications, such as DNA methylation, histone modifications, and noncoding RNA-based mechanisms, cause changes in the gene expression and genome-wide epigenetic alterations in cancer. DNA methylation, histone modifications, and posttranscriptional gene regulation by noncoding RNAs are not isolated events, but coordinated in higher-order chromatin structure. Thus, epigenetic modifications should not be interpreted independently, but only in combination with other modifications and within a context, leading to downstream transcriptional activation or repression

suppressor genes and oncogenes through modulation of DNA methylation and chromatin modification. These bioactive phytochemicals acting alone or in combination with other natural or synthetic agents showed promising results against various cancers (Shukla et al. 2014; Ullah and Khan 2008).

These recent advances have initiated significant interest in the use of natural, biological, or synthetic agents to prevent or delay the occurrence of cancer or its progression to invasive disease. The potential mechanisms of chemoprevention are the inhibition of cancer initiation with "blocking" agents and the inhibition of tumor progression with "suppressing" chemopreventive agents (Steward and Brown2013). Both mechanisms of cancer chemoprevention can be modified through epigenetic modulating agents, either natural or synthetic. Natural dietary compounds, including green tea polyphenols, soy isoflavones, isothiocyanates derived from cruciferous vegetables, and garlic-derived organosulfur compounds, have the strong potential to affect the gene expression via the epigenetic mechanisms, without the adverse toxic effects associated with synthetic epigenetic inhibitors used in chemotherapy. Another key aspect of the chemopreventive action of polyphenols and other dietary factors is their potential ability to selectively target cancer cells, while maintaining negligible cytotoxicity to normal cells (Khan et al. 2012).

2 Major Epigenetic Mechanisms in Cancer

2.1 DNA Methylation

The key epigenetic modification in mammals is the DNA methylation of cytosine, located 5′ to guanosine in the CpG dinucleotide (Szyf 2005; Herman and Baylin 2003). The covalent addition of a methyl group to the carbon-5 position of cytosine in DNA is catalyzed by the enzyme family of DNMTs, with *S*-adenosyl-methionine (SAM) acting as a universal methyl donor (Szyf 2005). While DNMT1 is mainly involved in the maintenance of DNA methylation after replication, DNMT3A and DNMT3B interact with transcription machinery and mediate de novo methylation (Szyf 2005). A number of studies have shown changes of DNMT expression (mainly DNMT1 and DNMT3B overexpression) in several cancer types (Girault et al. 2003; Agarwal et al. 2013; Yu et al. 2014).

CpG nucleotides are non-randomly distributed throughout the genome. Whereas solitary CpG dinucleotides are infrequent, CpG dinucleotides are often clustered in CpG-rich regions of DNA (CpG islands), with lengths from 0.5 to 4 kb. In normal cells, CpG islands are not methylated and are frequently associated with the transcription start site (Szyf 2005). During the process of carcinogenesis, paradoxical changes in DNA methylation patterns were observed. The "methylation paradox" is characterized by global hypomethylation followed by regional hypermethylation changes of tumor suppressor gene promoters. Global DNA hypomethylation may activate or "unlock" repetitive elements that could affect genome stability or could lead to transcriptional activation of latent viruses or oncogenes, whereas regional hypermethylation could lead to transcriptional silencing of tumor suppressor genes, which causes their inactivation, leading to malignant transformation (Herman and Baylin 2003). Patterns of tumor suppressor gene hypermethylation show tumor-type specificity (Esteller 2007). DNA methylation in cancer cells is now believed to be one of the major causes of the transcriptional silencing of tumor suppressor genes in carcinogenesis. Accumulating evidence demonstrates aberrant DNA methylation in most human cancers, including colon, breast, lung, and oral carcinomas (Esteller 2007; Belinsky et al. 2002; Supic et al. 2009, 2011a, b). A number of recent studies have demonstrated that dietary phytochemicals could have an important role in cancer chemoprevention by affecting DNA methylation (Shukla et al. 2014).

2.2 Histone Posttranslational Modifications

Histone modifications are posttranslational covalent modifications of histone tails, which result in changes to chromatin structure and gene activity. Histone tails can be modified by acetylation, methylation, phosphorylation, poly-ADP ribosylation, sumoylation, ubiquitination, citrullination, and proline isomerization (Jenuwein and Allis 2001; Tollefsbol 2009). Histone posttranslational modifications are complex, dynamic, and highly coordinated in chromatin remodeling and gene regulation. Different combinations of histone modification and histone variants, often referred as "histone code," determine the interactions of histones with DNA and regulate the chromatin structure and its accessibility to transcription factors (Margueron et al. 2005; Tollefsbol 2009).

Histone acetylation of lysine residues (K) by histone acetyltransferases (HATs) neutralizes the positive charge on lysine and releases the histone tails from the negatively charged DNA. Histone acetylation causes decondensation of chromatin, thus allowing its accessibility to transcriptional factors (Tollefsbol 2009). The reverse process is histone deacetylation, catalyzed by HDACs, which leads to chromatin condensation and the suppression of DNA transcription (Mahlknecht and Hoelzer 2000) (Fig. 2).

Histone methylation of lysine (K) and arginine (R) residues of histones H3 and H4 has been associated with both the activation and repression of transcription, depending on the modification target, type of amino acid, and its position in the histone tail (Jenuwein and Allis 2001; Tollefsbol 2009). While methylation of the residue of the fourth lysine on histone 3 (H3K4) leads to transcriptional activation, methylation of the ninth lysine on histone 3 (H3K9) leads to transcriptional repression. Histone methylation does not alter the charge of the histone tails but influences the chemical characteristics of histones and their affinity to transcription factors and other regulatory proteins. Histone methylation is catalyzed by a family of enzymes named histone methyltransferases (HMTs), whereas the removal of

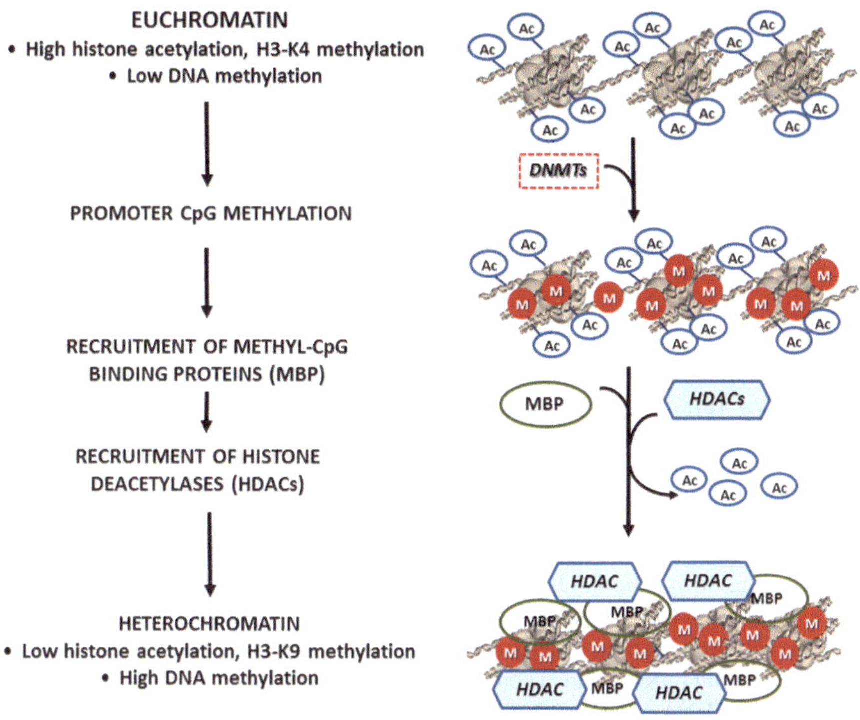

Fig. 2 The Epigenetic Control of Chromatin Organization. Euchromatin is characterized by low level of DNA methylation, high level of hyperacetylation of histones, and H3-K4 methylation. Promoter CpG methylation by DNMTs leads to the binding of MBPs that recruit histone deacetylases (HDACs) and histone methyltransferases (HMT). In contrast, heterochromatin shows hypermethylation of DNA, hypoacetylation of histones, and H3-K9 methylation that leads to the chromatin condensation and suppression of the DNA transcription

methyl groups is catalyzed by the histone demethylases (HDMs) (Margueron et al. 2005; Miremadi et al. 2007).

Histone phosphorylation is involved in diverse biological processes including mitosis, gene transcription, DNA repair, and cell cycle progression (Banerjee and Chakravarti 2011). The core histones and histone H1 undergo phosphorylation of serine and threonine residues by H1 and H3 kinases. Phosphorylation of histones during mitosis and meiosis is involved in chromosome condensation, whereas the same modification during interphase weakens H1 binding to DNA, thus promoting free access of transcriptional factors to the DNA and stimulating the gene expression. H3 phosphorylation at serine-10 has been associated with the transcriptional activation of the early response genes *c-fos* and *c-jun* (Kouzarides 2007).

Histone ubiquitination at lysine residues of histones H2A and H2B has a role in gene transcription control. Mono-ubiquitination of histone H2B is required for methylation of histone H3 at K4 and K79, where histone ubiquitination seems to promote methylation by recruiting proteasomal ATPases using ubiquitin-modified

H2B (Jenuwein and Allis 2001; Tollefsbol 2009). The global disruption of the histone acetylation and methylation, commonly found in cancer, has been associated with malignant transformation through transcriptional repression of the tumor suppressor genes (Jenuwein and Allis 2001; Tollefsbol 2009). Aberrant expression of histone-modifying enzymes (HDAC, HAT, HMT, and HDM) has also been observed in cancer cells (Mahlknecht and Hoelzer 2000; Tollefsbol 2009). A large number of dietary bioactive factors have been shown to have modifying effects on various histone-modifying enzymes (Tortorella et al. 2014).

2.3 RNA-Associated Silencing RNA-Interference and MicroRNAs

Noncoding RNAs, including microRNAs and small-interfering RNAs, have a very important role in the posttranscriptional regulation of gene expression. Noncoding RNAs act either by complete complementary base pairing, which results in mRNA degradation, or by a partial base pairing, which leads to translational inhibition of the targeted mRNA. MicroRNAs regulate genes with important cellular functions such as cell proliferation, differentiation, and apoptosis. Changes in the expression of genes coding miRNAs are a common event in cancer. Depending on their target, subsets of miRNAs that are downregulated in cancer may act as putative tumor suppressor genes, whereas upregulation of other miRNAs suggests that many miRNAs may act as oncogenes (Shivdasani 2006; Negrini et al. 2007).

Accumulating evidence suggests that epigenetic modifications cannot be interpreted independently, but only in combination with other modifications and within a context that leads to downstream transcriptional activation or repression. DNA methylation, histone modifications, and RNAi are not isolated events but coordinated in higher-order chromatin structures. DNA methylation leads to the binding of methylcytosine-binding proteins (MBPs), which recruit HDACs and HMTs (Herman and Baylin 2003; Tollefsbol 2009) (Fig. 2). Furthermore, noncoding miRNAs can regulate the expression of DNMTs and trigger locus-specific histone modifications and DNA methylation, causing gene silencing (Zilberman et al. 2003). In addition, the genes for miRNAs can be downregulated as a result of hypermethylation (Lujambio et al. 2007). Aberrant changes of miRNA expression appear to be one of the key epigenetic mechanisms involved in regulating gene expression during carcinogenesis (Shivdasani 2006; Negrini et al. 2007). In addition, accumulating evidence demonstrates that dietary factors can alter miRNA expression in cancer cells. Thus, targeting specific miRNAs with dietary phytochemicals could be a novel approach for cancer chemoprevention (Shah et al. 2012; Davis and Ross 2008).

3 Dietary Factors in Epigenetic Cancer Chemoprevention

Certain dietary factors, e.g., folate, tea polyphenols, phytoestrogens and isoflavones, curcumin, and resveratrol, are thought to have a chemoprotective effect on the development and the progression of cancer. Many bioactive phytochemicals could potentially alter the expression of key tumor suppressor genes or oncogenes through modulation of DNA methylation and chromatin modification in cancer (Figs. 3 and 4). Bioactive natural compounds appear to act through the decrease of the DNMTs or HDACs gene expression in cancer cell lines and in vivo. In addition, these bioactive dietary factors resulted in modulating tissue levels of miRNAs and

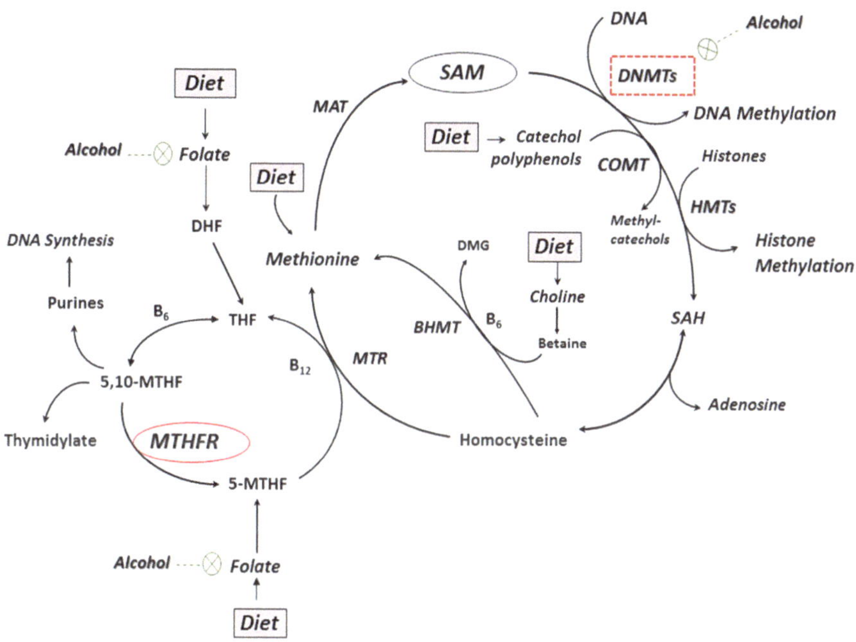

Fig. 3 A schematic representation of the one-carbon metabolism, transmethylation reactions, and steps that are inhibited by alcohol. Dietary folate is converted to 5 methyl tetrahydrofolate (5-MTHF) by the enzyme methylene tetrahydrofolate reductase (MTHFR). The transfer of methyl group from 5-MTHF to homocysteine results in the methionine synthesis. Methionine is the precursor for *S*-adenosylmethionine (SAM), the primary methyl donor for numerous reactions, including protein, RNA, DNA, and histone methylation. Methyl groups from SAM are transferred to DNA by DNA methyltransferases (DNMTs) and to histones by histone methyltransferases (HMTs). DNA methylation of CpG dinucleotides and histone methylation lead to the altered chromatin remodeling and gene expression. The MTHFR 677C$\rightarrow$T polymorphism reduces enzyme activity and could play a key role in interactions of one-carbon metabolism with alcohol, which could affect DNA methylation levels. *COMT* catechol-O-methyltransferase, *BHMT* betaine homocysteine methyltransferase, *DHF* dihydrofolate, *DHFR* dihydrofolate reductase, *MAT* methionine adenosyl transferase, *MT* methyltransferase, *MTR* methionine synthase, *SAH* S-adenosylhomocysteine, *THF* tetrahydrofolate, *TS* thymidylate synthase

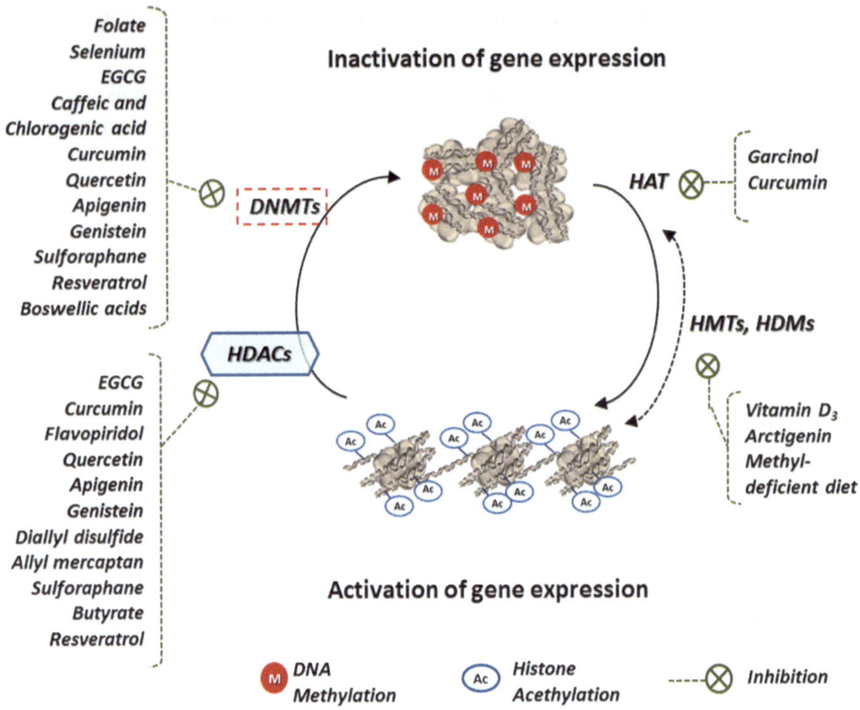

Fig. 4 The chemopreventive effects of dietary factors on specific epigenetic alterations. Dietary chemopreventive agents can affect DNMTs activity and the DNA promoter methylation status, as well as the HDAC activity and the pattern of histone modifications, thereby restoring the epigenetically silenced genes in cancer cells that regulate the cell cycle and apoptosis

their target genes (Shah et al. 2012). Most of the studies were performed in vitro using different cancer cell lines, or in animals, and few studies were intervention studies on human subjects.

The first study indicating this phenomenon showed that maternal diet supplemented with methyl donors, including folate, affected agouti gene expression in Avy/a mice, as a result of retrotransposon hypermethylation, and caused an altered coat phenotype (from a normal yellow to brown) in the genetically identical offspring (Wolff et al. 1998; Waterland and Jirtle 2003). Prenatal famine in humans influences phenotypic changes in offspring caused by DNA methylation changes that persist in the next generation offspring (Tobi et al. 2009; Heijmans et al. 2008). Individuals exposed to severe famine during childhood and adolescence, during the "Dutch Hunger Winter" of 1944–1945, had a decreased risk of developing colorectal cancer and a decreased methylation of a panel of cancer-related genes (Hughes et al. 2009). A reduced DNA methylation of the imprinted insulin-like growth factor 2 (IGF2), persisted six decades later, compared to their unexposed, same-sex siblings (Heijmans et al. 2008). A recent study showed that prenatal dietary supplementation with polyunsaturated fatty acid was associated with higher methylation levels in infants at IGF2/H19 imprinted regions. In addition, in the same study DNA methylation states in infants were associated with maternal body mass index (Lee et al. 2014). The data from these studies indicate that periconceptional, prenatal, and early-life conditions can cause epigenetic changes in humans that persist throughout life and could cause cancer.

Here we summarize the major phytochemicals that exert cancer-protective effects through modulation of epigenetic mechanisms, classified as essential micronutrients (folate and other nutrients of one-carbon metabolism, vitamin D, vitamin A, and selenium), polyphenol catechins (tea polyphenols—epigallocatechin gallate and epicatechin gallate, and coffee polyphenols—caffeic acid and chlorogenic acid), flavonoids (curcumin and difluorinated curcumin, garcinol, apigenin, quercetin, flavopiridol), isoflavonoids (genistein), phytoestrogen lignans (arctigenin), myco-strogens (zearalenone), organosulfur compounds(diallyl disulfide, *S*-allyl-mercaptocysteine, allyl mercaptan), isothiocyanates (sulforaphane and phenethyl-isothiocyanate), stilbenoids (resveratrol and pterostilbene), cyclic terpenoids (boswellic acids), plant alkaloids (mahanine, berberine), and short-chain fatty acids (butyrate).

4 Essential Micronutrients

Folate and other nutrients of one-carbon metabolism, such as vitamin B2, B6, and B12, are the main source of methyl groups or act as coenzymes for the one-carbon metabolism that regulates methyl transfer and DNA synthesis (Anderson et al. 2012). One-carbon metabolism is essential for the synthesis of *S*-adenosyl-L-methionine (SAM), universal methyl donor for various cellular reactions including DNA methylation and histone methylation (Fig. 3). Extensive evidence has accumulated suggesting that folate deficiency plays a significant role in developing several tumors including cancers of the colorectum, lung, pancreas, esophagus, stomach, cervix, and breast, as well as neuroblastoma and leukemia (Kim 1999). Head and neck cancer patients with the high dietary intake of micronutrients involved in one-carbon metabolism and antioxidant activity (folate, vitamin B12, and vitamin A) and cruciferous vegetable, compared with those in the lowest intake, showed significantly less tumor suppressor promoter methylation, assessed using the Illumina Goldengate Methylation Cancer Panel (Colacino et al. 2012). Low consumption of folate, vitamin A, vitamin B1, potassium, and iron in colorectal cancer patients was associated with the increased promoter hypermethylation of p16, p14 (ARF), or hMLH1 genes (Mas et al. 2007).

Several studies have established a connection between cancer susceptibility and methyl-group metabolism genes, including methylene tetrahydrofolate reductase (MTHFR), a key enzyme involved in folate metabolism and DNA synthesis (Fig. 3). MTHFRC677T genotype was associated with RASSF1A promoter hypermethylation in bladder and oral cancer (Cai et al. 2009; Supic et al. 2011a). Carriers of the 677 T allele of MTHFR gene in patients with colorectal, breast, or lung tumors had global hypomethylation, while patients with methionine synthase

2756GG genotype showed promoter hypermethylation in a large panel of tumor suppressor genes, including p16, p14, hMLH1, MGMT, APC, DAPK, GSTP1, BRCA1, RAR-β 2, CDH1, and RASSF1 (Paz et al. 2002). An interaction between low dietary folate and high alcohol intake in colorectal cancer patients resulted in concordant DNA methylation of tumor suppressor genes (van England et al. 2003). In addition, a significant interaction between heavy drinking and MTHFR667TT genotype, observed in oral cancer patients, resulted in the multiple DNA methylation of tumor suppressor genes (Supic et al. 2011a). These findings indicated that polymorphisms in genes encoding enzymes involved in folate metabolism could be an alternative mechanism that modulates the epigenetic effects of environmental factors. Interaction of folate intake or one-carbon metabolism-related polymorphisms with environmental factors, such as alcohol, could cause changes in DNA methylation (Fig. 3). Future investigations might predict individual susceptibility to cancer and provide science-based recommendations for methyl donors intake, depending on the individual genetic profile exposure for cancer prevention.

Retinoic acid (RA), generated via oxidative conversion from β-carotene absorbed from fruits and vegetables, binds to nuclear retinoic acid receptors (RAR) and heterodimerize with retinoid X receptors (RXR). Subsequently, RA modulates transcription through its response elements in the promoters of target genes, including p21 and AP-1, and exerts the pro-apoptotic actions (Stefanska et al. 2012a). It has been demonstrated that the treatment of noninvasive MCF-7 cells with RA caused the decrease in promoter methylation, consequent increase in the RARβ2 and PTEN (phosphatase and tensin homologue) expression, and the inhibition of breast cancer cell growth (Stefanska et al. 2012b). In the combined treatment, butyrate and RA inhibited proliferation of MCF-7 cells (Andrade et al. 2012). Thus, retinoids have been suggested as a potential epigenetic strategy for the cancer treatment, especially in breast cancers in which RAR β is epigenetically altered.

Vitamin D3, synthesized upon sun exposure and from the diet, binds to vitamin D receptors (VDR). Upon ligand binding, VDR heterodimerize with RXR or RAR, and regulate the transcription of more than a hundred genes, involved not only in calcium and phosphate homeostasis but also in cell proliferation, differentiation, and apoptosis (Chung et al. 2009). Accumulating results revealed the association between vitamin D deficiency and vitamin D-related genes with different cancer types, including breast, prostate, colorectal, oral, lung cancer, melanoma and acute myeloid leukemia (Feldman et al. 2014; Davis and Milner 2011; Zeljic et al. 2012, 2014, Puccetti et al. 2002). In addition, the gene expression of VDR and CYP24A1 gene, coding for 24-hydroxylase, enzyme involved in the vitamin D catabolism, and CYP27B1, coding for 1α-hydroxylase, involved in anabolism, is mediated by epigenetic modifications (Hobaus et al. 2013; Fetahu et al. 2014). In highly invasive MDA-MB-231 cells, exposure to vitamin D3 resulted in hypomethylation and induction of p21, PTEN, and RARβ2 expression (Stefanska et al. 2012a, b). Vitamin D3-mediated promoter demethylation induced the expression of E-cadherin and differentiation of aggressive triple-negative breast cancer cells (Lopes et al. 2012). Dietary vitamin D intake was strongly negatively associated with the Wnt antagonist gene DKK1 methylation in a large cohort of Canadian colorectal carcinoma patients (Rawson et al. 2012). In vitro studies demonstrated that calcitriol [1 alpha,25 Dihydroxyvitamin D(3)], an active metabolite of vitamin D, synergized the pro-apoptotic effect of HDAC inhibitors sodium butyrate (NaB), a natural short-chain fatty acid, and trichostatin A (TSA), a synthetic HDAC inhibitor, in the prostate cancer cells LNCaP, PC-3, and DU-145 (Rashid et al. 2001). Calcitriol inhibited the expression of several HDMs and induced the expression of others (Pereira et al. 2011, 2012). In the colon cancer SW480-ADH cells, calcitriol increased the expression of the HDM Jumonji JMJD3, which upregulated the epithelial-to-mesenchymal transition inducers SNAIL1 and ZEB1, while it downregulated the epithelial proteins, including E-cadherin (Pereira et al. 2011). Novel data indicate that calcitriol exerts its regulatory role via Jumonji C (JmjC) and lysine-specific demethylase (LSD) families of the HDMs (Pereira et al. 2012). In addition, JMJD3 knockdown decreases the expression of miR-200b and miR-200c, two microRNAs targeting ZEB1 RNA (Pereira et al. 2012). In another study, calcitriol upregulation of the expression of miR-627 in the colorectal cancer cells HT-29 and in the mice tumor xenografts led to lower levels of KDM2A, one of the direct targets of miR-627 (Padi et al. 2013). These findings indicate that the antiproliferative effect of calcitriol on the expression of HDMs may well be indirect and could be mediated by microRNAs.

Selenium is an essential micro-element with antioxidant and pro-apoptotic effect (Davis et al. 2000; Davis and Uthus 2002). In the rat colon and liver, selenium deficiency causes global hypomethylation and promoter methylation of p53 and p16gene (Davis et al. 2000). Selenium inhibits DNMT directly interacting with enzyme and indirectly influencing plasma homocysteine level and the SAM:SAH (*S*-adenosyl-L-homocysteine) ratio in a rat model (Davis and Uthus 2002; Uthus and Ross 2007). In an azoxymethane-induced rat colon carcinogenesis model, combination of selenium and green tea revealed more effective suppression of colorectal oncogenesis than either agent alone. Rats fed the combination diet showed marked reduction of DNMT1 expression and induction of histone H3 acetylation, which were accompanied by restoration of SFRP5, reduced ß-catenin nuclear translocation, Cyclin D1 expression, and cell proliferation (Hu et al. 2013a). In human colon cancer, selenium plays a role in chemoprevention by inhibiting DNMTs, thus suppressing DNA methylation (Fiala et al. 1998). However, in another study treatment of colorectal cancer cells Caco-2 and HCT116 with different concentrations of selenium methylselenocysteine and selenite, either alone or in combination with sulforaphane and iberin, did not impact changes in gene-specific methylation of p16 and ESR1, global methylation of LINE-1 elements, or DNMT expression (Barrera et al. 2013).

5 Catechol-Structured Polyphenols

Epigallocatechin-3-gallate (EGCG), the major green tea polyphenol catechin, was associated with the lower incidence of a number of cancers (Yang et al. 2001; Tollefsbol 2009). Various findings indicate that EGCG is the potent inhibitor of catechol-*O*-methyltransferase (COMT) and DNMT activity, in a dose-dependent manner (Lu et al. 2003; Fang et al. 2003). Treatment of human esophageal cells, colon cancer cells, and prostate cancer cells with EGCG inhibits DNMT1 activity in a concentration- and time-dependent manner, leading to the hypomethylation and restored gene expression of p16, RAR β, MGMT, and hMLH1 (Fang et al. 2003). Decreased activity of human telomerase reverse transcriptase (hTERT) in cancer cells is associated with increased DNA methylation of its promoter (Berletch et al. 2008). EGCG treatment inhibits expression of DNMTs leading to the suppression of hTERT, the suppression of cell viability, and the induction of apoptosis in human breast cancer cells (Mittal et al. 2004; Meeran et al. 2011; Berletch et al. 2008). The treatment with natural compounds, EGCG, genistein, withaferin A, curcumin, resveratrol, and guggulsterone, resulted in the decrease of the DNMTs gene expression and the methyl-binding proteins MeCP2 in the breast cancer cell lines (Mirza et al. 2013). EGCG decreased the expression and the levels of DNMTs and HDAC, which resulted in the re-expression of silenced tumor suppressor genes, p16INK4a and p21 in human skin cancer cells, and increased levels of histones acetylation in human skin cancer cells A431 in a dose-dependent manner (Nandakumar et al. 2011).

By miRNA microarray analysis, EGCG treatment was found to modify the expressions of a number of the miRNAs in human hepatocellular carcinoma cell line, as well as miRNA-16 and its anti-apoptotic target Bcl-2, that lead to the induction of apoptosis (Tsang and Kwok 2010). These findings indicate that natural tea polyphenols and EGCG could have the strong potential to reverse the epigenetic changes, without the adverse toxic effects associated with synthetic DNMT or HDAC inhibitors used in chemotherapy.

Caffeic acid and Chlorogenic acid are catechol-structures polyphenols from coffee or black tea that inhibit the DNMTs activity in various human cancer cell lines. Catechol polyphenols may indirectly inhibit DNMT through the increased formation of SAH, during the COMT-mediated O-methylation of these dietary agents, thus changing the SAM:SAH ratio (Lee and Zhu 2006) (Fig. 3). Treatment of human breast cancer cells MCF-7 and MAD-MB-231 with caffeic acid or chlorogenic acid inhibited general DNA methylation in a concentration-dependent manner, and the regional methylation of the RAR β gene promoter (Lee and Zhu 2006).

6 Flavonoids

Curcumin (diferuloylmethane), flavanoid from the rhizome of the plant *Curcuma longa*, has anticancer activity both in vitro and in vivo (Kunnumakkara et al. 2008). Genome-wide methylation microarrays revealed that in contrast to the generalized, nonspecific global hypomethylation observed with 5-aza-2′-deoxycytidine, curcumin treatment of colorectal cancer cells HCT116, HT29, and RKO caused methylation changes in selected, partially methylated loci, instead of fully methylated CpG sites (Link et al. 2013).

Curcumin upregulates or downregulates histone acetylation, depending on the cell type. In brain cancer cells treated with curcumin, H4 histones are hypoacetylated (Kang et al. 2006), as opposite of prostate cancer cells treated with curcumin, where H3 and H4 histones are hyperacetylated and where curcumin induces apoptosis by the involvement of Bcl-2 family genes and p53 (Shankar and Srivastava 2007). Curcumin inhibited HDACs and HPV expression, upregulated p53, pRb, p21, and p27 in cervical cancer cells SiHa and SiHaR, and resulted in sensitization of cervical cancer cell toward cisplatin, lowering the dose of the chemotherapy (Royt and Mukherjee 2014) In addition, curcumin sensitized tumor cells to the chemotherapeutic drugs cyclophosphamide and paclitaxel through the modulation of PKC, telomerase, NF-kappa B, and HDAC in breast cancer (Royt et al. 2011)

Combined administration of curcumin and emodin, a bioactive factor isolated from the root and rhizome of *Rheum palmatum*, widely used in traditional Chinese medicine, synergistically inhibited proliferation, survival, and invasion of breast cancer cells through upregulation of miR-34a (Guo et al. 2013). Treatment of colon cancer cells with curcumin and synthetic analogues of curcumin induced apoptosis and reactive oxygen species (ROS) and decreased specificity protein (Sp) transcription factors and Sp-regulated genes, including the epidermal growth factor receptor (EGFR), survivin, bcl-2, cyclin D1, and NFκB, by targeting microRNAs (miR-27a, miR-20a, and miR-17-5p) (Gandhy et al. 2012). The potential effects of curcumin treatment on miRNA expression profiles in a pancreatic cancer cell line showed altered expression, with miRNA-22 upregulated, while miRNA-199a downregulated (Sun et al. 2008). In addition, curcumin reduced the expression of Bcl-2 by upregulating miRNA-15a and miRNA-16 in MCF-7 breast cancer cell line (Yang et al. 2010), thereby inducing apoptosis. Curcumin exerted inhibitory effects on proliferation, migration, and invasion in nasopharyngeal carcinoma by inhibiting the expression of miR-125a-5p, which led to the upregulation of p53 expression (Gao et al. 2014). Another miRNA, MicroRNA-200a/b, was overexpressed after curcumin treatment, and this was accompanied with the increase of apoptotic Bcl-2, Bax, and Bad levels in hepatocellular carcinoma cell lines (Liang et al. 2013). Difluorinated curcumin, a novel analogue of the curcumin, restores tumor suppressor PTEN expression in chemo-resistant colon cancer cells HCT116 and HT-29 through downregulation of key oncomir miR-21

(Roy et al. 2013), which suggests that this bioactive agent could be potentially used in chemotherapy-resistant colorectal cancer treatment.

Garcinol is a flavonoid derived from the plant *Garcinia indica* fruit with anticancer activity (Ahmad et al. 2012). Garcinol sensitizes human pancreatic cancer cells to gemcitabine treatment, resulting in the inhibition of cell proliferation and inducement of apoptosis via modulation of microRNAs expression, including miR-21, miR-196a, miR-495, miR-605, miR-638, and miR-453 (Parasramka et al. 2013). The anticancer activity of garcinol against aggressive triple-negative breast cancer cells MB-231 and BT-549 is, in part, due to the reversion of epithelial-to-mesenchymal transition (EMT) mediated by E-cadherin, is associated with the upregulation of miR-200 and let-7 family (Ahmad et al. 2012).

Quercetin, a dietary flavonoid abundant in fruits and vegetables with antioxidant and antiproliferative activities, is a natural inhibitor of COMT and multidrug resistance proteins. In lung cancer A549 cells, in kidney 786-O cells, and in liver HepG2 cells quercetin increased the cellular absorption of EGCG and decreased the activity and protein expression of COMT (Wang et al. 2012a). Additionally, quercetin reduced tumor incidence and induced cell cycle arrest and apoptosis in hamster buccal pouch tumors, and these anticancer properties were correlated with the inhibition of HDAC-1 and DNMT1 (Priyadarsini et al. 2011). Combination therapy with quercetin and sodium butyrate suppressed human esophageal 9706 cancer cell (Eca9706) growth in a dose-dependent manner, via downregulation of DNMT1 and HDAC1 which resulted in the increased expression of p16 and E-cadherin (Zheng et al. 2014). In prostate cancer cells, quercetin increased anti-proliferative activity of EGCG by increasing the bioavailability and decreasing EGCG methylation (Wang et al. 2012b). In human leukemia HL-60 cells, quercetin induced Fas L-related apoptosis and induced histone acetylation by the activation of HAT and the inhibition of HADC (Lee et al. 2011).

Apigenin, a potent cancer chemopreventive phytoestrogen, reversed the nuclear factor erythroid 2-related factor 2 (Nrf2) promoter hypermethylation, followed by the increase of the Nrf2 expression, and reduced the expression of the DNMTs and HDACs in mouse skin epidermal JB6P+ cells (Paredes-Gonzalez et al. 2014). Synergistically with genistein, apigenin exerted a stimulatory effect on the proliferation of ERα-positive breast cancer cells MCF-7 and T47D by activating ERα (Seo et al. 2006). These findings indicate that, until comprehensive evaluation, phytoestrogens and concentrated phytoestrogen supplements should be used with caution in breast cancer patients.

7 Isoflavonoids

Genistein, an isoflavone found in soy and other legumes, has been shown to be a chemopreventive agent against various types of cancer cells, including cancers of the prostate, esophageal, and colon (Li and Tollefsbol 2010). Genistein has been associated with a lower incidence and mortality rate of breast cancer in Asian women, who daily consumed soy food (Fang et al. 2005). In vitro treatment of human uveal melanoma cells with genistein showed a significant inhibition of cell growth in a time- and dose-related manner, and in vivo study confirmed that genistein significantly inhibited the growth of xenografts (Sun et al. 2009a). The precise mechanism by which genistein suppresses carcinogenesis remains unrevealed, but potential mechanism includes modulating epigenetic gene regulation mechanisms such as DNA methylation and/or chromatin modifications (Pudenz et al. 2014). In clinically aggressive ERα-negative breast cancer, which does not respond to conventional estrogen target-directed therapies, genistein induced the epigenetic reactivation of the ERα promoter, which in turn increased tamoxifen-dependent sensitivity in vitro and in vivo (Li et al. 2013b). These findings suggest that a novel combined therapy with genistein and tamoxifen in refractory ERα-negative breast cancer could provide more effective strategy. However, the findings that genistein stimulates the proliferation of ERα-positive breast cancer cells MCF-7 and T47D, and antagonizes the anti-proliferative effect of tamoxifen (Seo et al. 2006), suggest that phytoestrogens could have detrimental effects in breast cancer patients. It has been shown that genistein inhibits DNMT activity and reversed aberrant DNA methylation in esophageal and prostate cancer cells, leading to the reactivation of p16, RAR β, and MGMT gene expression (Fang et al. 2005). Genistein treatment induces demethylation of glutathione *S*-transferase P1 (GSTP1) and ephrin B2 (EPHB2) tumor suppressor promoters, followed by activation of expression in prostate cancer cell lines (Vardi et al. 2010), which might be related to the protective effect of soy on prostate cancer. Although the inhibitory effect of genistein on DNMT is weaker than that of EGCG, genistein exerts greater stability in the cell culture medium than EGCG, and can reach to higher intracellular concentrations than does EGCG (Fang et al. 2003; Fang et al. 2005), leading to the reactivation of methylation-silenced genes.

The chemopreventive effect of genistein has additionally been associated with histone modifications. Genistein mediated histone acetylation and demethylation that activated tumor suppressor genes in prostate cancer cells (Kikuno et al. 2008). Long-term genistein treatment of MCF-7 breast cancer cell line reduced the acetylation of H3 and altered growth responses to mitogens and HDAC inhibitors (Jawaid et al. 2010). In colon tumor HT29 cells, combined therapy of EGCG and genistein inhibited HDACs activity (Groh et al. 2013). Genistein treated in breast cancer cell lines MDA-MB-231 and BT20 resulted in an increased kinase activity, accompanied by histone phosphorylation, transcriptional activation, and G2/M arrest (Cappelletti et al. 2000).

In addition, the expression level of miRNA-27a and its target gene *ZBTB10* (zinc finger and BTB domain containing 10) depended on the dose of genistein (Sun et al. 2009a). Another study reports that the genistein modulated miRNA-16 expression in a murine chronic lymphocytic leukemia B-1 cell line (Salerno et al. 2009). Genistein treatment of ovarian cancer cell lines induced differential expression of various miRNAs, with the induction of ER alpha and ER beta and a significant reduction in migration and invasion potential (Parker et al. 2009). A recent study showed a significant inverse relationship between downregulated tumor suppressor ARHI and miRNA-221 and miRNA-222, which were upregulated with the transfection of anti-miRNA-221 and anti-miRNA-222 in prostate cancer cells (Chen et al. 2011). These findings suggest that genistein could exert its chemopreventive effect, by modulating the microRNAs.

Arctigenin, a natural lignan phytoestrogen from *Arctium lappa L.*, induces apoptosis of breast cancer MDA-MB-231 cells via the ROS/p38 MAPK pathway and epigenetic silencing of Bcl-2 by histone H3K9 trimethylation (Hsieh et al. 2014).

However, all bioactive agents do not have a protective effect against cancer, and some phyto- or myco-estrogens or their metabolites showed a genotoxic activity in vitro (Stopper et al. 2005). *Zearalenone* is estrogenic mycotoxin contaminant derived from various Fusarium fungi and is present in high concentrations in moldy cereals and dairy products. Zearalenone acts as an antiapoptotic agent, increasing the expression of c-myc and cyclins, downregulating p27, phosphorylating retinoblastoma Rb gene, and increasing H3 phosphorylation in human breast carcinoma cell line MCF-7 (Ahamed et al. 2001). Therefore, the adverse health effects of phytoestrogens should not be overlooked (Stopper et al. 2005).

8 Organosulfur Compounds

Diallyl disulfide (DADS), the major organosulfur compound from garlic, induces cell cycle arrest in HT-29 human colon cancer cells, through p16 and p21, and this effect is mediated by the H3 and H4 histones acetylation (Myzak and Dashwood2006; Druesne et al. 2004a). When administrated as single treatments, the DADS antiproliferative effects were mediated by transient acetylation on histone H3, while repetitive treatment with DADS resulted in a prolonged hyperacetylation of histone H3 K14 in colon HT-29 cells (Druesne et al. 2004b). DADS treatment showed a dose-dependent induction of apoptosis in prostate cancer cells PC-3 by influencing histone acetylation (Arunkumar et al. 2007) DADS-induced apoptosis in MCF-7 breast cancer cells is caused by H4 hyperacetylation (Altonsy et al. 2012). All of these findings indicated that the DADS substantial antiproliferative and pro-apoptotic effect could be related to its ability to inhibit HDAC activity. In addition, DADS treatment suppresses proliferation and induces apoptosis in MGC-803 human gastric cancer cells, through the Wnt-1 pathway by upregulation of miR-200b and miR-22 (Tang et al. 2013).

Diallyl trisulfide, another garlic-derived organosulfur compounds, suppresses viability of human lung cancer cell lines H358 (a non-small cell lung cancer cell line) and H460 (a large cell lung cancer cell line) by causing cell cycle arrest and apoptosis (Xiao et al. 2009). It has been shown that diallyl trisulfide is considerably more effective than either diallyl sulfide or diallyl disulfide against lung cancer cells proliferation (Xiao et al. 2009), indicating that a subtle change in the structure of these bioactive agents could have a significant impact on its biological activity.

Allyl mercaptan is the most potent HDAC inhibitor among Allium family organosulfur compounds. Treatment with allyl mercaptan led to the HDAC inhibition and rapid and sustained hyperacetylation of histone H3 on the p21WAF1 gene promoter, which enhanced binding of the transcription factor Sp3, the induction of p21Waf1 protein expression, and the subsequent recruitment of p53 (Nian et al. 2008, 2009).

9 Isothiocyanates

Sulforaphane (SFN), isothiocyanates derived from cruciferous vegetables, cauliflower, cabbage, and particularly broccoli and broccoli sprouts, has been extensively studied due to its apparent anticancer properties. It has been shown that sulforaphane mediates a number of key cellular processes associated with malignant transformation, including the apoptosis, cell cycle arrest, and inhibition of NFκB. The significant decrease in the DNA strand breaks was observed in smokers and nonsmokers submitted to a controlled broccoli diet (Riso et al. 2009), indicating its protective effect. Sulforaphane may target the epigenetic alterations observed in specific cancers, reversing aberrant changes in gene transcription through mechanisms of HDAC inhibition, global demethylation, and microRNA modulation (Tortorella et al. 2014).

Sulforaphane is a promising chemopreventive agent that decreases DNMT expression in both normal PrEC and cancerous prostate epithelial cells, LnCAP and PC3, followed by widespread changes in promoter methylation, and reversed aberrantly methylated genes involved in cancer progression (Wong et al. 2014). Sulforaphane inhibited proliferation and induced apoptosis in MCF-7 and MDA-MB-231 breast cancer cells, inhibiting hTERT via promoter demethylation due to DNMTs downregulation. In addition, sulforaphane increased the level of histone acetylation, while decreasing the inactive chromatin markers trimethyl-H3K9 and trimethyl-H3K27 (Meeran et al. 2010). In prostate cancer TRAMP C1 cells, SFN exerts its chemopreventive effect by CpGs demethylation, decreasing the DNMT1, DNMT3a, HDACs levels, with subsequent induction of its downstream anti-oxidative system (Zhang et al. 2013). SFN strongly inhibited cell transformation and reduced promoter methylation of Nrf2, a transcription factor that plays key role in regulating the cellular antioxidant defense and detoxification enzymes, through decreasing the expression of DNMTs and HDAC in mouse skin JB6 P+ cells (Su et al. 2014).

Sulforaphane inhibits HDAC activity in vitro, in human colon, prostate, and breast cancer cells (Myzak et al. 2006a; Nian et al. 2009; Tortorella et al. 2014), and in vivo (Myzak et al. 2006b, 2007). In human colorectal and prostate cancer cells sulforaphane induces histone acetylation associated with the targeted p21 and Bax (Ho et al. 2009), thus inducing apoptosis. The first study demonstrating that natural dietary compounds from broccoli have a substantial effect on HDAC activity in human subjects showed that a single ingestion of one cup (68 g) of broccoli sprouts inhibited HDAC activity in circulating peripheral blood mononuclear cells early as 3 h after broccoli intake and returned to normal by 24 h, whereas histone hyperacetylation persisted for at least 48 h (Myzak et al. 2007). These findings suggest that HDAC activity in peripheral blood mononuclear cells could be used as future biomarker for the discovery and the evaluation of novel dietary HDAC inhibitors in human subjects. Phenethyl isothiocyanate, another isothiocyanate derived from cruciferous vegetables, attenuated proliferation of human colon tumor-derived SW480 cell line, in a concentration- and time-dependent manner, and induced changes to histone H3 in a gene-promoter-specific manner (Liu et al. 2013).

10 Stilbenoids

Resveratrol (Res) is an antioxidant phytoalexin from grapes, mulberries, and red wine. In breast carcinomas, resveratrol inhibited cancer proliferation by demethylation of tumor suppressor RASSF-1α gene promoter (Zhu et al. 2012). Aromatic hydrocarbon receptor (AhR) binds environmental xenobiotics and food compounds, and resveratrol acts as a potent dietary AhR antagonist. Recently, it has been shown that epigenetic silencing of the BRCA-1 gene by the AhR in MCF-7 breast cancer cells is preventable with resveratrol, which antagonizes the recruitment of AhR to the BRCA-1 promoter and reduced of BRCA-1 expression (Papoutsis et al. 2010). Resveratrol antagonized the physiologically relevant doses of the tetrachlorodibenzo-*p*-dioxin (TCDD)-induced repression of BRCA-1 protein, BRCA-1 promoter methylation, and the recruitment of the AhR, MBD2, and DNMTs in MCF-7 cells (Papoutsis et al. 2012). In murine model, maternal exposure to AhR agonists may increase the susceptibility to mammary carcinogenesis in offspring through epigenetic inhibition of BRCA-1 expression, whereas maternal pre-exposure to resveratrol, dietary antagonists of the AhR, exert protective effects (Papoutsis et al. 2013).

Resveratrol activates sirtuins (SIRT1), a Class III deacetylase, and increases NAD-dependent HDAC activity (Yeung et al. 2004). Resveratrol treatment induced cell cycle arrest and apoptosis, accompanied by downregulation of Sirt1 and its non-histone substrate p53 in bladder transitional cancer cells and in an experimental model (Wu et al. 2014). In prostate cancer, resveratrol treatment decreased Metastasis-associated protein 1 (MTA1), a part of the nucleosome remodeling deacetylation (NuRD) complex, that mediates posttranslational modifications of histones, thus enhancing p53 acetylation and subsequent activation of pro-apoptotic genes (Kai et al. 2010). Another stilbenoid, pterostilbene (PTER), found in blueberries, showed the superior potency over resveratrol as dietary epigenetic agent in the increase of MTA1-mediated p53 acetylation (Li et al. 2013a).

11 Cyclic Triterpenoids

Boswellic acids, an anti-inflammatory terpenoids from *Boswellia serrata*, inhibited DNMT activity and restored methylation-silenced tumor suppressor genes including SAMD14 and SMPD3, in colorectal cancer cells RKO, SW48, and SW480 (Shen et al. 2012). Boswellic acids may also exert their chemopreventive effects by modulating specific microRNAs. In various CRC cell lines, boswellic acid upregulated expression of the putative tumor suppressor let-7 and miR-200 family and the expression of their downstream targets CDK6, vimentin, and E-cadherin (Takahashi et al. 2012).

12 Plant Alkaloids

Mahanine, a carbazole alkaloid derived from the leaves of *Murraya koenigii*, commonly known as the curry leaf plant, inhibits ligand-dependent and ligand-independent androgen receptor signaling in human prostate cancer cells, leading to a prominent decline in AR target gene expression (Amin et al. 2014), and enhanced cisplatin-induced apoptosis and reduced its effective concentration in cervical cancer through STAT3 inhibition (Das et al. 2014). Mahanine reversed an epigenetically silenced tumor suppressor gene RASSF1A and induced its expression in both androgen-responsive (LNCaP) and androgen-negative (PC3) prostate cancer cells by inhibiting DNMTs activity (Jagadeesh et al. 2007; Agarwal et al. 2013). Thus, this plant-derived alkaloid could be a potential therapeutic agent for advanced prostate cancer in men when RASSF1A expression is epigenetically silenced.

Berberine is an anti-inflammatory and anti-oxidative isoquinoline alkaloid from the roots, rhizome, and stem bark of a number of plant species used in traditional Chinese medicine, including *Berberis vulgaris* (barberry), *Hydrastis canadensis* (goldenseal), and *Coptis chinensis* (Coptis or goldenthread) (Sun et al. 2009b). Berberine treatment suppressed proliferation via the NF-κB nuclear translocation, lysine methyltransferase Set9, and decreased expression of onco-miR miR21 and Bcl-2 (Hu et al. 2013b). Berberine induced apoptosis through hypomethylation of p53 promoter (Qing et al. 2014), in human multiple myeloma cells U266. In addition, berberine induced the epigenetic modifications, disrupted mitotic microtubules network, and modulated HPV-18 E6-E7 oncoproteins by targeting p53 in cervical cancer cells HeLa (Saha and Khuda-Bukhsh 2014), indicating its potential use as a natural agent in cervical cancer therapy.

13 Dietary Fibers, Short-Chain Fatty Acids, and Butyrate

Conflicting human epidemiologic findings suggest that dietary fibers could protect against colorectal cancer. Microbiota could have a key role in fiber fermentation into bioactive metabolite short-chain fatty acids; thus, their role should not be overlooked. In gnotobiotic mouse models colonized with wild-type or mutant strains of a butyrate-producing bacterium, it was shown that dietary fiber could have a potent tumor-suppressive effect in a microbiota- and butyrate-dependent manner (Donohoe et al. 2014).

Butyrate, a short-chain fatty acid, is a natural HDAC inhibitor, which promotes acetylation of histones, leading to the expression of genes involved in cellular differentiation and apoptosis (Myzak and Dashwood 2006; Scharlau et al. 2009). Butyrate induced promoter demethylation and reactivation of RARβ2 in colon cancer cells (Spurling et al. 2008).

In vitro studies demonstrated that low doses of sodium butyrate (NaB), and trichostatin A (TSA), a synthetic HDAC inhibitor, synergized with calcitriol [1 alpha,25 Dihydroxyvitamin D(3)], inhibited proliferation, and induced apoptosis in the prostate cancer cells LNCaP, PC-3, and DU-145 (Rashid et al. 2001). In a mouse model of colorectal cancer, sodium butyrate administration increased the expression of the p21 (WAF1) gene and P21 protein levels, and was associated with an accumulation of histone acetylation (Lu et al. 2008). Butyrate supplementation upregulated p21 expression and histone acetylation in vivo, in an azoxymethane-treated rat model of colon carcinogenesis, with either corn oil or fish oil as the lipid source. However, although butyrate enhanced p21 expression with both dietary lipid sources, the increase in p21 resulted in an increase in apoptosis and decrease in aberrant crypt foci formation with fish oil, but had no effect on apoptosis and ACF with corn oil (Crim et al. 2008). These findings indicate that butyrate can exert a chemoprotective or chemopromotive effect depending on the lipid component of the diet.

Gnotobiotic mouse models colonized with wild-type or mutant strains of a butyrate-producing bacterium demonstrated that dietary fiber protects against colorectal carcinoma in a microbiota-dependent and butyrate-dependent manner (Donohoe et al. 2014). Due to high aerobic glycolysis by malignant tumors (Warburg effect), butyrate is metabolized less in tumors where it accumulates and functions as an HDAC inhibitor, stimulating histone acetylation, inhibiting cell proliferation, and inducing apoptosis in cancer cells (Donohoe et al. 2014). These findings suggest that probiotic/prebiotic strategies could modulate endogenous natural HDAC inhibitors, such as butyrate, for anticancer chemoprevention. Their lack of toxicity makes these natural compounds promising candidates for the chemoprevention as opposed to synthetic HDAC inhibitors used in chemotherapy.

14 Conclusions

Many bioactive dietary components are known for a wide range of activities in the prevention of various cancers. Another key aspect of the chemopreventive action of dietary factors is their potential ability to selectively target cancer cells, while maintaining negligible cytotoxicity to normal cells. Recent studies provide substantial evidence that their protective roles are exerted through epigenetic mechanisms. Major epigenetic changes, including DNA methylation, chromatin modifications, and noncoding miRNA modification of gene expression, play important roles in carcinogenesis. The growing interest in cancer epigenetics is largely due to the reversible nature of epigenetic changes. Dietary components may affect DNA methylation, histone modifications, and miRNA expression in cancer. Thus, nutri-epigenetics and nutri-epigenomics have emerged as growing and promising fields in current cancer research in recent years. However, the precise mechanisms and their cellular targets in human cancers are not fully elucidated.

To provide safe dietary recommendations, it is necessary to identify the relevant bioactive dietary components and establish the optimal doses required for a chemopreventive effect. A key determination is the ability of bioactive dietary factors to distribute throughout the body and reach target tissues in concentrations that are sufficient to induce desirable epigenetic changes. Further studies are needed to determine effective doses and concentrations of bioactive dietary factors that are optimal for cancer prevention or treatment. Metabolism could play a pivotal role in generating intermediates with potential epigenetic effects. The interaction of dietary components with one another and with the body's metabolism, in addition to interactions with environmental factors, has made identifying key compounds even more difficult. It will be necessary for future studies to also characterize the tissue- and cell-type specificities of bioactive dietary compounds.

Another key determination to make is whether natural DNMT and HDAC inhibitors have only beneficial effects, or whether there are conditions when they might be harmful. Natural epigenetic inhibitors might cause unselective changes on global genome DNA methylation and impair genome stability. This could have a substantial effect on target genes involved in multiple signaling and cancer-related pathways, including the modulation of apoptosis and cell cycle arrest. Thus, the phytoestrogens genistein and apigenin have a stimulatory effect on the proliferation of ERα-positive breast cancer cells (Seo et al. 2006), suggesting that some bioactive dietary factors could have detrimental effects on specific cancer types. These findings indicate that comprehensive evaluations are warranted for long-term exposure and the use of concentrated phytoestrogen supplements in cancer patients.

Although observational studies have provided some insights into interactions between genetic or phenotypic variation and diet, and their impact on health, very few human dietary intervention studies have addressed these relationships. The first study demonstrating that natural dietary compounds from broccoli have a substantial effect on HDAC activity in human subjects showed that a single ingestion of one cup (68 g) of broccoli sprouts inhibited HDAC activity in circulating peripheral blood mononuclear cells early as 3 h after broccoli intake, whereas histone hyperacetylation persisted for at least 48 h (Myzak et al. 2007). These findings suggest that HDAC activity in peripheral blood mononuclear cells could be used as future biomarker for the discovery and the evaluation of novel dietary HDAC inhibitors in human subjects. An important area for future research will be developing high-throughput assays/methods for further elucidation of the complex interplay among nutrition, epigenetics, and cancer (Supic et al. 2013). Additional research is necessary to determine beneficial versus deleterious responses in healthy individuals and to provide personalized dietary recommendations (Lampe et al. 2013). The question as to whether nonhereditary cancers could be prevented or managed by controlled diet and lifestyle now arises (Toden and Goel 2014).

The critical question is prenatal exposure to dietary factors and caloric restriction. It has been shown that maternal diet and folate intake could affect long-term DNA methylation changes in offspring that occur later in life (Heijmans et al. 2008; Hughes et al. 2009). A recent study showed that prenatal dietary supplementation with polyunsaturated fatty acid was associated with higher methylation levels of imprinted regions in infants (Lee et al. 2014).

The complex interactions among environmental, genetic, and epigenetic factors in cancer development have not yet been fully identified. Elucidating the epigenetic mechanisms that underlie these modifications may serve as a tool to predict the individual genetic susceptibility to cancer, provide dietary recommendations, or provide therapeutic applications of natural compounds against cancer. Further characterization of the chemopreventive properties of bioactive compounds is warranted to potentially establish the clinical utility of dietary factors as anticancer compounds alone, or in combination with other dietary agents or well-known clinical therapeutics. Despite many unresolved questions, there is a promising future for dietary recommendations in cancer prevention and for therapeutic applications of natural dietary components in the future treatment of cancer.

References

Agarwal S, Amin KS, Jagadeesh S et al (2013) Mahanine restores RASSF1A expression by down-regulating DNMT1 and DNMT3B in prostate cancer cells. Mol Cancer 12(1):99

Ahamed S, Foster JS, Bukovsky A et al (2001) Signal transduction through the Ras/Erk pathway is essential for the mycoestrogen zearalenone-induced cell-cycle progression in MCF-7 cells. Mol Carcinog 30:88–98

Ahmad A, Sarkar SH, Bitar B et al (2012) Garcinol regulates EMT and Wnt signaling pathways in vitro and in vivo, leading to anticancer activity against breast cancer cells. Mol Cancer Ther 11:2193–2201

Altonsy MO, Habib TN, Andrews SC (2012) Diallyl disulfide-induced apoptosis in a breast-cancer cell line (MCF-7) may be caused by inhibition of histone deacetylation. Nutr Cancer 64:1251–1260

Amin KS, Jagadeesh S, Baishya G et al (2014) A naturally derived small molecule disrupts ligand-dependent and ligand-independent androgen receptor signaling in human prostate cancer cells. Mol Cancer Ther 13:341–352

Anderson OS, Sant KE, Dolinoy DC (2012) Nutrition and epigenetics: an interplay of dietary methyl donors, one-carbon metabolism and DNA methylation. J Nutr Biochem 23:853–859

Andrade FO, Nagamine MK, Conti AD et al (2012) Efficacy of the dietary histone deacetylase inhibitor butyrate alone or in combination with vitamin A against proliferation of MCF-7 human breast cancer cells. Braz J Med Biol Res 45:841–850

Arunkumar A, Vijayababu MR, Gunadharini N et al (2007) Induction of apoptosis and histone hyperacetylation by diallyl disulfide in prostate cancer cell line PC-3. Cancer Lett 251:59–67

Banerjee T, Chakravarti D (2011) A peek into the complex realm of histone phosphorylation. Mol Cell Biol 31:4858–4873

Barrera LN, Johnson IT, Bao Y et al (2013) Colorectal cancer cells Caco-2 and HCT116 resist epigenetic effects of isothiocyanates and selenium in vitro. Eur J Nutr 52:1327–1341

Belinsky SA, Palmisano WA, Gilliland FD et al (2002) Aberrant promoter methylation in bronchial epithelium and sputum from current and former smokers. Cancer Res 62:2370–2377

Berletch J, Liu C, Love W et al (2008) Epigenetic and genetic mechanisms contribute to telomerase inhibition by EGCG. J Cell Biochem 103:509–519

Cai DW, Liu XF, Bu RG et al (2009) Genetic polymorphisms of MTHFR and aberrant promoter hypermethylation of the RASSF1A gene in bladder cancer risk in a Chinese population. J Int Med Res 37:1882–1889

Cappelletti V, Fioravanti L, Miodini P et al (2000) Genistein blocks breast cancer cells in the G(2) M phase of the cell cycle. J Cell Biochem 79:594–600

Chen Y, Zaman MS, Deng G et al (2011) MicroRNAs 221/222 and genistein-mediated regulation of ARHI tumor suppressor gene in prostate cancer. Cancer Prev Res 4:76–86

Chung I, Han G, Seshadri M et al (2009) Role of vitamin D receptor in the antiproliferative effects of calcitriol in tumor-derived endothelial cells and tumor angiogenesis in vivo. Cancer Res 69:967–975

Colacino JA, Arthur AE, Dolinoy DC et al (2012) Pretreatment dietary intake is associated with tumor suppressor DNA methylation in head and neck squamous cell carcinomas. Epigenetics 7:883–891

Crim KC, Sanders LM, Hong MY et al (2008) Upregulation of p21Waf1/Cip1 expression in vivo by butyrate administration can be chemoprotective or chemopromotive depending on the lipid component of the diet. Carcinogenesis 29(7):1415–1420

Das R, Bhattacharya K, Samanta SK et al (2014) Improved chemosensitivity in cervical cancer to cisplatin: synergistic activity of mahanine through STAT3 inhibition. Cancer Lett 351:81–90

Davis CD, Milner JA (2011) Nutrigenomics, vitamin D and cancer prevention. J Nutrigenet Nutrigenomics 4:1–11

Davis CD, Ross SA (2008) Evidence for dietary regulation of microRNA expression in cancer cells. Nutr Rev 66:477–482

Davis C, Uthus E (2002) Dietary selenite and azadeoxycytidine treatments affect dimethylhydrazine-induced aberrant crypt formation in rat colon and DNA methylation in HT-29 cells. J Nutr 132:292–297

Davis C, Uthus E, Finley J (2000) Dietary selenium and arsenic affect DNA methylation in vitro in Caco-2 cells and in vivo in rat liver and colon. J Nutr 130:2903–2909

Donohoe DR, Holley D, Collins LB et al (2014) A gnotobiotic mouse model demonstrates that dietary fiber protects against colorectal tumorigenesis in a microbiota- and butyrate-dependent manner. Cancer Discov 4:1–10

Druesne N, Pagniez A, Mayeur C et al (2004a) Diallyl disulfide (DADS) increases histone acetylation and p21(waf1/cip1) expression in human colon tumor cell lines. Carcinogenesis 25:1227–1236

Druesne N, Pagniez A, Mayeur C et al (2004b) Repetitive treatments of colon HT-29 cells with diallyl disulfide induce a prolonged hyperacetylation of histone H3 K14. Ann N Y Acad Sci 1030:612–621

Esteller M (2007) Epigenetic gene silencing in cancer: the DNA hypermethylome. Hum Mol Genet 16:R50–R59

Fang M, Wang Y, Ai N et al (2003) Tea polyphenol (−)-epigallocatechin-3-gallate inhibits DNA methyltransferase and reactivates methylation-silenced genes in cancer cell lines. Cancer Res 63:7563–7570

Fang M, Chen D, Sun Y et al (2005) Reversal of hypermethylation and reactivation of p16INK4a, RARbeta, and MGMT genes by genistein and other isoflavones from soy. Cancer Res 11:7033–7041

Feldman D, Krishnan AV, Swami S et al (2014) The role of vitamin D in reducing cancer risk and progression. Nat Rev Cancer 14:342–357

Fetahu IS, Höbaus J, Kállay E (2014) Vitamin D and the epigenome. Front Physiol 5:164

Fiala E, Staretz M, Pandya G et al (1998) Inhibition of DNA cytosine methyltransferase by chemopreventive selenium compounds, determined by an improved assay for DNA cytosine methyltransferase and DNA cytosine methylation. Carcinogenesis 19:597–604

Gandhy SU, Kim K, Larsen L et al (2012) Curcumin and synthetic analogs induce reactive oxygen species and decreases specificity protein (Sp) transcription factors by targeting microRNAs. BMC Cancer 12:564

Gao W, Chan JY, Wong TS (2014) Curcumin exerts inhibitory effects on undifferentiated nasopharyngeal carcinoma by inhibiting the expression of miR-125a-5p. Clin Sci (Lond) 127:571–579

Girault I, Tozlu S, Lidereau R, Bieche I (2003) Expression analysis of DNA methyltransferases 1, 3A, and 3B in sporadic breast carcinomas. Clin Cancer Res 9:4415–4422

Groh IA, Chen C, Lüske C et al (2013) Plant polyphenols and oxidative metabolites of the herbal alkenylbenzene methyleugenol suppress histone deacetylase activity in human colon carcinoma cells. J Nutr Metab 2013:821082

Guo J, Li W, Shi H et al (2013) Synergistic effects of curcumin with emodin against the proliferation and invasion of breast cancer cells through upregulation of miR-34a. Mol Cell Biochem 382:103–111

Heijmans B, Tobi E, Stein A et al (2008) Persistent epigenetic differences associated with prenatal exposure to famine in humans. PNAS 105:17046–17049

Herman JG, Baylin SB (2003) Gene silencing in cancer in association with promoter hypermethylation. N Engl J Med 349:2042–2054

Ho E, Clarke JD, Dashwood RH (2009) Dietary sulforaphane, a histone deacetylases inhibitor for cancer prevention. J Nutr 139:2393–2396

Hobaus J, Fetahu IS, Khorchide M et al (2013) Epigenetic regulation of the 1,25-dihydroxyvitamin D(3) 24-hydroxylase (CYP24A1) in colon cancer cells. J Steroid Biochem Mol Biol 136:296–299

Hsieh CJ, Kuo PL, Hsu YC et al (2014) Arctigenin, a dietary phytoestrogen, induces apoptosis of estrogen receptor-negative breast cancer cells through the ROS/p38 MAPK pathway and epigenetic regulation. Free Radic Biol Med 67:159–170

Hu Y, McIntosh GH, Le Leu RK et al (2013a) Combination of selenium and green tea improves the efficacy of chemoprevention in a rat colorectal cancer model by modulating genetic and epigenetic biomarkers. PLoS One 8:e64362

Hu HY, Li KP, Wang XJ et al (2013b) Set9, NF-κB, and microRNA-21 mediate berberine-induced apoptosis of human multiple myeloma cells. Acta Pharmacol Sin 34:157–166

Hughes LA, van den Brandt PA, de Bruïne AP et al (2009) Early life exposure to famine and colorectal cancer risk: a role for epigenetic mechanisms. PLoS One 4:e7951

Jagadeesh S, Sinha S, Pal BC et al (2007) Mahanine reverses an epigenetically silenced tumor suppressor gene RASSF1A in human prostate cancer cells. Biochem Biophys Res Commun 362:212–217

Jawaid K, Crane SR, Nowers JL et al (2010) Long-term genistein treatment of MCF-7 cells decreases acetylated histone 3 expression and alters growth responses to mitogens and histone deacetylase inhibitors. J Steroid Biochem Mol Biol 120:164–171

Jenuwein T, Allis CD (2001) Translating the histone code. Science 293:1074–1080

Kai L, Samuel SK, Levenson AS (2010) Resveratrol enhances p53 acetylation and apoptosis in prostate cancer by inhibiting MTA1/NuRD complex. Int J Cancer 126:1538–1548
Kang S, Cha S, Jeon H (2006) Curcumin-induced histone hypoacetylation enhances caspase-3-dependent glioma cell death and neurogenesis of neural progenitor cells. Stem Cells Dev 15:165–169
Khan HY, Zubair H, Ullah MF et al (2012) A prooxidant mechanism for the anticancer and chemopreventive properties of plant polyphenols. Curr Drug Targets 13:1738–1749
Kikuno N, Shiina H, Urakami S et al (2008) Genistein mediated histone acetylation and demethylation activates tumor suppressor genes in prostate cancer cells. Int J Cancer 123:552–560
Kim Y (1999) Folate and carcinogenesis: evidence, mechanisms, and implications. J Nutr Biochem 10:66–88
Kouzarides T (2007) Chromatin modifications and their function. Cell 128:693–705
Kunnumakkara AB, Anand P, Aggarwal BB (2008) Curcumin inhibits proliferation, invasion, angiogenesis and metastasis of different cancers through interaction with multiple cell signaling proteins. Cancer Lett 269:199–225
Lampe JW, Navarro SL, Hullar MA, Shojaie A (2013) Inter-individual differences in response to dietary intervention: integrating omics platforms towards personalised dietary recommendations. Proc Nutr Soc 72:207–218
Lee WJ, Zhu BT (2006) Inhibition of DNA methylation by caffeic acid and chlorogenic acid, two common catechol-containing coffee polyphenols. Carcinogenesis 27:269–277
Lee WJ, Chen YR, Tseng TH (2011) Quercetin induces FasL-related apoptosis, in part, through promotion of histone H3 acetylation in human leukemia HL-60 cells. Oncol Rep 25:583–591
Lee HS, Barraza-Villarreal A, Biessy C et al (2014) Dietary supplementation with polyunsaturated fatty acid during pregnancy modulates DNA methylation at IGF2/H19 imprinted genes and growth of infants. Physiol Genomics 46(23):851–857. doi:10.1152/physiolgenomics.00061.2014
Li Y, Tollefsbol T (2010) Impact on DNA methylation in cancer prevention and therapy by bioactive dietary components. Curr Med Chem 17:2141–2151
Li K, Dias SJ, Rimando AM et al (2013a) Pterostilbene acts through metastasis-associated protein 1 to inhibit tumor growth, progression and metastasis in prostate cancer. PLoS One 8:e57542
Li Y, Meeran SM, Patel SN et al (2013b) Epigenetic reactivation of estrogen receptor-α (ERα) by genistein enhances hormonal therapy sensitivity in ERα-negative breast cancer. Mol Cancer 12:9–14
Liang HH, Wei PL, Hung CS et al (2013) MicroRNA-200a/b influenced the therapeutic effects of curcumin in hepatocellular carcinoma (HCC) cells. Tumour Biol 34:3209–3218
Link A, Balaguer F, Shen Y et al (2013) Curcumin modulates DNA methylation in colorectal cancer cells. PLoS One 8:e57709
Liu Y, Chakravarty S, Dey M (2013) Phenethylisothiocyanate alters site- and promoter-specific histone tail modifications in cancer cells. PLoS One 8:e64535
Lopes N, Carvalho J, Duraes C et al (2012) 1Alpha,25-dihydroxyvitamin D3 Induces de novo E-cadherin Expression in Triple-negative Breast Cancer Cells by CDH1-promoter Demethylation. Anticancer Res 32:249–257
Lu H, Meng X, Li C et al (2003) Glucuronides of tea catechins: enzymology of biosynthesis and biological activities. Drug Metab Dispos 31:452–461
Lu R, Wang X, Sun D et al (2008) Folic acid and sodium butyrate prevent tumorigenesis in a mouse model of colorectal cancer. Epigenetics 3:330–335
Lujambio A, Ropero S, Ballestar E et al (2007) Genetic unmasking of an epigenetically silenced microRNA in human cancer cells. Cancer Res 67(4):1424–1429
Magic Z, Supic G, Brankovic-Magic M (2009) Towards targeted epigenetic therapy of cancer. J BUON 14(Suppl 1):S79–S88
Mahlknecht U, Hoelzer D (2000) Histone acetylation modifiers in the pathogenesis of malignant disease. Mol Med 6:623–644

Margueron R, Trojer P, Reinberg D (2005) The key to development: interpreting the histone code? Cur Opin Genet Dev 15:163–176
Mas S, Lafuente MJ, Crescenti A et al (2007) Lower specific micronutrient intake in colorectal cancer patients with tumors presenting promoter hypermethylation in p16(INK4a), p4(ARF) and hMLH1. Anticancer Res 27:1151–1156
Meeran S, Patel S, Tollefsbol T (2010) Sulforaphane causes epigenetic repression of hTERT expression in human breast cancer cell lines. PLoS One 5:e11457
Meeran SM, Patel SN, Chan TH et al (2011) A novel prodrug of epigallocatechin-3-gallate: differential epigenetic hTERT repression in human breast cancer cells. Cancer Prev Res (Phila) 4:1243–1254
Miremadi A, Oestergaard M, Pharoah P et al (2007) Cancer genetics of epigenetic genes. Hum Mol Genet 16:28–49
Mirza S, Sharma G, Parshad R et al (2013) Expression of DNA methyltransferases in breast cancer patients and to analyze the effect of natural compounds on DNA methyltransferases and associated proteins. J Breast Cancer 16:23–31
Mittal A, Pate MS, Wylie RC et al (2004) EGCG downregulates telomerase in human breast carcinoma MCF-7 cells, leading to suppression of cell viability and induction of apoptosis. Int J Oncol 24:703–710
Myzak M, Dashwood R (2006) Histone deacetylases as targets for dietary cancer preventive agents: lessons learned with butyrate, diallyl disulfide, and sulforaphane. Curr Drug Targets 7:443–452
Myzak MC, Hardin K, Wang R et al (2006a) Sulforaphane inhibits histone deacetylase activity in BPH-1, LnCaP and PC-3 prostate epithelial cells. Carcinogenesis 27:811–819
Myzak MC, Dashwood WM, Orner GA et al (2006b) Sulforaphane inhibits histone deacetylase in vivo and suppresses tumorigenesis in Apc-minus mice. FASEB J 20:506–508
Myzak M, Tong P, Dashwood W et al (2007) Sulforaphane retards the growth of human PC-3 xenografts and inhibits HDAC activity in human subjects. Exp Biol Med (Maywood) 232:227–234
Nandakumar V, Vaid M, Katiyar SK (2011) (-)-Epigallocatechin-3-gallate reactivates silenced tumor suppressor genes, Cip1/p21 and p16INK4a, by reducing DNA methylation and increasing histones acetylation in human skin cancer cells. Carcinogenesis 32:537–544
Negrini M, Ferracin M, Sabbioni S et al (2007) MicroRNAs in human cancer: from research to therapy. J Cell Sci 120:1833–1840
Nian H, Delage B, Pinto JT et al (2008) Allyl mercaptan, a garlic-derived organosulfur compound, inhibits histone deacetylase and enhances Sp3 binding on the P21WAF1 promoter. Carcinogenesis 29:1816–1824
Nian H, Delage B, Ho E et al (2009) Modulation of histone deacetylases activity by dietary isothiocyanates and allyl sulfides: studies with sulforaphane and garlic organosulfur compounds. Environ Mol Mutagen 50:213–221
Padi SK, Zhang Q, Rustum YM et al (2013) MicroRNA-627 mediates the epigenetic mechanisms of vitamin D to suppress proliferation of human colorectal cancer cells and growth of xenograft tumors in mice. Gastroenterology 145:437–446
Papoutsis A, Lamore S, Wondrak G et al (2010) Resveratrol prevents epigenetic silencing of BRCA-1 by the aromatic hydrocarbon receptor in human breast cancer cells. J Nutr 140:1607–1614
Papoutsis AJ, Borg J, Selmin O et al (2012) BRCA-1 promoter hypermethylation and silencing induced by the aromatic hydrocarbon receptor-ligand TCDD are prevented by resveratrol in MCF-7 cells. J Nutr Biochem 23:1324–1332
Papoutsis AJ, Selmin OI, Borg JL et al (2013) Gestational exposure to the AhR agonist 2,3,7,8-tetrachlorodibenzo-p-dioxin induces BRCA-1 promoter hypermethylation and reduces BRCA-1 expression in mammary tissue of rat offspring: preventive effects of resveratrol. Mol Carcinog 54(4):261–269. doi:10.1002/mc.22095

Parasramka MA, Ali S, Banerjee S et al (2013) Garcinol sensitizes human pancreatic adenocarcinoma cells to gemcitabine in association with microRNA signatures. Mol Nutr Food Res 57:235–248
Paredes-Gonzalez X, Fuentes F, Su ZY et al (2014) Apigenin reactivates Nrf2 anti-oxidative stress signaling in mouse skin epidermal JB6P+ cells through epigenetics modifications. AAPS J 16:727–735
Parker L, Taylor D, Kesterson J et al (2009) Modulation of microRNA associated with ovarian cancer cells by genistein. Eur J Gynaecol Oncol 30:616–621
Paz M, Avila S, Fraga M et al (2002) Germ-line variants in methyl-group metabolism genes and susceptibility to DNA methylation in normal tissues and human primary tumors. Cancer Res 62:4519–4524
Pereira F, Barbachano A, Silva J et al (2011) KDM6B/JMJD3 histone demethylase is induced by vitamin D and modulates its effects in colon cancer cells. Hum Mol Genet 20:4655–4665
Pereira F, Barbachano A, Singh PK et al (2012) Vitamin D has wide regulatory effects on histone demethylase genes. Cell Cycle 11:1081–1089
Priyadarsini R, Vinothini G, Murugan R et al (2011) The flavonoid quercetin modulates the hallmark capabilities of hamster buccal pouch tumors. Nutr Cancer 63:218–226
Puccetti E, Obradovic D, Beissert T et al (2002) AML-associated translocation products block vitamin D(3)-induced differentiation by sequestering the vitamin D(3) receptor. Cancer Res 62:7050–7058
Pudenz M, Roth K, Gerhauser C (2014) Impact of soy isoflavones on the epigenome in cancer prevention. Nutrients 6:4218–4272
Qing Y, Hu H, Liu Y et al (2014) Berberine induces apoptosis in human multiple myeloma cell line U266 through hypomethylation of p53 promoter. Cell Biol Int 38:563–570
Rashid SF, Moore JS, Walker E et al (2001) Synergistic growth inhibition of prostate cancer cells by 1 alpha,25 Dihydroxyvitamin D(3) and its 19-nor-hexafluoride analogs in combination with either sodium butyrate or trichostatin A. Oncogene 20:1860–1872
Rawson JB, Sun Z, Dicks E et al (2012) Vitamin D intake is negatively associated with promoter methylation of the Wnt antagonist gene DKK1 in a large group of colorectal cancer patients. Nutr Cancer 64:919–928
Riso P, Martini D, Visioli F et al (2009) Effect of broccoli intake on markers related to oxidative stress and cancer risk in healthy smokers and nonsmokers. Nutr Cancer 61:232–237
Roy S, Yu Y, Padhye SB et al (2013) Difluorinated-curcumin (CDF) restores PTEN expression in colon cancer cells by down-regulating miR-21. PLoS One 8:e68543
Royt M, Mukherjee S (2014) Reversal of resistance towards cisplatin by curcumin in cervical cancer cells. Asian Pac J Cancer Prev 15:1403–1410
Royt M, Mukherjee S, Sarkar R et al (2011) Curcumin sensitizes chemotherapeutic drugs via modulation of PKC, telomerase, NF-kappaB and HDAC in breast cancer. Ther Deliv 2:1275–1293
Saha SK, Khuda-Bukhsh AR (2014) Berberine alters epigenetic modifications, disrupts microtubule network, and modulates HPV-18 E6-E7 oncoproteins by targeting p53 in cervical cancer cell HeLa: A mechanistic study including molecular docking. Eur J Pharmacol 744:132–146
Salerno E, Scaglione B, Coffman F et al (2009) Correcting miRNA-15a/16 genetic defect in New Zealand Black mouse model of CLL enhances drug sensitivity. Mol Cancer Ther 8:2684–2692
Scharlau D, Borowicki A, Habermann N et al (2009) Mechanisms of primary cancer prevention by butyrate and other products formed during gut flora-mediated fermentation of dietary fibre. Mutat Res 682:39–53
Seo HS, DeNardo DG, Jacquot Y et al (2006) Stimulatory effect of genistein and apigenin on the growth of breast cancer cells correlates with their ability to activate ER alpha. Breast Cancer Res Treat 99:121–134
Shah MS, Davidson LA, Chapkin RS (2012) Mechanistic insights into the role of microRNAs in cancer: influence of nutrient crosstalk. Front Genet 3:305

Shankar S, Srivastava R (2007) Involvement of Bcl-2 family members, phosphatidylinositol 30-kinase-AKT and mitochondrial p53 in curcumin (diferulolylmethane)-induced apoptosis in prostate cancer. Int J Oncol 30:905–918

Shen Y, Takahashi M, Byun HM et al (2012) Boswellic acid induces epigenetic alterations by modulating DNA methylation in colorectal cancer cells. Cancer Biol Ther 13:542–552

Shivdasani RA (2006) MicroRNAs: regulators of gene expression and cell differentiation. Blood 108:3646–3653

Shukla S, Meeran SM, Katiyar SK (2014) Epigenetic regulation by selected dietary phytochemicals in cancer chemoprevention. Cancer Lett 355:9–17

Spurling C, Suhl J, Boucher N et al (2008) The short chain fatty acid butyrate induces promoter demethylation and reactivation of RARβ2 in colon cancer cells. Nutr Cancer 60:692–702

Stefanska B, Karlic H, Varga F et al (2012a) Epigenetic mechanisms in anti-cancer actions of bioactive food components—the implications in cancer prevention. Br J Pharmacol 167:279–297

Stefanska B, Salamé P, Bednarek A et al (2012b) Comparative effects of retinoic acid, vitamin D and resveratrol alone and in combination with adenosine analogues on methylation and expression of phosphatase and tensin homologue tumour suppressor gene in breast cancer cells. Br J Nutr 107:781–790

Steward W, Brown K (2013) Cancer chemoprevention: a rapidly evolving field. Br J Cancer 109:1–7

Stopper H, Schmitt E, Kobras K (2005) Genotoxicity of phytoestrogens. Mutat Res 574:139–155

Su ZY, Zhang C, Lee JH et al (2014) Requirement and epigenetics reprogramming of Nrf2 in suppression of tumor promoter TPA-induced mouse skin cell transformation by sulforaphane. Cancer Prev Res (Phila) 7:319–329

Sun M, Estrov Z, Ji Y et al (2008) Curcumin (diferuloylmethane) alters the expression profiles of microRNAs in human pancreatic cancer cells. Mol Cancer Ther 7:464–473

Sun Q, Cong R, Yan H et al (2009a) Genistein inhibits growth of human uveal melanoma cells and affects microRNA-27a and target gene expression. Oncol Rep 22:563–567

Sun Y, Xun K, Wang Y et al (2009b) A systematic review of the anticancer properties of berberine, a natural product from Chinese herbs. Anti-Cancer Drugs 20:757–769

Supic G, Kozomara R, Branković-Magić M et al (2009) Gene hypermethylation in tumor tissue of advanced oral squamous cell carcinoma patients. Oral Oncol 45:1051–1057

Supic G, Jovic N, Kozomara R et al (2011a) Interaction between the MTHFR C677T polymorphism and alcohol—impact on oral cancer risk and multiple DNA methylation of tumor-related genes. J Dent Res 90:65–70

Supic G, Kozomara R, Jovic N et al (2011b) Prognostic significance of tumor-related genes hypermethylation detected in cancer-free surgical margins of oral squamous cell carcinomas. Oral Oncol 47:702–708

Supic G, Jagodic M, Magic Z (2013) Epigenetics: a new link between nutrition and cancer. Nutr Cancer 65:781–792

Szyf M (2005) DNA methylation and cancer therapy. Kluwer Academic, New York

Takahashi M, Sung B, Shen Y et al (2012) Boswellic acid exerts antitumor effects in colorectal cancer cells by modulating expression of the let-7 and miR-200 microRNA family. Carcinogenesis 33:2441–2449

Tang H, Kong Y, Guo J et al (2013) Diallyl disulfide suppresses proliferation and induces apoptosis in human gastric cancer through Wnt-1 signaling pathway by up-regulation of miR-200b and miR-22. Cancer Lett 340:72–81

Tobi EW, Lumey LH, Talens RP et al (2009) DNA methylation differences after exposure to prenatal famine are common and timing and sex-specific. Hum Mol Genet 18:4046–4053

Toden S, Goel A (2014) The importance of diets and epigenetics in cancer prevention: a hope and promise for the future? Altern Ther Health Med 20:6–11

Tollefsbol T (2009) Cancer epigenetics. CRC Press, Boca Raton

Tortorella SM, Royce SG, Licciardi PV et al (2014) Dietary sulforaphane in cancer chemoprevention: the role of epigenetic regulation and HDAC inhibition. Antioxid Redox Signal 22:1382–1424. doi:10.1089/ars.2014.6097

Tsang WP, Kwok TT (2010) Epigallocatechin gallate up-regulation of miRNA-16 and induction of apoptosis in human cancer cells. J Nutr Biochem 21:140–146
Ullah MF, Khan MW (2008) Food as medicine: potential therapeutic tendencies of plant derived polyphenolic compounds. Asian Pac J Cancer Prev 9:187–195
Uthus E, Ross S (2007) Dietary selenium affects homocysteine metabolism differently in Fisher-344 rats and CD-1 mice. J Nutr 137:1132–1136
van England M, Weijenberg MP, Roemen GM et al (2003) Effects of folate and alcohol intake on promoter methylation in sporadic colorectal cancer: the Netherlands cohort study on diet and cancer. Cancer Res 63:3133–3137
Vardi A, Bosviel R, Rabiau N et al (2010) Soy phytoestrogens modify DNA methylation of GSTP1, RASSF1A, EPH2 and BRCA1 promoter in prostate cancer cells. In Vivo 24:393–400
Wang P, Heber D, Henning S (2012a) Quercetin increased the antiproliferative activity of green tea polyphenol (-)-epigallocatechin gallate in prostate cancer cells. Nutr Cancer 64:580–587
Wang P, Heber D, Henning SM (2012b) Quercetin increased bioavailability and decreased methylation of green tea polyphenols in vitro and in vivo. Food Funct 3:635–642
Waterland RA, Jirtle RL (2003) Transposable elements: targets for early nutritional effects on epigenetic gene regulation. Mol Cell Biol 23:5293–5300
Wolff GL, Kodell RL, Moore SR et al (1998) Maternal epigenetics and methyl supplements affect agouti gene expression in Avy/a mice. FASEB J 12:949–957
Wong CP, Hsu A, Buchanan A et al (2014) Effects of sulforaphane and 3,3'-diindolylmethane on genome-wide promoter methylation in normal prostate epithelial cells and prostate cancer cells. PLoS One 9:e86787
Wu ML, Li H, Yu LJ et al (2014) Short-term resveratrol exposure causes in vitro and in vivo growth inhibition and apoptosis of bladder cancer cells. PLoS One 9:e89806
Xiao D, Zeng Y, Hahm ER et al (2009) Diallyl trisulfide selectively causes Bax- and Bak-mediated apoptosis in human lung cancer cells. Environ Mol Mutagen 50:201–212
Yang C, Landau J, Huang M et al (2001) Inhibition of carcinogenesis by dietary polyphenolic compounds. Annu Rev Nutr 21:381–406
Yang J, Cao Y, Sun J et al (2010) Curcumin reduces the expression of Bcl-2 by upregulating miRNA-15a and miRNA-16 in MCF-7 cells. Med Oncol 27:1114–1118
Yeung F, Hoberg JE, Ramsey CS et al (2004) Modulation of NF-kappaB-dependent transcription and cell survival by the SIRT1 deacetylase. EMBO J 23:2369–2380
Yu Z, Xiao Q, Zhao L et al (2014) DNA methyltransferase 1/3a overexpression in sporadic breast cancer is associated with reduced expression of estrogen receptor-alpha/breast cancer susceptibility gene 1 and poor prognosis. Mol Carcinog. doi:10.1002/mc.22133
Zeljic K, Supic G, Stamenkovic Radak M et al (2012) Vitamin D receptor, CYP27B1 and CYP24A1 genes polymorphisms association with oral cancer risk and survival. J Oral Pathol Med 41:779–787
Zeljic K, Kandolf-Sekulovic L, Supic G et al (2014) Melanoma risk is associated with vitamin D receptor gene polymorphisms. Melanoma Res 24:273–279
Zhang C, Su ZY, Khor TO et al (2013) Sulforaphane enhances Nrf2 expression in prostate cancer TRAMP C1 cells through epigenetic regulation. Biochem Pharmacol 85:1398–1404
Zheng NG, Wang JL, Yang SL et al (2014) Aberrant epigenetic alteration in Eca9706 cells modulated by nanoliposomal quercetin combined with butyrate mediated via epigenetic-NF-κB signaling. Asian Pac J Cancer Prev 15:4539–4543
Zhu W, Qin W, Zhang K et al (2012) Trans-resveratrol alters mammary promoter hyper-methylation in women at increased risk for breast cancer. Nutr Cancer 64:393–400
Zilberman D, Cao X, Jacobsen SE (2003) ARGONAUTE4 control of locus-specific siRNA accumulation and DNA and histone methylation. Science 299:716–719

Potential for Sesame Seed-Derived Factors to Prevent Colorectal Cancer

Shingo Miyamoto, Gen Fujii, Masami Komiya, Masaru Terasaki, and Michihiro Mutoh

Abstract Colorectal cancers (CRCs) are steadily increasing in most advanced countries, including Japan. The mechanisms of colon carcinogenesis have yet to be fully elucidated, but it is assumed that factors, such as insulin resistance, dyslipidemia, inflammation, and subsequent adipocytokine imbalance, might be involved in the promotion of colorectal carcinogenesis. In this chapter, we focus on the chemopreventive effects of natural compounds, especially sesame seed-derived factors on colorectal carcinogenesis, with the current status and future prospects for CRC chemoprevention. Furthermore, molecules suggested to be involved in CRC development are described, and the potential for cancer prevention by targeting NADPH oxidase is also discussed with respect to its inhibitors.

S. Miyamoto • M. Komiya
Epidemiology and Prevention Division, Research Center for Cancer Prevention and Screening, National Cancer Center, 5-1-1 Tsukiji, Chuo-ku, Tokyo 104-0045, Japan

G. Fujii
Carcinogenesis and Cancer Prevention Division, National Cancer Center Research Institute, 5-1-1, Tsukiji, Chuo-ku, Tokyo 104-0045, Japan

M. Terasaki
Department of Health and Environmental Sciences, School of Pharmaceutical Sciences, Health Sciences University of Hokkaido, 1757 Kanazawa, Ishikari-Tobetsu, Hokkaido 061-0293, Japan

M. Mutoh (✉)
Epidemiology and Prevention Division, Research Center for Cancer Prevention and Screening, National Cancer Center, 5-1-1 Tsukiji, Chuo-ku, Tokyo 104-0045, Japan

Carcinogenesis and Cancer Prevention Division, National Cancer Center Research Institute, 5-1-1, Tsukiji, Chuo-ku, Tokyo 104-0045, Japan
e-mail: mimutoh@ncc.go.jp

M.F. Ullah, A. Ahmad (eds.), *Critical Dietary Factors in Cancer Chemoprevention*,
DOI 10.1007/978-3-319-21461-0_8

1 Introduction

Colorectal cancer (CRC) is the third most common cancer worldwide. The prevalence of CRC is increasing and is expected to increase to 2.4 million annually by 2035 worldwide (Siegel et al. 2012). In particular, the prevalence of CRC is increasing in Eastern countries, including Japan. Many Eastern countries have undergone a two- to fourfold increase in CRC incidence over recent decades (Sung et al. 2005).

To control CRC, new strategies are necessary, such as preventative strategies using cancer chemopreventive agents. There are four reasons to explore this approach: (1) CRC mortality remains high, despite extensive efforts in developing anticancer drugs; (2) CRC risk is, to some extent, attributable to environmental factors or inherited predispositions (Tomasetti and Vogelstein 2015); (3) the evolution of sporadic CRC from normal mucosa spans on average 10–20 years; thus, there is time for effective prevention and intervention; and (4) the screening and surveillance strategies for CRC patient uptake, i.e., fecal occult blood testing and endoscopy, are often suboptimal and limit real effectiveness.

Because CRC development is affected by dietary habits and lifestyle, one approach to develop efficient cancer preventative strategies is the use of functional agents in foods or plants as supplements/medicines. Epidemiological data support the idea that using the functional agents contained in "functional foods" is a useful approach. It has been suggested that the intake of high dietary fruits is associated with reduced cancer risk (Riboli and Norat 2003). The other approach is chemopreventive medicines, particularly using available synthetic drugs in terms of "drug repositioning" (Temraz et al. 2013; Komiya et al. 2013).

The World Cancer Research Fund and American Institute for Cancer Research have evaluated and provided strong evidence that there are causal relationships between body fat and CRC (World Cancer Research Fund/American Institute for Cancer Research 2007). The metabolic syndrome and so-called "obesity-associated cancers" are extremely common in Western countries, and they are currently increasing in Eastern countries. The mechanisms underlying how the obesity is linked to colorectal carcinogenesis are not fully understood yet. However, it is assumed that factors, such as insulin resistance, dyslipidemia, inflammation, and subsequent adipocytokine imbalance, may be involved in the promotion of carcinogenesis (Fujii et al. 2011). Of note, such factors play an important role in promoting cell growth, cell survival, and production of mitochondrial/NADPH oxidase (NOX)-derived reactive oxygen species (ROS).

In this chapter, important aspects of the current status and future prospects for CRC chemoprevention, particularly using natural compounds (sesame seed-derived factors), are summarized. As discussed in the text, sesame seed-derived factors may provide health benefits, such as reduced inflammation. Moreover, the biological significance of NOX as an important target candidate for the chemoprevention of cancer is becoming clearer.

2 Sesame Plant

The sesame plant (*Sesamum indicum* L., Pedaliaceae family) is one of most prevalent edible seed and oil worldwide (Sugano and Akimoto 1993). Asian and African countries belonging to tropical and subtropical areas are the major producers (Abou-Gharbia et al. 2000). Sesame seed contains approximately 50 % oil, 20 % protein, 10 % carbohydrate, and unique flavors (Abou-Gharbia et al. 1997, 2000; Yoshida 1994). Sesame oil is used as nutritious food, cooking oil, pharmaceuticals, seasoning, shortening, margarine, soap, and insecticides (Xu et al. 2005; Doker et al. 2010). Components of sesame oil are characterized by the presence of fatty acids (arachidic, eicosenoic, linoleic, linolenic, oleic, palmitic, and stearic acids), oil-soluble lignans (asarinin, sesamin, sesaminol, sesamol, and sesamolin), phenol compounds (ferulic and *o*-Coumaric), phytosterols (β-sitosterol, campesterol, and stigmasterol), volatiles (hexanal, nonanal, pentanal, 2-pentylfuran, and terpene), and others (squalene, β and γ-tocopherol) (Haiyan et al. 2007; Ryan et al. 2007; Namiki 1995). Sesame oil shows strong antioxidant activity because it contains abundant amounts of antioxidants. γ-Tocopherol, sesamolin, and sesamin, potent fat-soluble antioxidants, are contained at approximately 0.3, 1.0–7.0, and 2.0–11.0 mg/g dry weight, respectively, in sesame oil (Namiki 1995; Wu 2007; Wang et al. 2013; Cooney et al. 2001). Moreover, plasma concentrations of γ-tocopherol and sesamolin are easily enhanced by moderate dietary intake of sesame seed additive food by a daily intake of several ten grams of sesame seeds weekly (γ-tocopherol: 1.5 μg/mL and sesamolin: average 35.9 ng/mL in plasma) (Cooney et al. 2001). Recently, multiple biological functions of sesame seeds, such as the inhibition of inflammation and carcinogenesis, have been elucidated (Hagiwara et al. 1996; Hirose et al. 1992; Salerno and Smith 1991; Kapadia et al. 2002). In the next section, we will describe recent findings of five sesame seeds constituents (ferulic acid, sesamin, sesamolin, γ-tocopherol, and sesamol) on its biological function, especially its cancer preventive potential (Fig. 1).

3 Bioactivities and Anticancer Effects of Sesame Seed Constituents

3.1 Ferulic Acid

Ferulic acid has been reported to improve glucose tolerance and lipid metabolism (El-Seedi et al. 2012; Ardiansyah et al. 2006). Recently, Wang et al. reported that ferulic acid administration alleviated high-fat and high-fructose diet-induced metabolic syndrome parameters, such as obesity, hyperglycemia, hyperlipidemia, and insulin resistance (Wang et al. 2015). Several studies have shown that ferulic acid acts as a potent antioxidant by scavenging free radicals in rats (Sudheer et al. 2005).

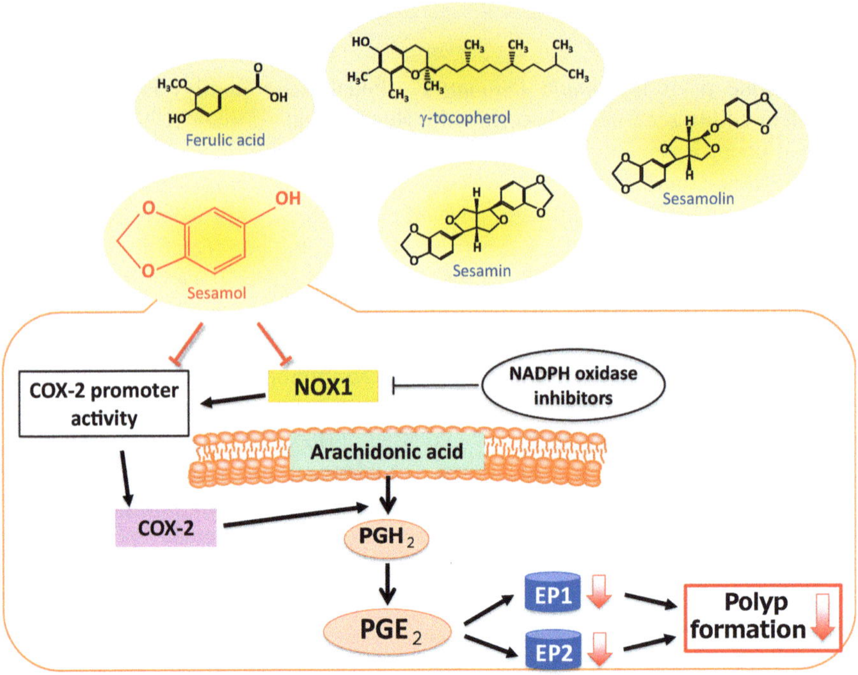

Fig. 1 Chemical structure of potential anticancer factors from sesame seed and proposed underlying mechanisms for the suppression of polyp formation in Min mice by Sesamol. Ferulic acid, sesamin, sesamolin, γ-tocopherol, and sesamol are the major sesame seed constituents that possess the potential anticancer effects. Indeed, in our experiments, sesamol suppressed intestinal polyp formation in Min mice. Interestingly, expression levels of PGE_2 receptor subtypes EP1 and EP2 were reduced in the polyp parts with sesamol administration. Furthermore, sesamol inhibited transcriptional activity of COX-2 promoter in colon cancer cells partly through the downregulation of NOX1 expression level. These results suggest that NADPH oxidase is an important target and sesamol could be a promising candidate for colorectal cancer chemoprevention

Antioxidants are considered potential inhibitors of cancer by protecting critical cellular molecules from oxidative damages. Indeed, ferulic acid suppresses chemically induced colon (Kawabata et al. 2000), skin (Asanoma et al. 1994), and lung carcinogenesis (Lesca 1983) in animals.

3.2 *Sesamin*

Sesamin is a furofuran-type lignan in sesame seed oil, which has potential benefits for health promotion (Pathak et al. 2014). Studies have shown that sesamin plays a significant role in lipid metabolism through the downregulation of lipogenic enzymes (Peñalvo et al. 2006), sterol regulatory element binding protein-1 (SREBP-1), acetyl-CoA carboxylase, and fatty acid synthase (Ide et al. 2001) in animals. In addition, sesamin inhibits cholesterol absorption and biosynthesis in humans (Hirose et al. 1991; Hirata et al. 1996). These bioactivities may be beneficial for preventing the obesity and atherosclerosis. Sesamin showed anti-inflammatory activities through the inhibition of $\Delta5$ desaturase, a key enzyme in arachidonic acid biosynthesis that leads to a lower level of pro-inflammatory mediators (Shimizu et al. 1991; Chavali et al. 1998). As inflammation plays an important role in carcinogenesis, sesamin could be a good candidate cancer preventive agent. Indeed, Hirose et al. reported that the administration of 0.2 % sesamin significantly reduced the number of 7,12-dimethylbenz[a]anthracene (DMBA)-induced palpable mammary cancers compared with control animals (Hirose et al. 1992).

3.3 Sesamolin

Sesamolin has been demonstrated to increase the activity and mRNA level of various enzymes involved in hepatic fatty acid oxidation in rats (Lim et al. 2007). Sesamolin is also known as an antioxidant and has been shown to have a protective effect in neuronal cells against hypoxic and lipopolysaccharide (LPS)-induced toxicity or excitotoxicity in vitro and in vivo (Hou et al. 2003a, b; Cheng et al. 2006). In addition, Miyahara et al. reported that sesamolin inhibited proliferation and induced apoptosis in human lymphoid leukemia Molt 4B cells (Miyahara et al. 2001).

3.4 γ-Tocopherol

γ-Tocopherol, the most abundant tocopherol in sesame seed oil, showed a very broad range of medicinal properties (including anticancer, antidiabetic, anti-inflammatory, and anti-oxidative effects) not only in preclinical studies but also in human intervention studies (Jiang 2014). In a preclinical model, γ-tocopherol administration attenuated dextran sulfate sodium (DSS)-induced colitis and azoxymethane (AOM)/DSS-induced colon tumorigenesis (Jiang et al. 2013), partly through the suppression of eicosanoids [prostaglandin (PG) E_2 and leukotriene B4] production (Ju et al. 2009). In addition, Takahashi et al. demonstrated that the supplementation of γ-tocopherol suppressed prostate tumor progression with the induction of apoptosis through caspase activation in the transgenic rats for adenocarcinoma of prostate (TRAP) model (Takahashi et al. 2009). Thus, γ-tocopherol exhibits strong anti-oxidative and anti-inflammatory effects in many studies, and it could be a good candidate as cancer preventive agent.

3.5 Sesamol

Sesamol is involved in the oil-soluble compartment as oil-soluble lignans. Sesamol possesses antioxidant (Hsu et al. 2006), anti-inflammatory (Chavali et al. 2001), and free radical scavenging activity (Parihar et al. 2006). As neutrophil-derived hydrogen peroxide (H_2O_2) plays an important role in the progression of inflammatory bowel disease (IBD), a previous report examined the sesamol protective effects on dinitrochlorobenzene (DNCB)-induced mucosal injury in a rat IBD model. Sesamol (100 mg/kg, po) treatment for 7 days significantly decreased the levels of myeloperoxidase, thiobarbituric acid reactive species, and nitrite in the colon tissue (Kondamudi et al. 2013). In a long-term animal experimental study, sesamol treatment at dietary levels up to 2 % for 2 years was shown to decrease the spontaneous development of preneoplastic hepatocytic foci in F344 rats (Hagiwara et al. 1996).

In our experiments, among the four sesame seed constituents (ferulic acid, sesamin, sesamol, and sesamolin), 100 μM sesamol treatment in a human colon cancer cell line, DLD-1 cells, for 48 h suppressed basal cyclooxygenase-2 (COX-2) promoter transcriptional activity as detected by a β-galactosidase reporter gene system (Mutoh et al. 2000; Shimizu et al. 2014). COX-2 is an inducible enzyme to produce PGE_2, and both COX-2 expression and PGE_2 levels are increased in colon carcinoma tissues compared with that of normal colonic mucosa. Accumulating evidence suggests that COX inhibitors suppress colon carcinogenesis in animal experiments and human trials (Komiya et al. 2013; Mutoh et al. 2006). It has also been reported that COX-2 gene knockout results in the reduction of intestinal polyp development in a model of human familial adenomatous polyposis, Min mice (Oshima et al. 1996). Thus, it is likely that agents that can suppress COX-2 expression at the transcriptional level may also suppress colon carcinogenesis in animal experiments and human trials.

We have shown the suppressive potential of sesamol on intestinal polyp development in Min mice (Shimizu et al. 2014). The administration of 500 ppm sesamol reduced the total number of intestinal polyp development compared with that of the untreated group. When the small intestine is divided into three parts, the proximal, middle, and distal parts, sesamol decreased the number of polyps in the middle part.

In the polyp parts of Min mice, sesamol suppressed COX-2 mRNA expression levels. Sesamol treatment also reduced cytosolic prostaglandin E synthase (cPGES) mRNA expression levels. Moreover, a tendency of suppression in the expression levels of PGE_2 receptor subtypes EP1 and EP2 in the polyp parts was observed. We confirmed the effect of sesamol on human EP1 and EP2 mRNA levels in DLD-1 cells and found that sesamol significantly suppressed EP1 and EP2 mRNA levels. PGE_2 receptor subtype-knockout mice have demonstrated that EP1, EP2, and EP4 are promotive receptors in colorectal carcinogenesis, and EP3 plays suppressive roles (Mutoh et al. 2006). Unfortunately, there are a few inhibitors for PGE_2 receptor subtypes. Thus, the novel potential of sesamol may be worthwhile from the aspect of developing chemopreventive agents.

In addition, we performed a preliminary experiment using intestinal polyp samples of Min mice to examine effects of sesamol on the expression levels of oxidative-related factors. We obtained the data showing a tendency toward the reduction of NOX1 mRNA by sesamol as described in the next section.

4 Possibility of NOX as a Novel Cancer Prevention Target

4.1 Nicotinamide Adenine Dinucleotide Phosphate Oxidase

Cancerous tissue is known to be under oxidative stress conditions. Distinct amounts of ROS are produced as a by-product from the mitochondrial respiratory chain, and a large amount of superoxide anion radical (O_2^-) is often generated by cancer cells due to a complex I dysfunction in mitochondria. The initial step in ROS formation is the generation of O_2^- and then proceeds to H_2O_2 and the hydroxyl radical (OH), which causes strong damage to cells (Halliwell 1978). At low ROS concentrations, intracellular signaling is initiated, whereas at high ROS concentrations, oxidative stress is induced. Extensive studies over the years have determined that high ROS conditions contribute to the progression of various human diseases, especially cancer. ROS targets regulate proliferation, including cellular signaling (phosphatases, AP1 and NF-κB) and cell cycle (CDC25, cyclin D, and forkhead proteins; G1, G2, respectively) proteins.

Another enzyme that generates ROS is NOX. Membrane-integrated NOX family oxidases, such as NOX1 and Duox2, are known to produce O_2^- or H_2O_2 (Sumimoto 2008). NOX is a multicomponent enzyme, which is formed of a complex, membrane-associated component (Nox1-5, Duox1, 2, and $p22^{phox}$), cytosolic components ($p47^{phox}$, Noxo1 (homologue of $p47^{phox}$), Noxa1 (homologue of $p67^{phox}$), and $p40^{phox}$), and the small GTP-binding protein Rac (Vulcano et al. 2004; Li and Shah 2001; Muzaffar et al. 2008; Brandes and Schroder 2008).

Correlating with activating mutations in *K-ras*, NOX1 is overexpressed in human colon cancers (Laurent et al. 2008). Other factors are also elevated in cancer cells and have been suggested to play an important role in carcinogenesis. The function of NOX2 and NOX3 in cancer is not well known. NOX4-generated ROS has been suggested to induce resistance of pancreatic cancer cells to apoptosis (Mochizuki et al. 2006), and its inhibition suppresses melanoma cell growth (Yamamura et al. 2009). On the other hand, Duox1 and Duox2 are remarkably suppressed in lung cancer cells due to the hypermethylation of CpG-rich regions of their promoters (Luxen et al. 2008).

4.2 NOX Inhibitors and Cancer/Carcinogenesis

As described in a previous section, many studies have indicated that the NOX family of genes appears to be required for survival and growth of a subset of human cancer cells. Thus, the NOX family should be a focus of attention in cancer etiology and cancer prevention studies (Kamata 2009). The significance of NOX in carcinogenesis has been shown in experiments using NOX inhibitors. NOX functional inhibitors are classified as (1) small molecule chemical NOX inhibitors and (2) biological inhibitors for NOX, such as neopterin and gp91ds-tat. In this section, we will review and discuss the relationship between NOX inhibitors (apocynin, diphenylene iodonium, vanillin, and methyl-vanillin) and carcinogenesis.

4.2.1 Apocynin (4′-Hydroxy-3′-Methoxyacetophenone; Acetovanillone)

Apocynin is a methoxy-substituted catechol, compound isolated from the traditional medicinal plant *P. kurroa*, and is structurally related to vanillin. Apocynin is commonly used as an inhibitor of NOX ($IC_{50} = 10$ μM) (Stefanska and Pawliczak 2008).

At 300 μM, it is effective in preventing the production of O_2^- in human white blood cells and neutrophilic granulocytes. Due to the selectivity of its inhibition, apocynin can be widely used as an NOX inhibitor without interfering in other systems. It has been used in the treatment of arthritis, bowel disease, asthma, atherosclerosis, and familial amyotrophic lateral sclerosis (Stefanska and Pawliczak 2008; Heumüller et al. 2008).

Studies have shown the ability of apocynin to decrease O_2^- generation in bovine pulmonary arteries as well as neutrophils and macrophages at 10 μM. In experimental rats, apocynin displayed anti-inflammatory activity and improved endothelial function by reducing oxidative stress. On the other hand, Heumüller et al. insisted that apocynin predominantly acts as an antioxidant in endothelial cells and vascular smooth muscle cells and should not be used as an NOX inhibitor in vascular systems (Heumüller et al. 2008).

Regarding carcinogenesis, Suzuki et al. noted that apocynin possesses chemopreventive potential against prostate cancer, using the TRAP model. The ratio and numbers of carcinomas in prostates were significantly reduced by apocynin treatment, with dose dependence (Suzuki et al. 2013a). The authors also found that apocynin significantly inhibited cell proliferation of the prostate cancer cell line PLS10 via inducing a G1 arrest of the cell cycle in vitro. Surprisingly, apocynin did not affect ROS production but inhibited phosphorylation of Rac1, a component of the NOX complex (Suzuki et al. 2013b).

In the same experiments, the expression and secretion of vascular endothelial growth factor (VEGF), important growth factor for malignant progression, were reduced by apocynin treatment (Suzuki et al. 2013b). In addition, it has been reported that ROS suppress adiponectin production in adipocytes, and treatment of obese mice with anti-oxidative agents improves insulin resistance and restores adiponectin production (Matsuda and Shimomura 2014). We previously discovered that mice with disruptions in adiponectin loci develop an increased number of intestinal tumors compared with wild-type mice (Mutoh et al. 2011). Therefore, we suggest that apocynin could be a direct and indirect chemopreventive reagent for carcinogenesis.

4.2.2 Diphenylene Iodonium

Diphenylene iodonium (DPI) is the most commonly used NOX inhibitor. DPI abstracts an electron from transporter and forms a radical, which inhibit the respective electron transport through a covalent binding step to flavin proteins. DPI is a very effective NOX inhibitor; however, it interferes with many other enzymes, such as nitric oxide synthase, xanthine oxidase, mitochondrial complex I, cytochrome P-450, etc. Therefore, DPI effectiveness could be due to effects other than its specific activity against NOX (Bedard and Krause 2007).

On that assumption, DPI could function in the malignant process. For example, DPI treatment strongly inhibits ROS generation and HIF-1α expression in MDA-MB-231 cells as well as cell migration and invasion. The inhibition of ROS production with DPI attenuates ERK1/2 activation (Liu et al. 2014).

4.2.3 Vanillin and Methyl-Vanillin

As noted above, apocynin is structurally related to vanillin, and apocynin powder has a fragrance similar to vanilla. Based on the structural resemblance, vanilla could function as an NOX inhibitor. Glutathione (GSH), cysteine, ovalbumin, and the coenzyme NADPH were chosen as potential target biomolecules that could be affected by transient free radicals from vanillin and vanillic acid (Castor et al. 2010).

Respiratory burst activity was suppressed by a previous infusion of 2 mM vanillin. Vanillin suppresses the respiratory burst activity of Kupffer cells as assessed in intact liver, which may be associated with the inhibition of macrophage NOX activity (Galgani et al. 2012).

Vanillin and apocynin inhibit cell migration, and both compounds selectively inhibit Akt phosphorylation of HGF signaling without affecting the phosphorylation of Met and Erk. Furthermore, vanillin and apocynin inhibit the enzymatic activity of phosphoinositide 3-kinase (PI3K), as revealed by an in vitro lipid kinase assay, suggesting that the inhibition of PI3K activity was a mechanism underlying the inhibitory effect on cancer cell migration, and the presence of an aldehyde or ketone group in the vanillin structure was important for this inhibition (Lirdprapamongkol et al. 2009).

Other small molecular chemicals, such as ABESF, Ebselen, ML171, VA2870, GKT137831, etc., function as NOX inhibitors in in vitro experiments; nevertheless, there are fewer reports of their effectiveness against carcinogenesis.

4.3 NOX and Sesamol

COX-2 is known to be induced by many stimuli, such as growth factors, mitogens, and pro-inflammatory cytokines (Mutoh et al. 2006). Thus, the downstream targets of protein-tyrosine kinases (PTKs), i.e., growth factor receptors, might be involved in the suppressive mechanisms of COX-2 promoter transcriptional activity by sesamol. Signals from activated PTKs are transduced to the downstream transcription factor NF-κB that regulates COX-2 expression. Based on this information, we further attempted to clarify the underlying suppressive mechanism of COX-2 promoter transcriptional activity by sesamol. However, NF-κB transcriptional activity is not suppressed by 100 μM sesamol in DLD-1 cells, which suggested that NF-κB is not a responsible target in this suppressive mechanism. Other responsible targets are the Ras and mitogen-activated protein kinases (MAPKs). Meanwhile, our preliminary experiment using intestinal polyp samples of Min mice showed that NOX might be one of the responsible targets.

Our preliminary results encouraged us to investigate the effects of NOX inhibitors, apocynin, benzaldehyde, and vanillin on COX-2 promoter transcriptional activity in DLD-1 cells. NOX inhibitors successfully demonstrated its potential to suppress COX-2 promoter transcriptional activity (Shimizu et al. 2015). It has been reported that LPS activates NOX and induces COX-2 expression, and these effects could be explained by ROS generation (Lin et al. 2011). It has been reported that ROS activates crucial components for mitogen signaling, such as p38 MAPK, Akt/PI3K, and tyrosine phosphatase (McCarty 2012). In our experiments using NOX inhibitors, we could not exclude the possibility that NOX inhibitors blocked ROS generation and thus suppressed COX-2 promoter transcriptional activity. The modulation of ROS generation explains this suppressive mechanism.

We also investigated the effects of sesamol on NOX1 and NOX2 mRNA expression levels in DLD-1 cells and found that NOX1 mRNA was strongly suppressed by sesamol treatment. Next, we knocked down NOX1 using NOX1-specific siRNAs and showed the suppression of COX-2 promoter transcriptional activity in DLD-1 cells. These data suggested that NOX1 plays a major role in the regulation of COX-2 promoter transcriptional activity. It is assumed that knocking down NOX1 can block complex formation of NOX components and result in NOX activity inhibition, as NOX inhibitors do. Of course, other factors, such as NOX2 and MAPK pathways, might be involved in the regulation of COX-2 expression, because we found that inhibitory effects of siRNA of NOX1 on COX-2 promoter transcriptional activity were not equal to those on NOX1 protein expression levels.

As mentioned, sesamol inhibits intestinal polyp development in *Apc*-mutant Min mice. *Apc* mutation results in β-catenin signaling activation and plays a pivotal role in the development of intestinal polyps. Recent studies have shown that β-catenin signaling could be inhibited by NOX1 ablation (Kajla et al. 2012). Thus, β-catenin signaling-induced COX-2 expression is another candidate pathway that explains the suppression of COX-2 promoter transcriptional activity by sesamol. Of note, it is worth mentioning that the downregulation of NOX1 by sesamol could be an additional approach against β-catenin signaling-dependent cancers, such as CRC.

5 Future Aspects

To control CRC, the challenge of the next decade will be using a double approach based on the development of innovative preventive strategies and anticancer therapies. Of note, preventative strategies using cancer chemopreventive agents might be a major approach for patients with a high cancer risk. Further means may be taken by combining two agents/drugs that target different pathway for effective prevention by safe medicines. From the aspects of health economics, there are financial benefits of using several drugs/combined medicine. For instance, it is recommended that clinical trials incorporate more than one agent or available synthetic drugs instead of a large and very expensive trial using one novel agent (Kaiser 2012).

Although the tools to accurately estimate CRC risk are improving, we still have to overcome some problems to achieve good CRC control: (1) we should further clarify the pathogenesis of CRC; (2) we should develop biomarkers to detect the early stages of CRC; and (3) we should identify or develop safe and effective chemopreventive agents against CRC. In this chapter, we described sesame seed-derived factors as examples of candidate chemopreventive agents derived from natural compounds and also suggested the biological significance of NOX as an important target candidate for the chemoprevention of CRC.

References

Abou-Gharbia HA, Shahidi F, Adel A, Shehata AAY, Youssef MM (1997) Effects of processing on oxidative stability of sesame oil extracted from intact and dehulled seeds. J Am Oil Chem Soc 74:215–221

Abou-Gharbia HA, Shehala AAY, Shahidi F (2000) Effect of processing on oxidative stability and lipid classes of sesame oil. Food Res Int 33:331–340

Ardiansyah SH, Koseki T, Ohinata K, Hashizume K, Komai M (2006) Rice bran fractions improve blood pressure, lipid profile, and glucose metabolism in stroke-prone spontaneously hypertensive rats. J Agric Food Chem 54:1914–1920

Asanoma M, Takahashi K, Miyabe M, Yamamoto K, Yoshimi N, Mori H, Kawazoe Y (1994) Inhibitory effect of topical application of polymerized ferulic acid, a synthetic lignin, on tumor promotion in mouse skin two-stage tumorigenesis. Carcinogenesis 15:2069–2071

Bedard K, Krause KH (2007) The NOX family of ROS-generating NADPH oxidases: physiology and pathophysiology. Physiol Rev 87:245–313

Brandes RP, Schroder K (2008) Differential vascular functions of Nox family NADPH oxidases. Curr Opin Lipidol 19:513–518
Castor LR, Locatelli KA, Ximenes VF (2010) Pro-oxidant activity of apocynin radical. Free Radic Biol Med 48:1636–1643
Chavali SR, Zhong WW, Forse RA (1998) Dietary alpha-linolenic acid increases TNF-alpha, and decreases IL-6, IL-10 in response to LPS: effects of sesamin on the delta-5 desaturation of omega6 and omega3fattyacids in mice. Prostaglandins Leukot Essent FattyAcids 58:185–191
Chavali SR, Utsunomiya T, Forse RA (2001) Increased survival after cecal ligation and puncture in mice consuming diets enriched with sesame seed oil. Crit Care Med 29:140–143
Cheng FC, Jinn TR, Hou RC, Tzen JT (2006) Neuroprotective effects of sesamin and sesamolin on gerbil brain in cerebral ischemia. Int J Biomed Sci 2:284–288
Cooney RV, Custer LJ, Okinaka L, Franke AA (2001) Effects of dietary sesame seeds on plasma tocopherol levels. Nutr Cancer 39:66–71
Doker O, Salgin U, Yieldiz N, Aydognus M, Calimi A (2010) Extraction of sesame seed oil using supercritical CO_2 and mathematical modeling. J Food Eng 97:360–366
El-Seedi HR, El-Said AM, Khalifa SA, Göransson U, Bohlin L, Borg-Karlson AK, Verpoorte R (2012) Biosynthesis, natural sources, dietary intake, pharmacokinetic properties, and biological activities of hydroxycinnamic acids. J Agric Food Chem 60:10877–10895
Fujii G, Yamamoto M, Takahashi M, Mutoh M (2011) Role of adipocytokines in colorectal carcinogenesis. Curr Res Cancer 5:39–48
Galgani JE, Núñez B, Videla LA (2012) Vanillin suppresses Kupffer cell-related colloidal carbon-induced respiratory burst activity in isolated perfused rat liver: anti-inflammatory implications. Food Funct 3:1319–1323
Hagiwara A, Kokubo Y, Takesada Y, Tanaka H, Tamano S, Hirose M, Shirai T, Ito N (1996) Inhibitory effects of phenolic compounds on development of naturally occurring preneoplastic hepatocytic foci in long-term feeding studies using male F344 rats. Teratog Carcinog Mutagen 16:317–325
Haiyan Z, Bedgood DR Jr, Bishop AG, Prenzler PD, Robards K (2007) Endogenous biphenol, fatty acid and volatile profiles of selected oils. Food Chem 100:1544–1551
Halliwell B (1978) Superoxide-dependent formation of hydroxyl radicals in the presence of iron salts. Its role in degradation of hyaluronic acid by a superoxide-generating system. FEBS Lett 96:238–242
Heumüller S, Wind S, Barbosa-Sicard E, Schmidt HH, Busse R, Schröder K, Brandes RP (2008) Apocynin is not an inhibitor of vascular NADPH oxidases but an antioxidant. Hypertension 51:211–217
Hirata F, Fujita K, Ishikura Y, Hosoda K, Ishikawa T, Nakamura H (1996) Hypocholesterolemic effect of sesame lignan in humans. Atherosclerosis 122:135–136
Hirose N, Inoue T, Nishihara K, Sugano M, Akimoto K, Shimizu S, Yamada H (1991) Inhibition of cholesterol absorption and synthesis in rats by sesamin. J Lipid Res 32:629–638
Hirose N, Doi F, Ueki T, Akazawa K, Chijiiwa K, Sugano M, Akimoto K, Shimizu S, Yamada H (1992) Suppressive effect of sesamin against 7, 12-dimethylbenz[a]-anthracene induced rat mammary carcinogenesis. Anticancer Res 12:1259–1265
Hou RC, Huang HM, Tzen JT, Jeng KC (2003a) Protective effects of sesamin and sesamolin on hypoxic neuronal and PC12 cells. J Neurosci Res 74:123–133
Hou RC, Chen HL, Tzen JT, Jeng KC (2003b) Effect of sesame antioxidants on LPS-induced NO production by BV2 microglial cells. Neuroreport 14:1815–1819
Hsu DZ, Chen KT, Li YH, Chuang YC, Liu MY (2006) Sesamol delays mortality and attenuates hepatic injury after cecal ligation and puncture in rats: role of oxidative stress. Shock 25:528–532
Ide T, Ashakumary L, Takahashi Y, Kushiro M, Fukuda N, Sugano M (2001) Sesamin, a sesame lignan, decreases fatty acid synthesis in rat liver accompanying the down-regulation of sterol regulatory element binding protein-1. Biochim Biophys Acta 1534:1–13

Jiang Q (2014) Natural forms of vitamin E: metabolism, antioxidant, and anti-inflammatory activities and their role in disease prevention and therapy. Free Radic Biol Med 72:76–90

Jiang Q, Jiang Z, Hall YJ, Jang Y, Snyder PW, Bain C, Huang J, Jannasch A, Cooper B, Wang Y, Moreland M (2013) Gamma-tocopherol attenuates moderate but not severe colitis and suppresses moderate colitis-promoted colon tumorigenesis in mice. Free Radic Biol Med 65:1069–1077

Ju J, Hao X, Lee MJ, Lambert JD, Lu G, Xiao H, Newmark HL, Yang CS (2009) A gamma-tocopherol-rich mixture of tocopherols inhibits colon inflammation and carcinogenesis in azoxymethane and dextran sulfate sodium-treated mice. Cancer Prev Res (Phila) 2:143–152

Kaiser J (2012) Profile: Bert Vogelstein. Cancer genetics with an edge. Science 337:282–284

Kajla S, Mondol AS, Nagasawa A, Zhang Y, Kato M, Matsuno K, Yabe-Nishimura C, Kamata T (2012) A crucial role for Nox 1 in redox-dependent regulation of Wnt-β-catenin signaling. FASEB J 26:2049–2059

Kamata T (2009) Roles of Nox1 and other Nox isoforms in cancer development. Cancer Sci 100:1382–1388

Kapadia GJ, Azuine MA, Tokuda H, Takasaki M, Mukainaka T, Konoshima T, Nishino H (2002) Chemopreventive effect of resveratrol, sesamol, sesame oil and sunflower oil in the Epstein-Barr virus early antigen activation assay and the mouse skin two-stage carcinogenesis. Pharmacol Res 45:499–505

Kawabata K, Yamamoto T, Hara A, Shimizu M, Yamada Y, Matsunaga K, Tanaka T, Mori H (2000) Modifying effects of ferulic acid on azoxymethane-induced colon carcinogenesis in F344 rats. Cancer Lett 157:15–21

Komiya M, Fujii G, Takahashi M, Iigo M, Mutoh M (2013) Prevention and intervention trials for colorectal cancer. Jpn J Clin Oncol 43:685–694

Kondamudi PK, Kovelamudi H, Mathew G, Nayak PG, Rao CM, Shenoy RR (2013) Modulatory effects of sesamol in dinitrochlorobenzene-induced inflammatory bowel disorder in albino rats. Pharmacol Rep 65:658–665

Laurent E, McCoy JW 3rd, Macina RA, Liu W, Cheng G, Robine S, Papkoff J, Lambeth JD (2008) Nox1 is over-expressed in human colon cancers and correlates with activating mutations in *K-Ras*. Int J Cancer 123:100–107

Lesca P (1983) Protective effects of ellagic acid and other plant phenols on benzo[a]pyrene -induced neoplasia in mice. Carcinogenesis 4:1651–1653

Li JM, Shah AM (2001) Differential NADPH- versus NADH-dependent superoxide production by phagocyte-type endothelial cell NADPH oxidase. Cardiovasc Res 52:477–486

Lim JS, Adachi Y, Takahashi Y, Ide T (2007) Comparative analysis of sesame lignans (sesamin and sesamolin) in affecting hepatic fatty acid metabolism in rats. Br J Nutr 97:85–95

Lin WN, Lin CC, Cheng HY, Yang CM (2011) Regulation of cyclooxygenase-2 and cytosolic phospholipase A_2 gene expression by lipopolysaccharide through the RNA-binding protein HuR: involvement of NADPH oxidase, reactive oxygen species and mitogen-activated protein kinases. Br J Pharmacol 163:1691–1706

Lirdprapamongkol K, Kramb JP, Suthiphongchai T, Surarit R, Srisomsap C, Dannhardt G, Svasti J (2009) Vanillin suppresses metastatic potential of human cancer cells through PI3K inhibition and decreases angiogenesis in vivo. J Agric Food Chem 57:3055–3063

Liu Y, Cui Y, Shi M, Zhang Q, Wang Q, Chen X (2014) Deferoxamine promotes MDA-MB-231 cell migration and invasion through increased ROS-dependent HIF-1α accumulation. Cell Physiol Biochem 33:1036–1046

Luxen S, Belinsky SA, Knaus UG (2008) Silencing of DUOX NADPH oxidases by promoter hypermethylation in lung cancer. Cancer Res 68:1037–1045

Matsuda M, Shimomura I (2014) Roles of adiponectin and oxidative stress in obesity-associated metabolic and cardiovascular diseases. Rev Endocr Metab Disord 15:1–10

McCarty MF (2012) Minimizing the cancer-promotional activity of cox-2 as a central strategy in cancer prevention. Med Hypotheses 78:45–57

Miyahara Y, Hibasami H, Katsuzaki H, Imai K, Komiya T (2001) Sesamolin from sesame seed inhibits proliferation by inducing apoptosis in human lymphoid leukemia Molt 4B cells. Int J Mol Med 7:369–371

Mochizuki T, Furuta S, Mitsushita J, Shang WH, Ito M, Yokoo Y, Yamaura M, Ishizone S, Nakayama J, Konagai A, Hirose K, Kiyosawa K, Kamata T (2006) Inhibition of NADPH oxidase 4 activates apoptosis via the AKT/apoptosis signal-regulation kinase 1 pathway in pancreatic cancer PANC-1 cells. Oncogene 25:3699–3707

Mutoh M, Takahashi M, Fukuda K, Matsushita-Hibiya Y, Mutoh H, Sugimura T, Wakabayashi K (2000) Suppression of cyclooxygenase-2 promoter-dependent transcriptional activity in colon cancer cells by chemopreventive agents with a resorcin-type structure. Carcinogenesis 21:959–963

Mutoh M, Takahashi M, Wakabayashi K (2006) Roles of prostanoids in colon carcinogenesis and their potential targeting for cancer chemoprevention. Curr Pharm Des 12:2375–2382

Mutoh M, Teraoka N, Takasu S, Takahashi M, Onuma K, Yamamoto M, Kubota N, Iseki T, Kadowaki T, Sugimura T, Wakabayashi K (2011) Loss of adiponectin promotes intestinal carcinogenesis in Min and wild-type mice. Gastroenterology 140:2000–2008

Muzaffar S, Jeremy JY, Sparatore A, Del Soldato P, Angelini GD, Shukla N (2008) H2S-donating sildenafil (ACS6) inhibits superoxide formation and gp91phox expression in arterial endothelial cells: role of protein kinases A and G. Br J Pharmacol 155:984–994

Namiki M (1995) The chemistry and physiological functions of sesame. Food Rev Int 11:281–329

Oshima M, Dinchuk JE, Kargman SL, Oshima H, Hancock B, Kwong E, Trzaskos JM, Evans JF, Taketo MM (1996) Suppression of intestinal polyposis in *Apc*^{delta716} knockout mice by inhibition of cyclooxygenase 2 (COX-2). Cell 87:803–809

Parihar VK, Prabhakar KR, Veerapur VP, Kumar MS, Reddy YR, Joshi R, Unnikrishnan MK, Rao CM (2006) Effect of sesamol on radiation-induced cytotoxicity in Swiss albino mice. Mutat Res 611:9–16

Pathak N, Rai AK, Kumari R, Bhat KV (2014) Value addition in sesame: a perspective on bioactive components for enhancing utility and profitability. Pharmacogn Rev 8:147–155

Peñalvo JL, Hopia A, Adlercreutz H (2006) Effect of sesamin on serum cholesterol and triglycerides levels in LDL receptor-deficient mice. Eur J Nutr 45:439–444

Riboli E, Norat T (2003) Epidemiologic evidence of the protective effect of fruit and vegetables on cancer risk. Am J Clin Nutr 78:559S–569S

Ryan E, Galvin K, O'Connor TP, Maguire AR, O'Brien NM (2007) Phytosterol, squalene, tocopherol content and fatty acid profile of selected seeds, grains, and legumes. Plant Foods Hum Nutr 62:85–91

Salerno JW, Smith DE (1991) The use of sesame oil and other vegetable oils in the inhibition of human colon cancer growth in vitro. Anticancer Res 11:209–215

Shimizu S, Akimoto K, Shinmen Y, Kawashima H, Sugano M, Yamada H (1991) Sesamin is a potent and specific inhibitor of delta 5 desaturase in polyunsaturated fatty acid biosynthesis. Lipids 26:512–516

Shimizu S, Fujii G, Takahashi M, Nakanaishi R, Komiya M, Shimura M, Noma N, Onuma W, Terasaki M, Yano T, Mutoh M (2014) Sesamol suppresses cyclooxygenase-2 transcriptional activity in colon cancer cells and modifies intestinal polyp development in *Apc*$^{Min/+}$ mice. J Clin Biochem Nutr 54:95–101

Shimizu S, Ishigamori R, Fujii G, Takahashi M, Onuma W, Terasaki M, Yano T, Mutoh M (2015) Involvement of NADPH oxidases in suppression of cyclooxygenase-2 promoter-dependent transcriptional activities by sesamol. J Clin Biochem Nutr 56(2):118–122

Siegel R, Naishadham D, Jemal A (2012) Cancer statistics, 2012. CA Cancer J Clin 62:10–29

Stefanska J, Pawliczak R (2008) Apocynin: molecular aptitudes. Mediators Inflamm 2008:106507

Sudheer AR, Chandran K, Marimuthu S, Menon VP (2005) Ferulic Acid modulates altered lipid profiles and prooxidant/antioxidant status in circulation during nicotine-induced toxicity: a dose-dependent study. Toxicol Mech Methods 15:375–381

Sugano M, Akimoto K (1993) Sesamin: a multifunctional gift from nature. J Chin Nutr Soc 18:1–11

Sumimoto H (2008) Structure, regulation and evolution of Nox-family NADPH oxidases that produce reactive oxygen species. FEBS J 275:3249–3277

Sung JJ, Lau JY, Goh KL, Leung WK, Asia Pacific Working Group on Colorectal Cancer (2005) Increasing incidence of colorectal cancer in Asia: implications for screening. Lancet Oncol 6:871–876

Suzuki S, Shiraga K, Sato S, Punfa W, Naiki-Ito A, Yamashita Y, Shirai T, Takahashi S (2013a) Apocynin, an NADPH oxidase inhibitor, suppresses rat prostate carcinogenesis. Cancer Sci 104:1711–1717

Suzuki S, Pitchakarn P, Sato S, Shirai T, Takahashi S (2013b) Apocynin, an NADPH oxidase inhibitor, suppresses progression of prostate cancer via Rac1 dephosphorylation. Exp Toxicol Pathol 65:1035–1041

Takahashi S, Takeshita K, Seeni A, Sugiura S, Tang M, Sato SY, Kuriyama H, Nakadate M, Abe K, Maeno Y, Nagao M, Shirai T (2009) Suppression of prostate cancer in a transgenic rat model via gamma-tocopherol activation of caspase signaling. Prostate 69:644–651

Temraz S, Mukherji D, Shamseddine A (2013) Potential targets for colorectal cancer prevention. Int J Mol Sci 14:17279–17303

Tomasetti C, Vogelstein B (2015) Cancer etiology. Variation in cancer risk among tissues can be explained by the number of stem cell divisions. Science 347:78–81

Vulcano M, Dusi S, Lissandrini D, Badolato R, Mazzi P, Riboldi E, Borroni E, Calleri A, Donini M, Plebani A, Notarangelo L, Musso T, Sozzani S (2004) Toll receptor-mediated regulation of NADPH oxidase in human dendritic cells. J Immunol 173:5749–5756

Wang L, Zhang Y, Li P, Zhang W, Wang X, Qi X, Zhang X (2013) Variation of sesamin and sesamolin contents in sesame cultivators from China. Pak J Bot 45:177–182

Wang O, Liu J, Cheng Q, Guo X, Wang Y, Zhao L, Zhou F, Ji B (2015) Effects of ferulic acid and γ-oryzanol on high-fat and high-fructose diet-induced metabolic syndrome in rats. PLoS One 10:e0118135

World Cancer Research Fund/American Institute for Cancer Research (2007) Food, nutrition, physical activity, and the prevention of cancer: a global perspective. AICR, Washington, DC

Wu W-H (2007) The contents of lignans in commercial sesame oils of Taiwan and their changes during heating. Food Chem 104:341–344

Xu J, Chen S, Hu Q (2005) Antioxidant activity of brown pigment and extracts from black sesame seed (*Sesamum indicum* L). Food Chem 91:79–83

Yamamura M, Mitsushita J, Furuta S, Kiniwa Y, Ashida A, Goto Y, Shang WH, Kubodera M, Kato M, Takata M, Saida T, Kamata T (2009) NADPH oxidase (Nox) 4 contributes to transformation phenotype of melanoma cells by regulating G2-M cell cycle progression. Cancer Res 69:2647–2654

Yoshida H (1994) Composition and quality characteristics of sesame seed (*Sesamum indicum*) oil roasted at different temperatures in an electric oven. J Sci Food Agric 65:331–336

Progress in the Development of Black Seed-Derived Anticancer Agents

Irfana Muqbil and Ramzi M. Mohammad

Abstract Black seeds, in some form or the other, have remained popular in folklore medicine throughout the history of mankind. This herb has been used for millenniums to strengthen the immune system, cleanse the body, purify the blood, protect against irritants, and support health longevity. Not only do the scriptures from three major religions of the world (Judaism, Christianity, and Islam) endorse their health benefits, the use of black seed oil has been emphasized in the Mesopotamian, Greek, Indus Valley, Egyptian, and other important civilizations. Despite the unequivocal medicinal use of black seeds since ancient times, little was known in terms of its major active ingredients. Modern molecular research has expanded the repertoire of biological effects elicited by these intriguing seeds compelling the research community to characterize the main element responsible for the health benefits. The development of high-performance purification techniques allowed the parsing of the constituents of Black seeds to a much deeper level. These studies have concluded in the identification of Thymoquinone as the major component in black seeds that is responsible for the various biological effects, particularly its anticancer mechanism. These findings drove intense research in different laboratories all across the globe leading to considerable enhancement of our knowledge of Thymoquinone's primary as well as interacting mechanisms against cancer cells. Despite the encouraging laboratory results in cancer cell lines and preclinical efficacy in animal tumor models, a major problem associated with Thymoquinone is its poor bioavailability. This serves as a major caveat and is therefore the chief hurdle blocking its translation as a therapeutic agent in the clinic. In order to overcome this problem, a number of novel analogues of Thymoquinone have been developed recently that have shown superior pharmacokinetic properties. These analogues show early promise at least in the preclinical setting and provide confidence for their future incorporation into clinical practice as single agent or part

I. Muqbil
Department of Oncology, Wayne State University School of Medicine, 4100 John R, HWCRC 732, Detroit, MI 48201, USA

R.M. Mohammad, Ph.D. (✉)
Department of Oncology, Wayne State University School of Medicine, 4100 John R, HWCRC 732, Detroit, MI 48201, USA

iTRI, Hamad Medical Corporation, Doha, Qatar
e-mail: mohammar@karmanos.org

M.F. Ullah, A. Ahmad (eds.), *Critical Dietary Factors in Cancer Chemoprevention*,
DOI 10.1007/978-3-319-21461-0_9

of a combination regimen for cancer treatment. Through this chapter, we bring forth a historical perspective on the different major milestones in Black seed anticancer research. The current knowledge on the progress of black seed-derived anticancer agents is highlighted along with a forward-looking view as to where the Thymoquinone-related research field might be heading.

1 Introduction

Black seeds are obtained from *Nigella sativa* (also known as *Kalonji* or simply *Nigella*) which is an annual flowering plant in the family *Ranunculaceae* that is native to south and southwest Asia (Khan 1999). It grows less than a foot tall, with finely divided linear leaves. The flowers are delicate and usually colored pale blue and white, with five to ten petals. The fruit is a large and inflated capsule composed of three to seven united follicles, each containing numerous black seeds which are used as a spice.

The journey of Black seed use began in ancient times and still continues to fascinate the research community as a promising anticancer and disease preventing agent. The use of Black seeds and its derivates has been documented in ancient, medieval, as well as modern era. Despite the appreciation of the health benefits from anecdotal studies, it was only in the last 20 years that modern molecular biology has been applied to Black seed research. Deeper exploration and multifaceted research approaches have led to the identification of Thymoquinone as the chief component responsible for the health benefits of Black seed. However, we are still a long way from witnessing their use as clinical agents in the treatment of cancer. Through this chapter, we unveil the long and slow journey of Black seed over 3000 years. We present some insights into the various ongoing strategies that are being utilized that hopefully will accelerate their entry in clinical trials for the management of different diseases and possibly cancer.

2 Historical Perspective on Black Seeds

Attesting to their use by various civilizations, Black seeds have been mentioned since ancient times in various scriptures over the course of history. Although, according to Zohary and Hopf (Domestication of plants in the Old World. Ed), the archaeological evidence about the earliest cultivation of *N. sativa* "is still scanty" (Zohary 1982), in their reports they do indicate that *N. sativa* seeds have been found in several sites from ancient Egypt, including Pharaoh Tutankhamun's tomb. Despite the lack of knowledge of its use in Egyptian culture, they do hold significance since it is recognized that items (including Black seeds) entombed with a pharaoh were carefully selected to assist him in the afterlife.

The earliest documented reference to Black seeds is thought to be in the book of Isaiah in the Old Testament, where the reaping of nigella and wheat is contrasted (Isaiah 28: 25, 27). Easton's Bible dictionary states the Hebrew word *ketsah* refers to *N. sativa* without doubt (although there are some disagreements to the true translation of Ketsah). Nevertheless, according to Zohary and Hopf, *N. sativa* was another traditional condiment of the Old World during classical times, and its black seeds were extensively used to flavor food. Seeds were found in a Hittite flask in Turkey from the second millennium BC which indicates their use across Europe and North Eastern parts of Asia (Salih et al. 2009).

A noted Greek herbalist Dioscorides discussed what he called melanthion in the third volume of his materia medica (Sect. 79) around the first century AD (Rothman 1972). His description unambiguously identifies the plant as Nigella sativa. Interestingly, Dioscorides' description also mentions the use of Black seed in the making of bread, a dietary practice still prevalent in parts of the current day Middle East. Dioscorides recommends the use of black seed for different ailments such as headaches, swellings, warts, toothaches, colds, dyspnea, and spider bites among other things. It is reputedly the most mentioned herb in the Islamic scriptures. It is discussed as a remedy to improve bodily energy in Avicenna's (980–1037) massive materia medica, Te Canon of Medicine (Qanun fi al-Tibb) (O'Sullivan 1928). The Prophet of Islam (PBUH) described black seed as a remedy for every disease except death (Sahih Bukhari 7:71:592). Primarily these scriptures mention the immune boosting properties of Black seeds that have been suggested to prevent disease development in early stages. Figure 1 gives a timeline description of discovery of Black seed over the course of different civilizations and how the field has progressed in modern times.

3 Black Seeds in Modern Times (Isolation and Characterization of Active Ingredients)

Black seed research has picked up pace in the last quarter of twentieth century and it is safe to say that most of the modern research has unfolded in the last 25 years or so. Table 1 shows the list of papers that are available on PubMed in relation to Black Cumin, Black seeds, Nigella Sativa, Thymoquinone, Black Seed Cancer, and Thymoquinone Cancer.

The first reported study showing some impact of dietary Black seed consumption on Esophageal cancer came from an Iranian group (Ghadirian 1987). In this report, the authors evaluated dietary habits (including the consumption of black seed in diet) of a total of 1501 individuals, in 197 households, from 35 Iranian villages in different regions and its causal link to Esophageal cancer. While these studies did not give a very clear picture of the roles played by Black seed in cancer

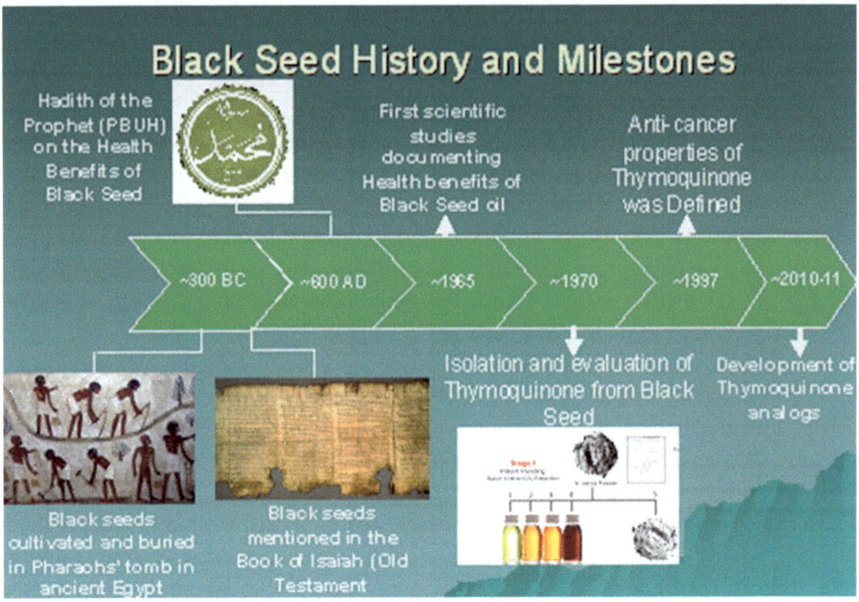

Fig. 1 Figure shows a timeline of the various periods (over the last 3000–4000 years) of Black seed use that has led to the discovery of Thymoquinone. The first description of Black seed can be dated back to the Egyptian civilization where Nigella seeds were widely cultivated and used. The seeds also find mention in the Old Testament and later on in the Hadith of the Prophet of Islam (PBUH). The first scientific studies demonstrating the health benefits of Black seed and its oil were published in the 1960s. Isolation of Thymoquinone was documented in the 1970s that was followed by the first publications on its anticancer properties in the late 1990s. In recent times, research has focused on the development of novel analogues of Thymoquinone with better efficacy and superior bioavailability parameters

Table 1 Current status of literature on black seed and related research topics: a PubMed search

PubMed search key	Words returned search hits
Black cumin	725
Black seed(s)	1100
Black seed cancer	95
Black seed oil	169
Black seed oil cancer	29
Thymoquinone	480
Thymoquinone cancer	166
Thymoquinone analogue(s)	29

development or prevention, they certainly paved the way for future studies on Black seeds. Later on, Corder and colleagues showed that apoptosis by Lipopolysaccharide (LPS) or cortisol can be prevented by Black seed extracts (Corder et al. 2003). In another study, Hansen and colleagues showed that metabolic deregulation caused by LPS can be reversed using black seed extracts (Hansen et al. 2003). Having established the protective and immune stimulatory roles of Black seeds in various models, the research community moved toward exploring their anticancer effects. Salim and Fukushima were among the first group to demonstrate the chemopreventive benefits of a volatile black seed oil against chemically induced colon carcinogenesis in rat models (Salim and Fukushima 2003). These investigations drove further analyses into the constituents responsible for the anticancer activity of Black seed oil and ultimately resulted in the discovery of Thymoquinone.

4 Purification and Evaluation of the Anticancer Activity of Thymoquinone

Thymoquinone is the major bioactive component (~25 %) in Nigella sativa volatile oil. Over the years, Nigella sativa oil and its bioactive compound, Thymoquinone, have been shown to possess multiple health-beneficial activities, which include antitumor, anti-inflammatory, antibacterial, antidiabetic, antihypertensive, hyperglycemic, anti-oxidative, and immuno-modulation activities (Schneider-Stock et al. 2014).

Due to its multiple health benefits, extraction of Thymoquinone from Nigella sativa seeds was considered of prime importance and thus has received continuous attention from researchers and nutraceutical industry worldwide. There have been a number of methods developed for the extraction of Thymoquinone from Black seed oil including solvent extractions and hydrodistillation (Ghosheh et al. 1999). Some of these methods are time-consuming and costly and are not very environment friendly. Further, most of the solvent extraction methods impose a threat to consumers' health if the organic solvents are not completely removed from the extractives. Improving on these methodologies, supercritical carbon dioxide fluid extraction (SFE) procedure has been patented recently that provides a better alternative for Nigella sativa seeds extraction US20120046366 A1. Advantageously, SFE offers the usage of nontoxic, nonexplosive, environmental friendly, cost-effective, time-saving, and selectivity-adjustable solvent (supercritical carbon dioxide fluid) in the extraction process. Furthermore, it also enables the oil extraction to be carried out under low temperature and oxygen-free condition. This feature is very crucial in the extraction of bioactive compounds that are highly susceptible to oxidative degradation, for instance, Thymoquinone. On the other hand, simultaneous fractionation by using SFE enables the concentration of targeted bioactive compound such as Thymoquinone to be conducted in a solvent free as well as time and cost saving manner.

Having identified Thymoquinone as the major active component in Black seeds, researchers shifted their focus toward understanding their anticancer and disease preventing benefits. Thymoquinone is recognized to impact inflammation (Woo et al. 2012) and other diseases for which there are numerous outstanding reviews (Butt and Sultan 2010). Here we only focus on the anticancer activities of Black seed-derived Thymoquinone. Early indications for their anticancer benefits were chance findings. For example, Badary and colleagues while evaluating the preventive activity of Thymoquinone against nephrotoxicity induced by cisplatin observed an enhancement in the antitumor activity of the chemotherapeutic agents in rodents (Badary et al. 1997). Similarly, Worthen and colleagues showed anticancer activity of Thymoquinone and di-Thymoquinone (DIM) in cellular models of cancer (Worthen et al. 1998). Later on al-shabanah and colleagues showed that Thymoquinone protects against doxorubicin-induced cardiotoxicity without compromising its antitumor activity (al-Shabanah et al. 1998). In other studies, Badary et al. have also showed inhibition of benzo(a)pyrene-induced forestomach carcinogenesis in mice (Badary et al. 1999), suppression of 20-methylcholanthrene-induced fibrosarcoma tumorigenesis (Badary and Gamal El-Din 2001), and anticlastogenic activity against benzo(a)pyrene-induced carcinogenesis (Badary et al. 2007). Adding on to these findings, in their study Ghali-Muhtasib and colleagues demonstrated that Thymoquinone could trigger apoptotic cell death in human colorectal cancer cells via a p53-dependent mechanism (Gali-Muhtasib et al. 2004). Since these initial pathbreaking studies, a number of groups independently evaluated the anticancer activity of Thymoquinone as single agent or in combination with various chemotherapeutic agents against different tumor models. Table 2 below lists the different studies on Black seeds, Black seed oil, and Thymoquinone (either alone or in combination with different standard chemotherapeutics) that have been evaluated preclinically in different cancers.

5 Progress in the Development of Thymoquinone Analogues as Anticancer Agents

Bioavailability of any drug to the target cells, whether in vitro or in vivo, is critical for its optimal efficacy. If an agent does not possess optimal half-life and cannot reach target site (i.e., tumors), it is bound to have limited effects. Similar to many other natural dietary chemopreventive agents, Thymoquinone also possesses poor pharmacokinetic parameters. This is specially highlighted by the fact that the doses required for Thymoquinone to show in vitro cell death are in high micromolar range (usually >25 μM range for most cancer cell types). Therefore, despite the promising behavior shown in preclinical in vitro and in vivo cancer models, there are a number of bioavailability related caveats that hinder the clinical translation of Thymoquinone.

There have been two distinct approaches to enhance the bioavailability of Thymoquinone: (a) nano-encapsulation and (b) development of Thymoquinone analogues with better efficacy and half-life. Effenberger and colleagues recently demonstrated that conjugates of thymoquinone with various monoterpenes, sesquiterpenes, and the cytotoxic triterpene betulinic acid possess anticancer activity (Effenberger et al. 2010). In these studies, the attachment of ester residues of various terpene alcohols to C(6) of Thymoquinone via spacers of variable length

Table 2 List of studies on black seed, black seed oil and thymoquinone in relation to cancer

Agent	Tumor models	Reference
Black seed	Esophageal cancer	Ghadirian (1987)
	Colon cancer cells	Kamei et al. (1997)
	Laryngeal cancer cells	Corder et al. (2003)
Black seed oil	Colon cancer	Salim and Fukushima (2003)
	Multi-organ carcinogenesis models	Salim (2010)
	Hepatic metastasis models	Sorenson et al. (2011)
Thymoquinone	Breast cancer	Woo et al. (2013), Velho-Pereira et al. (2011), Sutton et al. (2014), Rajput et al. (2013a, b, 2015), Motaghed et al. (2013, 2014), Effenberger-Neidnicht and Schobert (2011), and Arafa el et al. (2011)
	Cervical cancer	Ng et al. (2015), Ichwan et al. (2014), and Hafiza and Latifah (2014)
	Cholangiocarcinoma	Xu et al. (2014)
	Colon cancer	Chen et al. (2015), Kundu et al. (2014), Gali-Muhtasib et al. (2008), and Norwood et al. (2006, 2007)
	Gastric cancer	Lei et al. (2012)
	Hepatocellular cancer	Ashour et al. (2014) and Raghunandhakumar et al. (2013)
	Intestinal cancer	Kortum et al. (2014), Ghayur et al. (2012), and Kapan et al. (2012)
	Leukemias (ALL, AML, CML, and others)	El-Mahdy et al. (2005)
	Lymphomas	Hussain et al. (2011, 2013)
	Ovarian cancer	Nessa et al. (2011) and Wilson-Simpson et al. (2007)
	Pancreatic cancer	Mu et al. (2014), Yusufi et al. (2013), Al Wafai (2013), Wang (2011), Wu et al. (2011), Abdelmeguid et al. (2010), Torres et al. (2010), Chehl et al. (2009), Banerjee et al. (2009) and HIV-1 protease inhibitor induced oxidative stress in pancreatic beta-cells: protection with thymoquinone (2009)
	Prostate cancer	Kaseb et al. (2007), Dirican et al. (2014, 2015), and Koka et al. (2010)

enhanced the growth inhibitory potential in multiple tumor cell lines (e.g., HL-60 leukemia, 518A2 melanoma, MDR KB-V1/Vbl cervix carcinoma, and MCF-7/Topo breast adenocarcinoma and nonmalignant foreskin fibroblasts). Similarly, Nair and colleagues described the potential of using nanobased formulations to package Thymoquinone to enhance its biological activity (Nair et al. 2010). Working further in this direction, Ravindran et al. developed a formulation in which

Thymoquinone was encapsulated into biodegradable poly(lactide-co-glycolide) (PLGA) nanoparticulates and the stabilizer polyethylene glycol (termed Thymoquinone-nanoparticle or simply TQ-NP). The resultant formulation demonstrated enhanced antiproliferative, anti-inflammatory, and chemosensitization potential against different cellular cancer models (Ravindran et al. 2010). These nanobased Thymoquinone showed superior cell kill as well as demonstrated a marked increase in their potential as a sensitizing agent to paclitaxel-induced apoptosis. In another study, a focused approach toward COX-2 docking was taken to develop analogues of Thymoquinone (Yusufi et al. 2013). The identified Thymoquinone analogues appended with gallate and fluorogallate pharmacophores showed superior activity against pancreatic cancer cell lines and also synergized with standard chemotherapeutic gemcitabine.

Our laboratory took a distinct approach and developed Thymoquinone analogues with the hope to enhance its potency and bioavailability (Banerjee et al. 2010). Using single-pot synthesis, we developed and tested several Thymoquinone analogues for their anticancer activity. Out of 27 analogues synthesized, 3 compounds exhibited superior activity than Thymoquinone. These compounds were further evaluated toward improvement of sensitivity to oxaliplatin and gemcitabine in pancreatic cancer cells and again were found superior to parent Thymoquinone in causing reduced cell viability and inducing apoptosis. Most importantly, the analogues showed greater retention in target organ (here pancreas) as detected using HPLC.

Despite the efforts on elucidating mechanism of action of Thymoquinone or its analogues, no clear single mechanism of action is yet to emerge. With each passing year, newer molecular targets of Black seeds, Thymoquinone, or their analogues are being defined that include apoptosis regulation, suppression of pro-survival transcription factors, blocking inflammatory response, and immune stimulation [the reader is referred to the excellent reviews on this topic (Schneider-Stock et al. 2014)]. Being natural products, they are bound to have a promiscuous mechanism of action. Our laboratory has primarily focused on NF-kB and COX-2 inhibitory properties of Thymoquinone and its analogues. Figure 2 is a summary diagram of the different mechanism that is thought to be supporting the underlying anticancer actions of Thymoquinone or its analogues. It is recognized that more work needs to be done in order to validate these targets in a broad spectrum of tumor models.

6 Clinical Studies on Black Seeds

Despite the comprehensive amount of preclinical work in so many different cancer models, we are yet to see a clinical study that involves the use of Thymoquinone as an anticancer agent either in the preventive or therapeutic setting. Surfing the ClinicalTrials.gov website shows that most of the studies on Black seeds revolve around exploring its health benefits for diseases other than cancer. Conducted in

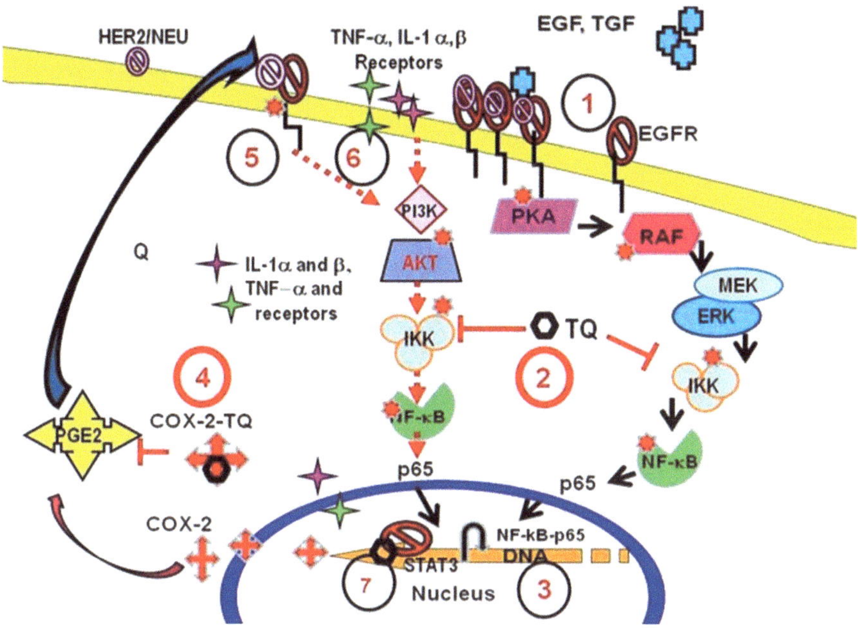

Fig. 2 Hypothesized inhibition of the COX-2–EGFR–NF-kB Loop by Thymoquinone and its Analogues (specific to pancreatic cancer). *Early events* in the initiation of pancreatic cancer (1) Autocrine/paracrine/endocrine ligands for the EGFR/HER2/NEU receptors activate the growth receptor survival pathway and induce overexpression of EGFR receptors in cancer cells. (2) EGFR ligands activated pathways include phosphorylation of protein kinase A (PKA) for Ras/Raf-MEK/ERK-induced IKK-NF-kB activation (*TQ inhibits IKK activity*). (3) NF-kBp65 transduction leads to transcription of COX-2, EGFR, EGFR ligands, as well as other survival factors such as IL-6, IL-1α and β, and TNF-α (*TQ inhibits NF-kB activity*). (4) COX-2 protein is encoded and the enzyme produced; COX-2 activity is required for the generation of PGE-2 (Direct *binding of TQ to COX-2 prevents COX-2 activity and generation of PGE-2*). (5) In the absence of PGE-2, phosphorylation of EGFR/HER2/Neu receptors for continuous autocrine EGFR loop is blocked. *Later events* for sustained survival and chemoresistance include (6) TQ-induced downregulation of NF-kB activation inhibiting transcription of autocrine survival factors, EGF, IL1α and β, and TNF-α, also downregulating the PI3K/Akt-NF-kB pathway. (7) Finally, *TQ-induced downregulation of EGFR/Her2/Neu* prevents nuclear EGFR-STAT3 regulation of Aurora Kinase A, E2F1, and cyclin D1, affecting cell cycle progression and Her2/Neu-DNA interaction, thereby regulating COX-2 expression

Indonesia, clinical trial NCT01531062 involves the determination whether Nigella sativa seed extracts are effective in the treatment of dyslipidemia in the elderly. Another clinical trial NCT02307344 to be initiated in Hillel Yaffe, Israel, proposes to investigate the effect on nonalcoholic steatohepatitis and liver steatosis by enhancing lipophagy in the liver tissue. In yet another clinical study from Bangladesh the effect of daily intake of Nigella sativa for 12 weeks in the treatment of palmer arsenical keratosis was evaluated (NCT01735097). A clinical study NCT01393054 proposes to conduct a randomized, double-blind, placebo-controlled trial to prove the effect of Nigella sativa seed extract in elderly patients with hypertension. The main hypothesis of this trial is that 300 mg Nigella sativa seed extract twice daily will have antihypertensive effect on the blood pressure of the elderly with hypertension. The Agha Khan University in Pakistan recently concluded a clinical study NCT00327054 evaluating the effectiveness of Nigella sativa (Kalonji) seed in dyslipidemia. However, the results are yet to be released for this study. The fact that clinical studies have taken place using Black Seeds is itself encouraging. These patient studies bring hope that in the near future we may witness cancer-related clinical trials involving either Black seeds, Thymoquinone, or some of the emerging novel promising analogues of this agent.

7 Conclusion and Future Directions

Black seeds have been used over 3000 years in different ways for their healing powers. While their health benefits are unquestionable and have been appreciated for long, the scientific research on Black seeds remained slow, stagnated, and anecdotal for several centuries. It is quite surprising to note that natural products such as resveratrol and curcumin received greater attention than Thymoquinone. It was only recently that modern molecular and chemical approaches were applied to investigate the underlying reasons for their disease preventive effects. The field has witnessed a spurt in research approaches evaluating the multifaceted health benefits possessed by these intriguing seeds. Despite a global focus that has led to the identification of Thymoquinone as the major component for the underlying health benefits, this knowledge could not be translated into clinical trials, especially for cancer. A major reason for the failure to translate the sizable in vitro and in vivo results in the clinic is poor bioavailability of Thymoquinone in humans. This puts to question whether the preclinical anticancer studies have been done with the correct perspective. One needs to be cautious of not over-interpreting the laboratory results as the effective doses (observed in ex vivo models) may be completely different from the pharmacological doses that are required for meaningful activity in humans. The future for Thymoquinone research relies on the development of more potent analogues that have superior bioavailability parameters. As presented in this chapter, some inroads have been made toward the development of novel analogues of Thymoquinone. Preliminary studies show that these agents hold promise as therapeutics for cancer treatment. Such agents may see the light at the end of the tunnel and hopefully will be incorporated into clinical evaluation for the treatment of cancer.

References

Abdelmeguid NE, Fakhoury R, Kamal SM, Al Wafai RJ (2010) Effects of Nigella sativa and thymoquinone on biochemical and subcellular changes in pancreatic beta-cells of streptozotocin-induced diabetic rats. J Diabetes 2(4):256–266. doi:10.1111/j.1753-0407.2010.00091.x

Al Wafai RJ (2013) Nigella sativa and thymoquinone suppress cyclooxygenase-2 and oxidative stress in pancreatic tissue of streptozotocin-induced diabetic rats. Pancreas 42(5):841–849. doi:10.1097/MPA.0b013e318279ac1c

al-Shabanah OA, Badary OA, Nagi MN, al-Gharably NM, al-Rikabi AC, al-Bekairi AM (1998) Thymoquinone protects against doxorubicin-induced cardiotoxicity without compromising its antitumor activity. J Exp Clin Cancer Res 17(2):193–198

Arafa el SA, Zhu Q, Shah ZI, Wani G, Barakat BM, Racoma I et al (2011) Thymoquinone up-regulates PTEN expression and induces apoptosis in doxorubicin-resistant human breast cancer cells. Mutat Res 706(1–2):28–35. doi:10.1016/j.mrfmmm.2010.10.007

Ashour AE, Abd-Allah AR, Korashy HM, Attia SM, Alzahrani AZ, Saquib Q et al (2014) Thymoquinone suppression of the human hepatocellular carcinoma cell growth involves inhibition of IL-8 expression, elevated levels of TRAIL receptors, oxidative stress and apoptosis. Mol Cell Biochem 389(1–2):85–98. doi:10.1007/s11010-013-1930-1

Badary OA, Gamal El-Din AM (2001) Inhibitory effects of thymoquinone against 20-methylcholanthrene-induced fibrosarcoma tumorigenesis. Cancer Detect Prev 25(4):362–368

Badary OA, Nagi MN, al-Shabanah OA, al-Sawaf HA, al-Sohaibani MO, al-Bekairi AM (1997) Thymoquinone ameliorates the nephrotoxicity induced by cisplatin in rodents and potentiates its antitumor activity. Can J Physiol Pharmacol 75(12):1356–1361

Badary OA, Al-Shabanah OA, Nagi MN, Al-Rikabi AC, Elmazar MM (1999) Inhibition of benzo (a)pyrene-induced forestomach carcinogenesis in mice by thymoquinone. Eur J Cancer Prev 8 (5):435–440

Badary OA, Abd-Ellah MF, El-Mahdy MA, Salama SA, Hamada FM (2007) Anticlastogenic activity of thymoquinone against benzo(a)pyrene in mice. Food Chem Toxicol 45(1):88–92. doi:10.1016/j.fct.2006.08.004

Banerjee S, Kaseb AO, Wang Z, Kong D, Mohammad M, Padhye S et al (2009) Antitumor activity of gemcitabine and oxaliplatin is augmented by thymoquinone in pancreatic cancer. Cancer Res 69(13):5575–5583. doi:10.1158/0008-5472.CAN-08-4235

Banerjee S, Azmi AS, Padhye S, Singh MW, Baruah JB, Philip PA et al (2010) Structure-activity studies on therapeutic potential of Thymoquinone analogs in pancreatic cancer. Pharm Res 27 (6):1146–1158. doi:10.1007/s11095-010-0145-3

Butt MS, Sultan MT (2010) Nigella sativa: reduces the risk of various maladies. Crit Rev Food Sci Nutr 50(7):654–665. doi:10.1080/10408390902768797

Chehl N, Chipitsyna G, Gong Q, Yeo CJ, Arafat HA (2009) Anti-inflammatory effects of the Nigella sativa seed extract, thymoquinone, in pancreatic cancer cells. HPB (Oxford) 11 (5):373–381. doi:10.1111/j.1477-2574.2009.00059.x

Chen MC, Lee NH, Hsu HH, Ho TJ, Tu CC, Hsieh DJ et al (2015) Thymoquinone induces caspase-independent, autophagic cell death in CPT-11-resistant lovo colon cancer via mitochondrial dysfunction and activation of JNK and p38. J Agric Food Chem 63(5):1540–1546. doi:10.1021/jf5054063

Corder C, Benghuzzi H, Tucci M, Cason Z (2003) Delayed apoptosis upon the treatment of Hep-2 cells with black seed. Biomed Sci Instrum 39:365–370

Dirican A, Erten C, Atmaca H, Bozkurt E, Kucukzeybek Y, Varol U et al (2014) Enhanced cytotoxicity and apoptosis by thymoquinone in combination with zoledronic acid in hormone- and drug-resistant prostate cancer cell lines. J BUON 19(4):1055–1061

Dirican A, Atmaca H, Bozkurt E, Erten C, Karaca B, Uslu R (2015) Novel combination of docetaxel and thymoquinone induces synergistic cytotoxicity and apoptosis in DU-145 human prostate cancer cells by modulating PI3K-AKT pathway. Clin Transl Oncol 17 (2):145–151. doi:10.1007/s12094-014-1206-6

Effenberger K, Breyer S, Schobert R (2010) Terpene conjugates of the Nigella sativa seed-oil constituent thymoquinone with enhanced efficacy in cancer cells. Chem Biodivers 7 (1):129–139. doi:10.1002/cbdv.200900328

Effenberger-Neidnicht K, Schobert R (2011) Combinatorial effects of thymoquinone on the anti-cancer activity of doxorubicin. Cancer Chemother Pharmacol 67(4):867–874. doi:10.1007/s00280-010-1386-x

El-Mahdy MA, Zhu Q, Wang QE, Wani G, Wani AA (2005) Thymoquinone induces apoptosis through activation of caspase-8 and mitochondrial events in p53-null myeloblastic leukemia HL-60 cells. Int J Cancer 117(3):409–417. doi:10.1002/ijc.21205

Gali-Muhtasib H, Diab-Assaf M, Boltze C, Al-Hmaira J, Hartig R, Roessner A et al (2004) Thymoquinone extracted from black seed triggers apoptotic cell death in human colorectal cancer cells via a p53-dependent mechanism. Int J Oncol 25(4):857–866

Gali-Muhtasib H, Ocker M, Kuester D, Krueger S, El-Hajj Z, Diestel A et al (2008) Thymoquinone reduces mouse colon tumor cell invasion and inhibits tumor growth in murine colon cancer models. J Cell Mol Med 12(1):330–342. doi:10.1111/j.1582-4934.2007.00095.x

Ghadirian P (1987) Food habits of the people of the Caspian Littoral of Iran in relation to esophageal cancer. Nutr Cancer 9(2–3):147–157. doi:10.1080/01635588709513922

Ghayur MN, Gilani AH, Janssen LJ (2012) Intestinal, airway, and cardiovascular relaxant activities of thymoquinone. Evid Based Complement Alternat Med 2012:305319. doi:10.1155/2012/305319

Ghosheh OA, Houdi AA, Crooks PA (1999) High performance liquid chromatographic analysis of the pharmacologically active quinones and related compounds in the oil of the black seed (Nigella sativa L.). J Pharm Biomed Anal 19(5):757–762

Hafiza WA, Latifah SY (2014) Potential implications of GRP58 expression and susceptibility of cervical cancer to cisplatin and thymoquinone-based therapy. Onco Targets Ther 7:1375–1387. doi:10.2147/OTT.S62928

Hansen JT, Benghuzzi H, Tucci M, Cason Z (2003) The role of black seed in the proliferation and biochemical marker levels of Hep-2 cells. Biomed Sci Instrum 39:371–376

HIV-1 protease inhibitor induced oxidative stress in pancreatic beta-cells: protection with thymoquinone (2009) Exp Biol Med (Maywood) 234(4):x

Hussain AR, Ahmed M, Ahmed S, Manogaran P, Platanias LC, Alvi SN et al (2011) Thymoquinone suppresses growth and induces apoptosis via generation of reactive oxygen species in primary effusion lymphoma. Free Radic Biol Med 50(8):978–987. doi:10.1016/j.freeradbiomed.2010.12.034

Hussain AR, Uddin S, Ahmed M, Al-Dayel F, Bavi PP, Al-Kuraya KS (2013) Phosphorylated IkappaBalpha predicts poor prognosis in activated B-cell lymphoma and its inhibition with thymoquinone induces apoptosis via ROS release. PLoS One 8(3):e60540. doi:10.1371/journal.pone.0060540

Ichwan SJ, Al-Ani IM, Bilal HG, Suriyah WH, Taher M, Ikeda MA (2014) Apoptotic activities of thymoquinone, an active ingredient of black seed (Nigella sativa), in cervical cancer cell lines. Chin J Physiol 57(5):249–255. doi:10.4077/CJP.2014.BAB190

Kamei H, Koide T, Hashimoto Y, Kojima T, Hasegawa M, Umeda T (1997) Effect of allomelanin on tumor growth suppression in vivo and on the cell cycle phase. Cancer Biother Radiopharm 12(4):273–276

Kapan M, Tekin R, Onder A, Firat U, Evliyaoglu O, Taskesen F et al (2012) Thymoquinone ameliorates bacterial translocation and inflammatory response in rats with intestinal obstruction. Int J Surg 10(9):484–488. doi:10.1016/j.ijsu.2012.06.006

Kaseb AO, Chinnakannu K, Chen D, Sivanandam A, Tejwani S, Menon M et al (2007) Androgen receptor and E2F-1 targeted thymoquinone therapy for hormone-refractory prostate cancer. Cancer Res 67(16):7782–7788. doi:10.1158/0008-5472.CAN-07-1483

Khan MA (1999) Chemical composition and medicinal properties of Nigella sativa Linn. Inflammopharmacology 7(1):15–35. doi:10.1007/s10787-999-0023-y

Koka PS, Mondal D, Schultz M, Abdel-Mageed AB, Agrawal KC (2010) Studies on molecular mechanisms of growth inhibitory effects of thymoquinone against prostate cancer cells: role of reactive oxygen species. Exp Biol Med (Maywood) 235(6):751–760. doi:10.1258/ebm.2010.009369

Kortum B, Campregher C, Lang M, Khare V, Pinter M, Evstatiev R et al (2014) Mesalazine and thymoquinone attenuate intestinal tumour development in Msh2loxP/loxP Villin-Cre mice. Gut. doi:10.1136/gutjnl-2014-307663

Kundu J, Choi BY, Jeong CH, Kundu JK, Chun KS (2014) Thymoquinone induces apoptosis in human colon cancer HCT116 cells through inactivation of STAT3 by blocking JAK2- and Src-mediated phosphorylation of EGF receptor tyrosine kinase. Oncol Rep 32(2):821–828. doi:10.3892/or.2014.3223

Lei X, Lv X, Liu M, Yang Z, Ji M, Guo X et al (2012) Thymoquinone inhibits growth and augments 5-fluorouracil-induced apoptosis in gastric cancer cells both in vitro and in vivo. Biochem Biophys Res Commun 417(2):864–868. doi:10.1016/j.bbrc.2011.12.063

Motaghed M, Al-Hassan FM, Hamid SS (2013) Cellular responses with thymoquinone treatment in human breast cancer cell line MCF-7. Pharmacognosy Res 5(3):200–206. doi:10.4103/0974-8490.112428

Motaghed M, Al-Hassan FM, Hamid SS (2014) Thymoquinone regulates gene expression levels in the estrogen metabolic and interferon pathways in MCF7 breast cancer cells. Int J Mol Med 33 (1):8–16. doi:10.3892/ijmm.2013.1563

Mu GG, Zhang LL, Li HY, Liao Y, Yu HG (2014) Thymoquinone pretreatment overcomes the insensitivity and potentiates the antitumor effect of gemcitabine through abrogation of Notch1, PI3K/Akt/mTOR regulated signaling pathways in pancreatic cancer. Dig Dis Sci. doi:10.1007/s10620-014-3394-x

Nair HB, Sung B, Yadav VR, Kannappan R, Chaturvedi MM, Aggarwal BB (2010) Delivery of antiinflammatory nutraceuticals by nanoparticles for the prevention and treatment of cancer. Biochem Pharmacol 80(12):1833–1843. doi:10.1016/j.bcp.2010.07.021

Nessa MU, Beale P, Chan C, Yu JQ, Huq F (2011) Synergism from combinations of cisplatin and oxaliplatin with quercetin and thymoquinone in human ovarian tumour models. Anticancer Res 31(11):3789–3797

Ng WK, Saiful Yazan L, Yap LH, Wan Nor Hafiza WA, How CW, Abdullah R (2015) Thymoquinone-loaded nanostructured lipid carrier exhibited cytotoxicity towards breast cancer cell lines (MDA-MB-231 and MCF-7) and cervical cancer cell lines (HeLa and SiHa). Biomed Res Int 2015:263131. doi:10.1155/2015/263131

Norwood AA, Tan M, May M, Tucci M, Benghuzzi H (2006) Comparison of potential chemotherapeutic agents, 5-fluoruracil, green tea, and thymoquinone on colon cancer cells. Biomed Sci Instrum 42:350–356

Norwood AA, Tucci M, Benghuzzi H (2007) A comparison of 5-fluorouracil and natural chemotherapeutic agents, EGCG and thymoquinone, delivered by sustained drug delivery on colon cancer cells. Biomed Sci Instrum 43:272–277

O'Sullivan PM (1928) The Canon medicine of Avicenna. Bull Med Libr Assoc 17(3):14–15

Raghunandhakumar S, Paramasivam A, Senthilraja S, Naveenkumar C, Asokkumar S, Binuclara J et al (2013) Thymoquinone inhibits cell proliferation through regulation of G1/S phase cell cycle transition in N-nitrosodiethylamine-induced experimental rat hepatocellular carcinoma. Toxicol Lett 223(1):60–72. doi:10.1016/j.toxlet.2013.08.018

Rajput S, Kumar BN, Sarkar S, Das S, Azab B, Santhekadur PK et al (2013a) Targeted apoptotic effects of thymoquinone and tamoxifen on XIAP mediated Akt regulation in breast cancer. PLoS One 8(4):e61342. doi:10.1371/journal.pone.0061342

Rajput S, Kumar BN, Dey KK, Pal I, Parekh A, Mandal M (2013b) Molecular targeting of Akt by thymoquinone promotes G(1) arrest through translation inhibition of cyclin D1 and induces apoptosis in breast cancer cells. Life Sci 93(21):783–790. doi:10.1016/j.lfs.2013.09.009

Rajput S, Kumar BN, Banik P, Parida S, Mandal M (2015) Thymoquinone restores radiation-induced TGF-beta expression and abrogates EMT in chemoradiotherapy of breast cancer cells. J Cell Physiol 230(3):620–629. doi:10.1002/jcp.24780

Ravindran J, Nair HB, Sung B, Prasad S, Tekmal RR, Aggarwal BB (2010) Thymoquinone poly (lactide-co-glycolide) nanoparticles exhibit enhanced anti-proliferative, anti-inflammatory, and chemosensitization potential. Biochem Pharmacol 79(11):1640–1647. doi:10.1016/j.bcp.2010.01.023

Rothman T (1972) De Laguna's commentaries on hallucinogenic drugs and witchcraft in Dioscorides' Materia Media. Bull Hist Med 46(6):562–567

Salih B, Sipahi T, Donmez EO (2009) Ancient nigella seeds from Boyali Hoyuk in north-central Turkey. J Ethnopharmacol 124(3):416–420. doi:10.1016/j.jep.2009.05.039

Salim EI (2010) Cancer chemopreventive potential of volatile oil from black cumin seeds, Nigella sativa L., in a rat multi-organ carcinogenesis bioassay. Oncol Lett 1(5):913–924. doi:10.3892/ol_00000162

Salim EI, Fukushima S (2003) Chemopreventive potential of volatile oil from black cumin (Nigella sativa L.) seeds against rat colon carcinogenesis. Nutr Cancer 45(2):195–202. doi:10.1207/S15327914NC4502_09

Schneider-Stock R, Fakhoury IH, Zaki AM, El-Baba CO, Gali-Muhtasib HU (2014) Thymoquinone: fifty years of success in the battle against cancer models. Drug Discov Today 19(1):18–30. doi:10.1016/j.drudis.2013.08.021

Sorenson BS, Banton KL, Augustin LB, Leonard AS, Saltzman DA (2011) Antioxidant oils and Salmonella enterica Typhimurium reduce tumor in an experimental model of hepatic metastasis. Onco Targets Ther 4:59–69. doi:10.2147/OTT.S17081

Sutton KM, Greenshields AL, Hoskin DW (2014) Thymoquinone, a bioactive component of black caraway seeds, causes G1 phase cell cycle arrest and apoptosis in triple-negative breast cancer cells with mutant p53. Nutr Cancer 66(3):408–418. doi:10.1080/01635581.2013.878739

Torres MP, Ponnusamy MP, Chakraborty S, Smith LM, Das S, Arafat HA et al (2010) Effects of thymoquinone in the expression of mucin 4 in pancreatic cancer cells: implications for the development of novel cancer therapies. Mol Cancer Ther 9(5):1419–1431. doi:10.1158/1535-7163.MCT-10-0075

Velho-Pereira R, Kumar A, Pandey BN, Jagtap AG, Mishra KP (2011) Radiosensitization in human breast carcinoma cells by thymoquinone: role of cell cycle and apoptosis. Cell Biol Int 35(10):1025–1029. doi:10.1042/CBI20100701

Wang YM (2011) Inhibitory effects of thymoquinone on human pancreatic carcinoma orthotopically implanted in nude mice. Zhonghua Yi Xue Za Zhi 91(44):3111–3114

Wilson-Simpson F, Vance S, Benghuzzi H (2007) Physiological responses of ES-2 ovarian cell line following administration of epigallocatechin-3-gallate (EGCG), thymoquinone (TQ), and selenium (SE). Biomed Sci Instrum 43:378–383

Woo CC, Kumar AP, Sethi G, Tan KH (2012) Thymoquinone: potential cure for inflammatory disorders and cancer. Biochem Pharmacol 83(4):443–451. doi:10.1016/j.bcp.2011.09.029

Woo CC, Hsu A, Kumar AP, Sethi G, Tan KH (2013) Thymoquinone inhibits tumor growth and induces apoptosis in a breast cancer xenograft mouse model: the role of p38 MAPK and ROS. PLoS One 8(10):e75356. doi:10.1371/journal.pone.0075356

Worthen DR, Ghosheh OA, Crooks PA (1998) The in vitro anti-tumor activity of some crude and purified components of blackseed, Nigella sativa L. Anticancer Res 18(3A):1527–1532

Wu ZH, Chen Z, Shen Y, Huang LL, Jiang P (2011) Anti-metastasis effect of thymoquinone on human pancreatic cancer. Yao Xue Xue Bao 46(8):910–914

Xu D, Ma Y, Zhao B, Li S, Zhang Y, Pan S et al (2014) Thymoquinone induces G2/M arrest, inactivates PI3K/Akt and nuclear factor-kappaB pathways in human cholangiocarcinomas both in vitro and in vivo. Oncol Rep 31(5):2063–2070. doi:10.3892/or.2014.3059

Yusufi M, Banerjee S, Mohammad M, Khatal S, Venkateswara Swamy K, Khan EM et al (2013) Synthesis, characterization and anti-tumor activity of novel thymoquinone analogs against pancreatic cancer. Bioorg Med Chem Lett 23(10):3101–3104. doi:10.1016/j.bmcl.2013.03.003

Zohary M (1982) Plants of the Bible: a complete handbook to all the plants with 200 full-color plates taken in the natural habitat. Cambridge University Press, Cambridge

Soy Isoflavones in the Breast Cancer Risk: From Preclinical Findings to Clinical Strategy

P. Kubatka, J. Mojžiš, M. Pilátová, M. Péč, and P. Kruzliak

Abstract There has been considerable interest about the potential of soy products to decrease risk of cancer, in particular cancer of the breast. Soy products are a unique dietary source of isoflavones, which bind to estrogen receptors and exhibit weak estrogen-like effects under certain experimental conditions. Based mostly on in vitro and rodent results, the relationship between soy foods/isoflavone supplements and breast cancer has become controversial. Several research groups observed that soy isoflavones may promote the growth of estrogen receptor-positive breast cancer cells, and in this regard, it is essential to evaluate the relevance of the preclinical data to the human disease. On the other hand, there are only limited clinical results with no evidence that soy isoflavones increase breast cancer risk in healthy women or worsen the prognosis of breast cancer patients. The epidemiologic data are generally consistent with the clinical results, with no association between increased breast cancer risk and regular consumption of soy products. It is important to determine if and when isoflavones are beneficial or detrimental in breast cancer patients and identify their role in the molecular mechanisms of mammary carcinogenesis.

This book chapter focuses on the biological effects of soy isoflavones in breast tissue, as well as preclinical research and clinical/epidemiologic data with recommendations required in human investigation.

P. Kubatka • M. Péč
Jessenius Faculty of Medicine in Martin, Department of Medical Biology, Comenius University, Bratislava, Slovak Republic

J. Mojžiš • M. Pilátová
Faculty of Medicine, Department of Pharmacology, P. J. Šafárik University, Košice, Slovak Republic

P. Kruzliak (✉)
Department of Cardiovascular Diseases, International Clinical Research Centre, St. Anne's University Hospital and Masaryk University, Brno, Czech Republic
e-mail: peter.kruzliak@savba.sk

M.F. Ullah, A. Ahmad (eds.), *Critical Dietary Factors in Cancer Chemoprevention*,
DOI 10.1007/978-3-319-21461-0_10

1 Introduction

Cancer remains one of the leading causes of morbidity and mortality worldwide. Based on the GLOBOCAN 2008 estimates, about 12.7 million cancer cases and 7.6 million cancer deaths are estimated to have occurred in 2008. By 2030, it is projected that there will be approximately 26 million new cancer cases and 17 million cancer deaths per year (Ferlay et al. 2010; Thun et al. 2010). Breast cancer is the most frequently diagnosed cancer and the leading cause of cancer death among females, accounting for 1.38 million of the total cancer cases and 458,400 of the cancer deaths in 2008 (Jemal et al. 2011).

Although the direct causes of breast cancer are not known, a number of well-established risk factors have been identified. Some of them such as family history, lactation, menstrual history, and reproductive history are, however, generally difficult to modify. On the other hand, it has been documented that vegetable diet (Cho et al. 2010; Ronco et al. 2010; Shin et al. 2010) may reduce breast cancer risk and it is estimated that approximately one-third of cases could be prevented by dietary modification. It is well known that Asian populations have historically lower rates of breast cancer than in Western populations (Dong and Qin 2011; Xie et al. 2013). One possible explanation of this phenomenon is a high consumption of soy foods in Asia (Shu et al. 2009). Soybeans and soy foods contain several compounds with the ability to inhibit malignant transformation. Among them, phytoestrogens attract great interest because of a wide range of biological actions (Kwon and Song 2011; Valeri et al. 2012; Zhang et al. 2012a) including chemopreventive activity in some malignancies such as breast and prostate cancer (Constantinou et al. 2001; Horie 2012; Wada et al. 2013).

Breast cancer is known to be influenced by several hormones. Approximately two-thirds of breast cancers are positive for estrogen receptors (ER) and estrogens are hormonal risk factors for breast cancer (Lim et al. 2012). Soy phytoestrogens including genistein, daidzein, and glycitein are isoflavonoids with structural similarity to human 17β-estradiol (Hooper et al. 2009). They exhibit estrogen-like properties but bind more weakly to ER than 17β-estradiol (Dixon 2004). Genistein and daidzein preferentially activate the binding of ERβ to estrogen-response element than ERα (Kostelac et al. 2003) and induce distinct changes in ER conformation (Pike et al. 1999). These findings lead to a speculation that isoflavones may function as a selective estrogen receptor modulator. Nowadays, there are hundreds of scientific publications focused on the ability of soy isoflavonoids to modify the processes of carcinogenesis including initiation, promotion, and progression. Numerous potential mechanisms have been proposed for this cancer-preventing activity of isoflavonoids. They may inhibit different signaling pathways associated with the growth of cancer cells (e.g., PTK, Akt, NF-κB, MAPK, COX-2, AP-1), angiogenesis (HIF-1α, VEGF), adhesion, and metastasis (FAK, MMPs), or inhibit topoisomerases I and II, 5α-reductase, and protein histidine kinase (Sarkar and Li 2002; Nagaraju et al. 2013). Moreover, genistein also antagonizes estrogen-mediated signaling pathways in the processes of carcinogenesis (Banerjee et al. 2008).

Since the cancer-promoting effects of soy isoflavones in preclinical research were found (Hsieh et al. 1998; Ju et al. 2001; Allred et al. 2001, 2004), several clinical studies have been conducted to clarify the effect of soy isoflavones on breast cancer risk (Fang et al. 2005; Kang et al. 2010; Nechuta et al. 2012; Conroy et al. 2013; Chi et al. 2013). In above noted clinical research, however, soy consumption did not adversely affect breast cancer risk or survival in women. Recent research has shown that since diagnosis of breast cancer, 17 % of women started or stopped soy foods (Boucher et al. 2012). On the other hand, phytoestrogens including soy isoflavones were found to have potentially positive effects in the prevention of menopausal symptoms. Nevertheless, there is insufficient evidence to recommend the use of phytoestrogens in place of traditional estrogen replacement therapy, or to make recommendations to women about specific phytoestrogen products (Glazier and Bowman 2001). For that reasons, it is necessary to establish whether intake of soy foods or isoflavones should be avoided in breast cancer patients or high-risk individuals, or on the other hand, may have potentially positive effects in women. Based on the results from preclinical and clinical research, we summarize the current knowledge regarding the effects of soy isoflavones in the breast and the needs for improving clinical strategies about the use of these phytoestrogens.

2 In Vitro Studies

A number of studies suggest that soy isoflavones, mainly genistein, may suppress growth of different cancer cells including breast cancer cells (Chen and Chien 2014; Choi and Kim 2013; Lepri et al. 2014; Li et al. 2011; Mukherjee et al. 2010). As it was mentioned above genistein displays structural similarities with estradiol and may act as an agonist or antagonist of ER. This biphasic effect on the growth of breast cancer cells is strictly dependent on its concentrations. It is well documented that soy isoflavones possess pleiotropic effects in the cell which are involved in the processes of breast carcinogenesis.

2.1 Effect of Isoflavones on Cell Proliferation

As it has been documented, genistein at low concentrations (up to 10^{-6} M) stimulated growth of ER-positive (ER+) breast cancer cells (MCF-7) but not ER-negative (ER−) breast cancer (MDA-MB-435) cells, whereas at higher concentrations (>10 mM) growth of both MCF-7 and MDA-MB-435 cells was inhibited (Hsieh et al. 1998; Maggiolini et al. 2001; Li et al. 1999a; Zava and Duwe 1997). These data indicated that genistein may modulate cell proliferation by different mechanisms of action; ER-mediated mechanism is important for low concentrations, whereas other mechanisms of action are suggested for higher genistein concentrations. Genistein, apart from its estrogenic and anti-estrogenic activity, inhibits also growth of different hormone non-dependent cancer cells. The possible explanation of this effect is the ability of genistein to influence mechanisms involved in cell proliferation and growth.

It is well known that activation of receptor-associated tyrosine kinases (RTKs) may result in abnormal cell proliferation, abundant angiogenesis, or inhibition of apoptotic pathways (Jones and Kazlauskas 2001). In 1987, Akiyama and coworkers (1987) documented ability of genistein to inhibit protein-tyrosine kinase (PTK) associated with the epidermal growth factor receptor (EGFR). As they documented, genistein competitively inhibits the ATP catalytic sites on this RTK. On the other hand, the study of Peterson and Barnes (1996) showed that anti-proliferative effect of genistein may not be related to RTK inhibition. They found no inhibition of EGFR-tyrosine phosphorylation by genistein in MGF-7 cells at concentration of $\leq$20 mg/ml.

In addition to PTK-inhibitory activity of isoflavones, genistein has also been shown to inhibit DNA topoisomerase II. Topoisomerases are nuclear enzymes that alter the DNA topology required for the replication, transcription, recombination, and segregation of daughter chromosomes (Wang 1996). Furthermore, both topoisomerase I (TOPO I) and topoisomerase II (TOPO II) are target molecules for potent anticancer drugs such as irinotecan and topotecan (TOPO I) (Pommier 2006) or etoposide, teniposide, and doxorubicin (TOPO II) (Martincic and Hande 2005). Genistein may inhibit a wide range of cancer cells, and its cytotoxicity is considered to involve an inhibitory effect of TOPO II. Recently, Mizushina and coworkers (2013) studied the inhibitory activity of daidzein, genistein, and glycitein and their glycosides (daidzin, genistin, and glycitin) on purified TOPO I and TOPO II. They found that only genistein selectively inhibited human TOPO II at $IC_{50} = 37.5\ \mu M$. Activity of TOPO I was not influenced. Humans encode two isoforms of topoisomerase II—α and β (Wang 1996). TOPO IIα is essential to the survival of all proliferating cells and increases dramatically during the S and G2/M phases of cell cycle (Mandraju et al. 2008). On the other hand, TOPO IIβ is associated with non-proliferating function and believed to maintain the integrity of nuclear chromatin. Perrin et al. (1998) compared the effects of a series of compounds on the activity of the α and β forms of recombinant human TOPO II. According to their results, genistein showed equivalent effects on both enzymes. On the other hand, data of Salti et al. (2000) strongly suggest that the preferred enzymatic target of genistein is TOPO IIα. Furthermore, genistein not only inhibits enzyme activity but also suppresses TOPO IIα expression through the regulation of Specificity protein 1 and Specificity protein 3 (Zhou et al. 2009). In contrast, transgenic cells lacking DNA topoisomerase IIβ are resistant to genistein (López-Lazaro et al. 2007). Higher affinity of genistein to TOPO IIβ has also been confirmed by Bandele and Osheroff (2007). These data suggest that TOPO IIβ has important function in genistein-induced anti-proliferative effect.

It was well known that the growth and proliferation of mammalian cells are mediated via cell cycle progression and the growth inhibition of cancer cells could be due to cell cycle arrest, which ultimately results in cessation of cell proliferation. It has been documented that genistein may induce a G2/M arrest in different cancer cell lines (Liu et al. 2013b; Han et al. 2013) or arrest mouse fibroblast at an G0/G1 phase of the cell cycle (Kuzumaki et al. 1998). Pagliacci et al. (1994) have shown that genistein at low dose causes a reversible G2/M arrest in MCF-7 cells whereas higher dose results in a marked fall in number of cells in S phase associated with a persistent arrest in the G2/M phase. As documented recently, this effect is irrespective of the cell line's ER status (Liu et al. 2013a). Moreover, genistein also blocks G2/M cell cycle progression in non-cancer human mammary epithelial cells (Frey et al. 2001). Cell cycle is tightly regulated by different cyclins, cyclin-dependent kinases (CDKs), and cyclin-dependent kinase inhibitors (CDKIs) in different phases of the cell cycle. Genistein was found to decrease the expression of cyclin B, an important regulator of CDK activity which is necessary for forming cyclin B/CDK complex during the G2/M phase procession (Davis et al. 1998; Liao et al. 2004). Cell cycle progression is also affected by the p21WAF1 and p27KIP1, CDK inhibitors. Several in vivo and in vitro studies showed significant upregulation of both inhibitors in breast cancer cells after genistein treatment (Shao et al. 1998; Eto 2006; Lian et al. 1998).

Another soy isoflavonoid, daidzein, also significantly increased percentage of cells in G2/M phase in both MCF-7 and MDA-MB-453 cells. This effect was associated with decrease in cyclin D and cyclin-dependent kinases (CDK2 and CDK4), whereas the expression of CDK6 and cyclin E was unchanged. Furthermore, the protein expression of CDK1 related to the G2/M phase decreased markedly after incubation of cells with daidzein. Moreover, daidzein also increased the expression of the CDK inhibitors p21Cip1 and p57Kip2 (Choi and Kim 2008).

2.2 *The Impact on Apoptosis*

Defective apoptosis is one of the hallmark characteristic that is required for cells to become cancerous. Drugs that can restore the apoptotic signaling pathways toward normality have the potential to eliminate cancer cells. A number of studies suggest that genistein may induce apoptosis in breast cancer cell lines either alone or in combination with other anticancer drugs. Although the precise molecular mechanism of genistein's effect on apoptosis has not been identified, most studies indicate its effect on the expression of the various pro-apoptotic and anti-apoptotic proteins. Major regulators of apoptosis are different members of the Bcl-2 family of proteins and the regulation of Bcl-2 and/or Bax is probably the key element of the pro-apoptotic mechanism of genistein. Li et al. (2008) have found that treatment of MDA-MB-231 cells for 48 h with genistein caused a dose-dependent increase in the level of the pro-apoptotic Bax protein as well as reduction of anti-apoptotic Bcl-2 in a dose-dependent manner. Different effect of genistein on Bax and Bcl-2 expression in MCF-7 cells was documented by Xu and Loo (2001). Bax levels were not influenced significantly whereas Bcl-2 decreased slightly at 24 h but then increased considerably after 48 h. Increased apoptosis and reduced Bcl-2/Bax ratio were also observed in MCF-7 cells treated with glycitein (Sakamoto et al. 2010).

The role of caspases in genistein-induced apoptosis has been emphasized. Ability of genistein to modulate activity of caspases depends on the cell lines. MDA-MB-231 cells express functional caspase-3 (Li et al. 1999b), whereas MCF-7 cells are caspase-3 deficient (Xu and Loo 2001). In the study of Li et al. (2008), cleavage of procaspase-3 and induction of caspase-3 activity occurred following exposure of MDA-MB-231 cells to genistein. On the other hand, activation of caspase-7 (Shim et al. 2007) and caspase-12 (Sergeev 2004) has been observed in MCF-7 cells after incubation with genistein.

Nuclear factor-κB (NF-κB) is a transcription factor which controls expression of several genes involved in cell proliferation, invasion, transformation, and angiogenesis (Shishodia and Aggarwal 2004). Moreover, it has been demonstrated that the activation of NF-κB may suppress apoptosis (Bharti and Aggarwal 2002). Thus, inhibition of NF-κB activity in cancer cells may provide a target for either prevention or treatment of cancer. Recently, Yamasaki and coworkers (2013) showed that genistein induced apoptosis in T-cell leukemia cells. This effect was associated with decreased nuclear p65 translocation and IκBα phosphorylation, and downregulation of the anti-apoptotic proteins, XIAP, cIAP, and survivin, NF-κB-responsive gene products. Pro-apoptotic effect of genistein mediated by inactivation of NF-kB signaling pathway has also been presented in MDA-MB-231 breast cancer cells. As authors documented, inactivation of NF-kB was mediated via downregulation of Akt pathway (Gong et al. 2003). Later, Li et al. (2008) observed dose-dependent effect of genistein on the MEK5/ERK5/NF-κB pathway in MDA-MB-231 breast cancer. Genistein decreased NF-κB/p65 protein levels and DNA-binding activity of NF-κB. Suppressive effect of genistein on ERK5 expression with accompanied increase of Bax expression and caspase-3 activity MDA-MB-231 breast cancer cells was also reported (Li et al. 2006). Recently, the study of Pan et al. (2012) also demonstrated downregulation of the expression of cyclin B1, Bcl-2, and Bcl-xL. As it was suggested, these effects were mediated by inhibition of NF-κB activity. Furthermore, it has also been found that genistein through regulation of NF-κB can potentiate the antitumor activity of chemotherapeutic agents. Several anticancer drugs (e.g., cis-platin, doxorubicin, 5-fluorouracil, paclitaxel) can activate NF-κB in cancer cells and this has been believed to be responsible in part for drug resistance in cancer cells (Chuang et al. 2002; Yeh et al. 2002). Li et al. (2005) studied effect of genistein on anti-proliferative activity of three anticancer drugs. They found that pretreatment of prostate, breast, lung, and pancreas cancer cells with genistein resulted in significantly greater anti-proliferative and pro-apoptotic effect of cis-platin, docetaxel, and doxorubicin. Moreover, they found that the anticancer drug-stimulated NF-κB activity was completely abrogated in cells pretreated with genistein. Genistein also potentiated pro-apoptotic effect of irinotecan and topotecan in different cancer cell lines and this action may be consequence of inhibition of nuclear translocation of NF-κB (Papazisis et al. 2006).

2.3 *Isoflavones and BRCA1/BRCA2 Genes*

The breast cancer-associated gene 1 (BRCA1) is frequently mutated tumor-suppressor gene found in familial breast cancers and BRCA1 mutation carriers have a risk of developing breast cancer (Lee et al. 2010). It was reported that genistein induces the expression of breast tumor suppressors (BRCA1 and BRCA2) in hormone-dependent breast cancer cells (Fan et al. 2006). As authors suggested, genistein may induce BRCA expression via activation of endoplasmic reticulum stress response signaling. In other studies, genistein has also been shown to inhibit BRCA1-mutant mammary tumor cells (Tominaga et al. 2007; Privat et al. 2010). Data from these experiments indicated that BRCA1-mutant cells were more sensitive to genistein than some other types of cancer cells expressing wild-type BRCA1 protein. This finding highlights a good therapeutic potential of genistein for BRCA1-associated breast cancer whereby p21 (WAF1/CIP1) and Akt could be genistein potential targets in these cells. Moreover, Bosviel et al. (2012) suggested that treatment of MCF-7, MDA-MB 231, and MCF10a cell lines with genistein or daidzein might reverse DNA hypermethylation and restore the expression of the oncosuppressor genes BRCA1 and BRCA2. Authors provided new evidence on potential epigenetic mechanisms by which genistein and daidzein might contribute to regulation of the BRCA1 and BRCA2. Finally, Satih et al. (2010) observed that the significant expression decrease of apoptosis-related genes, such as Bax, and the expression increase of Bcl-2, under BRCA1 knockdown condition in MCF-7, MDA-MB 231, and MCF10a cell lines, were completely reversed after genistein or daidzein treatments. Figure 1 summarizes the molecular targets of genistein on cancer cells.

3 Animal Studies

Because sexual maturation is similar among species, animal models provide a practical design for the study of variety endocrine functions. Numerous endocrine-mediated functions in mice or rats, for example, are comparable to other mammalian species including humans. Due to these species-related similarities, rodents may provide high reproducibility model for investigation in humans (Russo et al. 1996; Medina 2007). In the years since, there has been considerable investigation of the potential anticancer effects of soy products against breast cancer in animal studies. Soy foods have been suggested to have both positive health effects and potentially adverse effects as a consequence of the content of isoflavones—a natural phytoestrogen with potential hormonal activity due to their

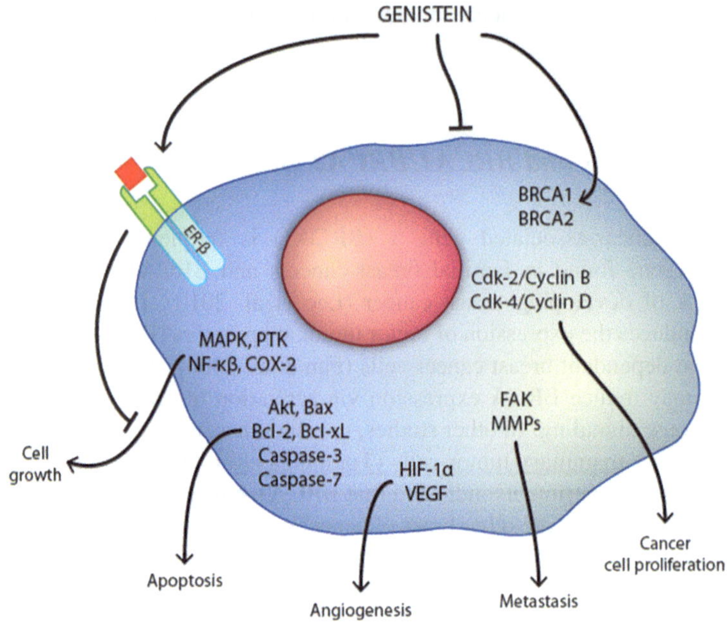

Fig. 1 Molecular targets of genistein on cancer cells. Genistein exhibits either stimulatory or inhibitory effects on different signaling pathways. Abbreviations: *COX-2* cyclooxygenase-2, *FAK* focal adhesion kinase, *HIF-1α* hypoxia-inducible factor 1α, *MAPK* mitogen-activated protein kinase, *MMPs* matrix metalloproteinases, *NF-κβ* nuclear factor κβ, *PTK* protein-tyrosine kinase, *VEGF* vascular endothelial growth factor

similar chemical structure to 17-β-estradiol. In this regard, there are two recent experiments which suggested that soy protein isolate fails to recruit appropriate co-activators at estradiol-inducible genes and behaves like selective estrogen receptor modulator rather than weak estrogen in the developing rat mammary gland (Miousse et al. 2013; Ronis et al. 2012). Long-term administration of isoflavones to rats (24 months) led to substantial increase in gene expression in the mammary gland and thus these natural compounds significantly influence cell signaling (Chalabi et al. 2010). Molzberger et al. (2013) found that isoflavone exposure to female rats during puberty is sufficient to reduce the proliferative response of the adult mammary gland to estradiol but not to reduce the response of progesterone receptor (PR). Importantly, studies focused on the detailed analysis of the soy isoflavones' estrogenicity in mammary carcinogenesis are still lacking.

There are some scientific approaches investigating antitumor efficacy of soy products or isolated soy isoflavones in breast cancer animal models. Numerous experiments realized in this research were based on the ovariectomized athymic mouse model; on the other hand, it is the chemically induced rat mammary carcinogenesis.

3.1 ER-Positive Breast Cancer Model in Ovariectomized Athymic Mice

A variety of studies have found that soy isoflavones stimulate estrogen receptor-positive (ER+) human breast cancer cell xenoplasts in ovariectomized athymic mice that first raised fear that soy isoflavones might be contraindicated for breast cancer patients. The Helferich's group demonstrated that the isoflavone, genistein, stimulates the growth of estrogen-dependent human breast cancer (MCF-7) cells in vivo (Hsieh et al. 1998). In this study, MCF-7 cells were implanted s.c. in ovariectomized athymic mice, and the growth of the estrogen-dependent tumors was measured weekly. Tumors were larger in the genistein-treated group than they were in the untreated control group. The same group using the same model investigated whether consumption of genistein from soy protein will have similar effects on estrogen-dependent tumor growth as pure genistein (Allred et al. 2001). Soy protein diets containing varying amounts of genistein increased estrogen-dependent tumor growth in a dose-dependent manner. Similar results with stimulatory effects of isoflavones on ER+ breast cancer cells xenoplasts in ovariectomized mice were confirmed also in other experiments (Ju et al. 2001; Allred et al. 2004). Furthermore, using the same model, dietary genistein negated the inhibitory effect of tamoxifen on MCF-7 tumor growth, lowered estradiol levels in plasma, and increased expression of estradiol-responsive genes (e.g., pS2, progesterone receptor, and cyclin D1) (Ju et al. 2002). The same group evaluated the interaction of dietary genistein and an aromatase inhibitor, letrozole, on the growth of tumors in an aromatase-expressing breast cancer xenograft model (MCF-7Ca) in the presence and absence of the substrate androstenedione. Dietary genistein increased the growth of MCF-7Ca tumors implanted in ovariectomized mice, and in the presence of androstenedione and letrozole, dietary genistein reversed the inhibitory effect of letrozole on MCF-7Ca tumor growth in a dose-dependent manner (Ju et al. 2008).

Other research using athymic mouse model has found that more processed soy products result in faster tumor growth than mice exposed to less processed soy product even if the amount of genistein in both groups was the same (Allred et al. 2004). There are some explanations for this finding. Soy foods' processing causes greater increase of serum genistein levels in animals. Food processing can remove non-nutritive components of soy products which are able to inhibit the tumor-stimulatory effects of isoflavones. These changes in the diet composition may increase circulating (and probably target tissue) concentrations of genistein, which activates ER-mediated processes required for tumor growth stimulation in the mouse postmenopausal breast cancer model (Allred et al. 2005). Using a similar rodent model of breast cancer, the Thompson's group also observed stimulatory effects of isolated soy protein on tumor growth (Saarinen et al. 2006).

Daidzein, the second most prominent isoflavone from soy, has been shown to have only modest stimulatory effect on the growth of MCF-7 cells in the athymic ovariectomized mouse model. Daidzein can be further metabolized to equol by bacterial microflora in the rodent intestine. Equol is structurally similar to estrogen and it is a potent ligand for ERβ. Thus, it has a potential to exert a greater estrogenic effect in comparison with the parent molecule—daidzein (Setchell et al. 2005; Setchell and Clerici 2010). Ju et al. (2006) evaluated the estrogenic potential of daidzein and synthetic equol to affect the growth of MCF-7 cells in vitro and in vivo. Similarly, dietary daidzein had a slight but significant stimulatory effect on MCF-7 tumor growth in ovariectomized athymic mice. However, no significant induction of pS2 mRNA (an estrogen-responsive marker) in tumors by dietary daidzein was found. On the other hand, dietary equol treatment did not stimulate MCF-7 tumor growth in this mouse model. No statistical differences in tumor size, proliferation, and pS2 expression among any treatment groups were found. Total daidzein or equol plasma levels in mice fed with the isoflavones were in the range that stimulated in vitro MCF-7 cell growth. The results of Ju et al. (2006) suggested that pharmacokinetic and/or metabolic factors attenuate the estrogenic effects of soy isoflavones in vivo.

There is, however, warrantable debate about the merits of using athymic ovariectomized mouse model of breast cancer to evaluate effects in humans. There are several limitations and weaknesses of abovementioned studies (Messina et al. 2006a; Messina and Wood 2008). A specific criticism is that unlike pre- and postmenopausal women, these mice do not produce sufficient endogenous estrogen to promote development and growth or to even maintain estrogen-dependent tumors. Therefore, the effects of soy isoflavones on MCF-7 cells xenoplasts were evaluated in an estrogen-deficient environment that does not adequately reflect conditions in both pre- and postmenopausal women. It has been debated that estrogenic effect of isoflavones characterized by stimulatory effects on tumor growth may be evident only in this model with hypoestrogenic environment. Nevertheless, there are some rodent studies in which estrogen levels were more reflective of the hormonal status of postmenopausal women and, however, tumor stimulation caused by isoflavonoids was found. It is the mouse model with implanted MCF-7a cells which serve as an autocrine source of estrogen in the ovariectomized, immune-suppressed animals (Ju et al. 2008) and model with silastic implants in mice that yield low circulating plasma estradiol levels similar to those observed in postmenopausal women (Ju et al. 2006). Another critic of abovementioned studies is the use of high oral doses of isoflavonoids. Isoflavones are relatively weak estrogen agonist compared to estradiol, but the markedly higher circulating concentrations of biologically active (unconjugated) genistein in certain strains of mice cast doubt on the value of the use of these rodents for gaining insight into the effects of isoflavones in humans (Setchell et al. 2011). In most of in vivo studies, the doses of isoflavonoids (750 ppm) were at least 15 times higher than the amounts found in traditional Asian diets (30–40 ppm) (Messina et al. 2006b). In addition, serum isoflavonoid molar ratios differ between rodents and humans also due to the rodent intestinal bacteria which effectively convert daidzein to equol, whereas only 30–50 % of humans are carriers of this specific bacterium (Gu et al. 2006). Even in human equol producers, genistein is the predominant serum isoflavone after the ingestion of soy products, whereas equol predominates in most other species including rodents. Importantly, from the clinical point of view, the isoflavone doses required for estrogen-stimulatory effects in women have not been identified yet. Furthermore, the important feature of this model is the lack of immune function that may eliminate possible mechanisms by which soy isoflavones suppress carcinogenesis. Guo et al. (2007) analyzed whether genistein modulation of the immune responses might contribute to the increased host resistances to tumors in adult female B6C3F1 mice. Pretreatment with genistein by gavage enhanced host resistances to the B16F10 tumors and DMBA-induced carcinogenesis. In addition, the exposure of mice to genistein increased the activities of in vivo cytotoxic T lymphocytes and natural killer cells. Another possible limitation of this model may be the extent how existing MCF-7 xenoplasts in nude mice reflect tumors in patients with breast cancer. These model tumors are transformed and consist of cells that are very sensitive to proliferative effects of estrogen or even genistein with weak estrogenic properties. Finally, there are other relevant rodent models (e.g., chemically induced rat mammary carcinogenesis) that have shown the suppression rather than stimulation of mammary tumor growth (Ma et al. 2014; Ronis et al. 2012; Dave et al. 2010).

3.2 Chemically Induced ER-Positive Tumors in Rats

Rat mammary carcinogenesis in female rats induced by 7,12-dimethylbenz[a] anthracene(DMBA) is well-established hormone-dependent breast cancer model which tremendously increased the understanding of chemically induced tumors in the mammary gland. The conversion of normal mammary epithelial cells to adenocarcinomas by DMBA is relevant to the events leading to breast cancer in women. This model is favored by the National Cancer Institute for the evaluation of breast cancer chemopreventive agents (Kelloff 2000). There are numerous recent studies which investigated whether soy isoflavones have any effect on the chemoprevention and suppression of experimental rat mammary gland cancer development induced by DMBA. Ma et al. (2014) found that soy isoflavone intake inhibited the development of DMBA-induced mammary tumors in normal and ovariectomized rats. In this study, mRNA and protein expression of ER was significantly higher in treated groups. Moreover, isoflavone treatment significantly decreased 8-hydroxydeoxyguanosine content and increased superoxide dismutase level in normal rats and decreased malondialdehyde concentrations in ovariectomized rats. In another study of this group, isoflavone or equol intake significantly inhibited the incidence and lengthened the latency period of DMBA-induced mammary tumors in ovariectomized rats probably due to increased antioxidant and estrogenic activities (Ma et al. 2014). In another study, the supplementation of genistin alone or with selenium provided antioxidant defense with high-potential chemopreventive activity against DMBA-induced mammary tumors more than selenium alone. These positive effects of genistein were characterized with decreasing levels of tumorigenicity, endocrine derangement, and oxidative stress in premenopausal breast cancer model (Hamdy et al. 2012).

The status of glycoconjugates (protein-bound hexose, hexosamine, sialic acid, and fucose) in plasma or serum serves as potential biomarkers for assessing tumor progression and therapeutic interventions. Pugalendhi et al. (2011) observed that genistein and daidzein in combination protected the structural integrity of the cell surface and membranes during DMBA-induced rat mammary tumorigenesis. The same combination of isoflavones showed anti-lipid peroxidative efficacy and modulatory effect on phase I and phase II detoxification cascade during DMBA-induced rat mammary carcinogenesis (Pugalendhi and Manoharan 2010). In addition to genistein and daidzein combination in DMBA breast cancer model, Aidoo and Manjanatha (2011) suggested that consuming diets containing more than one soy isoflavones as opposed to taking supplements in isolation could impart some benefits.

There are also recent studies, which evaluated the efficacy of two equol enantiomers S-(−)equol and R-(+)equol dietary administered in animal model of DMBA-induced mammary gland cancer. In the first study, S-(−)equol had no chemopreventive action, nor was it stimulatory. In contrast, R-(+)equol significantly decreased tumor frequency and lengthened tumor latency and tumors were less invasive. Both enantiomers had no effect on absolute uterine weight (Brown et al. 2010a). In the second study, rats were exposed to S-(−)equol or R-(+)equol during the neonatal (0–21 days) or prepubertal (21–35 days) periods only. The exposure of both equol enantiomers resulted in a decrease in immature terminal end structures and an increase in mature lobules. Despite these morphological changes to the mammary gland, neonatal and prepubertal exposure to equol had no long-term chemopreventive effects in DMBA-induced mammary carcinogenesis (Brown et al. 2010b). In addition, significant tumor-suppressive effects of soy isoflavones in hormone-dependent rat mammary carcinoma model induced by ethyl methanesulfonate (Ono et al. 2012) or *N*-methyl-*N*-nitrosourea (NMU) (Dave et al. 2010) were found. However, in the experiment with NMU, soy-rich diet may influence the development of more aggressive carcinomas by enhancing progesterone receptor-A-dependent signaling.

In contrast to plentiful above noted results with significant antitumor effects of isoflavones in chemically induced rat breast cancer model, there is the study where postpubertal exposure of Donryu rats to isoflavones at an estrogenic dose resulted in promotion of mammary and uterine carcinogenesis induced by DMBA and *N*-ethyl-*N*′-nitro-*N*-nitrosoguanidine. Authors suggested that this result might be caused by the activation of ER-dependent signaling and alteration of the molecular tumor environment in the target organs (Kakehashi et al. 2012). Possible explanation for this relatively isolated negative result in rat model may be the use of different strain of Donryu rats with different genetic background when compared to often investigated Sprague-Dawley rats. In conclusion, however, findings noted above demonstrated clear chemopreventive and tumor-suppressive effects of soy isoflavones in a well-established chemically induced breast cancer model.

3.3 Effects on ER-Negative Breast Cancer Model

The effects of genistein on hormone-independent breast cancer model in vivo have been less investigated. To evaluate the effect of dietary genistein on tumor growth in vivo, genistein was fed to female athymic mice inoculated with ER-negative MDA-MB-231 cells. After solid tumor masses had formed, mice were fed genistein at a dose of 750 mg/kg. This dose of genistein did not significantly alter tumor development (Santell et al. 2000). Similarly, genistein (at the same dose) fed 3 days before cells were inoculated into mice did not significantly inhibit tumor formation or growth. However, another study reported that lower dose of genistein (250 mg/kg) suppressed the growth of MDA-MB-231 cells implanted into female nude mice orthotopically (Li et al. 2013). Possible explanation of this discrepancy in results may be the orthotopic mouse model used by Li et al. that provides probably better physiological conditions in comparison with subcutaneous implantation of cancer cells as realized by Santell et al. In addition, Li et al. (2013) in the same experiment suggested that soybean genistein can epigenetically restore ERα expression probably through the inhibition of expression and activity of enzymes that regulate chromatin structure in MDA-MB-231 breast cancer cells. These changes in turn increase tamoxifen-dependent anti-estrogen therapeutic sensitivity of MDA-MB-231 cells in vitro and in vivo. ER-negative breast cancers are unresponsive to tamoxifen therapy and more aggressive, resulting in a poorer prognosis. Therefore, novel therapeutic combination approach using bioactive soybean product and tamoxifen therapy in refractory ERα-negative breast cancer might be a good option but needs to be evaluated further (Li et al. 2013).

In preclinical research, the effects of daidzein on ER-negative breast cancer are insufficient and inconsistent. Athymic female mice with ER-negative MDA-MB-435 xenoplasts were treated orally with 10 mg/kg genistein or daidzein. Results showed that daidzein increased while genistein decreased mammary tumor growth. Daidzein increased lung and heart metastases while genistein decreased bone and liver metastases. Combined soy isoflavones did not affect primary tumor growth but increased metastasis to all organs tested (Martínez-Montemayor et al. 2010). Daidzein alone significantly upregulated 9 of 84 genes that regulate proliferation and protein synthesis (e.g., EIF4G1, eIF4E, and survivin). On the other hand, metastatic effects of eqoul on MDA-MB-435 cells were not confirmed in vitro (Magee et al. 2014). In this regard, however, the identity of MDA-MB-435 as breast cancer cells was questioned (Lacroix 2009), and it will be necessary to verify the relevance of this cell line for future breast cancer research.

4 Soy and Breast Cancer: Results from Clinical Research

Soy and soy isoflavones' consumption has been studied in relation to breast cancer. Decrease in disease incidence was noted likely as a result of their ability to mimic natural estrogens, which are known to play a role in breast cancer progression (Pavese et al. 2010). Wu et al. study (2008) showed 18 % lower breast cancer risk in Asian women with the highest isoflavone intake (≥10.6 mg/day). However, Dong and Qin (2011) described only 11 % decrease in risk of breast cancer incidence. They documented that the risk of breast cancer incidence decreased, on average, by 4 % for every 10 mg/day increase of soy isoflavones intake. No significant effects were found in Western population. The Westerners' results may largely be attributed to the different amount of soy consumption which is obviously far below even the lower levels of intake in an Asian population (Xie et al. 2013; Dong and Qin 2011). In Asian women, the lowest risk was noticed in the category of the highest of isoflavone intake. The risk in the low- and medium-dose category was similar (Table 1).

The fact that increased prevalence of clinical cancer may occur within a single generation after migration from the East to the West points out that cancer is not entirely genetic and that it can be pharmacologically altered by dietary constituents such as soy (Pavese et al. 2010). In Western diet, the majority of isoflavone intake comes from non-soy foods, such as soy additives in baked goods, tuna, or coffee. Asian people's isoflavone consumption is through soy foods, such as tofu, soy milk, miso, etc., in which the isoflavone content is similar (Xie et al. 2013; Horn-Ross et al. 2000). Early isoflavone exposure can protect against breast cancer as they may exert their putative protective effects by stimulating breast cell differentiation so isoflavone intake since childhood or adolescence may influence the risk of breast cancer incidence in adulthood (Messina and Wu 2009). One of the factors affecting the bioavailability of isoflavones may be frequency of ingestion. Relatively small doses of soy throughout the day can keep an optimum steady-state serum isoflavone level, as opposed to a single dose at once. Also interindividual differences in daidzein metabolism may play important role in the soy and breast cancer association. Isoflavan equol, a bacterially active derived metabolite of daidzein that is produced only by 25 % of Westerners, has been proposed as an especially beneficial compound. Equol binds with greater affinity to both ERs, with a higher binding affinity for ERβ having pro-apoptotic properties, than its parent compound

Table 1 The doses of isoflavones in humans

Asian women	
The highest dose category	>25 mg/day
Medium-dose category	15–25 mg/day
The low-dose category	5–15 mg/day
Western women	
High-dose category	>1000 μg/day
Low-dose category	500–1000 μg/day

daidzein. Clinical response is usually limited to people who are "equol producers," and its production varies across individuals and populations, equol-producer status should be considered as it may modify the estrogenic potency of isoflavones (Dong and Qin 2011; Nagata 2010; Setchell et al. 2002; Setchell and Cole 2006; Goodman et al. 2009; Ward et al. 2008). Until now limited clinical research has been done about association between the intake of soy isoflavones and its effect in breast cancer patients. As mentioned above, early life exposure to isoflavone in Asian women has protective effect on breast cancer risk (Lee et al. 2009; Xie et al. 2013) and has been associated with lower Her2/neu and proliferating cell nuclear antigen expression in malignant compared to benign breast tissue (Maskarinec et al. 2009). Clinical research studied mainly focus on determination of association between the intake of soy food and menopausal status, ER status and effect on adjuvant therapy, recurrence and survival among breast cancer patients.

4.1 Menopausal Status and Exposure to Soy Isoflavones

Endogenous estrogen levels in premenopausal women are greatly different from postmenopausal women. Since isoflavones possess estrogen-like effects it was assumed that menopausal status may play a modifying role in the isoflavone intake and breast cancer risk association (Chen et al. 2014; Dong and Qin 2011). Many epidemiological studies explored this association but inconclusive results were obtained. Lee et al. (2009) noted protective effect of isoflavone intake against premenopausal breast cancer, but no significant association between isoflavone intake and postmenopausal breast cancer. Isoflavone consumption did not affect estradiol or estrone, but it reduced FSH and LH in premenopausal women (Hooper et al. 2009). Other epidemiologic analyses suggest that high soy intake is associated with an approximate one-third reduction in the risk of both pre- and postmenopausal breast cancer among Asian women (Messina and Wu 2009). Stronger inverse association of isoflavone consumption with breast cancer incidence in postmenopausal women than in premenopausal women was presented in more studies (Xie et al. 2013; Nagata 2010; Dong and Qin 2011; Wu et al. 2008; Yamamoto et al. 2003).

Shike et al. (2014) described that after short-term soy administration (7–30 days) to premenopausal and early postmenopausal women with a diagnosis of breast cancer, three times more frequent beneficial responses in women over the age of 60 years than in those under that age. This fact may support the finding that the objective remission rate from estrogen replacement therapy in patients with metastatic breast cancer was higher in women more than 5 years past menopause (35 %) when compared with women who were less than five years postmenopause (9 %) or to patients who took estrogen replacement therapy straight after menopause where increase in breast cancer was noted (Anderson et al. 2012; Beral et al. 2011; Stoll 1977). Gene expression analysis associated with soy intake done on premenopausal and early postmenopausal breast cancer patients showed overexpression of protumorigenic growth factor receptor *FGFR2* and genes that drive and regulate G1/S and G2/M cell cycle processes, such as E2F5, BUB1, CCNB2 (Cyclin B2), MYBL2, CDK1, and CDC20, and proliferation pathways (Shike et al. 2014). The insufficient effect of estrogens and phytoestrogens in premenopausal women suggests that these compounds may be effective only at low sex hormone concentrations as in postmenopausal women (Dong and Qin 2011). This theory can be supported by physiologic estrogen-induced apoptosis in cells adapted to long-term estrogen deprivation when estrogen is not considered as survival signal for cell replication but as a trigger of apoptosis (Shike et al. 2014).

Sartippour et al. (2004) failed to find an effect of short-term isoflavone supplement administration on breast cancer growth. It is important to consider that this study was limited by the small number of patients and menopausal status of patients was not defined. No significant differences between premenopausal and postmenopausal women were found in Western population (Xie et al. 2013; Dong and Qin 2011).

4.2 ER Status of the Tumor

It is well known that soy isoflavones are structurally similar to estrogen and bind to ER so it was suggested that soy isoflavones may influence breast cancer risk and may play a differential role according to hormonal receptor status (Zhang et al. 2010; Kang et al. 2010). ER status is a prognostic factor as ER-positive tumors are associated with better survival and can be treated with hormone therapy (Bentzon et al. 2008). Results from studies evaluated the association between the intake of soy food and the risk of breast cancer by receptor status found that a stronger protective effect was associated with ER-positive tumors than with ER-negative tumors (Linseisen et al. 2004; Guha et al. 2009; Zhang et al. 2010). In The Shanghai Breast Cancer study stronger protective effect of soy was noted for both ER- and PR-positive patients (Dai et al. 2001; Zhang et al. 2009). The studies of Boyapati et al. (2005) and Shu et al. (2009) focused on the association between soy food intake and prognosis of breast cancer; however, it did not differ by ER/PR status.

4.3 Adjuvant Therapy, Recurrence, and Breast Cancer Survival

Tamoxifen, a selective estrogen receptor modulator, and anastrozole, third-generation nonsteroidal aromatase inhibitor, are commonly used as adjuvant endocrine therapy for hormone-sensitive breast cancer, and these drugs are effective in preventing recurrence and prolonging survival (Colozza et al. 2008; Ingle 2001).

Little is known about the potential effects of soy isoflavones intake in breast cancer patients receiving adjuvant endocrine therapy (Kang et al. 2010). As isoflavonoids exert estrogenic effects and play a competitive role with endogenous estrogens in the binding to ERs and breast cancer treatments is focused to a decrease in the endogenous estrogen supply, the question arose whether soy consumption interferes with the efficacy of tamoxifen and anastrozole in breast cancer patients (Zhang et al. 2012b; Kang et al. 2010). Although in some preclinical studies the inhibitory effects of tamoxifen on growth of implanted mammary tumors were negated by dietary administration of soy isoflavones (Liu et al. 2005; Ju et al. 2002), studies done on breast cancer patients did not confirm these assumptions. No adverse associations of soy consumption on breast cancer prognosis, recurrence, or total mortality either alone or in combination with tamoxifen was noted even at levels similar to those consumed in Asian populations (Caan et al. 2011; Guha et al. 2009; Shu et al. 2009). Several studies reported that consumption of soy foods may be associated with a reduced risk of recurrence among patients with tamoxifen treatment in postmenopausal women (Kang et al. 2010; Guha et al. 2009) but not in premenopausal women (Dong and Qin 2011). In Kang et al.'s (2010) study, the statistically significant inverse association between soy food intake and breast cancer recurrence was seen among Chinese, US, and US non-Asian postmenopausal women treated with tamoxifen. Soy isoflavones most likely acted as estrogen antagonists in postmenopausal breast cancer patients (Shu et al. 2009). More detailed analysis showed that the statistically significant inverse associations were restricted to ER- and PR-positive breast cancers (Kang et al. 2010). Shu et al. (2009) found that intake of soy foods was associated with improved survival regardless of tamoxifen use. High intake of soy isoflavones during anastrozole treatment reduced the risk of recurrence which could be explained by synergistic inhibitory effects of isoflavones and anastrozole on the synthesis of estrogen as isoflavones inhibit the activity of aromatase and 17β-hydroxysteroid dehydrogenases and increase clearance of steroids from the circulation (Kang et al. 2010; Taylor et al. 2009; Trock et al. 2006; Lacey et al. 2005; Brooks and Thompson 2005). Other studies showed that the high intake of soy food was positively associated with better prognosis, reduced mortality, recurrence, and longer survival among breast cancer patients (Conroy et al. 2013; Zhang et al. 2012b; Shu et al. 2009). Shu et al. (2009) observed that the benefit appears to reach the isoflavone dose of 36.6–62.7 mg/day and a further increase in intake does not confer greater benefit. Nechuta et al. (2012) in cohort studies of US and Chinese women found that the inverse association of soy isoflavone intake and recurrence appeared only among women with ER-negative breast cancer.

4.4 *Other Factors to Consider in Risk Assessment*

The results of published studies on soy intake and breast cancer risk in women are variable and showed risk-enhancing as well as risk-reducing effects. They suggest that soy may play a role in initial cancer prevention and/or in cancer progression. It was documented that early life is the critical period for soy exposure to decrease breast cancer risk. It was documented that consumption of soy is generally much lower in Western than in Asian women especially in early life which is the critical period for soy exposure to decrease breast cancer risk. Therefore the evaluation of exposure to soy food in adulthood or in different later periods of life may be more significant when evaluating its effect on analyzing breast cancer risk in Western women. Another reason supporting the need to take account of this fact is that soy food consumption is increasing in Western societies (Trock et al. 2006). Key enzymes involved in estrogen metabolism and their polymorphisms may also play an important role in the effect of isoflavones as they may modify the activity of these enzymes. Wang et al. (2011) observed that *CYP1B1* susceptible genotypes (Val/Leu or Leu/Leu) also contribute to increased breast cancer risk, regardless of menopausal status, but high soy isoflavone intake may reduce this risk. Recent research suggests benefit from high soy isoflavone intake especially for women who are at increased risk of breast cancer due to polymorphisms in genes associated with the disease (Magee and Rowland 2012).

Limitations and inconsistent results of provided studies complicate interpretation of the summary. Current clinical data have shown that no estrogen is good around menopause (Jordan 2014; Shike et al. 2014). Very important finding is that pharmacokinetic parameters were not affected after chronic dosing (Fischer et al. 2004) and it does not appear that soy negatively interfere with tamoxifen or anastrozole therapy (Magee and Rowland 2012).

5 Conclusion

Based on available in vitro data, genistein possesses pleiotropic molecular mechanisms of action. It can modulate processes such as cell cycle, cell growth, apoptosis, invasion, and metastasis. These effects may be primarily due to specific effects on different signaling pathways including Akt, NF-κB, MEK5/ERK5, proteins involved in apoptosis or cell cycle regulators. However, more in vitro and in vivo studies are required to fully elucidate the mechanism of action of soy isoflavones, particularly genistein on breast cancer cells.

Estrogenic effects of soy products observed in athymic ovariectomized mouse model are considerably debated by oncologists. There is a doubt about the merits of using this breast cancer model to predict effects in humans. On the other hand, numerous experimental studies demonstrated significant antitumor effects of soy isoflavones in chemically induced rat mammary carcinogenesis. Since DMBA-induced rat mammary gland carcinomas are reported to be similar to human breast cancers in several aspects, including histopathology, the origin of the cancers from ductal epithelial cells, and the dependency on ovarian hormones for tumor development, it is anticipated to have comparable effects of soy isoflavones on the suppression of human breast cancer development.

Lower breast cancer risk was noted in Asian women with the highest isoflavone intake (>25 mg/day). Early isoflavone exposure can protect against breast cancer as they may exert their putative protective effects by stimulating breast cell differentiation. No significant differences were found in Western population where amount of soy intake is far below even the lower levels of intake in an Asian population. Clinical research dealing with determination of association between the intake of soy food and menopausal status and ER status among breast cancer patients demonstrated inconsistent results. Current clinical data have shown that no estrogen is good around the menopause; therefore, isoflavone intake in this time is not recommended. Further clinical trials are needed to validate the usefulness of these agents either alone or in combination with existing therapy. Then it is important to evaluate the amount of isoflavone intake and timing of isoflavone exposure to clarify and to determine what a safe and acceptable level of isoflavone intake is in women with breast cancer given the potential biphasic effect of isoflavone exposure.

Acknowledgments This work was supported by the Scientific Grant Agency of the Ministry of Education of the Slovak Republic (No. VEGA 11/0322/14 and VEGA 1/0071/13) and by the grant FNUSA-ICRC (No. CZ.1.05/1.1.00/02.0123) co-funded from EU sources and European Regional Development Fund. The authors declare no conflict of interest.

References

Aidoo A, Manjanatha MG (2011) Influence of dietary soy isoflavones genistein and daidzein on genotoxicity and mammary carcinogenicity in rats exposed to the model carcinogen 7,12-dimethylbenz[a]anthracene (DMBA). In: Mutanen M, Pajari AM (eds) Vegetables, whole grains, and their derivates in cancer prevention: Diet and cancer, vol 2. Springer, Dordrecht, pp 143–171

Akiyama T, Ishida J, Nakagawa S et al (1987) Genistein, a specific inhibitor of tyrosine-specific protein kinases. J Biol Chem 262:5592–5595

Allred CD, Allred KF, Ju YH et al (2001) Soy diets containing varying amounts of genistein stimulate growth of estrogen-dependent (MCF-7) tumors in a dose-dependent manner. Cancer Res 61:5045–5050

Allred CD, Allred KF, Ju YH et al (2004) Soy processing influences growth of estrogen-dependent breast cancer tumors. Carcinogenesis 25:1649–1657

Allred CD, Twaddle NC, Allred KF et al (2005) Soy processing affects metabolism and disposition of dietary isoflavones in ovariectomized BALB/c mice. J Agric Food Chem 53:8542–8550

Anderson GL, Chlebowski RT, Aragaki AK et al (2012) Conjugated equine oestrogen and breast cancer incidence and mortality in postmenopausal women with hysterectomy: extended follow-up of the Women's Health Initiative randomised placebo-controlled trial. Lancet Oncol 13:476–486

Bandele OJ, Osheroff N (2007) Bioflavonoids as poisons of human topoisomerase IIα and IIβ. Biochemistry 46:6097–6108

Banerjee S, Li Y, Wang Z, Sarkar FH (2008) Multi-targeted therapy of cancer by genistein. Cancer Lett 269:226–422

Bentzon N, Düring M, Rasmussen BB et al (2008) Prognostic effect of estrogen receptor status across age in primary breast cancer. Int J Cancer 122:1089–1094

Beral V, Reeves G, Bull D et al (2011) Breast cancer risk in relation to the interval between menopause and starting hormone therapy. J Natl Cancer Inst 103:296–305

Bharti AC, Aggarwal BB (2002) Nuclear factor-kappa B and cancer: its role in prevention and therapy. Biochem Pharmacol 64:883–888

Bosviel R, Dumollard E, Déchelotte P et al (2012) Can soy phytoestrogens decrease DNA methylation in BRCA1 and BRCA2 oncosuppressor genes in breast cancer? OMICS 16:235–244

Boucher BA, Cotterchio M, Curca IA et al (2012) Intake of phytoestrogen foods and supplements among women recently diagnosed with breast cancer in Ontario, Canada. Nutr Cancer 64:695–703

Boyapati SM, Shu XO, Ruan ZX et al (2005) Soyfood intake and breast cancer survival: a follow up of the Shanghai Breast Cancer Study. Breast Cancer Res Treat 92:11–17

Brooks JD, Thompson LU (2005) Mammalian lignans and genistein decrease the activities of aromatase and 17β-hydroxysteroid dehydrogenase in MCF-7 cells. J Steroid Biochem Mol Biol 94:461–467

Brown NM, Belles CA, Lindley SL et al (2010a) The chemopreventive action of equol enantiomers in a chemically induced animal model of breast cancer. Carcinogenesis 31:886–893

Brown NM, Belles CA, Lindley SL et al (2010b) Mammary gland differentiation by early life exposure to enantiomers of the soy isoflavone metabolite equol. Food Chem Toxicol 48:3042–3050

Caan BJ, Natarajan L, Parker B et al (2011) Soy food consumption and breast cancer prognosis. Cancer Epidemiol Biomarkers Prev 20:854–858

Chalabi N, Coxam V, Satih S et al (2010) Gene signature of rat mammary glands: influence of lifelong soy isoflavones consumption. Mol Med Rep 3:75–81

Chen FP, Chien MH (2014) Phytoestrogens induce apoptosis through a mitochondria/caspase pathway in human breast cancer cells. Climacteric 17:385–392

Chen M, Rao Y, Zheng Y et al (2014) Association between soy isoflavone intake and breast cancer risk for pre- and post-menopausal women: a meta-analysis of epidemiological studies. PLoS One 9:e89288

Chi F, Wu R, Zeng YC et al (2013) Post-diagnosis soy food intake and breast cancer survival: a meta-analysis of cohort studies. Asian Pac J Cancer Prev 14:2407–2412

Cho YA, Kim J, Shin A et al (2010) Dietary patterns and breast cancer risk in Korean women. Nutr Cancer 62:1161–1169

Choi EJ, Kim GH (2008) Daidzein causes cell cycle arrest at the G1 and G2/M phases in human breast cancer MCF-7 and MDA-MB-453 cells. Phytomedicine 15:683–690

Choi EJ, Kim GH (2013) Antiproliferative activity of daidzein and genistein may be related to ERα/c-erbB-2 expression in human breast cancer cells. Mol Med Rep 7:781–784

Chuang SE, Yeh PY, Lu YS et al (2002) Basal levels and patterns of anticancer drug-induced activation of nuclear factor-kappaB (NF-kappaB), and its attenuation by tamoxifen, dexamethasone, and curcumin in carcinoma cells. Biochem Pharmacol 63:1709–1716

Colozza M, Califano R, Minenza E et al (2008) Aromatase inhibitors: a new reality for the adjuvant endocrine treatment of early-stage breast cancer in postmenopausal women. Mini Rev Med Chem 8:564–574

Conroy SM, Maskarinec G, Park SY et al (2013) The effects of soy consumption before diagnosis on breast cancer survival: the Multiethnic Cohort Study. Nutr Cancer 65:527–537

Constantinou A, Xu H, Cunningham E et al (2001) Consumption of soy products may enhance the breast cancer-preventive effects of tamoxifen. Proc Am Assoc Cancer Res 42:826–827

Dai Q, Shu XO, Jin F et al (2001) Population-based case-control study of soyfood intake and breast cancer risk in Shanghai. Br J Cancer 85:372–378

Dave B, Wynne R, Su Y et al (2010) Enhanced mammary progesterone receptor-A isoform activity in the promotion of mammary tumor progression by dietary soy in rats. Nutr Cancer 62:774–782

Davis JN, Singh B, Bhuiyan M et al (1998) Genistein-induced upregulation of p21WAF1, downregulation of cyclin B, and induction of apoptosis in prostate cancer cells. Nutr Cancer 32:123–131

Dixon RA (2004) Phytoestrogens. Annu Rev Plant Biol 55:225–261

Dong JY, Qin LQ (2011) Soy isoflavones consumption and risk of breast cancer incidence or recurrence: a meta-analysis of prospective studies. Breast Cancer Res Treat 125:315–323

Eto I (2006) Nutritional and chemopreventive anti-cancer agents up-regulate expression of p27Kip1, a cyclin-dependent kinase inhibitor, in mouse JB6 epidermal and human MCF7, MDA-MB-321 and AU565 breast cancer cells. Cancer Cell Int 6:1–19

Fan S, Meng Q, Auborn K et al (2006) BRCA1 and BRCA2 as molecular targets for phytochemicals indole-3-carbinol and genistein in breast and prostate cancer cells. Br J Cancer 94:407–426

Fang CY, Tseng M, Daly MB (2005) Correlates of soy food consumption in women at increased risk for breast cancer. J Am Diet Assoc 105:1552–1558

Ferlay J, Shin HR, Bray F et al (2010) Estimates of worldwide burden of cancer in 2008: GLOBOCAN 2008. Int J Cancer 127:2893–2917

Fischer L, Mahoney C, Jeffcoat AR et al (2004) Clinical characteristics and pharmacokinetics of purified soy isoflavones: multiple-dose administration to men with prostate neoplasia. Nutr Cancer 48:160–170

Frey RS, Li J, Singletary KW (2001) Effects of genistein on cell proliferation and cell cycle arrest in nonneoplastic human mammary epithelial cells: involvement of Cdc2, p21(waf/cip1), p27 (kip1), and Cdc25C expression. Biochem Pharmacol 61:979–989

Glazier MG, Bowman MA (2001) A review of the evidence for the use of phytoestrogens as a replacement for traditional estrogen replacement therapy. Arch Intern Med 161:1161–1172

Gong L, Li Y, Nedeljkovic-Kurepa A, Sarkar FH (2003) Inactivation of NF-kappaB by genistein is mediated via Akt signaling pathway in breast cancer cells. Oncogene 22:4702–4709

Goodman MT, Shvetsov YB, Wilkens LR et al (2009) Urinary phytoestrogen excretion and postmenopausal breast cancer risk: the multiethnic cohort study. Cancer Prev Res (Phila) 2:887–894

Gu L, House SE, Prior RL et al (2006) Metabolic phenotype of isoflavones differ among female rats, pigs, monkeys, and women. J Nutr 136:1215–1221

Guha N, Kwan ML, Quesenberry CP Jr et al (2009) Soy isoflavones and risk of cancer recurrence in a cohort of breast cancer survivors: the Life After Cancer Epidemiology study. Breast Cancer Res Treat 118:395–405

Guo TL, Chi RP, Hernandez DM et al (2007) Decreased 7,12-dimethylbenz[a]anthracene-induced carcinogenesis coincides with the induction of antitumor immunities in adult female B6C3F1 mice pretreated with genistein. Carcinogenesis 28:2560–2566

Hamdy SM, Latif AK, Drees EA, Soliman SM (2012) Prevention of rat breast cancer by genistin and selenium. Toxicol Ind Health 28:746–757

Han J, Kurita Y, Isoda H (2013) Genistein-induced G2/M cell cycle arrest of human intestinal colon cancer Caco-2 cells is associated with Cyclin B1 and Chk2 down-regulation. Cytotechnology 65:973–978

Hooper L, Ryder JJ, Kurzer MS et al (2009) Effects of soy protein and isoflavones on circulating hormone concentrations in pre- and post-menopausal women: a systematic review and meta-analysis. Hum Reprod Update 15:423–440

Horie S (2012) Chemoprevention of prostate cancer: soy isoflavones and curcumin. Korean J Urol 53:665–672

Horn-Ross PL, Lee M, John EM et al (2000) Sources of phytoestrogen exposure among non-Asian women in California, USA. Cancer Causes Control 11:299–302

Hsieh CY, Santell RC, Haslam SZ et al (1998) Estrogenic effects of genistein on the growth of estrogen receptor-positive human breast cancer (MCF-7) cells in vitro and in vivo. Cancer Res 58:3833–3838

Ingle JN (2001) Current status of adjuvant endocrine therapy for breast cancer. Clin Cancer Res 7:4392–4396

Jemal A, Bray F, Center MM et al (2011) Global cancer statistics. CA Cancer J Clin 61:69–90

Jones SM, Kazlauskas A (2001) Growth factor-dependent signaling and cell cycle progression. FEBS Lett 490:110–116

Jordan VC (2014) Avoiding the bad and enhancing the good of soy supplements in breast cancer. J Natl Cancer Inst 4:106–109

Ju YH, Allred CD, Allred KF et al (2001) Physiological concentrations of dietary genistein dose-dependently stimulate growth of estrogen-dependent human breast cancer (MCF-7) tumors implanted in athymic nude mice. J Nutr 131:2957–2962

Ju YH, Doerge DR, Allred KF et al (2002) Dietary genistein negates the inhibitory effect of tamoxifen on growth of estrogen-dependent human breast cancer (MCF-7) cells implanted in athymic mice. Cancer Res 62:2474–2477

Ju YH, Fultz J, Allred KF et al (2006) Effects of dietary daidzein and its metabolite, equol, at physiological concentrations on the growth of estrogen-dependent human breast cancer (MCF-7) tumors implanted in ovariectomized athymic mice. Carcinogenesis 27:856–863

Ju YH, Doerge DR, Woodling KA et al (2008) Dietary genistein negates the inhibitory effect of letrozole on the growth of aromatase-expressing estrogen-dependent human breast cancer cells (MCF-7Ca) in vivo. Carcinogenesis 29:2162–2168

Kakehashi A, Tago Y, Yoshida M et al (2012) Hormonally active doses of isoflavone aglycones promote mammary and endometrial carcinogenesis and alter the molecular tumor environment in Donryu rats. Toxicol Sci 126:39–51

Kang X, Zhang Q, Wang S et al (2010) Effect of soy isoflavones on breast cancer recurrence and death for patients receiving adjuvant endocrine therapy. CMAJ 182:1857–1862

Kelloff GJ (2000) Perspectives on cancer chemoprevention research and drug development. Adv Cancer Res 78:199–334

Kostelac D, Rechkemmer G, Briviba K (2003) Phytoestrogens modulate binding response of estrogen receptors alpha and beta to the estrogen response element. J Agric Food Chem 51:7632–7635

Kuzumaki T, Kobayashi T, Ishikawa K (1998) Genistein induces p21(Cip1/WAF1) expression and blocks the G1 to S phase transition in mouse fibroblast and melanoma cells. Biochem Biophys Res Commun 251:291–295

Kwon SJ, Song BH (2011) Meta-analysis for effect of dietary isoflavones on breast density and hot flush suppression. Korean J Microbiol Biotechnol 39:224–237

Lacey M, Bohday J, Fonseka SM et al (2005) Dose–response effects of phytoestrogens on the activity and expression of 3β-hydroxysteroid dehydrogenase and aromatase in human granulosa-luteal cells. J Steroid Biochem Mol Biol 96:279–286

Lacroix M (2009) MDA-MB-435 cells are from melanoma, not from breast cancer. Cancer Chemother Pharmacol 63:567

Lee SA, Shu XO, Li H et al (2009) Adolescent and adult soy food intake and breast cancer risk: results from the Shanghai Women's Health Study. Am J Clin Nutr 89:1920–1926

Lee EH, Park SK, Park B et al (2010) Effect of BRCA1/2 mutation on short-term and long-term breast cancer survival: a systematic review and meta-analysis. Breast Cancer Res Treat 122:11–25

Lepri SR, Zanelatto LC, da Silva PB et al (2014) Effects of genistein and daidzein on cell proliferation kinetics in HT29 colon cancer cells: the expression of CTNNBIP1 (β-catenin), APC (adenomatous polyposis coli) and BIRC5 (survivin). Hum Cell 27:78–84

Li Y, Bhuiyan M, Sarkar FH (1999a) Induction of apoptosis and inhibition of c-erbB-2 in MDA-MB-435 cells by genistein. Int J Oncol 15:525–533

Li Y, Upadhyay S, Bhuiyan M et al (1999b) Induction of apoptosis in breast cancer cells MDA-MB-231 by genistein. Oncogene 18:3166–3172

Li YW, Ahmed F, Ali S et al (2005) Inactivation of nuclear factor kappa B by soy isoflavone genistein contributes to increased apoptosis mduced by chemotherapeutic agents in human cancer cells. Cancer Res 65:6934–6942

Li J, Li Z, Mo BQ (2006) Effects of ERK5 MAPK signaling transduction pathway on the inhibition of genistein to breast cancer cells. Wei Sheng Yan Jiu 35:184–186

Li Z, Li J, Mo B et al (2008) Genistein induces cell apoptosis in MDA-MB-231 breast cancer cells via the mitogen-activated protein kinase pathway. Toxicol In Vitro 22:1749–1753

Li YS, Wu LP, Li KH et al (2011) Involvement of nuclear factor κB (NF-κB) in the downregulation of cyclooxygenase-2 (COX-2) by genistein in gastric cancer cells. J Int Med Res 39:2141–2150

Li Y, Meeran SM, Patel SN et al (2013) Epigenetic reactivation of estrogen receptor-α (ERα) by genistein enhances hormonal therapy sensitivity in ERα-negative breast cancer. Mol Cancer 12:9

Lian FR, Bhuiyan M, Li YW et al (1998) Genistein-induced G(2)-M arrest, p21(WAF1) upregulation, and apoptosis in a non-small-cell lung cancer cell line. Nutr Cancer 31:184–191

Liao CH, Pan SL, Guh JH et al (2004) Genistein inversely affects tubulin-binding agent-induced apoptosis in human breast cancer cells. Biochem Pharmacol 67:2031–2038

Lim E, He HH, Chi D et al (2012) Estrogen receptor signaling in normal, BRCA (B) 1 and B2 mutation associated, and ER-positive breast cancer (BC) mammary cells. J Clin Oncol 30 (Suppl):576

Linseisen J, Piller R, Hermann S et al (2004) German case-control study. Dietary phytoestrogen intake and premenopausal breast cancer risk in a German case-control study. Int J Cancer 110:284–290

Liu B, Edgerton S, Yang X et al (2005) Low-dose dietary phytoestrogen abrogates tamoxifen-associated mammary tumor prevention. Cancer Res 65:879–886

Liu X, Sun C, Jin X et al (2013a) Genistein enhances the radio sensitivity of breast cancer cells via G2/M cell cycle arrest and apoptosis. Molecules 18:13200–13217

Liu YL, Zhang GQ, Yang Y et al (2013b) Genistein induces G2/M arrest in gastric cancer cells by increasing the tumor suppressor PTEN expression. Nutr Cancer 65:1034–1041

López-Lazaro M, Willmore E, Austin CA (2007) Cells lacking DNA topoisomerase IIβ are resistant to genistein. J Nat Prod 70:763–767

Ma D, Zhang Y, Yang T et al (2014) Isoflavone intake inhibits the development of 7,12-dimethylbenz(a)anthracene(DMBA)-induced mammary tumors in normal and ovariectomized rats. J Clin Biochem Nutr 54:31–38

Magee PJ, Rowland I (2012) Soy products in the management of breast cancer. Curr Opin Clin Nutr Metab Care 15:586–591

Magee PJ, Allsopp P, Samaletdin A, Rowland IR (2014) Daidzein, R-(+)equol and S-(-)equol inhibit the invasion of MDA-MB-231 breast cancer cells potentially via the down-regulation of matrix metalloproteinase-2. Eur J Nutr 53:345–350

Maggiolini M, Bonofiglio D, Marsico S et al (2001) Estrogen receptor alpha mediates the proliferative but not the cytotoxic dose-dependent effects of two major phytoestrogens on human breast cancer cells. Mol Pharmacol 60:595–602

Mandraju RK, Kannapiran P, Kondapi AK (2008) Distinct roles of Topoisomerase II isoforms: DNA damage accelerating α, double strand break repair promoting β. Arch Biochem Biophys 470:27–34

Martincic D, Hande KR (2005) Topoisomerase II inhibitors. Cancer Chemother Biol Response Modif 22:101–121

Martínez-Montemayor MM, Otero-Franqui E, Martinez J et al (2010) Individual and combined soy isoflavones exert differential effects on metastatic cancer progression. Clin Exp Metastasis 27:465–480

Maskarinec G, Erber E, Verheus M et al (2009) Soy consumption and histopathologic markers in breast tissue using tissue microarrays. Nutr Cancer 61:708–716

Medina D (2007) Chemical carcinogenesis of rat and mouse mammary glands. Breast Dis 28:63–68

Messina MJ, Wood CE (2008) Soy isoflavones, estrogen therapy, and breast cancer risk: analysis and commentary. Nutr J 7:17
Messina M, Wu AH (2009) Perspectives on the soy-breast cancer relation. Am J Clin Nutr 89:1673S–1679S
Messina M, McCaskill-Stevens W, Lampre JW (2006a) Addressing the soy and breast cancer relationship: review, commentary, and workshop proceedings. J Natl Cancer Inst 98:1275–1284
Messina M, Nagata C, Wu AH (2006b) Estimated Asian adult soy protein and isoflavone intakes. Nutr Cancer 55:1–12
Miousse IR, Sharma N, Blackburn M et al (2013) Feeding soy protein isolate and treatment with estradiol have different effects on mammary gland morphology and gene expression in weanling male and female rats. Physiol Genomics 45:1072–1083
Mizushina Y, Shiomi K, Kuriyama I et al (2013) Inhibitory effects of a major soy isoflavone, genistein, on human DNA topoisomerase II activity and cancer cell proliferation. Int J Oncol 43:1117–1124
Molzberger AF, Soukup ST, Kulling SE, Diel P (2013) Proliferative and estrogenic sensitivity of the mammary gland are modulated by isoflavones during distinct periods of adolescence. Arch Toxicol 87:1129–1140
Mukherjee S, Acharya BR, Bhattacharyya B et al (2010) Genistein arrests cell cycle progression of A549 cells at the G(2)/M phase and depolymerizes interphase microtubules through binding to a unique site of tubulin. Biochemistry 49:1702–1712
Nagaraju GP, Zafar SF, El-Rayes BF (2013) Pleiotropic effects of genistein in metabolic, inflammatory, and malignant diseases. Nutr Rev 71:562–572
Nagata C (2010) Factors to consider in the association between soy isoflavone intake and breast cancer risk. J Epidemiol 20:83–89
Nechuta SJ, Caan BJ, Chen WY et al (2012) Soy food intake after diagnosis of breast cancer and survival: an in-depth analysis of combined evidence from cohort studies of US and Chinese women. Am J Clin Nutr 96:123–132
Ono M, Koga T, Ueo H, Nakano S (2012) Effects of dietary genistein on hormone-dependent rat mammary carcinogenesis induced by ethyl methanesulphonate. Nutr Cancer 64:1204–1210
Pagliacci MC, Smacchia M, Migliorati G et al (1994) Growth-inhibitory effects of the natural phyto-oestrogen genistein in MCF-7 human breast cancer cells. Eur J Cancer 30A:1675–1682
Pan H, Zhou W, He W et al (2012) Genistein inhibits MDA-MB-231 triple-negative breast cancer cell growth by inhibiting NF-κB activity via the Notch-1 pathway. Int J Mol Med 30:337–343
Papazisis KT, Kalemi TG, Zambouli D et al (2006) Synergistic effects of protein tyrosine kinase inhibitor genistein with camptothecins against three cell lines in vitro. Cancer Lett 233:255–264
Pavese JM, Farmer RL, Bergan RC (2010) Inhibition of cancer cell invasion and metastasis by genistein. Cancer Metastasis Rev 29:465–482
Perrin D, van Hille B, Hill BT (1998) Differential sensitivities of recombinant human topoisomerase IIα and β various classes of topoisomerase II-interacting agents. Biochem Pharmacol 56:503–507
Peterson G, Barnes S (1996) Genistein inhibits both estrogen and growth factor-stimulated proliferation of human breast cancer cells. Cell Growth Differ 7:1345–1351
Pike AC, Brzozowski AM, Hubbard RE et al (1999) Structure of the ligand-binding domain of oestrogen receptor beta in the presence of a partial agonist and a full antagonist. EMBO J 18:4608–4618
Pommier Y (2006) Topoisomerase I inhibitors: camptothecins and beyond. Nat Rev Cancer 6:789–802
Privat M, Aubel C, Arnould S et al (2010) (2010) AKT and p21 WAF1/CIP1 as potential genistein targets in BRCA1-mutant human breast cancer cell lines. Anticancer Res 30:2049–2054
Pugalendhi P, Manoharan S (2010) Chemopreventive potential of genistein and daidzein in combination during 7,12-dimethylbenz[a]anthracene (DMBA) induced mammary carcinogenesis in Sprague-Dawley rats. Pak J Biol Sci 13:279–286

Pugalendhi P, Manoharan S, Suresh K, Baskaran N (2011) Genistein and daidzein, in combination, protect cellular integrity during 7,12-dimethylbenz[a]anthracene (DMBA) induced mammary carcinogenesis in Sprague-Dawley rats. Afr J Tradit Complement Altern Med 8:91–97

Ronco AL, de Stefani E, Aune D et al (2010) Nutrient patterns and risk of breast cancer in Uruguay. Asian Pac J Cancer Prev 11:519–524

Ronis MJ, Shankar K, Gomez-Acevedo H et al (2012) Mammary gland morphology and gene expression differ in female rats treated with 17β-estradiol or fed soy protein isolate. Endocrinology 153:6021–6032

Russo IH, Ruso J et al (1996) Mammary gland neoplasia in long-term rodent studies. Environ Health Perspect 104:938–967

Saarinen NM, Power K, Chen J, Thompson LU (2006) Flaxseed attenuates the tumor growth stimulating effect of soy protein in ovariectomized athymic mice with MCF-7 human breast cancer xenografts. Int J Cancer 119:925–931

Sakamoto T, Horiguchi H, Oguma E et al (2010) Effects of diverse dietary phytoestrogens on cell growth, cell cycle and apoptosis in estrogen-receptor-positive breast cancer cells. J Nutr Biochem 21:856–864

Salti GI, Grewal S, Mehta RR, Das Gupta TK, Boddie AW Jr, Constantinou AI (2000) Genistein induces apoptosis and topoisomerase II-mediated DNA breakage in colon cancer cells. Eur J Cancer 36:796–802

Santell RC, Kieu N, Helferich WG (2000) Genistein inhibits growth of estrogen-independent human breast cancer cells in culture but not in athymic mice. J Nutr 130:1665–1669

Sarkar FH, Li YW (2002) Mechanisms of cancer chemoprevention by soy isoflavone genistein. Cancer Metastasis Rev 21:265–280

Sartippour MR, Rao JY, Apple S et al (2004) A pilot clinical study of short term isoflavone supplements in breast cancer patients. Nutr Cancer 49:59–65

Satih S, Chalabi N, Rabiau N et al (2010) Transcriptional profiling of breast cancer cells exposed to soy phytoestrogens after BRCA1 knockdown with a whole human genome microarray approach. Nutr Cancer 201062:659–667

Sergeev IN (2004) Genistein induces Ca2+-mediated, calpain/caspase-12-dependent apoptosis in breast cancer cells. Biochem Biophys Res Commun 321:462–467

Setchell KD, Clerici C (2010) Equol: pharmacokinetics and biological actions. J Nutr 140:1363–1368

Setchell KD, Cole SJ (2006) Method of defining equol-producer status and its frequency among vegetarians. J Nutr 136:2188–2193

Setchell KD, Brown NM, Lydeking-Olsen E (2002) The clinical importance of the metabolite equol-a clue to the effectiveness of soy and its isoflavones. J Nutr 132:3577–3584

Setchell KD, Clerici C, Lephart ED et al (2005) S-equol, a potent ligand for estrogen receptor beta, is the exclusive enantiomeric form of the soy isoflavone metabolite produced by human intestinal bacterial flora. Am J Clin Nutr 81:1072–1079

Setchell KD, Brown NM, Zhao X et al (2011) Soy isoflavone phase II metabolism differs between rodents and humans: implications for the effect on breast cancer risk. Am J Clin Nutr 94:1284–1294

Shao ZM, Wu J, Shen ZZ et al (1998) Genistein exerts multiple suppressive effects on human breast carcinoma cells. Cancer Res 58:4851–4857

Shike M, Doane A, Russo L et al (2014) The effects of soy supplementation on gene expression in breast cancer: a randomized placebo-controlled study. J Natl Cancer Inst 106(9):dju189. doi:10.1093/jnci/dju189

Shim HY, Park JH, Paik HD et al (2007) Genistein-induced apoptosis of human breast cancer MCF-7 cells involves calpain-caspase and apoptosis signaling kinase 1-p38 mitogen-activated protein kinase activation cascades. Anticancer Drugs 18:649–657

Shin A, Kim J, Lim SY et al (2010) Dietary mushroom intake and the risk of breast cancer based on hormone receptor status. Nutr Cancer 62:476–483

Shishodia S, Aggarwal BB (2004) Nuclear factor-kappaB activation mediates cellular transformation, proliferation, invasion angiogenesis and metastasis of cancer. Cancer Treat Res 119:139–173

Shu XO, Zheng Y, Cai H et al (2009) Soy food intake and breast cancer survival. JAMA 302:2437–2443

Stoll B (1977) Palliation by castration or hormone ablation. In: Stoll BA (ed) Breast cancer management early and late. London: William Herman Medical Books Ltd, pp 135–149

Taylor CK, Levy RM, Elliott JC et al (2009) The effect of genistein aglycone on cancer and cancer risk: a review of in vitro, preclinical, and clinical studies. Nutr Rev 67:398–415

Thun MJ, DeLancey JO, Center MM et al (2010) The global burden of cancer: priorities for prevention. Carcinogenesis 31:100–110

Tominaga Y, Wang A, Wang RH et al (2007) Genistein inhibits Brca1 mutant tumor growth through activation of DNA damage checkpoints, cell cycle arrest, and mitotic catastrophe. Cell Death Differ 14:472–479

Trock BJ, Hilakivi-Clarke L, Clarke R (2006) Meta-analysis of soy intake and breast cancer risk. J Natl Cancer Inst 98:459–471

Valeri A, Fiorenzani P, Rossi R et al (2012) The soy phytoestrogens genistein and daidzein as neuroprotective agents against anoxia-glucopenia and reperfusion damage in rat urinary bladder. Pharmacol Res 66:309–316

Wada K, Nakamura K, Tamai Y et al (2013) Soy isoflavone intake and breast cancer risk in Japan: from the Takayama study. Int J Cancer 133:952–960

Wang JC (1996) DNA topoisomerases. Annu Rev Biochem 65:635–692

Wang Q, Li H, Tao P et al (2011) Soy isoflavones, CYP1A1, CYP1B1, and COMT polymorphisms, and breast cancer: a case-control study in southwestern China. DNA Cell Biol 30:585–595

Ward H, Chapelais G, Kuhnle GG et al (2008) Breast cancer risk in relation to urinary and serum biomarkers of phytoestrogen exposure in the European Prospective into Cancer-Norfolk cohort study. Breast Cancer Res 10:R32

Wu AH, Koh WP, Wang R et al (2008) Soy intake and breast cancer risk in Singapore Chinese Health Study. Br J Cancer 99:196–200

Xie Q, Chen ML, Qin Y et al (2013) Isoflavone consumption and risk of breast cancer: a dose-response meta-analysis of observational studies. Asia Pac J Clin Nutr 22:118–127

Xu J, Loo G (2001) Different effects of genistein on molecular markers related to apoptosis in two phenotypically dissimilar breast cancer cell lines. J Cell Biochem 82:78–88

Yamamoto S, Sobue T, Kobayashi M et al (2003) Soy, isoflavones, and breast cancer risk in Japan. J Natl Cancer Inst 95:906–913

Yamasaki M, Mine Y, Nishimura M et al (2013) Genistein induces apoptotic cell death associated with inhibition of the NF-κB pathway in adult T-cell leukemia cells. Cell Biol Int 37:742–747

Yeh PY, Chuang SE, Yeh KH et al (2002) Increase of the resistance of human cervical carcinoma cells to cisplatin by inhibition of the MEK to ERK signaling pathway partly via enhancement of anticancer drug-induced NF kappa B activation. Biochem Pharmacol 63:1423–1430

Zava DT, Duwe G (1997) Estrogenic and antiproliferative properties of genistein and other flavonoids in human breast cancer cells in vitro. Nutr Cancer 27:31–40

Zhang M, Yang H, Holman CD (2009) Dietary intake of isoflavones and breast cancer risk by estrogen and progesterone receptor status. Breast Cancer ResTreat 118:553–563

Zhang C, Ho SC, Lin F et al (2010) Soy product and isoflavone intake and breast cancer risk defined by hormone receptor status. Cancer Sci 101:501–507

Zhang X, Gao YT, Yang G et al (2012a) Urinary isoflavonoids and risk of coronary heart disease. Int J Epidemiol 41:1367–1375

Zhang YF, Kang HB, Li BL et al (2012b) Positive effects of soy isoflavone food on survival of breast cancer patients in China. Asian Pac J Cancer Prev 3:479–482

Zhou N, Yan Y, Li W et al (2009) Genistein inhibition of topoisomerase IIα expression participated by Sp1 and Sp3 in HeLa cell. Int J Mol Sci 10:3255–3268

Pharmacological Role of Dietary Polyphenols in Prostate Cancer Chemoprevention

Sebastiano Cimino, Giorgio Ivan Russo, Giulio Reale, Daniele Urzì, Tommaso Castelli, Vincenzo Favilla, and Giuseppe Morgia

Abstract Prostate cancer (PCa) is the most common solid neoplasm and it is now recognized as one of the most important medical problems facing the male population. Due to its long latency and its identifiable pre-neoplastic lesions, prostate cancer is an ideal target tumor for chemoprevention. Different compounds of dietary origin are available on the market and certainly polyphenols such as epigallocatechin-3-gallate, curcumin, resveratrol, and the flavonoids quercetin and genistein represent those with supposed efficacy against PCa. As shown by many reports on PCa, the use of natural compounds could act against oxidative stress chronic inflammation. Basic research studies have revealed that polyphenols appear to act not only against oxidative stress but also impede pro-neoplastic cancer cell signaling. Although the current studies are limited, mechanisms of action of polyphenols have been confirmed, showing a promising future strategy in prostate cancer chemoprevention.

1 Epidemiology

Prostate cancer (PCa) is one of the most common cancers in men as reported by SEER statistics: in 2011 in the USA, there were more than 2.7 million people affected by prostate cancer with 233,000 new cases estimated during 2014 (Siegel et al. 2015). The trend in mortality for this cancer, due to amelioration of the diagnosis and treatment strategies, decreased during the last three decades and in 2014 it was about 5 % (Siegel et al. 2015).

PCa etiology has been not yet demonstrated, but several reports have linked chronic inflammation to its onset, and, in particular, the increase in oxidative stress could lead to higher expression of pro-inflammatory cytokines and growth factors. These mechanisms resulted in higher rates of cell division and therefore enhancing the possibility of incurring mutations (De Nunzio et al. 2011). Furthermore, the presence of proliferative inflammatory atrophy (PIA), precursor HGPIN, and prostate cancer may involve the presence of abnormal values of gene coding for

S. Cimino, MD (✉) • G.I. Russo • G. Reale • D. Urzì • T. Castelli • V. Favilla • G. Morgia
Department of Urology, School of Medicine Policlinico Hospital, University of Catania, Catania, Italy
e-mail: ciminonello@hotmail.com

M.F. Ullah, A. Ahmad (eds.), *Critical Dietary Factors in Cancer Chemoprevention*,
DOI 10.1007/978-3-319-21461-0_11

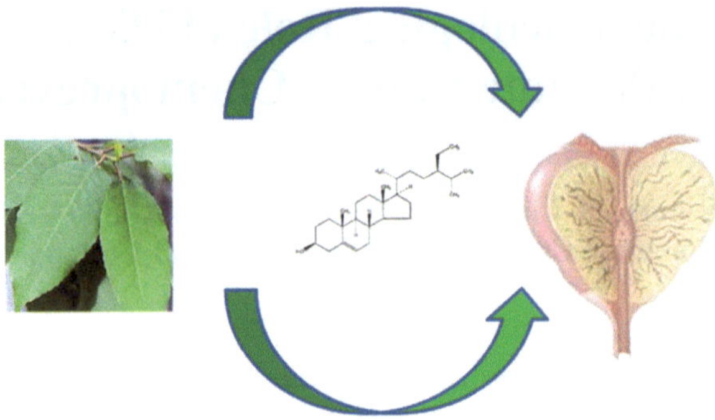

Fig. 1 Polyphenolic phytochemicals in prevention of prostate cancer

glutathione *S*-transferase (GSTP1), gene coding for glutathione *S*-transferase A1 (GSTA1), and COX-2 (enzyme determining the conversion of arachidonic acid (AA) into the prostaglandin endoperoxide H2 precursors of PGD2, PGE2, PGF2α, PGI2, and thromboxane A2) (Cimino et al. 2014).

Based on these premises, polyphenols assume significance as constituents of chemopreventive fruits and vegetables worldwide for reducing the risk of cancer of various kinds including that of prostate (Fig. 1). Polyphenols occur naturally in different foods, and today there are more than 8000 divided into different subclasses of which the most represented are flavonoids, stilbenes, phenolic acids, and lignans (Ramos 2007). The importance of the polyphenols as anticancer substances shall be represented by the fact that they possess properties that act at different levels of molecular and cellular signaling.

2 Epigallocatechin-3-Gallate

Epigallocatechin-3-gallate (EGCG) represents the major polyphenol constituent present in green tea, the most popular beverage next to water. The tea plant (*Camellia sinensis*) has been cultivated in Asia for thousands of years and green tea has been used for centuries in China, Japan, and Thailand as a traditional medicine with a variety of applications (Abbas et al. 2013). Over the last two decades, many epidemiological studies have evaluated the chemopreventive properties of green tea, suggesting that increasing intake of green tea is correlated with significant decrease in the development of prostate cancer. The anticarcinogenic effects could be related to the inhibition of growth proliferation, induction of apoptosis, induction of phase II detoxifying enzymes, and reduction of oxidative damage to DNA as revealed by various in vitro and in vivo studies resulting in decreased risk and/or slower progression of prostate cancer with consumption of green tea (Khan et al. 2009). According to cell-culture studies, EGCG induced apoptosis and cell cycle arrest in many cancer cells without affecting normal cells. Particularly in PCa cells, EGCG activates growth arrest and apoptosis primarily via p53-dependent pathway that involves the function of both p21 and Bax such that downregulation of either molecule confers a growth advantage to the cells. In androgen-sensitive LNCaP and androgen-insensitive PC-3 human prostate carcinoma cells, EGCG inhibited COX-2 (inducible enzymatic isoform rapidly induced by growth factors, tumor promoters, oncogenes, and carcinogens) without affecting COX-1 expression at both the mRNA and protein levels (Khan et al. 2009). A study published in 2007 tested the effect of EGCG alone and in combination with specific COX-2 inhibitors on the growth and apoptosis induction of human prostate cancer cells both in vitro and in vivo. This study demonstrated a synergic action and an increased efficacy of selective COX-2 inhibitors in combination with polyphenols from green tea, inhibiting the growth of human prostate cancer cells. It was observed that this effect was mainly due to increased apoptosis from enhanced activation of caspase-6 and caspase-9 (Adhami et al. 2007). It has been shown that ester bond-containing green tea polyphenols, such as EGCG, potently and specifically inhibit the chymotrypsin-like activity of the proteasome in vitro and in vivo at the concentrations found in the serum on consumption of green tea, causing growth arrest in the G(1) phase of the cell cycle (Khan et al. 2009). In a study published in 2006, the combination treatment with EGCG, green tea extract, water extract of black tea, and theaflavins was shown to reduce gene expression and protein expression of androgen receptor in the athymic nude mice implanted with androgen-sensitive human CaP CWR22Rν1 cells that resulted in induction of apoptosis, decrease in the levels of VEGF protein, reduction in the level of serum PSA, and a reduced tumor volume (Khan et al. 2009; Siddiqui et al. 2006). Furthermore, this polyphenolic compound also seems to inhibit tumor expression of matrix metalloproteases (MMP-2 and MMP-9) and vascular endothelial growth factor (VEGF), which are overexpressed in angiogenesis and thereby prevent the invasion and the metastatic spread of cancer (Adhami et al. 2003). In a mouse model of orthotopic androgen-sensitive human PCa, the combination of soy phytochemical concentrate, black tea, and green tea significantly reduced tumor activity. This association synergistically inhibited tumor angiogenesis, final tumor weight, and metastasis and significantly reduced serum concentrations of both testosterone and dihydrotestosterone in vivo (Zhou et al. 2003). A prospective, double-blind, placebo-controlled study, using a defined product of green tea in capsule form in men with HGPIN, observed a 90 % reduction in developing PCa. This was the first study that has shown the effectiveness of green tea polyphenols for the treatment of premalignant lesions of prostate cancer (Bettuzzi et al. 2006). In the Japan Public Health Center-based prospective study, 49,950 men aged 40–69 completed a questionnaire on the basis of their green tea consumption habit. Consumption was associated with a dose-dependent decrease in the risk of advanced PCa. The multivariate relative risk was 0.52 for men drinking 5 or more cups/day compared with less than 1 cup/day (Kurahashi et al. 2008). However, further studies are needed so that the EGCG can be safely considered as potent chemopreventive agent for prostate cancer.

3 Curcumin

Curcumin (diferuloylmethane) is a major chemical component of turmeric (*Curcuma longa* Linn.) and it is used as a spice to give a specific flavor and yellow color to food in the Indian subcontinent (Khan et al. 2010). It has been used for centuries throughout Asia not only as a food additive but also as cosmetic and as a traditional herbal medicine to treat a variety of inflammatory conditions and chronic diseases. Over the past decades, several studies have substantiated the potential prophylactic or therapeutic value of curcumin and have unequivocally supported reports of its anticarcinogenic properties, such as its ability to influence a diverse range of molecular targets within cells. To date, no studies have reported any toxicity associated with the use of curcumin in either animals or humans (Goel and Aggarwal 2010). The chemopreventive properties of curcumin are attributed to its effect on several targets including transcription factors, growth regulators, adhesion molecules, apoptotic genes, angiogenesis regulators, and cellular signaling molecules. It has been shown that curcumin has the ability to induce apoptosis in both androgen-dependent and androgen-independent prostate cancer cells acting through the downregulating apoptosis suppressor proteins and other crucial proteins such as the androgen receptor. In PC-3 (hormone-independent line possessing dysfunctional androgen receptors) and LNCaP (hormone-sensitive cells), curcumin significantly altered microfilament organization and cell motility. In PC-3, human prostate cancer cell line, curcumin reduced MDM2 protein and mRNA and enhanced the expression of the tumor suppressor p21/WAF1, a gene that encodes a potent cyclin-dependent kinase inhibitor of cyclin–CDK2 and cyclin–CDK4 complexes, inducing apoptosis and inhibiting proliferation. Furthermore, curcumin inhibited androgen receptor-mediated induction of NKX3.1 expression and decreased the expression of androgen receptors and the binding activity to antioxidant response element directly (Khan et al. 2008). NKX3.1, a gene located nearly on 8p21.2, is involved in the initiation stage of prostatic tumorgenesis. There is considerable evidence that loss of NKX3.1 expression, along with PTEN heterozygosity, a gene that codes for a lipid phosphatase and functions as a negative regulator of phosphoinositol-3-kinase (PI3K) signaling, is found at high frequency in CaP (Syed et al. 2007). NKX3.1 gene encodes a homeobox-containing transcription factor that functions as a negative regulator of epithelial cell growth in prostate tissue. Thus, cellular NKX3.1 protein levels are critical for the maintenance of the prostate epithelial phenotype. Experiments conducted on LNCaP and PC-3 cells demonstrated that inflammation and in particular overproduction of TNF-α and IL-β lead to rapid ubiquitination and proteasomal degradation of NKX3.1 protein through phosphorylation of serine-196 (Markowski et al. 2008). In a study, it was found that treatment of prostate cancer cells with curcumin (1–100 μM) suppresses both constitutive (DU145) and inducible (LNCaP) NF-κB activation and potentiates TNF-induced apoptosis. Curcumin treatment (50–100 μM) induced apoptosis in both cell types, which correlated with the downregulation of the expression of Bcl-2 and Bcl-xL and the activation of procaspase-3 and -8 (Mukhopadhyay et al. 2001). Moreover, a study previously showed that curcumin blocked the activation of L-mimosine or dimethyloxalylglycine treatment on PSA expression in human prostate carcinoma LNCaP cells (Chung et al. 2011).

In hormone refractory PCa, it was found that curcumin, in addition to conventional treatment, may decrease PCa aggressive proliferation and potentiate activity of taxane therapy increasing cytotoxicity and delaying prostate cancer cell resistance to these chemotherapeutic drugs (Cabrespine-Faugeras et al. 2010; Choi et al. 2008; Hour et al. 2002). In combination with radiation, curcumin (2–5 μM) showed significant enhancement of radiation-induced clonogenic inhibition and apoptosis in PC-3 cells and significant activation of cytochrome c and caspases-9 and -3. These mechanisms suggest that this natural compound acts by overcoming the effects of radiation-induced pro-survival gene expression in prostate cancer (Chendil et al. 2004). Others in vitro and in vivo studies have also demonstrated the inhibitory effects exerted by treatment with only curcumin against the growth and invasiveness of DU-145 prostate cancer cells. The inhibition of tumor cell invasion was due to reductions in MMP-2 and MMP-9. Curcumin was also shown to induce a marked reduction of tumor volume. This compound may therefore have a role as a chemopreventive agent and/or adjuvant therapy in the treatment of prostate cancer, probably as a nontoxic dietary supplement (Hong et al. 2006; Sharma et al. 2001). Until now, only few clinical data about curcumin have been obtained in humans, despite the large number of studies in in vitro and in animal models. In a pilot study of a standardized oral *Curcuma* extract, doses up to 180 mg of curcumin per day were administered to patients with advanced colorectal cancer for up to 4 months without overt toxicity (Sharma et al. 2001). A subsequent study has suggested that doses up to 8 g could be administered daily to patients with premalignant lesions for 3 months without overt toxicity (Chung et al. 2011). In a phase I clinical trial of oral curcumin, 15 patients with colorectal cancer refractory to standard chemotherapy consumed a capsule with a dose escalation between 0.4 g and 3.6 g daily for up to 4 months. A daily dose of 3.6 g curcumin was found to reduce 57–62 % of inducible PGE-2, suggesting a possible use of this compound for chemoprevention (Sharma et al. 2004).

4 Resveratrol

Resveratrol (*trans*-3,4,5-trihydroxystilbene, $C_{14}H_{12}O_3$) is a plant-derived polyphenolic phytoalexin produced by the enzyme stilbene synthase in response to infection by the pathogen *Botrytis cinerea* and to a variety of stress conditions, such as vicissitudes in climate, exposure to ozone, sunlight, and heavy metals. It exists in two isoforms: *trans*-resveratrol and *cis*-resveratrol where the trans isomer is the more stable form. Resveratrol is present in red grapes, peanuts, some common drinks, and dietary supplements. It has broad-spectrum beneficial health effects including anti-infective, antioxidant, and cardioprotective functions, but it has gained considerable attention because of its potential cancer chemopreventive properties (Cimino et al. 2012). To this regard, resveratrol represents an ideal molecule, due to its relatively low toxicity and capacity to target multiple signaling molecules that collectively promote cancer cell survival and tumor growth. It was demonstrated that this natural compound can modulate many intracellular cancer targets, which affect cell growth, inflammation, apoptosis, angiogenesis, invasion, and metastasis. It is also able to potentiate the apoptotic effects of cytokines, such as TRAIL, chemotherapeutic agents, and gamma radiation (Cimino et al. 2012). Many in vitro studies have investigated the antiproliferative or proapoptotic effects of resveratrol in human prostate cancer cells, and its mechanism of action. Resveratrol was found to inhibit the growth of LNCaP cells (hormone sensitive cells), DU-145 (androgen-independent cells), and PC-3 (hormone-independent line possessing dysfunctional androgen receptors) in a concentration-dependent manner. It has also been shown to exert a strong inhibitory effect on the formation of free radicals in human macrophages, reducing oxidative stress within premalignant cells, and to reduce growth and spread of prostate cancer (Ratan et al. 2002). With regard to its proapoptotic effects, it has been shown to induce apoptosis in LNCaP and DU145 prostate cancer cell lines through different PKC-mediated and MAPK-dependent pathways (Shih et al. 2004). Furthermore, resveratrol-mediated apoptosis has been associated with p53 activation and also occurs via the death receptor Fas/CD95/APO-1 in various human cancer cells (Cimino et al. 2012). It is also possible that resveratrol exerts its chemopreventive action in part by modulating the expression or function of androgen receptor (Ratan et al. 2002). Another interesting chemopreventive mechanism related to this compound is represented by sensitization effect. Research from in vitro and in vivo studies indicates that resveratrol can overcome chemoresistance in tumor cells by modulating apoptotic pathways, downregulating drug transporters, modulating proteins involved in tumor cell proliferation, and inhibiting NF-κB and STAT-3 pathway (Cimino et al. 2012).

However, despite previous considerations, absorption of compounds should be evaluated before supposing a clinical effectiveness on human. In this context, Goldberg et. al. reported that after an oral dose of resveratrol (25 mg/70 kg), catechin (25 mg/70 kg), and quercetin (10 mg/70 kg) to healthy human subjects, these compounds appeared in serum and urine predominantly as glucuronide and sulfate conjugates and free polyphenols accounted for 1.7–1.9 % (resveratrol), 1.1–6.5 % (catechin), and 17.2–26.9 % (quercetin) of the peak serum concentrations and more than 80 % is absorbed. The absorption of transresveratrol was the most efficient as judged by peak serum concentration (16–17 % of dose consumed) (Goldberg et al. 2003; Vijayababu et al. 2006a).

These results support the hypothesis to use resveratrol as potentially chemopreventive drugs in prostate cancer patients, but clinical studies should be conducted to assess the real efficacy in humans.

5 Quercetin

Quercetin is the main representative of the flavonol class and antioxidant found in a variety of fruits and vegetables, highly concentrated in onions, broccoli, apples, grapes (red wine), and in soybeans (Vijayababu et al. 2006a). This flavonoid, besides having antioxidant and antiinflammatory activities, has been shown to possess potent antiproliferative effects against various malignant cells, although its molecular mechanism involved in chemoprevention of prostate cancer remains unclear in many respects (Vijayababu et al. 2006a). Quercetin treatment has been associated with selective antiproliferative effects and induction of cell death, predominantly through an apoptotic mechanism, in cancer cell lines. This compound seems to be able to induce apoptosis through multiple mechanisms: causing arrest in the G1 phase of the cell cycle or through interaction with cell cycle-regulated proteins, like cyclin D1 and CDK4; releasing cytochrome c and activating caspase-9 and caspase-3; through inhibition of PI3K, an enzyme involved in the pivotal cell survival pathway; and synergizing the effect of EGCG (Vijayababu et al. 2006a). Epidemiological studies and preliminary data have shown that quercetin inhibits the onset/growth of prostate cancer. It was noted that there is a 27 % risk reduction for prostate cancer for those who consume at least 24 μg of quercetin a day (Tang et al. 2010). In human prostate carcinoma LNCaP cells, quercetin inhibited the PI3K/Akt pathway, suppressed the phosphorylation of Bad, proapoptotic Bcl-2 family member, and subsequently altered the interaction between Bcl-xL and Bax, leading to cytochrome c release, activation of caspases, and consequently apoptotic death (Lee et al. 2008). It was also found that quercetin inhibits the proliferation of PC-3 cells causing a significant decrease in Cdc2/Cdk-1 and cyclin B1 protein expressions and increasing hypo-phosphorylated level of pRb and this may be attributed to decreased expression of growth responsive genes and subsequent growth inhibition of PC-3 cells (Vijayababu et al. 2005). Another important chemopreventive activity of quercetin might be to reduce the risk of prostate cancer metastasis. Tumor invasion and metastasis represent a multistep process that depends on the activity of many proteins. Proteolytic degradation of the extracellular matrix components is a central event of this process, primarily due to the action of matrix metalloproteinases. A study showed that this natural compound inhibits the expression of MMP-2 and -9 in prostate cancer cells (PC-3). As it has been detected that MMP-2 and -9 expressions were regulated by MAP kinase signaling pathways and quercetin is an inhibitor of several kinases including MAP kinases and tyrosine kinases, it is reasonable to speculate that quercetin might have downregulated the expression of MMP 2 and -9 through inhibition of protein kinases (Vijayababu et al. 2006b). In addition, quercetin appears to have the ability to suppress the function of androgen receptor, pivotal molecule in normal development of the prostate and in the development and progression of prostate cancer. Quercetin-mediated inhibition of the androgen receptor transcription activity in prostate cancer cells may be caused, at least in part, by the formation of a protein complex containing c-Jun, Sp1, and androgen receptor, but further investigation will be necessary to examine whether other factors are also involved in this protein complex (Yuan et al. 2010).

6 Genistein

Genistein (4,5,7-trihydroxyisoflavone), the predominant isoflavone in human nutrition, is derived mainly from soybeans but also from other legumes, including peas, lentils, or beans (Perabo et al. 2008). Genistein has many important health benefits, such as lowering the incidence of cardiovascular diseases, prevention of osteoporosis, attenuation of postmenopausal problems, and reduction of body mass and fat tissue. It also has chemopreventive properties, and in particular genistein has been shown to inhibit growth of both androgen-dependent and -independent prostate cancer cells in vitro. Several mechanisms have been proposed for genistein-induced anticarcinogenic activity: inhibition of protein-tyrosine kinase, with the result of alleviating the growth of cancer cells by inhibiting PTK-mediated signaling mechanisms; inhibition of topoisomerases I and II and protein histidine kinase with antiproliferative or proapoptotic effects; antioxidant effects, through inhibition of the expression of stress response-related genes; inhibition of NF-κB and Akt signaling pathways, both of which are important for cell survival; the inhibition of angiogenesis; the downregulation of transforming growth factor-beta (TGF-β); and the inhibition of epidermal growth factor (EGF) (Zhao et al. 2009; Banerjee et al. 2008). In vitro studies have also demonstrated that this natural compound downregulates the androgen receptor of PCa cells via the estrogen receptor β, resulting in a modified response to hormonal stimuli, inhibits several steroid-metabolizing enzymes such as 5-α-reductase or aromatase creating a more favorable hormonal milieu and a protective effect against prostate cancer, blocks the cell cycle progression at G1, and inhibits PSA expression (Perabo et al. 2008). With regard to its modulation of antioxidant activity, a study examined the effect of genistein on human prostate cancer (LNCaP and PC-3) cells. The analysis of this study has shown that while the expression of many genes, including apoptosis inhibitor (survivin), DNA topoisomerase II, cell division cycle 6 (CDC6), and mitogen-activated protein kinase 6 (MAPK 6), was downregulated, the glutathione peroxidase (GPx)-1 gene expression level was upregulated with a subsequent increase of GPx enzyme activities (Suzuki et al. 2002). These results strengthen the hypothesis of a potential use of genistein in prostate cancer chemoprevention.

The tumor initiation and progression are often attributed to oxidative stress and the generations of ROS, which exceed cell ability to metabolize and detoxify them. In addition to causing genetic changes, ROS may lead to epigenetic alterations that affect the genome and play a key role in the development of human carcinogenesis (Campos et al. 2007). More specifically, ROS production is associated with alterations in DNA methylation patterns. Furthermore, ROS-induced oxidative stress can contribute to gene silencing by mechanisms that involve aberrant hypermethylation of tumor suppressor gene promoter regions and thus lead toward progression to a malignant phenotype (Ziech et al. 2011). Oxygen radicals may cause damage to DNA and chromosomes, induce epigenetic alterations, interact with oncogenes or tumor suppressor genes, and impart changes in immunological mechanisms, like mutation of nuclear encoded genes, such as TP53, promotes carcinogenesis (Campos et al. 2007; Colotta et al. 2009). ROS are further determinant for the activation of inflammatory pathways that play a key role in cancer progression. Inflammation in cancer involves a close interplay between tumor-associated immune cells and the tumor cells themselves. Activation of NF-κB and AP-1 in immune cells, induced by ROS, determines production of inflammatory cytokines such as TNFα and IL-6 that have been demonstrated to be important in tumor progression (Wellen and Thompson 2010). Since ROS are considered key participants in the progression of cancer, the antioxidant effect of genistein might prevent tumor invasion or metastasis in prostate cancer cells by inhibiting production of matrix metalloproteinase, cell motility, and degradation of the basement membrane (Suzuki et al. 2002). The anti-metastatic potential of genistein was evaluated by a study through the development of an animal model, a murine model of human PCa metastasis. It has been demonstrated that genistein inhibits initial steps in the metastatic cascade, namely, cell detachment and cell invasion, and for the first time induces flattening of cell nuclei in vivo, a measure of increased cell attachment. Furthermore, genistein, through inhibition of phosphorylation, has been shown to inhibit activation of p38 MAPK and FAK (pro-motility proteins) in vivo, blocking cell motility. Genistein decreased metastases by 96 % and induced nuclear morphometric changes in PC3-M cells indicative of increased adhesion (i.e., decreased detachment) but did not alter tumor growth. This study showed for the first time that dietary concentrations of genistein can inhibit prostate cancer cell metastasis, but more specific analysis on the genistein effects upon human prostate cells is needed (Lakshman et al. 2008; Harper et al. 2009). Another interesting study has investigated the potential additive and synergistic effects of genistein and resveratrol for suppressing prostate cancer in the Simian Virus-40 Tantigen (SV-40 Tag)-targeted probasin promoter rat model, a transgenic model of spontaneously developing prostate cancer. It has been shown that high-dose genistein and resveratrol treatments, reducing cell proliferation and increasing apoptosis mainly through the modulation of sex steroid receptor and growth factor signaling, suppress the most severe grade of prostate cancer in these transgenic animals (Harper et al. 2009). In a randomized, placebo-controlled, double-blind phase II clinical trial, 54 study subjects were recruited and randomized to treatment with genistein 30 mg ($n = 23$) or placebo ($n = 24$) for 3–6 weeks prior to prostatectomy. It was shown that serum prostate-specific antigen (PSA) decreased by 7.8 % in the genistein arm and increased by 4.4 % in the placebo arm, without adverse events and with beneficial effect on blood cholesterol (Lazarevic et al. 2011).

7 Conclusion

In conclusion, the chemopreventive properties of dietary polyphenols are directed toward different molecular levels in prostate cancer. The primary action of these molecules may be reflected against oxidative stress. Furthermore, other evidences have confirmed that these compounds influence the growth of the prostate cancer by modulating cell survival signals and aiding in cell death pathways. Although a large number of studies have been conducted in vitro and in murine models, few clinical trials with well-defined concentrations of these compounds have been performed. Therefore, since the use of the polyphenols seems to have good perspectives, comprehensive randomized clinical trials are warranted in patients with prostate cancer to substantiate their benefits. However, regular consumption of diet rich in these polyphenols as reflected by the abovementioned studies presumably has the potential to lower the risk of prostate cancer.

References

Abbas A, Patterson W 3rd, Georgel PT (2013) The epigenetic potentials of dietary polyphenols in prostate cancer management. Biochem Cell Biol 91(6):361–368. doi:10.1139/bcb-2012-0044

Adhami VM, Ahmad N, Mukhtar H (2003) Molecular targets for green tea in prostate cancer prevention. J Nutr 133(7 Suppl):2417S–2424S

Adhami VM, Malik A, Zaman N, Sarfaraz S, Siddiqui IA, Syed DN, Afaq F, Pasha FS, Saleem M, Mukhtar H (2007) Combined inhibitory effects of green tea polyphenols and selective cyclooxygenase-2 inhibitors on the growth of human prostate cancer cells both in vitro and in vivo. Clin Cancer Res 13(5):1611–1619. doi:10.1158/1078-0432.CCR-06-2269

Banerjee S, Li Y, Wang Z, Sarkar FH (2008) Multi-targeted therapy of cancer by genistein. Cancer Lett 269(2):226–242. doi:10.1016/j.canlet.2008.03.052

Bettuzzi S, Brausi M, Rizzi F, Castagnetti G, Peracchia G, Corti A (2006) Chemoprevention of human prostate cancer by oral administration of green tea catechins in volunteers with high-grade prostate intraepithelial neoplasia: a preliminary report from a one-year proof-of-principle study. Cancer Res 66(2):1234–1240. doi:10.1158/0008-5472.CAN-05-1145

Cabrespine-Faugeras A, Bayet-Robert M, Bay JO, Chollet P, Barthomeuf C (2010) Possible benefits of curcumin regimen in combination with taxane chemotherapy for hormone-refractory prostate cancer treatment. Nutr Cancer 62(2):148–153. doi:10.1080/01635580903305383

Campos AC, Molognoni F, Melo FH, Galdieri LC, Carneiro CR, D'Almeida V, Correa M, Jasiulionis MG (2007) Oxidative stress modulates DNA methylation during melanocyte anchorage blockade associated with malignant transformation. Neoplasia 9(12):1111–1121

Chendil D, Ranga RS, Meigooni D, Sathishkumar S, Ahmed MM (2004) Curcumin confers radiosensitizing effect in prostate cancer cell line PC-3. Oncogene 23(8):1599–1607. doi:10.1038/sj.onc.1207284

Choi BH, Kim CG, Lim Y, Shin SY, Lee YH (2008) Curcumin down-regulates the multidrug-resistance mdr1b gene by inhibiting the PI3K/Akt/NF kappa B pathway. Cancer Lett 259(1):111–118. doi:10.1016/j.canlet.2007.10.003

Chung LC, Tsui KH, Feng TH, Lee SL, Chang PL, Juang HH (2011) Curcumin provides potential protection against the activation of hypoxia and prolyl 4-hydroxylase inhibitors on prostate-

specific antigen expression in human prostate carcinoma cells. Mol Nutr Food Res 55 (11):1666–1676. doi:10.1002/mnfr.201100328
Cimino S, Sortino G, Favilla V, Castelli T, Madonia M, Sansalone S, Russo GI, Morgia G (2012) Polyphenols: key issues involved in chemoprevention of prostate cancer. Oxidative Med Cell Longev 2012:632959. doi:10.1155/2012/632959
Cimino S, Favilla V, Russo GI, Galvano F, Li Volti G, Barbagallo I, Giofre SV, D'Orazio N, Di Rosa A, Madonia M, Morgia G (2014) Oxidative stress and body composition in prostate cancer and benign prostatic hyperplasia patients. Anticancer Res 34(9):5051–5056
Colotta F, Allavena P, Sica A, Garlanda C, Mantovani A (2009) Cancer-related inflammation, the seventh hallmark of cancer: links to genetic instability. Carcinogenesis 30(7):1073–1081. doi:10.1093/carcin/bgp127
De Nunzio C, Kramer G, Marberger M, Montironi R, Nelson W, Schroder F, Sciarra A, Tubaro A (2011) The controversial relationship between benign prostatic hyperplasia and prostate cancer: the role of inflammation. Eur Urol 60(1):106–117. doi:10.1016/j.eururo.2011.03.055
Goel A, Aggarwal BB (2010) Curcumin, the golden spice from Indian saffron, is a chemosensitizer and radiosensitizer for tumors and chemoprotector and radioprotector for normal organs. Nutr Cancer 62(7):919–930. doi:10.1080/01635581.2010.509835
Goldberg DM, Yan J, Soleas GJ (2003) Absorption of three wine-related polyphenols in three different matrices by healthy subjects. Clin Biochem 36(1):79–87
Harper CE, Cook LM, Patel BB, Wang J, Eltoum IA, Arabshahi A, Shirai T, Lamartiniere CA (2009) Genistein and resveratrol, alone and in combination, suppress prostate cancer in SV-40 tag rats. Prostate 69(15):1668–1682. doi:10.1002/pros.21017
Hong JH, Ahn KS, Bae E, Jeon SS, Choi HY (2006) The effects of curcumin on the invasiveness of prostate cancer in vitro and in vivo. Prostate Cancer Prostatic Dis 9(2):147–152. doi:10.1038/sj.pcan.4500856
Hour TC, Chen J, Huang CY, Guan JY, Lu SH, Pu YS (2002) Curcumin enhances cytotoxicity of chemotherapeutic agents in prostate cancer cells by inducing p21(WAF1/CIP1) and C/EBPbeta expressions and suppressing NF-kappaB activation. Prostate 51(3):211–218. doi:10.1002/pros.10089
Khan N, Afaq F, Mukhtar H (2008) Cancer chemoprevention through dietary antioxidants: progress and promise. Antioxid Redox Signal 10(3):475–510. doi:10.1089/ars.2007.1740
Khan N, Adhami VM, Mukhtar H (2009) Review: green tea polyphenols in chemoprevention of prostate cancer: preclinical and clinical studies. Nutr Cancer 61(6):836–841. doi:10.1080/01635580903285056
Khan N, Adhami VM, Mukhtar H (2010) Apoptosis by dietary agents for prevention and treatment of prostate cancer. Endocr Relat Cancer 17(1):R39–R52. doi:10.1677/ERC-09-0262
Kurahashi N, Sasazuki S, Iwasaki M, Inoue M, Tsugane S (2008) Green tea consumption and prostate cancer risk in Japanese men: a prospective study. Am J Epidemiol 167(1):71–77. doi:10.1093/aje/kwm249
Lakshman M, Xu L, Ananthanarayanan V, Cooper J, Takimoto CH, Helenowski I, Pelling JC, Bergan RC (2008) Dietary genistein inhibits metastasis of human prostate cancer in mice. Cancer Res 68(6):2024–2032. doi:10.1158/0008-5472.CAN-07-1246
Lazarevic B, Boezelijn G, Diep LM, Kvernrod K, Ogren O, Ramberg H, Moen A, Wessel N, Berg RE, Egge-Jacobsen W, Hammarstrom C, Svindland A, Kucuk O, Saatcioglu F, Tasken KA, Karlsen SJ (2011) Efficacy and safety of short-term genistein intervention in patients with localized prostate cancer prior to radical prostatectomy: a randomized, placebo-controlled, double-blind Phase 2 clinical trial. Nutr Cancer 63(6):889–898. doi:10.1080/01635581.2011.582221
Lee DH, Szczepanski M, Lee YJ (2008) Role of Bax in quercetin-induced apoptosis in human prostate cancer cells. Biochem Pharmacol 75(12):2345–2355. doi:10.1016/j.bcp.2008.03.013
Markowski MC, Bowen C, Gelmann EP (2008) Inflammatory cytokines induce phosphorylation and ubiquitination of prostate suppressor protein NKX3.1. Cancer Res 68(17):6896–6901. doi:10.1158/0008-5472.CAN-08-0578

Mukhopadhyay A, Bueso-Ramos C, Chatterjee D, Pantazis P, Aggarwal BB (2001) Curcumin downregulates cell survival mechanisms in human prostate cancer cell lines. Oncogene 20 (52):7597–7609. doi:10.1038/sj.onc.1204997

Perabo FG, Von Low EC, Ellinger J, von Rucker A, Muller SC, Bastian PJ (2008) Soy isoflavone genistein in prevention and treatment of prostate cancer. Prostate Cancer Prostatic Dis 11 (1):6–12. doi:10.1038/sj.pcan.4501000

Ramos S (2007) Effects of dietary flavonoids on apoptotic pathways related to cancer chemoprevention. J Nutr Biochem 18(7):427–442. doi:10.1016/j.jnutbio.2006.11.004

Ratan HL, Steward WP, Gescher AJ, Mellon JK (2002) Resveratrol—a prostate cancer chemopreventive agent? Urol Oncol 7(6):223–227

Sharma RA, McLelland HR, Hill KA, Ireson CR, Euden SA, Manson MM, Pirmohamed M, Marnett LJ, Gescher AJ, Steward WP (2001) Pharmacodynamic and pharmacokinetic study of oral Curcuma extract in patients with colorectal cancer. Clinl Cancer Res 7(7):1894–1900

Sharma RA, Euden SA, Platton SL, Cooke DN, Shafayat A, Hewitt HR, Marczylo TH, Morgan B, Hemingway D, Plummer SM, Pirmohamed M, Gescher AJ, Steward WP (2004) Phase I clinical trial of oral curcumin: biomarkers of systemic activity and compliance. Clin Cancer Res 10(20):6847–6854. doi:10.1158/1078-0432.CCR-04-0744

Shih A, Zhang S, Cao HJ, Boswell S, Wu YH, Tang HY, Lennartz MR, Davis FB, Davis PJ, Lin HY (2004) Inhibitory effect of epidermal growth factor on resveratrol-induced apoptosis in prostate cancer cells is mediated by protein kinase C-alpha. Mol Cancer Ther 3(11):1355–1364

Siddiqui IA, Zaman N, Aziz MH, Reagan-Shaw SR, Sarfaraz S, Adhami VM, Ahmad N, Raisuddin S, Mukhtar H (2006) Inhibition of CWR22Rnu1 tumor growth and PSA secretion in athymic nude mice by green and black teas. Carcinogenesis 27(4):833–839. doi:10.1093/carcin/bgi323

Siegel RL, Miller KD, Jemal A (2015) Cancer statistics, 2015. CA Cancer J Clin 65:5–29. doi:10.3322/caac.21254

Suzuki K, Koike H, Matsui H, Ono Y, Hasumi M, Nakazato H, Okugi H, Sekine Y, Oki K, Ito K, Yamamoto T, Fukabori Y, Kurokawa K, Yamanaka H (2002) Genistein, a soy isoflavone, induces glutathione peroxidase in the human prostate cancer cell lines LNCaP and PC-3. Int J Cancer 99(6):846–852. doi:10.1002/ijc.10428

Syed DN, Khan N, Afaq F, Mukhtar H (2007) Chemoprevention of prostate cancer through dietary agents: progress and promise. Cancer Epidemiol Biomarkers Prev 16(11):2193–2203. doi:10.1158/1055-9965.EPI-06-0942

Tang SN, Singh C, Nall D, Meeker D, Shankar S, Srivastava RK (2010) The dietary bioflavonoid quercetin synergizes with epigallocathechin gallate (EGCG) to inhibit prostate cancer stem cell characteristics, invasion, migration and epithelial-mesenchymal transition. J Mol Signal 5:14. doi:10.1186/1750-2187-5-14

Vijayababu MR, Kanagaraj P, Arunkumar A, Ilangovan R, Aruldhas MM, Arunakaran J (2005) Quercetin-induced growth inhibition and cell death in prostatic carcinoma cells (PC-3) are associated with increase in p21 and hypophosphorylated retinoblastoma proteins expression. J Cancer Res Clin Oncol 131(11):765–771. doi:10.1007/s00432-005-0005-4

Vijayababu MR, Kanagaraj P, Arunkumar A, Ilangovan R, Dharmarajan A, Arunakaran J (2006a) Quercetin induces p53-independent apoptosis in human prostate cancer cells by modulating Bcl-2-related proteins: a possible mediation by IGFBP-3. Oncol Res 16(2):67–74

Vijayababu MR, Arunkumar A, Kanagaraj P, Venkataraman P, Krishnamoorthy G, Arunakaran J (2006b) Quercetin downregulates matrix metalloproteinases 2 and 9 proteins expression in prostate cancer cells (PC-3). Mol Cell Biochem 287(1–2):109–116. doi:10.1007/s11010-005-9085-3

Wellen KE, Thompson CB (2010) Cellular metabolic stress: considering how cells respond to nutrient excess. Mol Cell 40(2):323–332. doi:10.1016/j.molcel.2010.10.004

Yuan H, Young CY, Tian Y, Liu Z, Zhang M, Lou H (2010) Suppression of the androgen receptor function by quercetin through protein-protein interactions of Sp1, c-Jun, and the androgen receptor in human prostate cancer cells. Mol Cell Biochem 339(1–2):253–262. doi:10.1007/s11010-010-0388-7

Zhao R, Xiang N, Domann FE, Zhong W (2009) Effects of selenite and genistein on G2/M cell cycle arrest and apoptosis in human prostate cancer cells. Nutr Cancer 61(3):397–407. doi:10.1080/01635580802582751

Zhou JR, Yu L, Zhong Y, Blackburn GL (2003) Soy phytochemicals and tea bioactive components synergistically inhibit androgen-sensitive human prostate tumors in mice. J Nutr 133(2):516–521

Ziech D, Franco R, Pappa A, Panayiotidis MI (2011) Reactive oxygen species (ROS)-induced genetic and epigenetic alterations in human carcinogenesis. Mutat Res 711(1–2):167–173. doi:10.1016/j.mrfmmm.2011.02.015

Effects of Garcinol from Kokum (*Garcinia indica*) on the Prevention and Treatment of Cancer

Bernhard Biersack

Abstract Kokum (*Garcinia indica*) has been applied for dishes of the Konkan region of Western India for centuries. There is growing evidence that its major ingredients like hydroxycitric acid (HCA) and garcinol have beneficial health effects. While HCA is considered to be a suitable tool to manage obesity, the polyisoprenylated benzophenone garcinol has revealed potent anticancer, antibacterial, anti-inflammatory, and anti-ulcer effects. This chapter provides an overview of the latest developments of garcinol and its derivatives concerning the prevention and treatment of various cancer diseases. After a short introduction, important chemical aspects of garcinol are discussed followed by an overview of inflammation-related targets of garcinol such as NF-κB, 5-LOX, and STAT proteins playing also a big role in cancer progression. Interference of chromatin regulation and HAT substrate stability by the HAT inhibitor garcinol and a final comment on the anti-ulcer activity of garcinol complete this chapter. Pertinent literature is covered up to 2014.

1 Introduction

The prevention and treatment of cancer is one of the biggest challenges of our time. Despite the improved prognosis of certain cancer diseases during the last decades due to new therapy concepts, inexpensive and effective treatment options are still strongly demanded. Many dietary components such as curcumin (from turmeric), gingerol (from ginger), capsaicin (from chilli peppers), sulforaphane and 3,3-′-diindolylmethane (from broccoli), resveratrol (from grapes), or genistein (from soy) have exhibited distinct activity in the prevention and treatment of various cancer types. Most of these natural compounds from dietary plants have low side effects and the importance of these compounds as anticancer agents is growing. The role of another Indian spice called kokum (*Garcinia indica*) and of its component

B. Biersack (✉)
Organic Chemistry Laboratory, University of Bayreuth, Universitätsstr. 30, 95447 Bayreuth, Germany
e-mail: bernhard.biersack@uni-bayreuth.de

M.F. Ullah, A. Ahmad (eds.), *Critical Dietary Factors in Cancer Chemoprevention*, DOI 10.1007/978-3-319-21461-0_12

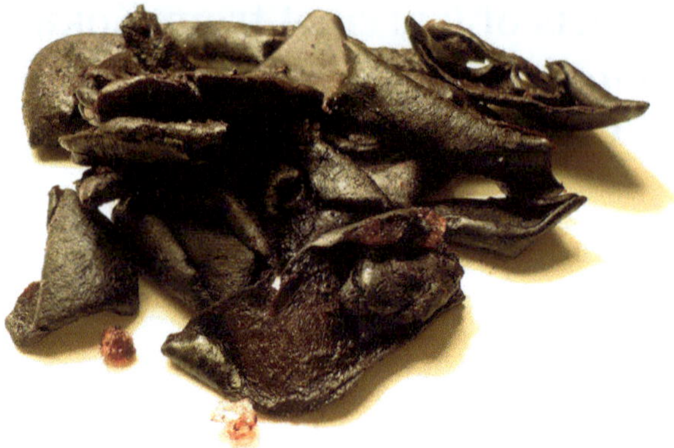

Fig. 1 Dried kokum plums (amsool)

garcinol is the matter of this chapter since garcinol appears to be underrated compared with curcumin, though both compounds share some similarities.

The kokum tree (*Garcinia indica*) belongs to the genus of *Garcinia* plants (ca. 300 species of trees and shrubs) growing in tropical regions of Africa, Asia, and the Pacific (Hemshekhar et al. 2011). The kokum tree is abundant in Western India, the Konkan, Malabar, and Kanara regions, blessed with fertile soils and sufficient rainfall and sunshine periods. Dried kokum plums (Fig. 1) are particularly popular in the Konkan region as a sour spice for the preparation of traditional local dishes, curries, and refreshing drinks. Kokum-based remedies have also been applied in Ayurvedic medicine for the treatment of infections and edema for centuries (Padhye et al. 2009; Saadat and Gupta 2012). Aside from high contents of hydroxycitric acid which is considered a magic bullet against obesity, the rind of the kokum plums contains certain polyisoprenylated benzophenones like garcinol and isogarcinol which are responsible for the immense antibiotic and anti-inflammatory activity of the kokum fruit. Garcinol possesses a β-diketone and a phenolic fragment like curcumin, and due to these structural similarities garcinol is able to bind to many curcumin targets as well. However, in some cases garcinol even exceeds the anticancer activity of curcumin which makes it a valuable alternative for cancer treatment (Pan et al. 2001).

In the following, an overview is presented of the miscellaneous biological activities of garcinol as obtained from preclinical evaluations concerning the treatment and prevention of cancer and metastases.

2 Chemical Aspects of Garcinol

Garcinol (also called camboginol, **1**) is a benzophenone derivative with five isoprenyl side chains attached to the central phloroglucinol ring (Fig. 2). Chemically, it belongs to the class of type B polycyclic polyprenylated acylphloroglucinols (PPAPs) (Ciochina and Grossman 2006). To date, there are more than

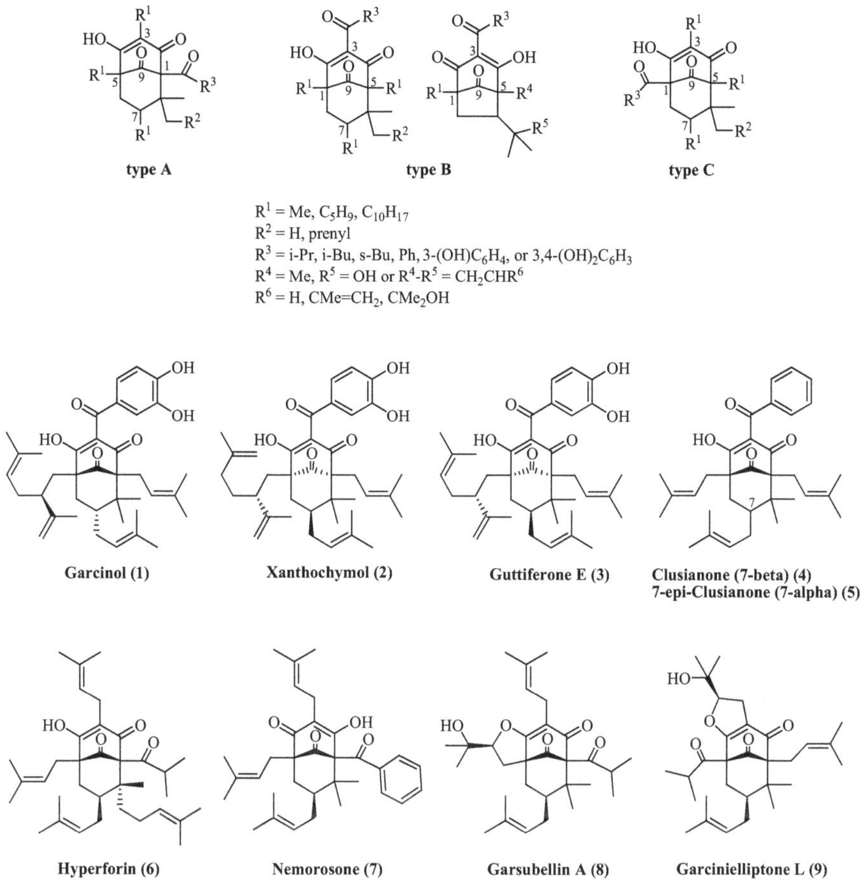

Fig. 2 Structures of natural type A, B, and C PPAPs

100 known PPAPs subdivided into three different types A, B, and C depending on the position of the acyl group. Other natural products of type B PPAPs isolated from *Garcinia* and *Clusia* species are xanthochymol (**2**), the guttiferones A–E (**3**), and the clusianones (**4**, **5**). For comparison purposes, hyperforin (**6**) from St. John's wort (*Hypericum perforatum*) features a type A PPAP with a well-documented antidepressant and anxiolytic activity. Nemorosone (**7**, from *Clusia* species) and garsubellin A (**8**, from *Garcinia subelliptica*) are further important type A PPAPs with antimicrobial and anti-inflammatory activity. The group of type C PPAPs is rather small and represented by garcinielliptones K, L (**9**), and M from *Garcinia subelliptica* (Ciochina and Grossman 2006).

From the biosynthetic point of view, it was initially assumed that garcinol/cambogniol and its close analogues might be derived from the benzophenone maclurin (2,3′,4,4′,6-pentahydroxybenzophenone) which is considered as a precursor for several xanthones in higher plants (Rao et al. 1980; Locksley et al. 1967).

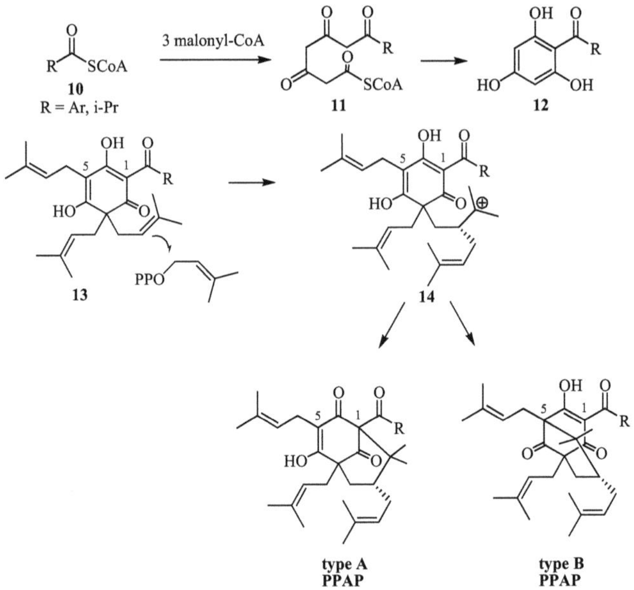

Fig. 3 Biosynthesis of type A and B PPAPs

Indeed, there is evidence that PPAPs are offsprings of the less complex monocyclic polyprenylated acylphloroglucinols (MPAP) which are mainly discovered in plants of the *Myrtaceae* and *Cannabinaceae* families (e.g., in hops, *Humulus lupulus*) (Zhao et al. 2005). A polyketide-type biosynthesis involving one acyl-CoA (**10**) and three malonyl-CoA molecules was elucidated as to labelling and enzymologic experiments (Fig. 3). The formed tetraketide **11** undergoes Dieckmann cyclisation to acylphloroglucinol **12** (catalysed by benzophenone synthase in case of benzoyl derivatives), followed by enzyme-catalysed prenylation/geranylation with prenyl/geranyl pyrophosphate to MPAPs (**13**). Attack of one of the geminal prenyl groups of the MPAP molecule to another prenyl pyrophosphate generates a carbocation (**14**) which is ready to undergo cyclisation to type A (after C1 attack) or type B (after C5 attack) PPAP derivatives (Ciochina and Grossman 2006). In contrast to that, formation of the rare PPAPs of type C probably requires a quaternary centre adjacent to the acyl group (at C1).

Interestingly, optically active garcinol/camboginol (**1**, $[\alpha]^{30}$ −132.9°C, 1 % in $CHCl_3$) was first described upon isolation from the latex of another *Garcinia* species, *Garcinia cambogia* (thus, the name camboginol is also casually applied for garcinol) (Rao et al. 1980). Despite this, garcinol is very abundant in the rinds of kokum plums and can be easily isolated from dried kokum/*Garcinia indica* fruits (also called amsool) in reasonable amounts yielding, for instance, up to 5 g of pure garcinol from 500 g of dried kokum fruits. In brief, commercially available dried kokum plums are chopped and extracted with methanol by stirring a methanolic kokum suspension with a mechanical stirrer. After filtration and removal of the

Fig. 4 Structures of the enantiomers isogarcinol (**15**) and isoxanthochymol (**16**)

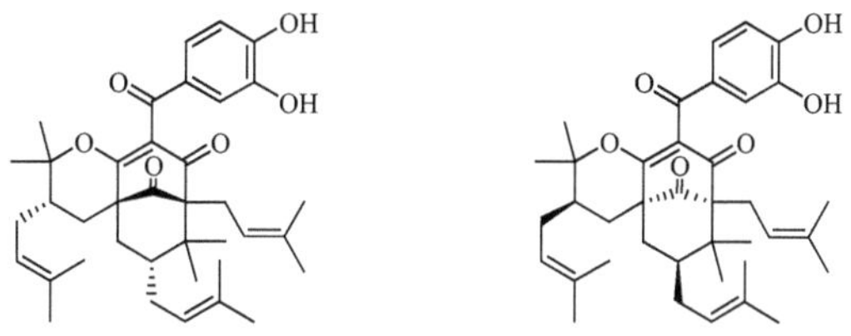

Isogarcinol (15)
(-)-enantiomer

Isoxanthochymol (16)
(+)-enantiomer

solvent, water is added and the aqueous phase extracted with ethyl acetate. Purification of the ethyl acetate extract by column chromatography (silica gel 60, ethyl acetate/*n*-hexane 1:2) gives crude garcinol which is finally recrystallised from *n*-hexane as a pure yellow solid. The colorless pyrano-isomer isogarcinol (**15**, cambogin) is easily obtained from garcinol under acidic conditions and features the (−)-enantiomer ($[\alpha]^{30}$ −209.9°C, 1 % in MeOH) of the natural product isoxanthochymol (**16**, Fig. 4). An efficient thermal conversion of garcinol to isogarcinol (at 200 °C for 5 min) was likewise reported (Rao et al. 1980).

Garcinol (**1**) possesses significant radical-scavenging properties due to its structure (catechol and β-diketone fragments). The oxidation products of garcinol have been identified and possess themselves significant biological properties. Mechanistically, the treatment of garcinol with AIBN or DPPH leads to abstraction of a hydrogen radical from garcinol forming a conjugated garcinol radical (**17**, Fig. 5). This garcinol radical converts to isogarcinol (**15**), to a hydroperoxide metabolite (**18**), or to xanthone derivatives garcim-1 (**19**) and garcim-2 (**20**) (Sang et al. 2001, 2002; Hong et al. 2007).

Although garcinol is readily available from its biological sources, total synthetic approaches toward PPAPs are generally of importance in order to obtain less abundant derivatives and for the design of new PPAP compounds with improved biological properties. The first total syntheses of PPAPs were accomplished for garsubellin A, a type A PPAP, by Shibasaki (2005) and Danishefsky (2006) (Kuramochi et al. 2005; Siegel and Danishefsky 2006). Meanwhile, total syntheses of additional PPAPs are available, including type B derivatives such as clusianones and guttiferone A. Simpkins and coworkers have disclosed the total synthesis of racemic clusianone in 2006 using an Effenberger cyclisation key step to generate the bicyclic trione fragment (Fig. 6) (Rodeschini et al. 2006; Schönwälder et al. 1984). Starting from the vinylogous ester **21** repeated prenylation gave a mixture of enol ethers **22** and **23**, which underwent Effenberger cyclisation forming the bicycle[3.3.1]nonane-2,4,9-trione **24**. Regioselective lithiation reactions led to the final product, racemic clusianone (**4**). A similar approach was applied by Marazano and coworkers starting from an enol silyl ether which was reacted with malonyl chloride under Effenberger conditions (Nuhant et al. 2007).

In contrast to that, Danishefsky and coworkers applied a iodonium-catalysed carbocyclisation to build up the bicycle **27** starting from commercially available 3,5-dimethoxyphenol (**25**, Fig. 7). Though the yield of the cyclisation step is low,

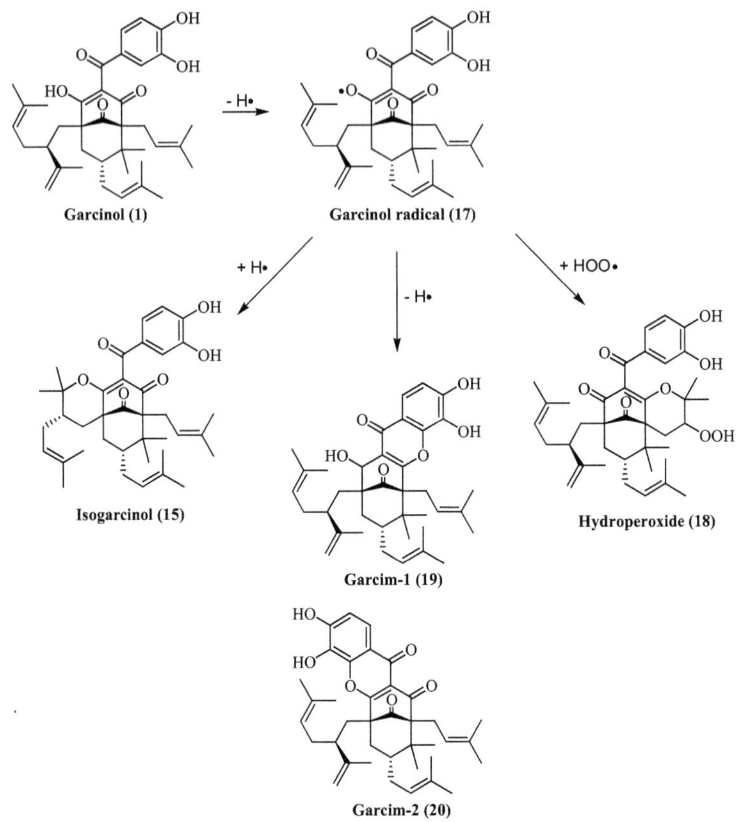

Fig. 5 Radical reaction of garcinol (**1**)

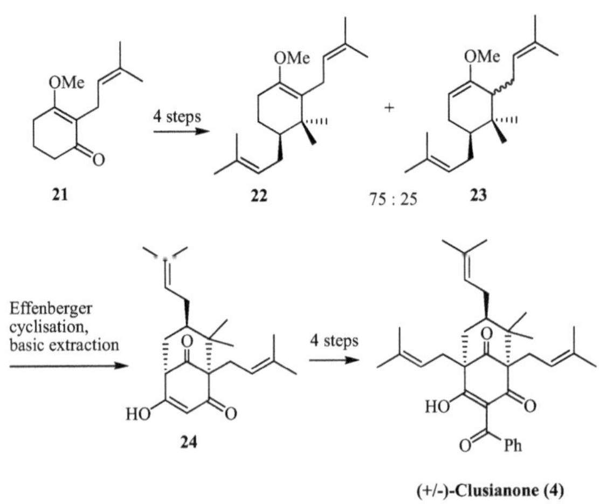

Fig. 6 Total synthesis of (+/−)-clusianone (**4**) by Simpkins

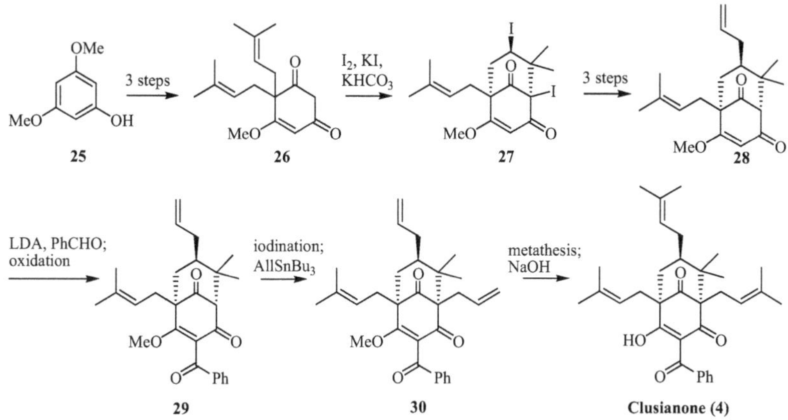

Fig. 7 Total synthesis of clusianone (**4**) by Danishefsky

the isolated side products can be recycled to the precursor **26**. After introduction of the allyl and benzoyl groups, cross-metathesis of **30** with 2-methylpropene using a Grubbs second-generation catalyst and final methyl ether cleavage with aq. NaOH gives clusianone (**4**) (Tsukano et al. 2007).

Recently, Boyce and Porco Jr. have disclosed a six-step asymmetric synthesis of (−)-clusianone (**4**) from 5-methoxyresorcinol via benzophenones **31** and **32** using a biomimetic cationic cyclisation procedure (Boyce and Porco 2014). Allylation and Claisen rearrangement forms diallyl benzophenone **32** which is alkylated with the chiral alkyl *O*-triflate **33** to intermediate **34** (Fig. 8). Cationic cyclisation under acidic conditions generates the precursor (−)-**35**, which is converted to (−)-clusianone (**4**) via cross-metathesis using a Grubbs II catalyst. The same group has recently reported a quick route to PPAPs (both type A and type B) by Pd-catalysed dearomative conjunctive allylic alkylation of allyl deoxyhumulones (Grenning et al. 2014).

A different route was chosen by Plietker and coworkers to accomplish the total synthesis of the type B PPAPs epi-clusianone (**5**), oblongifolin A (**40a**), hyperpapuanone (**40b**), and hyperibone L (**40c**) (Biber et al. 2011). Starting from acetylacetone **36** the ketones **37** were prepared (Fig. 9). After Michael addition and Knoevenagel condensation followed by alkylation the cyclohexenones **38** were obtained. Subsequent alkylation (cuprate addition) gives the cyclohexenones **39** which were converted to the acylated bicyclo-nonatriones **40a–c** and **5** via Dieckmann condensation and acylation in one step. Overall yields of this synthetic method ranged from 6 to 22 %. Meanwhile, the same group has disclosed the total synthesis of guttiferone A in a similar way (Horeischi et al. 2014).

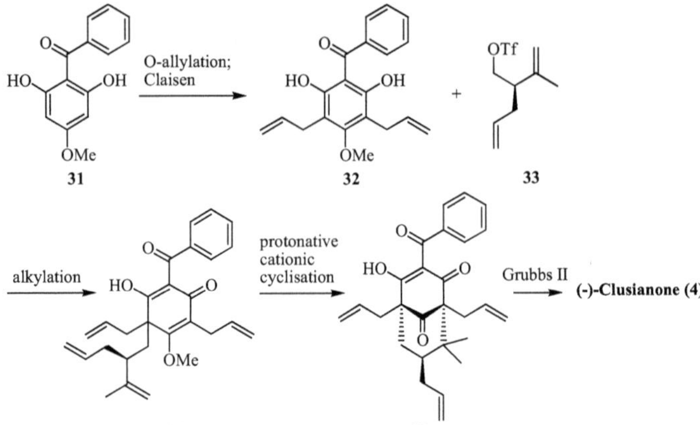

Fig. 8 Asymmetric total synthesis of (−)-clusianone (**4**) by Porco Jr

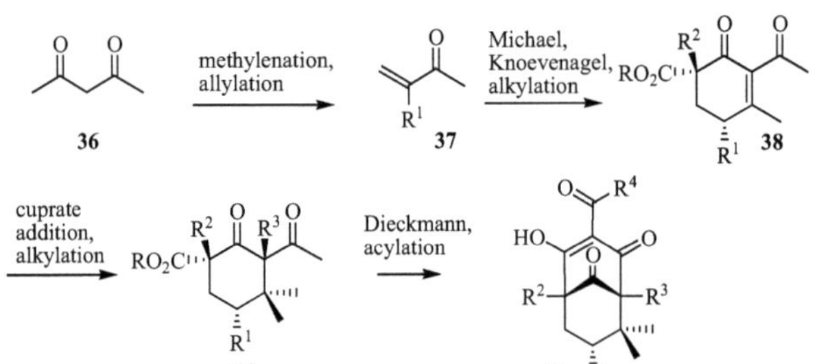

Oblongifolin A (40a): R^1 = geranyl; R^2, R^3 = prenyl; R^4 = 3,4-$(OH)_2$-C_6H_3
Hyperpapuanone (40b): R^1 = prenyl; R^2 = methyl; R^3 = prenyl;tR^4 = i-Pr
epi-Clusianone (5): R^1, R^2, R^3 = prenyl; R^4 = Ph
Hyperibone L (40c): R^1, R^2 = prenyl; R^3 = methyl; R^4 = Ph

Fig. 9 Total syntheses of oblongifolin A (**40a**), hyperpapuanone (**40b**), epi-clusianone (**5**), and hyperibone L (**40c**) by Plietker

3 Garcinol, Inflammation, and Cancer

Much of the chemopreventive activity of garcinol (**1**) can be assigned to its radical scavenging properties against superoxide anions, hydroxyl radicals, and methyl radicals and, thus, protection of cellular components from lethal damage. Garcinol showed superoxide anion scavenging activity comparable with DL-α-tocopherol, a threefold higher 2,2-diphenyl-1-picrylhydrazyl (DPPH) scavenging activity than DL-α-tocopherol, and saved indomethacin-treated rats from acute ulceration (Yamaguchi et al. 2000). In addition, garcinol also inhibited protein glycation (Yamaguchi et al. 2000). F344 rats were protected from azoxymethane (AOM)-induced colonic aberrant crypt foci (ACF) by treatment with garcinol which caused decreased proliferating cell nuclear antigen (PCNA) index in ACF and increased liver glutathione *S*-transferase (GST) and quinone reductase (QR) activities (Tanaka et al. 2000). The expression of iNOS and COX-2 enzymes was significantly downregulated in the ACF of the garcinol cohort. Hence, pre-neoplastic progression in rat colons is efficiently suppressed by garcinol. Recently, Tsai and coworkers have shown that garcinol inhibits inflammation-associated colon carcinogenesis in mice induced by dextran sodium sulphate and azoxymethane by downregulation of iNOS, COX-2, and PCNA basing on inhibition of ERK1/2, PI3K/Akt, and Wnt/β-catenin signalling (Tsai et al. 2014). Oral carcinogenesis caused by 4-nitroquinoline-1-oxide (4NQO) was likewise silenced in F344 rats by feeding with garcinol which reduced cell proliferation rate and COX-2 levels in affected tongue tissues (Yoshida et al. 2005).

Neuroprotective effects of garcinol were also observed as well as reduction of nitric oxide (NO) radical levels in astrocytes treated with lipopolysaccharides (LPS) (Liao et al. 2005a). Indeed, formation of NO radicals seems to play a key role concerning inflammation and carcinogenesis processes. LPS-stimulated macrophages (murine RAW264.7 cells) and intestinal cells treated with garcinol revealed reduced arachidonic acid metabolism and NO synthesis (Hong et al. 2006). While treatment with garcinol after LPS stimulation might be conferred to inhibition of $cPLA_2$ and ERK1/2 which are involved in arachidonic acid release from membrane phospholipids, garcinol treatment before macrophage stimulation with LPS might inhibit toll-like receptors. Again, suppression of COX-2 and of NF-κB proteins was observed which feature crucial factors of inflammation processes (Hong et al. 2006; Liao et al. 2004). In fact, blocked NF-κB signalling is involved in induction of apoptosis by garcinol in highly metastatic MDA-MB-231 breast cancer cells as well as in prostate and pancreatic cancer cells (Ahmad et al. 2010, 2011). The close garcinol analogue isogarcinol (**15**) also displayed anti-inflammatory activity by downregulation of iNOS, COX-2, and NF-κB and suppressed xylene-induced mouse ear edema and collagen-induced arthritis in vivo (Fu et al. 2014).

5-Lipoxygenase (5-LOX) and microsomal prostaglandin E2 synthase-1 feature additional important targets of garcinol (Koeberle et al. 2009). Suppression of 5-LOX and PGE2 was observed in human neutrophils and interleukin-stimulated human lung cancer cells after garcinol treatment. Inhibition of 5-LOX activity seems to be a particularly efficient strategy to combat metastases, and COX-2 catalysed PGE2 formation is often related with enhanced metastasis by upregulation of matrix metalloproteinases such as MMP-2 (Flavin 2007; Ito et al. 2004). 5-LOX inhibition by topical garcinol treatment suppressed 7,12-dimethylbenz[a]anthracene (DMBA)-induced hamster cheek pouch carcinogenesis by inhibition of leukotriene B4 (LTB4) biosynthesis (Xin et al. 2012). Inflammation and carcinogenesis in the oral epithelium were efficiently prevented by garcinol.

Hong and coworkers have shown that garcinol-based anti-inflammatory activity was observed due to inhibition of Janus kinase/signal transducer and activator of transcription (JAK/STAT)-dependent pathways in LPS-stimulated macrophages (Hong et al. 2006). Recently, a direct interaction of garcinol with the transcription factor STAT-1 was disclosed as well as inhibition of cytokine signalling by blocking STAT-1 transfer into the nucleus and STAT-1 binding to DNA (Masullo et al. 2014). STAT-3 features another STAT protein known for its cross talk with NF-κB in cancers leading to increased tumour progression and dissemination (Grivennikov and Karin 2010; Bollrath and Greten 2009). Thus, inactivation of STAT-3 has become a promising target for cancer therapy. There are already some curcuminoid derivatives which are able to inhibit the phosphorylation of the SH2 domain of STAT-3 by binding to the SH2 domain and, thus, suppress the dimerisation of STAT-3 to functional transcription factors (Bill et al. 2012; Lin et al. 2011). Due to the structural similarity to curcuminoids, it is not surprising that garcinol has exhibited similar effects. Ahmad and coworkers disclosed STAT-3 inhibition by garcinol in metastatic breast cancer as well as in prostate and pancreatic cancer cells (Ahmad et al. 2012a). STAT-3 inhibition was also documented in vivo from tumour remnants after oral application of garcinol (5 mg/kg/day) which likewise reduced MDA-MB-231 breast tumour growth significantly. Recently, garcinol treatment led to STAT-3 inhibition and suppressed in vivo tumour growth in human head and neck squamous cell carcinoma (HNSCC) xenografts and human hepatocellular carcinoma (HCC) xenografts, in the latter case also by inhibition of STAT-3 acetylation (see next Chapter “Effects of Garcinol on Chromatin-Regulating Proteins”) (Li et al. 2013; Sethi et al. 2014).

The chaperone Hsp90 (heat-shock protein 90) is involved in inflammation and cancer since it is critical for the stability of its client proteins such as IKK and iNOS. Recently, the Hsp90 inhibitory activity of garcinol was identified by a high-throughput screening of natural product libraries and the effects of garcinol on NF-κB activity and NO formation can be partially mediated via Hsp90 inhibition as well (Davenport et al. 2014). However, further tests are necessary to validate the initial experiments on Hsp90 inhibition by garcinol.

Apoptosis induction and interference with mitosis in proliferating cancer cells have been reported for garcinol featuring additional hallmarks of garcinol-mediated anticancer activity. In HL-60 leukaemia cells, garcinol induced apoptosis via cytochrome c release from mitochondria and activation of caspase-9, caspase-3, and caspase-2 and surpassed the pro-apoptotic activity of curcumin (Pan et al. 2001). PARP cleavage and DNA fragmentation were observed from garcinol-treated cells as well as upregulation of proapoptotic Bad and Bax. In garcinol-treated hepatocellular carcinoma cells, formation of ROS led to mitochondrial apoptosis induction and significant increase in the Bax/Bcl-2 ratio (Cheng et al. 2010). Autoxidation of garcinol to xanthones with enhanced anticancer activity was also observed; the derivatives garcim-1 (**19**) and garcim-2 (**20**) (Fig. 5) revealed an even higher activity than garcinol in colon cancer cells (Hong et al. 2007). Garcinol appears to be a selective anticancer agent. Distinctly stronger caspase-3-dependent apoptosis induction was discovered in intestinal cancer cells than in nonmalignant cells (Hong et al. 2007). A similar effect was observed in breast cancer cells (Ahmad et al. 2010). Interestingly, at low doses below 1 μM garcinol promotes cell growth, and, thus, the cell killing effect of garcinol depends on its dosage (Hong et al. 2007). Ahmad and coworkers have disclosed that apoptosis induction by garcinol in cancer cells is supported by blocked NF-κB signalling leading to reduced activation of anti-apoptotic Bcl-2

(Ahmad et al. 2008, 2010). Suppression of TGF-activated kinase 1 (TAK1) and inhibitor of IκB kinase (IKK) by garcinol seems to play a role for NF-κB downregulation by garcinol (Ahmad et al. 2010; Li et al. 2013). In addition, garcinol is able to activate the death receptors DR4 and DR5 and, thus, to enhance apoptosis induced by TRAIL, a cytokine in advanced clinical trials, solely in malignant cells (Prasad et al. 2010). Suppression of anti-apoptotic proteins such as survivin, XIAP, and cFLIP was observed after garcinol treatment, while garcinol-mediated apoptosis induction or sensitisation to TRAIL could not be detected in nonmalignant cells, which underscores the tumour-selective character of garcinol once again.

Nicotine-induced breast cancer cell growth was blocked by garcinol via downregulation of the nicotinic acetylcholine receptor (α9-nAChR) and cyclin D3 proteins inducing cell cycle arrest and accumulation of garcinol-treated breast cancer cells in the G0/G1 phase (Chen et al. 2011). Recently, garcinol was reported to induce G1 cell cycle arrest by activation of $p21^{CIP1/WAF1}$ and suppression of p38-MAPK signalling in p53-independent H1299 lung carcinoma cells, while apoptosis was predominant in p53-wild-type H460 lung cancer cells (Yu et al. 2014). Levels of cyclin-dependent kinases such as CDK2 and CDK4 as well as cyclin D1 and cyclin D3 were decreased in garcinol-treated H1299 cells. Inhibition of p38 synergistically increased garcinol-mediated expression of p21. Isogarcinol (**15**) has caused selective S-phase arrest and apoptosis in medulloblastoma cells (Daoy MB cells) expressing platelet-derived growth factor receptors (PDGFR) via suppression of cyclin A and cyclin E and activation of caspases (Tian et al. 2011). The garcinol-related PPAPs xanthochymol and guttiferone E inhibit microtubule disassembly (IC_{50} values between 1.5 and 2 μM) comparable with the approved anticancer drug paclitaxel ($IC_{50} = 0.5$ μM) (Roux et al. 2000). Interestingly, like garcinol paclitaxel induces G1 arrest at very low doses rather than mitotic arrest in certain cancer cell lines (Giannakakou et al. 2001).

Aside from cell cycle inhibition and apoptosis induction in cancer cells, there is evidence of distinct anti-metastatic and anti-angiogenic activities of garcinol. Focal adhesion kinase (FAK) is a cytoplasmic tyrosine kinase involved in the transduction of integrin-mediated cell-matrix signalling pathways which are relevant for metastasis formation and cancer cell survival. Garcinol was able to suppress activation (tyrosine phosphorylation) of FAK in colon cancer cells followed by apoptosis and downregulation of Src, ERK, and Akt signalling needed for cell survival (Liao et al. 2005b). Ahmad and coworkers have described a reversal of the epithelial-to-mesenchymal transition (EMT) in aggressive MDA-MB-231 breast cancer cells treated with garcinol which was associated with an upregulation of the epithelial marker E-cadherin and suppression of mesenchymal markers vimentin, ZEB-1, and ZEB-2 (Ahmad et al. 2012b). In addition, expression of let-7 family microRNAs and miR-200 was observed after garcinol treatment. Hints at inhibition of Wnt signalling (reduced nuclear β-catenin levels) characteristic of cancer stem-like cells were also visible in the garcinol-treated breast cancer cells.

Due to the manifold anticancer targets of garcinol, sensitisation of cancer cells to other anticancer drugs is another feature of garcinol. Gupta and coworkers observed

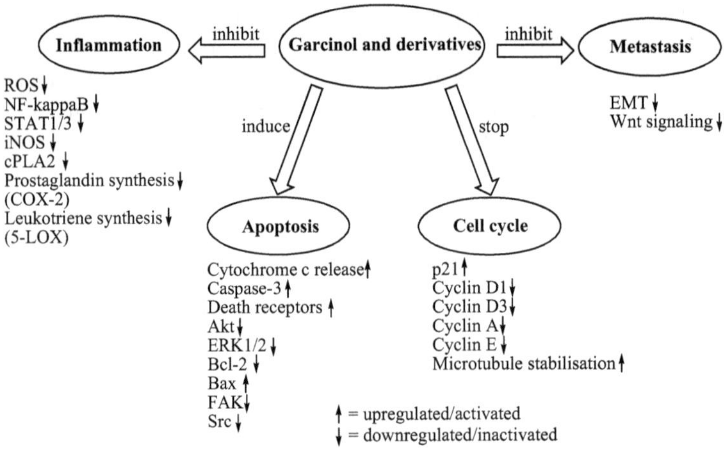

Fig. 10 Anticancer effects caused by garcinol

a synergistic effect of garcinol and curcumin in pancreatic cancer cells and the activity of the single agents was raised up to tenfold in the combination regimen (Parasramka and Gupta 2012). In this way, the active dose of the single agents could be reduced drastically. The same group has recently disclosed a garcinol-induced sensitisation of pancreatic cancer cells to the clinically applied drug gemcitabine which is used in first-line treatment of pancreatic cancer (Parasramka et al. 2013). Modulation of key regulators of pancreatic cancer cells was observed (PARP, VEGF, MMPs, ILs, caspases, NF-κB). In addition, expression of several microRNAs (miR-453, miR-638, miR21, miR-196a, and miR-605) was influenced by garcinol in the pancreatic cancer cells likely playing an important role in the anticancer effects of garcinol. Figure 10 gives an overview of the manifold anticancer-related effects of garcinol and its close derivatives.

4 Effects of Garcinol on Chromatin-Regulating Proteins

Together with histone deacetylases (HDACs), histone acetyl transferases (HATs) play a crucial role in the epigenetic control of cancer and other diseases (Roth et al. 2001; Oike et al. 2014). Histone acetylation is involved in chromatin remodelling leading to transcription of genes. However, acetylation and deacetylation are not restricted to histones, various non-histone proteins such as p53, tubulin, Hsp90, c-Myc, FOXO, and the androgen receptor can likewise be substrates of HDACs and HATs with consequences on function and stability of these non-histone substrates (Roth et al. 2001; Sterner and Berger 2000; Dal Piaz et al. 2011). Meanwhile, several PPAP-type HAT inhibitors have been identified including garcinol and its derivatives (Dal Piaz et al. 2011). Garcinol (**1**) and isogarcinol (**15**) inhibit various HATs such as p300-HAT (IC_{50} ca. 7 μM) and

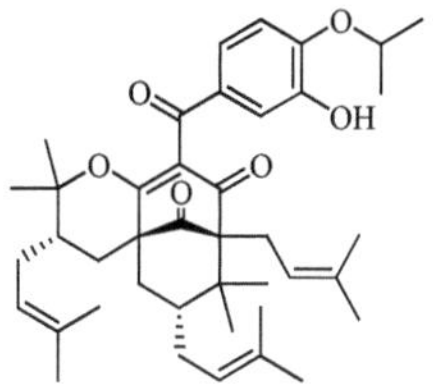

LTK-13 (41)

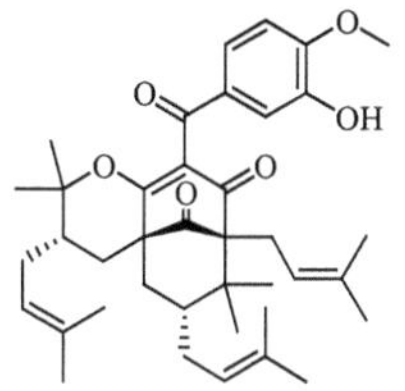

LTK-14 (42)

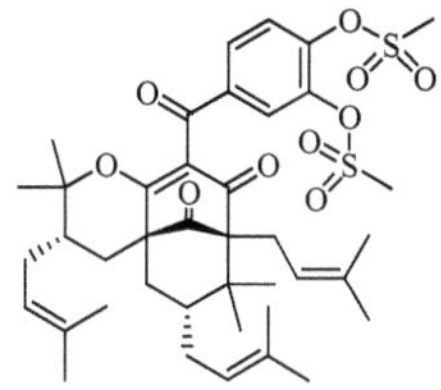

LTK-19 (43)

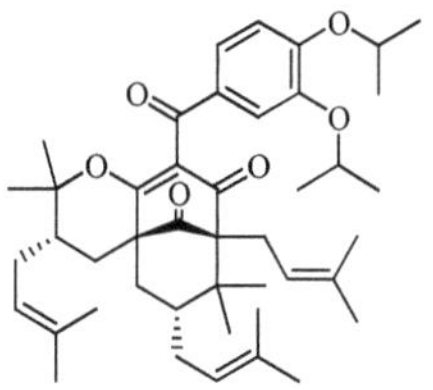

LTK-13A (44)

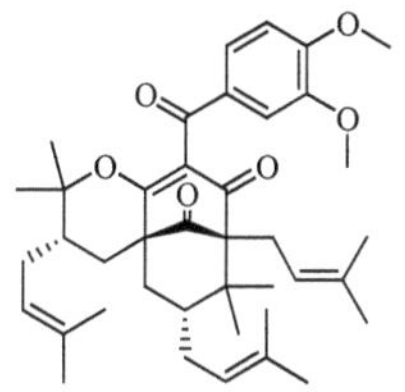

LTK-14A (45)

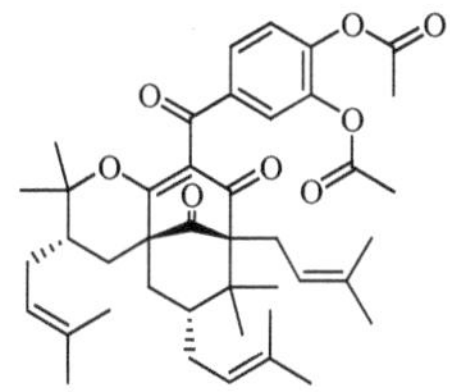

LTK-15 (46)

Fig. 11 Structures of the isogarcinol derivatives **41–46** prepared for HAT inhibition

PCAF (IC_{50} ca. 5 μM) both in vitro and in vivo leading to repression of chromatin transcription, changed global gene expression (mainly downregulation), and apoptosis induction in HeLa cancer cells (Balasubramaniam et al. 2004; Mantelingu et al. 2007). 4-*O*-Isopropyl (LTK-13, **41**) and 4-*O*-methyl (LTK-14, **42**) ethers of isogarcinol as well as the bis-methylsulfonate (LTK-19, **43**) of isogarcinol inhibited p300 specifically (IC_{50} between 5 and 7 μM) but remained nontoxic to cells in these experiments (Fig. 11) (Mantelingu et al. 2007). The corresponding bis-alkyl (LTK-13A, **44**; LTK-14A, **45**) and bis-acetyl (LTK-15, **46**) derivatives were inactive and lost HAT inhibitory activity completely. By the way, though the LTK series of compounds was prepared semi-synthetically from isogarcinol, LTK-14 (**42**) was also isolated from natural sources (*Garcinia assigu*) and exhibited distinct cancer chemopreventive activity (Ito et al. 2003).

LTK-14 (**42**) and garcinol (**1**) revealed growth inhibitory effects in MCF-7 breast cancer cells, in the case of garcinol by changes in histone and p53 acetylation (Collins et al. 2013). Garcinol reduced H3K18 acetylation in MCF-7 cells and two osteosarcoma cell lines U2OS and SaOS2, which is required for S-phase progression, and suppressed p300-dependent p53 acetylation at the C-terminal activation domain. In contrast, increases of H4K16 and trimethylated H4K20 were observed after garcinol treatment as well as p53K120 acetylation and accumulation of p53 in the cytoplasm. In addition, several DNA-damage signalling markers were more strongly upregulated in garcinol-treated cells than in curcumin-treated ones. Recently, garcinol was shown to reduce H3 acetylation and NF-κB/p65 acetylation induced by estradiol in hormone-sensitive MCF-7 breast cancer cells (Ye et al. 2014). Thus, translocation of NF-κB/p65 was blocked, and expression of cyclin D1, Bcl-2, and Bcl-xl was suppressed leading to G0/G1 cell cycle arrest of MCF-7 cells treated with garcinol. The garcinol-mediated inhibition of STAT-3 acetylation mentioned above is likely related to HAT inhibition as well (Sethi

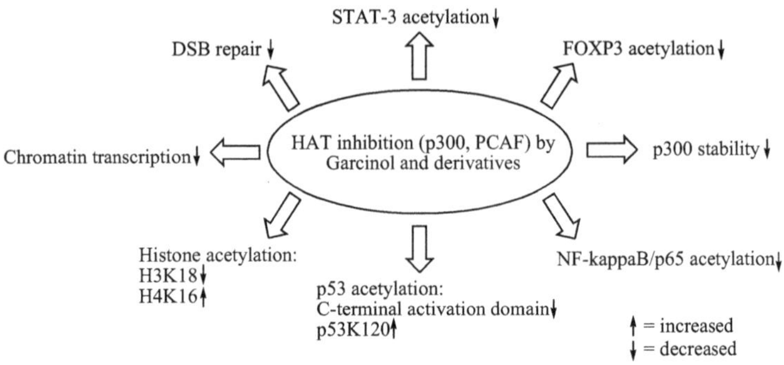

Fig. 12 Effects of garcinol-mediated HAT inhibition

et al. 2014). Garcinol is also involved in regulation of FOXP3 acetylation and stability by induction of p300 degradation (Du et al. 2013). Garcinol leads to dissociation of p300 from FOXP3 followed by reduced acetylation of FOXP3. Subsequent FOXP3 degradation cannot be prevented by the proteasome inhibitor MG132. Suppression of regulatory T cells by garcinol finally enhanced HER2-targeted tumour therapy in vivo. Garcinol is also able to radiosensitise tumour cells via inhibition of DNA repair (Oike et al. 2012). Suppression of double-strand break (DSB) repair including nonhomologous end joining (NHEJ) and radiosensitisation of A549 lung and HeLa cervical cancer cells was observed after garcinol treatment. Since functional DSB repair requires chromatin-remodelling at damaged sites, it is assumed that HAT inhibitory activity of garcinol plays a crucial role in silencing DSB repair. An overview of garcinol effects via HAT inhibition is given in Fig. 12.

5 Anti-ulcer Activity of Garcinol

Gastritis or stomach ulcer is caused by stress, drugs, and bacterial infections (*Helicobacter pylori*) and features itself the main cause of gastric cancer. Thus, garcinol (**1**) is able to suppress gastric cancer via its anti-ulcer activity. On the one hand, the anti-ulcer activity of garcinol can be explained by the radical-scavenging and anti-inflammatory properties of garcinol, in particular in case of indomethacin-induced acute ulceration (see above) (Yamaguchi et al. 2000). On the other hand, garcinol is likewise an efficient killer of the peptic ulcer-causing *Helicobacter pylori* bacteria. Garcinol inhibits *H. pylori* both time and dose dependently (Chatterjee et al. 2003, 2005). Garcinol was much more potent in *H. pylori* than other antioxidants, such as resveratrol and vitamin E, and reached or exceeded the antibiotic activity of the approved drug clarithromycin. Thus, garcinol or dried kokum plums are valuable means for the treatment of peptic ulcers.

By the way, the potent antibacterial effect of garcinol is not surprising since it has also displayed distinct activity in methicillin-resistant *Staphylococcus aureus* (MRSA) strains (Rukachaisirikul et al. 2005).

6 Conclusions

The polyisoprenylated benzophenone garcinol (**1**) and its derivatives revealed significant selective anticancer activity based on various antioxidant, anti-inflammation, and chromatin regulating properties. Garcinol reduces ROS and NO levels and prevents carcinogenesis efficiently. Inflammation-related cancer progression involving NF-κB signalling, prostaglandin synthesis, or STAT pathways, for instance, is suppressed either by direct binding or by indirect influences via HAT inhibition. Caspase-induced apoptosis and cell cycle arrest in G0/G1 and S phases have been discovered as garcinol-based modes of action in cancer cells, as well as sensitisation of cancer cells to approved drugs and therapies. Due to its antibacterial properties, garcinol also prevents peptic ulcer caused by *H. pylori* more efficiently than other antioxidants leading to reduced gastric cancer risk. High tumour selectivity combined with low side effects makes garcinol a valuable and easily available alternative or supplement to currently approved anticancer therapies.

References

Ahmad A, Banerjee S, Wang Z, Kong D, Sarkar FH (2008) Plumbagin-induced apoptosis of human breast cancer cells is mediated by inactivation of NF-kappaB and Bcl-2. J Cell Biochem 105:1461–1471

Ahmad A, Wang Z, Ali R, Maitah MY, Kong D, Banerjee S, Padhye S, Sarkar FH (2010) Apoptosis-inducing effect of garcinol is mediated by NF-kB signalling in breast cancer. J Cell Biochem 109:1134–1141

Ahmad A, Wang Z, Wojewoda C, Ali R, Kong D, Maitah MY, Banerjee S, Bao B, Padhye S, Sarkar FH (2011) Garcinol-induced apoptosis in prostate and pancreatic cancer cells is mediated by NF-κB signaling. Front Biosci 3:1483–1492

Ahmad A, Sarkar SH, Aboukameel A, Ali S, Biersack B, Seibt S, Li Y, Bao B, Kong D, Banerjee S, Schobert R, Padhye SB, Sarkar FH (2012a) Anticancer action of garcinol in vitro and in vivo is in part mediated through inhibition of STAT-3 signaling. Carcinogenesis 33:2450–2456

Ahmad A, Sarkar SH, Bitar B, Ali S, Aboukameel A, Sethi S, Li Y, Bao B, Kong D, Banerjee S, Padhye SB, Sarkar FH (2012b) Garcinol regulates EMT and Wnt signaling pathways in vitro and in vivo, leading to anticancer activity against breast cancer cells. Mol Cancer Ther 11:2193–2201

Balasubramaniam K, Altaf M, Varier RA, Swaminathan V, Ravindran A, Sadhale PP, Kundu TK (2004) Polyisoprenylated benzophenone, garcinol, a natural histone acetyltransferase inhibitor, represses chromatin transcription and alters global gene expression. J Biol Chem 279:33716–33726

Biber N, Möws K, Plietker B (2011) The total synthesis of hyperpapuanone, hyperibone L, epi-clusianone and oblongifolin A. Nat Chem 3:938–942

Bill MA, Nicholas C, Mace TA, Etter JP, Li C, Schwartz EB, Fuchs JR, Young GS, Lin L, Lin J, He L, Phelps M, Li P-K, Lesinski GB (2012) Structurally modified curcumin analogs inhibit STAT3 phosphorylation and promote apoptosis of human renal cell carcinoma and melanoma cell lines. PLoS One 7:e40724

Bollrath J, Greten FR (2009) IKK/NF-kappaB and STAT3 pathways: central signalling hubs in inflammation-mediated tumour progression and metastasis. EMBO Rep 10:1314–1319

Boyce JH, Porco JA Jr (2014) Asymmetric, stereodivergent synthesis of (-)-clusianone utilizing a biomimetic cationic cyclization. Angew Chem 126:7966–7971

Chatterjee A, Yaasmin T, Bagchi D, Stohs SJ (2003) The bactericidal effects of *Lactobacillus acidophilus*, garcinol and Protykin® compared to clarithromycin, on *Helicobacter pylori*. Mol Cell Biochem 243:29–35

Chatterjee A, Bagchi D, Yasmin T, Stohs SJ (2005) Antimicrobial effects of antioxidants with and without clarithromycin on *Helicobacter pylori*. Mol Cell Biochem 270:125–130

Chen C-S, Lee C-H, Hsieh C-D, Ho C-T, Pan M-H, Huang C-S, Tu S-H, Wang Y-J, Chen L-C, Chang Y-J, Wei P-L, Yang Y-Y, Wu C-H, Ho Y-S (2011) Nicotine-induced human breast cancer cell proliferation attenuated by garcinol through down-regulation of the nicotinic receptor and cyclin D3 proteins. Breast Cancer Res Treat 125:73–87

Cheng A-C, Tsai M-L, Liu C-M, Lee M-F, Nagabhushanam K, Ho C-T, Pan M-H (2010) Garcinol inhibits cell growth in hepatocellular carcinoma Hep3B cells through induction of ROS-dependent apoptosis. Food Funct 1:301–307

Ciochina R, Grossman RB (2006) Polycyclic polyprenylated acylphloroglucinols. Chem Rev 106:3963–3986

Collins HM, Abdelghany MK, Messmer M, Yue B, Deeves SE, Kindle KB, Mantelingu K, Aslam A, Winkler GS, Kundu TK, Heery DM (2013) Differential effects of carcinol and curcumin on histone and p53 modifications in tumour cells. BMC Cancer 13:37

Dal Piaz F, Vassallo A, Rubio OC, Castellano S, Sbardella G, De Tommasi N (2011) Chemical biology of histone acetyltransferase natural compounds modulators. Mol Divers 15:401–416

Davenport J, Balch M, Galam L, Girgis A, Hall J, Blagg BSJ, Matts RL (2014) High-throughput screen of natural product libraries for Hsp90 inhibitors. Biology 3:101–138

Du T, Nagai Y, Ciao Y, Greene MI, Zhang H (2013) Lysosome-dependent p300/FOXP3 degradation and limits T_{reg} cell functions and enhances targeted therapy against cancers. Exp Mol Pathol 95:38–45

Flavin DF (2007) A lipoxygenase inhibitor in breast cancer brain metastases. J Neurooncol 82:91–93

Fu Y, Zhou H, Wang M, Cen J, Wei Q (2014) Immune regulation and anti-inflammatory effects of isogarcinol extracted from *Garcinia mangostana* L. against collagen-induced arthritis. J Agric Food Chem 62:4127–4134

Giannakakou P, Robey R, Fojo T, Blagosklonny MV (2001) Low concentrations of paclitaxel induce cell type-dependent p53, p21 and G1/G2 arrest instead of mitotic arrest: molecular determinants of paclitaxel-induced cytotoxicity. Oncogene 20:3806–3813

Grenning AJ, Boyce JH, Porco JA Jr (2014) Rapid synthesis of polyprenylated acylphloroglucinol analogs via dearomative conjunctive allylic annulation. J Am Chem Soc 136:11799–11804

Grivennikov SI, Karin M (2010) Dangerous liaisons: STAT3 and NF-kappaB collaboration and crosstalk in cancer. Cytokine Growth Factor Rev 21:11–19

Hemshekhar M, Sunitha K, Santhosh MS, Devaraja S, Kemparaju K, Vishwanath BS, Niranjana SR, Girish KS (2011) An overview on genus *Garcinia*: phytochemical and therapeutical aspects. Phytochem Rev 10:325–351

Hong J, Sang S, Park HJ, Kwon SJ, Suh N, Huang MT, Ho CT, Yang CS (2006) Modulation of arachidonic acid metabolism and nitric oxide synthesis by garcinol and its derivatives. Carcinogenesis 27:278–286

Hong J, Kwon SJ, Sang S, Ju J, Zhou J-N, Ho C-T, Huang M-T, Yang CS (2007) Effects of garcinol and its derivatives on intestinal cell growth: inhibitory effects and autoxidation-dependent growth-stimulatory effects. Free Radic Biol Med 42:1211–1221

Horeischi F, Biber N, Plietker B (2014) The total synthesis of guttiferone A and 6-epi-guttiferone A. J Am Chem Soc 136:4026–4030

Ito C, Itoigawa M, Miyamoto Y, Onoda S, Rao KS, Mukainaka T, Tokuda H, Nishino H, Furukawa H (2003) Polyprenylated benzophenones from *Garcinia assigu* and their potential cancer chemopreventive activities. J Nat Prod 66:206–209

Ito H, Duxburry M, Benoit E, Clancy TE, Zinner MJ, Ashley SW, Whang EE (2004) Prostaglandin E2 enhances pancreatic cancer invasiveness through an Ets-1-dependent induction of matrix metalloproteinase-2. Cancer Res 64:7439–7446

Koeberle A, Northoff H, Werz O (2009) Identification of 5-lipoxygenase and microsomal prostaglandin E2 synthase-1 as functional targets of the anti-inflammatory and anti-carcinogenic garcinol. Biochem Pharmacol 77:1513–1521

Kuramochi A, Usada H, Yamatsugu K, Kanai M, Shibasaki M (2005) Total synthesis of (+/−)-garsubellin A. J Am Chem Soc 127:14200–14201

Li F, Shanmugam MK, Chen L, Chatterjee S, Basha J, Kumar AP, Kundu TK, Sethi G (2013) Garcinol, a polyisoprenylated benzophenone modulates multiple proinflammatory signalling cascades leading to the suppression of growth and survival of head and neck carcinoma. Cancer Prev Res 6:843–854

Liao C-H, Sang S, Liang Y-C, Ho C-T, Lin J-K (2004) Suppression of inducible nitric oxide synthase and cyclooxygenase-2 in downregulating nuclear factor-kappa B pathway by garcinol. Mol Carcinog 41:140–149

Liao CH, Ho CT, Lin JK (2005a) Effects of garcinol on free radical generation and NO production in embryonic rat cortical neurons and astrocytes. Biochem Biophys Res Commun 329:1306–1314

Liao C-H, Sang S, Ho C-T, Lin J-K (2005b) Garcinol modulates tyrosine phosphorylation of FAK and subsequently induces apoptosis through down-regulation of Src, ERK, and Akt survival signalling in human colon cancer cells. J Cell Biochem 96:155–169

Lin L, Liu Y, Li P-K, Fuchs J, Shibata H, Iwabuchi Y, Lin J (2011) Targeting colon cancer stem cells using a new curcumin analogue, GO-Y030. Br J Cancer 105:212–220

Locksley HD, Moore I, Scheinmann F (1967) Extractives from guttiferae-VI. The significance of maclurin in xanthone biosynthesis. Tetrahedron 23:2229–2234

Mantelingu K, Reddy BAA, Swaminathan V, Kishore AH, Siddappa NB, Kumar GVP, Nagashankar G, Natesh N, Roy S, Sadhale PP, Ranga U, Narayana C, Kundu TK (2007) Specific inhibition of p300-HAT alters global gene expression and represses HIV replication. Chem Biol 14:645–657

Masullo M, Menegazzi M, Di Micco S, Beffy P, Bifulco G, Dal Bosco M, Novelli M, Pizza C, Masiello P, Piacente S (2014) Direct interaction of garcinol and related polyisoprenylated benzophenones of *Garcinia cambogia* fruits with the transcription factor STAT-1 as a likely mechanism of their inhibitory effect on cytokine signaling pathways. J Nat Prod 77:543–549

Nuhant P, David M, Pouplin T, Delpech B, Marazano C (2007) α, α'-Annulation of 2,6-prenyl-substituted cyclohexanone derivatives with malonyl chloride: application to a short synthesis of (+/−)-clusianone. Formation and rearrangement of a biogenetic-like intermediate. Org Lett 9:287–289

Oike T, Ogiwara H, Torikai K, Nakano T, Yokota J, Kohno T (2012) Garcinol, a histone acetyltransferase inhibitor, radiosensitizes cancer cells by inhibiting non-homologous end joining. Int J Radiat Oncol Biol Phys 84:815–821

Oike T, Ogiwara H, Amornwichet N, Nakano T, Kohno T (2014) Chromatin-regulating proteins as targets for cancer therapy. J Radiat Res 55:613–628

Padhye S, Ahmad A, Oswal N, Sarkar FH (2009) Emerging role of garcinol, the antioxidant chalcone from *Garcinia indica* Choisy and its synthetic analogs. J Hematol Oncol 2:38

Pan M-H, Chang W-L, Lin-Shiau S-Y, Ho C-T, Lin J-K (2001) Induction of apoptosis by garcinol and curcumin through cytochrome c release and activation of caspases in human leukemia cells. J Agric Food Chem 49:1464–1474
Parasramka MA, Gupta SV (2012) Synergistic effect of garcinol and curcumin on antiproliferative and apoptotic activity in pancreatic cancer cells. J Oncol 2012:709739
Parasramka MA, Ali S, Banerjee S, Deryavoush T, Sarkar FH, Gupta SV (2013) Garcinol sensitizes human pancreatic adenocarcinoma cells to gemcitabine in association with microRNA signatures. Mol Nutr Food Res 57:235–248
Prasad S, Ravindran J, Sung B, Pandey MK, Aggarwal BB (2010) Garcinol potentiates TRAIL-induced apoptosis through modulation of death receptors and antiapoptotic proteins. Mol Cancer Ther 9:856–868
Rao AVR, Venkatswamy G, Pendse AD (1980) Camboginol and cambogin. Tetrahedron Lett 21:1975–1978
Rodeschini V, Ahmad NM, Simpkins NS (2006) Synthesis of (+/−)-clusianone: high yielding bridgehead and diketone substitutions by regioselective lithiation of enol ether derivatives of bicyclo[3.3.1]nonane-2,4,9-triones. Org Lett 8:5283–5285
Roth SY, Denu JM, Allis CD (2001) Histone acetyltransferases. Annu Rev Biochem 70:81–120
Roux D, Hadi HA, Thoret S, Guénard D, Thoison O, Pais M, Sévenet T (2000) Structure-activity relationship of polyisoprenyl benzophenones from *Garcinia pyrifera* on the tubulin/microtubule system. J Nat Prod 63:1070–1076
Rukachaisirikul V, Naklue W, Sukpondma Y, Phongpaichit S (2005) An antibacterial biphenyl derivative from *Garcinia bancana* MIQ. Chem Pharm Bull 53:342–343
Saadat N, Gupta SV (2012) Potential role of garcinol as an anticancer agent. J Oncol 2012:647206
Sang S, Pan M-H, Cheng X, Bai N, Stark RE, Rosen RT, Lin-Shiau S-Y, Lin J-K, Ho CT (2001) Chemical studies on antioxidant mechanism of garcinol: analysis of radical reaction products of garcinol and their antitumor activities. Tetrahedron 57:9931–9938
Sang S, Liao C-H, Pan M-H, Rosen RT, Lin-Shiau S-Y, Lin J-K, Ho C-T (2002) Chemical studies on antioxidant mechanism of garcinol: analysis of radical reaction products of garcinol with peroxyl radicals and their antitumor activities. Tetrahedron 58:10095–10102
Schönwälder K-H, Kollat P, Stezowski JJ, Effenberger F (1984) Synthese und Struktur von [n](2.4)Phloroglucinophanen. Chem Ber 117:3280–3296
Sethi G, Chatterjee S, Rajendran P, Li F, Shanmugam MK, Wong KF, Kumar AP, Senapati P, Behera AK, Hui KM, Basha J, Natesh N, Luk JM, Kundu TK (2014) Inhibition of STAT3 dimerisation and acetylation by garcinol suppresses the growth of human hepatocellular carcinoma in vitro and in vivo. Mol Cancer 13:66
Siegel DR, Danishefsky SJ (2006) Total synthesis of garsubellin A. J Am Chem Soc 128:1048–1049
Sterner DE, Berger SL (2000) Acetylation of histones and transcription-related factors. Microbiol Mol Biol Rev 64:435–459
Tanaka T, Kohno H, Shimada R, Kagami S, Yamaguchi F, Kataoka S, Ariga T, Murakami A, Koshimizu K, Ohigashi H (2000) Prevention of colonic aberrant crypt foci by dietary feeding of garcinol in male F344 rats. Carcinogenesis 21:1183–1189
Tian Z, Shen J, Wang F, Xiao P, Yang J, Lei H, Kazlauskas A, Kohane IS, Wi E (2011) Cambogin is preferentially cytotoxic to cells expressing PDGFR. PLoS One 6:e21370
Tsai M-L, Chiou Y-S, Ho C-T, Pan M-H (2014) Garcinol suppresses inflammation-associated colon carcinogenesis in mice. Mol Nutr Food Res 58:1820–1829
Tsukano C, Siegel DR, Danishefsky SJ (2007) Differentiation of nonconventional "carbanions"—the total synthesis of nemorosone and clusianone. Angew Chem 119:8996–9000
Xin C, Zhang X, Lu Y, Shim J-Y, Sang S, Sun Z, Chen X (2012) Chemoprevention of 7,12-dimethylbenz[a]anthracene (DMBA)-induced hamster cheek pouch carcinogenesis by a 5-lipoxygenase inhibitor, garcinol. Nutr Cancer 64:1211–1218
Yamaguchi F, Saito M, Ariga T, Yoshimura Y, Nakazawa H (2000) Free radical scavenging activity and antiulcer activity of garcinol from fruit rind. J Agric Food Chem 48:2320–2325

Ye X, Yuan L, Zhang L, Zhao J, Zhang C-M, Deng H-Y (2014) Garcinol, an acetyltransferase inhibitor, suppresses proliferation of breast cancer cell line MCF-7 promoted by 17β-estradiol. Asian Pac J Cancer Prev 15:5001–5007

Yoshida K, Tanaka T, Hirose Y, Yamaguchi F, Kohno H, Toida M, Hara A, Sugie S, Shibata T, Mori H (2005) Dietary garcinol inhibits 4-nitroquinoline 1-oxide-induced tongue carcinogenesis in rats. Cancer Lett 221:29–39

Yu S-Y, Liao C-H, Chien M-H, Tsai T-Y, Lin J-K, Weng M-S (2014) Induction of $p21^{Waf1/Cip1}$ by garcinol via downregulation of p38-MAPK signaling in p53-independent H1299 lung cancer. J Agric Food Chem 62:2085–2095

Zhao F, Watanabe Y, Nozawa H, Daikonnya A, Kondo K, Kitanaka S (2005) Prenylflavonoids and phloroglucinol derivatives from hops (*Humulus lupulus*). J Nat Prod 68:43–49

Modulation of Key Signaling Pathways in Cancer Cells by Dietary Factors

Amrah Ali and Aamir Ahmad

Abstract The World Health Organization has predicted new cancer rates to increase by 70 % within the next two decades. With rates expected to continue increasing in cancer incidence and mortality, chemoprevention and early diagnosis are the keys to decreasing cancer mortality. Chemoprevention is the use of natural or synthetic agents to inhibit, reverse, or prevent carcinogenesis. Studies have suggested there is a significant difference in cancer incidence among population groups with different lifestyle factors, especially diet. Phytochemicals or "nutraceuticals," the substances present in fruits, vegetables, and plants, have beneficial effects targeting multiple key signaling molecules and perturbing the carcinogenesis process. Studies have demonstrated curcumin, resveratrol, 3,3-′-diindolylmethane (DIM), and many others to hold inhibitory effects on cancer cells. There is overwhelming evidence that these nutraceuticals modulate key signaling pathways including cell cycle signaling and p53, transcription and inflammatory mediators such as NF-κB and PI3K/Akt/mTOR, and angiogenic pathways in cancer cells. Through regulation of cell signaling pathways, these dietary factors can induce cell arrest and apoptosis, and suppress proliferation and inflammation, resulting in inhibition of carcinogenesis. In this chapter, we review the effects of these nutraceuticals on some of the key signaling cellular and molecular pathways and highlight their roles as chemopreventive agents.

1 Introduction

Cancer is responsible for one of every four deaths in the United States (http://www.cdc.gov/cancer/dcpc/data/types.htm 2014) and is a leading cause of death globally causing 8.2 million deaths in 2012 (http://www.who.int/mediacentre/factsheets/fs297/en/2014). Annual cancer rates are predicted to increase to 22 million within

A. Ali
Department of Pathology, Karmanos Cancer Institute, Wayne State University School of Medicine, 707 HWCRC Bldg, 4100 John R. Street, Detroit, MI 48201, USA

A. Ahmad, Ph.D. (✉)
Department of Pathology, Karmanos Cancer Institute, Wayne State University-740 HWCRC, Detroit, Michigan, USA
e-mail: ahmada@karmanos.org

M.F. Ullah, A. Ahmad (eds.), *Critical Dietary Factors in Cancer Chemoprevention*,
DOI 10.1007/978-3-319-21461-0_13

the next two decades from 14 million in 2012, with new cancer rates growing by about 70 % according to the World Health Organization (http://www.who.int/mediacentre/factsheets/fs297/en/2014). Carcinogenesis is the process by which normal cells turn into cancer cells. Through an interplay of different factors extrinsically (such as diet, radiation exposure, chemicals, viruses) and intrinsically (cellular mutations, hormones), cells undergo several mutations which can result in uncontrolled cell growth.

With the growing numbers in cancer incidence and mortality, there is a strong interest in cancer chemoprevention and early diagnosis. Chemoprevention is the use of agents to inhibit, reverse, or prevent carcinogenesis (Bilecova-Rabajdova et al. 2013). Key molecular signaling events responsible for cancer initiation and progression are being targeted in the development of chemopreventive therapeutics (Kangwan et al. 2014). In particular, dietary derived chemopreventive agents with multi-targeted molecular effects on the carcinogenic process have been an area of great focus (Ahmad et al. 2013a, b, c, 2015; Steward and Brown 2013).

Cancer has been associated to certain lifestyle habits such as a low fruit and vegetable diet, alcohol use, low physical activity, tobacco use, and high body mass index. According to the WHO, approximately 30 % of cancer deaths could be prevented by modifying these lifestyle factors (http://www.who.int/mediacentre/factsheets/fs297/en/2014). Diet and its association with cancer has been increasingly receiving attention with studies, for example, that suggest a Mediterranean diet, rich in fruits and vegetables, showed a significant decreased risk in cancer (La 2009). Fruits, vegetables, grains, and legumes have important nutrients and other cancer-fighting phytochemicals. Phytochemicals are nonessential nutrients that are found in plants. They can be classified into phytoestrogens, polyphenols, sulfur-containing compounds, and other categories based on their chemical structure and effects (Bilecova-Rabajdova et al. 2013). Phytochemicals with chemopreventive abilities have different mechanisms of actions targeting several key cell signaling pathways to inhibit cell proliferation, tumor vascularization and inflammation, and modulate cell growth and survival (Bilecova-Rabajdova et al. 2013).

2 Nutraceuticals in Cancer Research

A number of nutraceuticals are under investigation in laboratories worldwide for their putative anticancer properties, and it will be beyond this chapter's scope to comment on most of them. To keep this chapter focused, we will discuss the three promising nutraceuticals—curcumin, resveratrol, and 3,3′-Diindolylmethane (DIM) and their reported beneficial effects against multiple human cancers.

2.1 Curcumin

Curcumin is a polyphenolic phytochemical found in the rhizomes of the turmeric plant (*Curcuma longa*) (Jiang et al. 2014). Turmeric is a spice commonly used in

Southeast Asia and also used as a yellow food coloring agent. Studies suggest that the increased intake of curcumin contributes to decreased risk of cancer in Southeast Asian populations compared to industrialized western nations (Parasramka and Gupta 2012). Curcumin has been shown to have anti-inflammatory and antitumor properties including inducing apoptosis, inhibiting angiogenesis and inhibiting cell proliferation in cancer cells (Jiang et al. 2014).

2.1.1 Cell Cycle

Progression through the cell cycle and proliferation are tightly controlled in normal cells. Curcumin regulates cell cycle signaling molecules, including cyclins, cyclin dependent kinases (CDK), and CDK inhibitors to induce cycle arrest, apoptosis, or inhibit proliferation (Liu et al. 2007; Choudhuri et al. 2005; Wilken et al. 2011; Cao et al. 2014). Curcumin treatment of human gastric carcinoma cells resulted in G2/M arrest, upregulation of cyclin B1, and a decreased expression of cyclin D1 (Choudhuri et al. 2005; Cao et al. 2014). The tumor suppressor gene, p53, is a critical checkpoint in cell cycle regulation and apoptosis, thus playing a protective role against tumorigenesis. Several studies have shown curcumin to induce apoptosis by the overexpression of p53 in various cancer cells (Jiang et al. 2014; Liu et al. 2007; Choudhuri et al. 2005; Wilken et al. 2011). Curcumin has also been shown to induce apoptosis by stimulation of the mitochondrial apoptotic pathway via downregulation of anti-apoptotic protein Bcl-2, increased Bax expression and cytochrome c release (Jiang et al. 2014; Choudhuri et al. 2005; Wilken et al. 2011), as well as its effects on the extrinsic apoptotic pathway by increasing activation of caspase-8 and caspase-3 (Jiang et al. 2014; Bush et al. 2001).

2.1.2 Transcription Factors and Inflammation

Curcumin also exerts anti-tumorigenic and anti-inflammatory properties through its effect on different transcription factors. It is known to suppress NF-κB (nuclear factor-kappaB), AP-1 (activator protein), STAT (Signal Transducer and Activator of Transcription) proteins, but also activate others including ATF3 (activating transcription factor), PPAR-γ (Peroxisome proliferator-activated receptor gamma), and Nrf2, the transcription factor that regulates the antioxidant response (Zhou et al. 2011). Unlike normal, healthy cells, NF-κB and STAT3 are found to be constitutively activated in many types of cancers (Wilken et al. 2011; Zhou et al. 2011; Orr et al. 2013; Shakibaei et al. 2013; Ravindran et al. 2009). NF-κB regulates DNA transcription involving cell survival and proliferation. Curcumin has been known to suppress the activation of NF-κB and its gene products such as cyclin D1, COX-2, MMP-9, and Bcl-2, consequently inhibiting tumor cell proliferation, inflammation, metastasis and promoting apoptosis, respectively (Jiang et al. 2014; Zhou et al. 2011; Orr et al. 2013; Shakibaei et al. 2013). Studies suggest that curcumin inhibits NF-κB via suppression of IκBα phosphorylation and degradation (Zhou et al. 2011; Orr et al. 2013; Shakibaei et al. 2013). Thus, NF-κB remains sequestered in the cytoplasm, inactive and unable to bind to the promoter of target genes. Similar to NF-κB, STAT3, a pro-inflammatory transcription factor, is involved in cell proliferation, survival, tumor invasion, and angiogenesis. Many studies have demonstrated the potent inhibitory effects of curcumin on the activation of STAT3 (Orr et al. 2013; Ravindran et al. 2009).

2.1.3 PI3K/Akt/mTOR Pathway

Activation of cell surface receptors like insulin receptor, EGFR, and others stimulates the enzyme phosphatidylinositol-3-kinase (PI3K) (Beevers et al. 2013). PI3K phosphorylates and activates the serine/threonine protein kinase Akt associating it to the plasma membrane. mTOR (mammalian target of rapamycin), a key downstream target of Akt, is a critical regulator of cell growth, proliferation, and survival. The PI3K/Akt/mTOR intracellular signaling pathway are dysregulated in many cancers (Zhou et al. 2011; Ravindran et al. 2009). PI3K/Akt activation leads to cell proliferation and survival with mTOR signaling playing a crucial role in tumorigenesis. mTOR functions as two signaling complexes, mTORC1 and mTORC2. Findings from studies have demonstrated that curcumin inhibits both mTORC1 and mTORC2 through a concentration-dependent manner (Beevers et al. 2013) and have also shown an inhibition of Akt phosphorylation in certain cancer cells (Zhou et al. 2011).

2.1.4 Angiogenesis

Angiogenesis, the stimulation of new blood vessel growth, is critical for tumor growth and metastasis. Angiogenesis is upregulated by a variety of signaling molecules including vascular endothelial growth factor (VEGF), fibroblast growth factor (FGF), and epidermal growth factor (EGF). Curcumin has demonstrated anti-angiogenic effects through inhibition of these pro-angiogenic growth factors (Cao et al. 2014; Zhou et al. 2011).

2.2 CDF

Despite the many beneficial anti-tumorigenic effects of curcumin on various signaling pathways, its therapeutic use is limited by its bioavailability and rapid metabolism. Curcumin is poorly absorbed and up to 75 % of it is excreted via fecal matter (Vyas et al. 2013). Research has focused on developing new synthetic curcumin analogs to increase curcumin's efficacy and tackle its shortcomings. One curcumin analog, difluorinated-curcumin (CDF), has emerged as a promising breakthrough for increasing bioavailability and tissue distribution (Vyas et al. 2013). CDF also demonstrates superior anticancer ability, as demonstrated in studies that suggest that CDF binds and inhibits COX-2 better than curcumin and suppresses expression of NF-κB at lower concentrations (Vyas et al. 2013). In addition to NF-κB and COX-2, CDF has shown to inhibit the Akt signaling pathway and increase expression of tumor-suppressive microRNAs (miRNA) (Bao et al. 2012). CDF is a comparatively new compound but extensive investigations in our laboratory do suggest a promising anticancer activity against multiple cancers (Vyas et al. 2013; Dandawate et al. 2012; Ali et al. 2010, 2012).

2.3 *Resveratrol*

Resveratrol, also a polyphenolic phytochemical, is an antioxidant found in several food and drink items such as red wine, grapes, berries, and nuts (Bilecova-Rabajdova et al. 2013; Bishayee 2009). The presence of resveratrol has emerged as a leading hypothesis to explain the lower incidence of cardiovascular disease in the French population, also known as the French paradox (Bishayee 2009; Kulkarni and Canto 2014). In addition to demonstrating cardiovascular health benefits, resveratrol has shown to hold many anti-tumorigenic properties mediated through several cell signaling pathways. Studies have shown resveratrol to inhibit inflammation, proliferation, angiogenesis, and metastasis, induce apoptosis, and regulate cell growth (Bishayee 2009; Kulkarni and Canto 2014; Athar et al. 2009).

2.3.1 Cell Cycle

Resveratrol has been found to modulate many cell cycle signaling factors resulting in cell cycle arrest or apoptosis. Resveratrol upregulates the CDK inhibitor p21 and downregulates cyclin D1 causing G1/S cell cycle arrest (Khan et al. 2014a; Liu et al. 2014). It has also been shown to increase the expression of the apoptosis-associated proteins caspase-7, caspase-9, and cleaved PARP (Liu et al. 2014). Similar to curcumin, resveratrol upregulates p53 expression and activity, inducing apoptosis (Athar et al. 2009; Khan et al. 2014a). It also increases expression of pro-apoptotic factors such as Bax, induces cytochrome c release, and downregulates anti-apoptotic factors like Bcl-2 and directly stimulates the mitochondrial apoptotic pathway (Bishayee 2009; Athar et al. 2009; Khan et al. 2014a).

2.3.2 Transcription Factors and Inflammation

In 1997, a study by the Pezzuto lab generated interest in resveratrol as a chemopreventive agent. They demonstrated the chemopreventive effects of resveratrol on mice skin via COX inhibition (Kulkarni and Canto 2014). COX catalyzes the formation of prostaglandins from arachidonic acid. Prostaglandins act as pro-inflammatory agents and are crucial for immune function and even carcinogenesis by stimulating cell proliferation (Athar et al. 2009). COX-2 is found to be highly expressed in premalignant and malignant cancerous conditions. Studies have shown resveratrol to inhibit COX-2 activity directly (Kulkarni and Canto 2014; Athar et al. 2009) and indirectly, such as by downregulating MAPK, AP-1, and NF-κB pathways (Athar et al. 2009), reducing inflammation and tumorigenesis.

Many studies have demonstrated the inhibition of resveratrol on NF-κB activity, but the mechanism through which this inhibition may occur is still unclear (Kulkarni and Canto 2014). Recent studies suggest resveratrol blocks the phosphorylation and degradation of IκBα, thus inhibiting the nuclear translocation and activation of NF-κB (Hsieh and Wu 2010; Kang et al. 2009). Resveratrol decreases IκB phosphorylation induced by pro-inflammatory stimuli, such as tumor necrosis factor α (TNF-α) and lipopolysaccharide (LPS) (Kulkarni and Canto 2014; Athar et al. 2009). It is suggested that TRAF6 (TNF receptor associated factor) plays a role in resveratrol blocking LPS-induced IκBα degradation. Resveratrol was also shown to inhibit LPS-induced TRAF6 expression in human mast cells (Jakus et al. 2013).

2.3.3 PI3K/Akt/mTOR Pathway

The chemopreventive activity of resveratrol is also attributed to its inhibition of PI3K/Akt/mTOR signaling (Kulkarni and Canto 2014; Khan et al. 2014a). Resveratrol directly binds and inhibits PI3K, suppresses PI3K downstream targets (Frojdo et al. 2007), downregulates Akt while also increasing the expression of PTEN, the inhibitor of PI3K and Akt (Khan et al. 2014a). This downregulation of PI3K/Akt results in suppression of cell growth (Khan et al. 2014a). Inactivation of Akt and its downstream targets was shown to result in ROS (reactive oxygen species) release causing apoptosis of diffuse large B cell lymphoma (DLBCL) cell lines (Hussain et al. 2011). Interestingly, our earlier work established a prooxidant action of resveratrol in the copper-enriched environment, leading to ROS generation and the anticancer activity (Ahmad et al. 2000, 2005; Hadi et al. 2000, 2010; Khan et al. 2014b).

As mentioned earlier, mTOR plays a crucial role in tumorigenesis, controlling cell growth, proliferation, metabolism, and angiogenesis (Kulkarni and Canto 2014). Studies suggest resveratrol stimulates AMPK which results in downregulation of mTOR activity (Kulkarni and Canto 2014; Liu et al. 2010). Another study shows that resveratrol inhibits mTOR signaling by promoting the association between mTOR and DEPTOR, an inhibitor of mTOR (Liu et al. 2010). Resveratrol has also been shown to increase the effect of mTOR inhibitor, rapamycin, on cell apoptosis and proliferation (Khan et al. 2014a).

2.4 3, 3′ Diindolylmethane

3,3′-Diindolylmethane (DIM) is a phytochemical and an active metabolite of indole 3-carbinol (I3C) (Tadi et al. 2005; Higdon et al. 2007). Indole-3-carbinol is hydrolyzed from glucosinolate glucobrassicin, a sulfur-containing phytochemical, found abundantly in cruciferous vegetables such as cabbage, cauliflower, broccoli, brussel sprouts, bok choy, turnips, and kale (Higdon et al. 2007). Many studies have shown a negative correlation between consumption of cruciferous vegetables and incidence of cancer in the prostate, breast, colon and lungs (Higdon et al. 2007; Bosetti et al. 2012). DIM has been intensely studied for its anticarcinogenic properties such as inducing apoptosis and cell cycle arrest and inhibiting inflammation, proliferation, and angiogenesis (Zhang et al. 2014).

2.4.1 Cell Cycle

DIM triggers G1/S cell cycle arrest through downregulation of cell cycle regulators like cyclin D1, cyclin E, cyclin B, CDK4, and CDK6, as well as upregulation of cell cycle inhibitors like p21 and p27, and activating p38 MAPK pathways (Zhang et al. 2014; Weng et al. 2012). Studies have also shown DIM to cause G2/M cell cycle arrest (Weng et al. 2012; Choi et al. 2009). DIM causes apoptosis by inducing p53 and other pro-apoptotic factors like Bax, cytochrome C, and caspases 9 and 3. DIM also suppresses anti-apoptotic factors such as Bcl-2, Bcl-xL and survivin (Zhang et al. 2014).

2.4.2 Transcription Factors and Inflammation

DIM exerts anti-inflammatory and chemopreventive effects through suppressing the NF-κB signaling pathway in cancer cells (Ahmad et al. 2013a; Weng et al. 2012; Maruthanila et al. 2014). DIM, or the formulated BR-DIM treatment, has been shown to inhibit NF-κB DNA-binding activity in prostate, breast, and pancreatic cancer cells (Weng et al. 2012; Ahmad et al. 2009a, b). Evidence suggests that DIM inhibits the translocation of NF-κB to the nucleus (Ahmad et al. 2013a; Maruthanila et al. 2014) by suppressing the expression of the RelA/p65 subunit of NF-κB and thus inhibiting RelA nuclear translocation activation (Weng et al. 2012). DIM also blocks the phosphorylation of IKBα, keeping NF-κB in an inactive state. This results in decreased expression of NF-κB downstream gene products such as Bcl-2, survivin, c-Myc, and COX-2, inhibiting cell growth and inducing apoptosis (Weng et al. 2012).

Inflammatory mediators COX-2 and iNOS were suppressed with DIM pretreatment, and their suppression was observed to be in part responsible for the inhibition of TPA (2-O-tetradecanoylphorbol-13-acetate)-induced tumor formation and inflammation in mouse skin (Kim et al. 2010).

2.4.3 PI3K/Akt/mTOR

DIM also inhibits cancer cell growth and induces apoptosis by its inhibition of PI3K and Akt signaling (Ahmad et al. 2013a; Banerjee et al. 2011). Studies have also demonstrated DIM to block invasion and angiogenesis of cancer cells by inhibiting mTOR and Akt (Ahmad et al. 2013a; Banerjee et al. 2011). Rapamycin, known suppressor of mTOR, has been shown to activate Akt through reverse feedback from a suppressed mTOR. In this regard, DIM, with its ability to suppress both, proves to be a superior therapeutic agent in malignant cells (Ahmad et al. 2013a; Banerjee et al. 2011). Furthermore, DIM was shown to suppress crosstalk between NF-κB and the PI3K/Akt/mTOR pathway in tumor cells. Inhibition of the crosstalk between Akt and NF-κB by DIM in oral squamous cell carcinoma cells was shown to trigger cell cycle arrest and apoptosis (Weng et al. 2012). The inhibitory effect of DIM on NF-κB-Akt crosstalk is also thought to increase chemo-sensitization of cancer cells to chemotherapeutic drugs (Ahmad et al. 2013a).

2.4.4 Angiogenesis

In addition to mTOR and Akt, DIM exhibits inhibitory activity on angiogenesis through other signaling pathways. DIM was found to inhibit neovascularization by inhibiting endothelial cell cycle progression. Results show high sensitivity of vascular endothelial cells, as compared to tumor cells, to DIM inhibition of cell cycle progression and growth (Chang et al. 2005). B-DIM was shown to inhibit VEGF in cancer cells by suppressing MMP-9 and uPA (urokinase plasminogen activator), via the inhibition of NF-κB DNA binding activity (Kong et al. 2007). VEGF, uPA, MMP-9, and IL-8 are downstream targets of NF-κB and modulate angiogenesis and metastasis. This resulted in the inhibition of angiogenesis and invasion of prostate cancer cells (Kong et al. 2007).

3 Conclusions

With the increasing rates in cancer incidence and mortality, focus is growing on developing cancer chemopreventive agents and methods to diagnose cancer early. There have been many encouraging developments in nutraceuticals stemming from naturally occurring substances found in our diet. Many studies have proven the potential and value of nutraceuticals as chemopreventive substances with their pleiotropic beneficial health effects, including antioxidant, anti-inflammatory, and other anti-tumorigenic properties. These effects are mediated by cell signaling pathways including p53, NF-κB, Akt, mTOR, and angiogenic pathways, through which chemopreventive agents activate apoptosis, inhibit proliferation, block metastasis, and induce cell cycle arrest.

Despite the chemoprotective benefits of healthy diets as suggested by studies, many challenges remain. Low bioavailability makes it difficult to ingest phytochemicals in adequate amounts for chemopreventive benefits. The complexities of the molecular pathways of these phytochemicals are still not clearly understood. More comprehensive in vivo and in vitro studies are needed to develop better treatment and prevention strategies. These findings have important implications for dietary agents as cancer therapeutics or as agents that can be used to improve chemotherapy efficacy through combination treatment.

References

Ahmad A, Farhan AS, Singh S, Hadi SM (2000) DNA breakage by resveratrol and Cu(II): reaction mechanism and bacteriophage inactivation. Cancer Lett 154:29–37

Ahmad A, Syed FA, Singh S, Hadi SM (2005) Prooxidant activity of resveratrol in the presence of copper ions: mutagenicity in plasmid DNA. Toxicol Lett 159:1–12

Ahmad A, Kong D, Wang Z, Sarkar SH, Banerjee S, Sarkar FH (2009a) Down-regulation of uPA and uPAR by 3,3′-diindolylmethane contributes to the inhibition of cell growth and migration of breast cancer cells. J Cell Biochem 108:916–925

Ahmad A, Kong D, Sarkar SH, Wang Z, Banerjee S, Sarkar FH (2009b) Inactivation of uPA and its receptor uPAR by 3,3′-diindolylmethane (DIM) leads to the inhibition of prostate cancer cell growth and migration. J Cell Biochem 107:516–527

Ahmad A, Biersack B, Li Y, Kong D, Bao B, Schobert R, Padhye SB, Sarkar FH (2013a) Targeted regulation of PI3K/Akt/mTOR/NF-kappaB signaling by indole compounds and their derivatives: mechanistic details and biological implications for cancer therapy. Anticancer Agents Med Chem 13:1002–1013

Ahmad A, Biersack B, Li Y, Kong D, Bao B, Schobert R, Padhye SB, Sarkar FH (2013b) Deregulation of PI3K/Akt/mTOR signaling pathways by isoflavones and its implication in cancer treatment. Anticancer Agents Med Chem 13:1014–1024

Ahmad A, Biersack B, Li Y, Bao B, Kong D, Ali S, Banerjee S, Sarkar FH (2013c) Perspectives on the role of isoflavones in prostate cancer. AAPS J 15:991–1000

Ahmad A, Ginnebaugh KR, Li Y, Padhye SB, Sarkar FH (2015) Molecular targets of naturopathy in cancer research: bridge to modern medicine. Nutrients 7:321–334

Ali S, Ahmad A, Banerjee S, Padhye S, Dominiak K, Schaffert JM, Wang Z, Philip PA, Sarkar FH (2010) Gemcitabine sensitivity can be induced in pancreatic cancer cells through modulation of miR-200 and miR-21 expression by curcumin or its analogue CDF. Cancer Res 70:3606–3617

Ali S, Ahmad A, Aboukameel A, Bao B, Padhye S, Philip PA, Sarkar FH (2012) Increased Ras GTPase activity is regulated by miRNAs that can be attenuated by CDF treatment in pancreatic cancer cells. Cancer Lett 319:173–181

Athar M, Back JH, Kopelovich L, Bickers DR, Kim AL (2009) Multiple molecular targets of resveratrol: anti-carcinogenic mechanisms. Arch Biochem Biophys 486:95–102

Banerjee S, Kong D, Wang Z, Bao B, Hillman GG, Sarkar FH (2011) Attenuation of multi-targeted proliferation-linked signaling by 3,3′-diindolylmethane (DIM): from bench to clinic. Mutat Res 728:47–66

Bao B, Ali S, Banerjee S, Wang Z, Logna F, Azmi AS, Kong D, Ahmad A, Li Y, Padhye S, Sarkar FH (2012) Curcumin analogue CDF inhibits pancreatic tumor growth by switching on suppressor microRNAs and attenuating EZH2 expression. Cancer Res 72:335–345

Beevers CS, Zhou H, Huang S (2013) Hitting the golden TORget: curcumin's effects on mTOR signaling. Anticancer Agents Med Chem 13:988–994

Bilecova-Rabajdova M, Birkova A, Urban P, Gregova K, Durovcova E, Marekova M (2013) Naturally occurring substances and their role in chemo-protective effects. Cent Eur J Public Health 21:213–219

Bishayee A (2009) Cancer prevention and treatment with resveratrol: from rodent studies to clinical trials. Cancer Prev Res (Phila) 2:409–418

Bosetti C, Filomeno M, Riso P, Polesel J, Levi F, Talamini R, Montella M, Negri E, Franceschi S, La VC (2012) Cruciferous vegetables and cancer risk in a network of case-control studies. Ann Oncol 23:2198–2203

Bush JA, Cheung KJ Jr, Li G (2001) Curcumin induces apoptosis in human melanoma cells through a Fas receptor/caspase-8 pathway independent of p53. Exp Cell Res 271:305–314

Cao AL, Tang QF, Zhou WC, Qiu YY, Hu SJ, Yin PH (2014) Ras/ERK signaling pathway is involved in curcumin-induced cell cycle arrest and apoptosis in human gastric carcinoma AGS cells. J Asian Nat Prod Res 17(1):56–63

Chang X, Tou JC, Hong C, Kim HA, Riby JE, Firestone GL, Bjeldanes LF (2005) 3,3-′-Diindolylmethane inhibits angiogenesis and the growth of transplantable human breast carcinoma in athymic mice. Carcinogenesis 26:771–778

Choi HJ, Lim DY, Park JH (2009) Induction of G1 and G2/M cell cycle arrests by the dietary compound 3,3′-diindolylmethane in HT-29 human colon cancer cells. BMC Gastroenterol 9:39

Choudhuri T, Pal S, Das T, Sa G (2005) Curcumin selectively induces apoptosis in deregulated cyclin D1-expressed cells at G2 phase of cell cycle in a p53-dependent manner. J Biol Chem 280:20059–20068

Dandawate PR, Vyas A, Ahmad A, Banerjee S, Deshpande J, Swamy KV, Jamadar A, Dumhe-Klaire AC, Padhye S, Sarkar FH (2012) Inclusion complex of novel curcumin analogue CDF and beta-cyclodextrin (1:2) and its enhanced in vivo anticancer activity against pancreatic cancer. Pharm Res 29:1775–1786

Frojdo S, Cozzone D, Vidal H, Pirola L (2007) Resveratrol is a class IA phosphoinositide 3-kinase inhibitor. Biochem J 406:511–518

Hadi SM, Asad SF, Singh S, Ahmad A (2000) Putative mechanism for anticancer and apoptosis-inducing properties of plant-derived polyphenolic compounds. IUBMB Life 50:167–171

Hadi SM, Ullah MF, Azmi AS, Ahmad A, Shamim U, Zubair H, Khan HY (2010) Resveratrol mobilizes endogenous copper in human peripheral lymphocytes leading to oxidative DNA breakage: a putative mechanism for chemoprevention of cancer. Pharm Res 27:979–988

Higdon JV, Delage B, Williams DE, Dashwood RH (2007) Cruciferous vegetables and human cancer risk: epidemiologic evidence and mechanistic basis. Pharmacol Res 55:224–236

Hsieh TC, Wu JM (2010) Resveratrol: biological and pharmaceutical properties as anticancer molecule. Biofactors 36:360–369

Hussain AR, Uddin S, Bu R, Khan OS, Ahmed SO, Ahmed M, Al-Kuraya KS (2011) Resveratrol suppresses constitutive activation of AKT via generation of ROS and induces apoptosis in diffuse large B cell lymphoma cell lines. PLoS One 6:e24703

Jakus PB, Kalman N, Antus C, Radnai B, Tucsek Z, Gallyas F Jr, Sumegi B, Veres B (2013) TRAF6 is functional in inhibition of TLR4-mediated NF-kappaB activation by resveratrol. J Nutr Biochem 24:819–823

Jiang AJ, Jiang G, Li LT, Zheng JN (2014) Curcumin induces apoptosis through mitochondrial pathway and caspases activation in human melanoma cells. Mol Biol Rep 42(1):267–275

Kang OH, Jang HJ, Chae HS, Oh YC, Choi JG, Lee YS, Kim JH, Kim YC, Sohn DH, Park H, Kwon DY (2009) Anti-inflammatory mechanisms of resveratrol in activated HMC-1 cells: pivotal roles of NF-kappaB and MAPK. Pharmacol Res 59:330–337

Kangwan N, Park JM, Kim EH, Hahm KB (2014) Chemoquiescence for ideal cancer treatment and prevention: where are we now? J Cancer Prev 19:89–96

Khan A, Aljarbou AN, Aldebasi YH, Faisal SM, Khan MA (2014a) Resveratrol suppresses the proliferation of breast cancer cells by inhibiting fatty acid synthase signaling pathway. Cancer Epidemiol 38:765–772
Khan HY, Zubair H, Faisal M, Ullah MF, Farhan M, Sarkar FH, Ahmad A, Hadi SM (2014b) Plant polyphenol induced cell death in human cancer cells involves mobilization of intracellular copper ions and reactive oxygen species generation: a mechanism for cancer chemopreventive action. Mol Nutr Food Res 58:437–446
Kim EJ, Park H, Kim J, Park JH (2010) 3,3′-diindolylmethane suppresses 12-O-tetradecanoylphorbol-13-acetate-induced inflammation and tumor promotion in mouse skin via the downregulation of inflammatory mediators. Mol Carcinog 49:672–683
Kong D, Li Y, Wang Z, Banerjee S, Sarkar FH (2007) Inhibition of angiogenesis and invasion by 3,3′-diindolylmethane is mediated by the nuclear factor-kappaB downstream target genes MMP-9 and uPA that regulated bioavailability of vascular endothelial growth factor in prostate cancer. Cancer Res 67:3310–3319
Kulkarni SS, Canto C (2014) The molecular targets of resveratrol. Biochim Biophys Acta 1852:1114–1123
La VC (2009) Association between Mediterranean dietary patterns and cancer risk. Nutr Rev 67 (Suppl 1):S126–S129
Liu E, Wu J, Cao W, Zhang J, Liu W, Jiang X, Zhang X (2007) Curcumin induces G2/M cell cycle arrest in a p53-dependent manner and upregulates ING4 expression in human glioma. J Neurooncol 85:263–270
Liu M, Wilk SA, Wang A, Zhou L, Wang RH, Ogawa W, Deng C, Dong LQ, Liu F (2010) Resveratrol inhibits mTOR signaling by promoting the interaction between mTOR and DEPTOR. J Biol Chem 285:36387–36394
Liu B, Zhou Z, Zhou W, Liu J, Zhang Q, Xia J, Liu J, Chen N, Li M, Zhu R (2014) Resveratrol inhibits proliferation in human colorectal carcinoma cells by inducing G1/Sphase cell cycle arrest and apoptosis through caspase/cyclinCDK pathways. Mol Med Rep 10:1697–1702
Maruthanila VL, Poornima J, Mirunalini S (2014) Attenuation of carcinogenesis and the mechanism underlying by the influence of indole-3-carbinol and its metabolite 3,3-′-diindolylmethane: a therapeutic marvel. Adv Pharmacol Sci 2014:832161
Orr WS, Denbo JW, Saab KR, Ng CY, Wu J, Li K, Garner JM, Morton CL, Du Z, Pfeffer LM, Davidoff AM (2013) Curcumin potentiates rhabdomyosarcoma radiosensitivity by suppressing NF-kappaB activity. PLoS One 8:e51309
Parasramka MA, Gupta SV (2012) Synergistic effect of garcinol and curcumin on antiproliferative and apoptotic activity in pancreatic cancer cells. J Oncol 2012:709739
Ravindran J, Prasad S, Aggarwal BB (2009) Curcumin and cancer cells: how many ways can curry kill tumor cells selectively? AAPS J 11:495–510
Shakibaei M, Mobasheri A, Lueders C, Busch F, Shayan P, Goel A (2013) Curcumin enhances the effect of chemotherapy against colorectal cancer cells by inhibition of NF-kappaB and Src protein kinase signaling pathways. PLoS One 8:e57218
Steward WP, Brown K (2013) Cancer chemoprevention: a rapidly evolving field. Br J Cancer 109:1–7
Tadi K, Chang Y, Ashok BT, Chen Y, Moscatello A, Schaefer SD, Schantz SP, Policastro AJ, Geliebter J, Tiwari RK (2005) 3,3′-Diindolylmethane, a cruciferous vegetable derived synthetic anti-proliferative compound in thyroid disease. Biochem Biophys Res Commun 337:1019–1025
Vyas A, Dandawate P, Padhye S, Ahmad A, Sarkar F (2013) Perspectives on new synthetic curcumin analogs and their potential anticancer properties. Curr Pharm Des 19:2047–2069
Weng JR, Bai LY, Chiu CF, Wang YC, Tsai MH (2012) The dietary phytochemical 3,3-′-diindolylmethane induces G2/M arrest and apoptosis in oral squamous cell carcinoma by modulating Akt-NF-kappaB, MAPK, and p53 signaling. Chem Biol Interact 195:224–230

Wilken R, Veena MS, Wang MB, Srivatsan ES (2011) Curcumin: a review of anti-cancer properties and therapeutic activity in head and neck squamous cell carcinoma. Mol Cancer 10:12

Zhang WW, Feng Z, Narod SA (2014) Multiple therapeutic and preventive effects of 3,3-′-diindolylmethane on cancers including prostate cancer and high grade prostatic intraepithelial neoplasia. J Biomed Res 28:339–348

Zhou H, Beevers CS, Huang S (2011) Targets of curcumin. Curr Drug Targets 12:332–347

Pivotal Role of Chemokine Receptor Signaling Axis and Natural Bioactive Chemopreventive Agents in Metastasis of Breast Cancer

Sanjeev Banerjee, Shivani B Paruthy, Paul R Rajamani, and Bin Bao

Abstract Breast cancer ranks as one of the most frequently diagnosed malignant neoplasm in women embracing multiple genomic alterations that influence tumor growth, progression, and metastasis. Despite significant advancements in systemic adjuvant chemotherapy for breast cancer, manifestations of distant metastasis raise significant clinical problems with worst prognosis. Therefore, defining molecular events underlying metastasis alongside well defined strategic abrogation of these molecular events is crucial for improving patient survival and better clinical management. The classic "seed and soil" hypothesis of tumor metastasis has been redefined in light of emerging evidence revealing chemokine [CXCL12 (SDF-1α)] and its cognate receptor (CXCR4) orchestrating signaling events that guide chemotaxis of tumor cells to site of metastasis. CXCR4 is a transmembrane G protein-coupled receptor reportedly overexpressed in primary and metastatic breast tumors compared to normal breast tissue, and its chemokine ligand (SDF-1α) presents peak expression in common metastatic sites. CXCR4-SDF-1α signaling has earned considerable attention underscoring its role in cancer metastasis including activation of focal clusters of integrin and adhesion kinase (Rho/ROCK) and multiple signaling entities (Cdc42, PI3K-Akt, p38 MAPK) that allow tumor cells to attain a migratory phenotype. Hypoxia, vascular endothelial growth factor (VEGF), transcription factor NF-κB, and estrogen receptor status upregulates CXCR4 expression in tumor microenvironment. A growing body of evidence suggests that natural chemo-dietary agents hold prospect targeting CXCR4-SDF-1α axis to prevent metastasis of breast cancer. This chapter presents a succinct overview about

S. Banerjee, PhD (✉) • B. Bao
Department of Pathology, Barbara Ann Karmanos Cancer Institute, Wayne State University School of Medicine, Room-715 HWCRC Bldg., 4100 John R Street, Detroit, MI 48201, USA
e-mail: sbanerjee@wayne.edu; sbanerjee341@hotmail.com

S.B. Paruthy
Department of Surgery, VM Medical College and Safdarjung Hospital, New Delhi 110062, India

P.R. Rajamani
Radiation Oncology Lab., School of Environmental Sciences, Jawaharlal Nehru University, New Delhi 110067, India

M.F. Ullah, A. Ahmad (eds.), *Critical Dietary Factors in Cancer Chemoprevention*, DOI 10.1007/978-3-319-21461-0_14

CXCR4 receptor signaling in breast cancer and related mechano-transductive pathways, microenvironmental cues, and current status and knowledge regarding efficacy of bioactive natural products on metastasis and homing of malignant tumor cells.

1 Introduction

Breast cancer is second most common cancer afflicting women in both developed and developing countries worldwide and leading cause of morbidity and mortality from this disease. According to recent reports, ~12 % of women in USA will develop breast cancer during life time and out of an estimated 231,840 new cases expected to be diagnosed this year, 15 % of women will succumb to this disease despite availability of advanced treatment modalities (Siegel et al. 2015). A vast majority of breast cancer related deaths result from systemic dissemination (metastasis) of tumor cells to organ specific secondary sites such as lungs, lymph nodes, liver, and bone marrow. Notwithstanding therapeutic challenges, the etiology of breast cancer involves a complex interplay of genetic, hormonal, and probably dietary factors as well. <25 % of the familial breast cancer patients express cancer susceptibility genes—*BRCA1* and *BRCA2*. Moreover, estrogen plays an important role in the pathogenesis and development of breast cancer; increased cumulative estrogen exposure has been hypothesized to accentuate breast cancer risk factors along with early age at menarche, late age at menopause, nulliparity, post-menopausal obesity, and possibly other factors (Kelsey and Bernstein 1996). Nevertheless, early detection accompanied by favorable clinical–pathological parameters with aggressive surgical and nonsurgical treatment interventions have shown an effect on improved survival and quality of life; it is the almost unpredictable tumor metastasis to preferential secondary sites that becomes a pervasive clinical problem culminating in high rate of mortality. Currently, the mechanisms guiding metastasis are emerging resulting in efficient and palliative approach for management of metastatic late-stage breast cancer.

Metastasis of cancer cells to distant sites, which occurs in as many as 90 % of cancer-associated deaths, is a highly organized, multistep, and organ selective dynamic process imitating leukocyte trafficking to specific anatomical sites. The process of metastasis involves tumor cells to dissociate from one another and acquire features for motility, ability to survive in circulation, and attach to a distant target organ. Emerging underlying mechanistic explanations driving these events are the small chemo-attracting proteins—chemokines and their receptors. Chemokines are a superfamily of small soluble peptides (MW: 8–12 kDa) sharing common biological activity in stimulating the migration of hematopoietic stem cells and chemotactic activity (Smith et al. 2012; Viola and Luster 2008). They are divided into four subfamilies (C, CC, CXC, and CX3C) based on the arrangement of their first two conserved cysteine residues at the amino terminus (Rollins 1997). Stromal cell-derived factor-1α (SDF-1α; also known as CXCL12) is a member of the CXC chemokine subfamily and appears to be the only ligand for chemokine receptor CXCR4. About 50 chemokines and 20 chemokine receptors have been identified till date. The previous much acclaimed Paget's seminal "seed and soil" hypothesis for tumor metastasis has been amended in light of new revelations that chemokines and their cognate receptors are critical regulators of cell trafficking and adhesion, and their expression correlates with unfavorable prognosis and metastasis of several malignant tumors. Accordingly, it has now been conceptualized that cancer cells with high expression of chemokine receptors will spread unambiguously where the ligand is highly secreted. Mueller and colleagues were the first to describe increased SDF-1α chemokine levels in organs of breast cancer metastasis, underpinning "CXCR4/SDF-1α chemotactic gradient" model accounting for preferential homing of circulating tumor cells to distant metastatic sites (Muller et al. 2001). Thereafter, an increasing body of evidence corroborate the fact that breast cancer cells display distinct pattern of chemokine receptor expression, and SDF-1α is highly expressed in the most common destinations of breast cancer metastasis—the lymph nodes, lungs, liver, and bone marrow. In breast cancer patients, meta-analysis for prognostic impact of CXCR4 expression revealed that elevated CXCR4 expression was significantly associated with poor overall survival (OS) and disease free survival (DFS) (Xu et al. 2013; Zhang et al. 2014).

Over the last decade, CXCR4 has been extensively reported to be overexpressed in most human solid tumors and have earned considerable attention elucidating its role in cancer metastasis (Balkwill 2004; Helbig et al. 2003; Kang et al. 2003; Phillips et al. 2003; Singh et al. 2013). Furthermore, bioactive compounds derived from natural dietary sources have been investigated and shown to downregulate or block SDF-1α/CXCR4 interaction or SDF-1α-induced chemotaxis in preclinical models inhibiting metastasis. This chapter presents a succinct and integrated overview of SDF-1α/CXCR4 signaling related events and effect of bioactive natural compounds in context of breast cancer metastasis leveraging possibility of novel therapeutic interventions especially in triple negative and HER2/neu breast tumors that metastasize and associated with least favorable prognosis.

2 Biology of SDF-1α and Its Receptor-CXCR4

The chemokine ligand stromal cell-derived factor-1α (SDF-1α) is a splice variant of a small homeostatic chemokine-CXCL-12, being first cloned by Tashiro et al. in 1993(Janowski 2009; Tashiro et al. 1993). The gene encoding CXCL12 is highly conserved and located on chromosome 10q11.21 and expressed for paracrine signaling in different organs including the brain, lung, colon, heart, kidney, liver stromal cells within solid tumors, and autocrine signaling within tumor cells but undergoes rapid degradation in the blood. The crystal structure of SDF-1α confirms it consists of two monomers that form an asymmetrical dimer (Dealwis et al. 1998). SDF-1α functions as a pleiotropic chemokine that has been studied mainly in hematopoietic cells, chemo-attracting progenitor and mature hematopoietic cells into the bone marrow and performing important role in inflammation, immune surveillance and homing of tumor cells. It is the known ligand for CXCR4 (Bleul et al. 1996). CXCL12 knockout mice die perinatally (embryonic day 18.5) with significantly reduced progenitor B-cells as well as, cardiovascular defects indicating critical role in lymphopoiesis, myelopoiesis, and development (Gangadhar et al. 2010; Nagasawa et al. 1996). Mice lacking CXCR4 exhibit identical defects, but in addition abnormal neuronal cell migration during development (Gangadhar et al. 2010; Zou et al. 1998).

Gene encoding CXCR4 is located on chromosome 2 band q22.1, clustered with genes for other CXC chemokine receptors. The crystal structure shows CXCR4 is a member of the G protein-coupled chemokine receptor family having seven transmembrane alpha helices that are bundled together to form an extracellular binding pocket (Muller et al. 2001). The extracellular loops (ECLs) and amino acids within the alpha helices bind with SDF-1α ligand. In normal and noninvasive breast cancer cell lines, CXCR4 gene expression is downregulated, but highly expressed both in primary and metastatic breast tumors (Muller et al. 2001). Additionally, CXCR4 is found to be expressed on diverse array of cancer cell types, including those of lung, prostate, kidney, ovary, etc. (Steeg 2003). Most potent inducers of CXCR4 gene expression are TNFα and TGF-β signaling and transcriptional activator HIF-1α (Rahimi et al. 2010). In breast cancer, HER-2/neu receptor tyrosine kinase has been shown to upregulate the expression and function of CXCR4 by inhibiting CXCR4 degradation (Li et al. 2004). Furthermore, CXCR4 relies on the molecular chaperone- heat shock protein 90 (Hsp90) for proper folding and delivery into the lipid bilayer (Mandawat et al. 2010). Once SDF-1α is bound, the receptor mediates actin polymerization, pseudopod formation, and directed cell migration (Gangadhar et al. 2010). At least 23 different cancers have been reported to express this receptor (Balkwill 2012). Silencing CXCR4 by siRNA and monoclonal antibodies (mAbs) to CXCR4, significantly inhibits breast cancer metastasis (Liang et al. 2005; Muller et al. 2001). Genetically knockout mice experiments displayed significant defects in the development of cardiovascular and CNS organs, and in case of dual SDF-1α and CXCR-4 ablation, embryos died in utero implying SDF-1α/CXCR4 axis to have a fundamental physiological role in normal tissue development.

3 The SDF-1α–CXCR4 Signaling Pathway

The engagement of CXCR4 receptor by the ligand SDF-1α forms an important signaling axis, and cross talk between tumor cells and the surrounding activated stroma (microenvironment) guide a "homing route" for migratory tumor cells to sites of metastasis. Importantly, this interaction provides growth advantage to cancer cells, both at the primary and metastatic sites, and stimulates chemotactic and invasive behavior of tumor cells. Upon ligand binding, chemokine receptors undergo homo- or hetero-dimerization resulting in divergent downstream signaling pathways (Fig.1). It was earlier assumed that SDF-1α binds primarily only to its

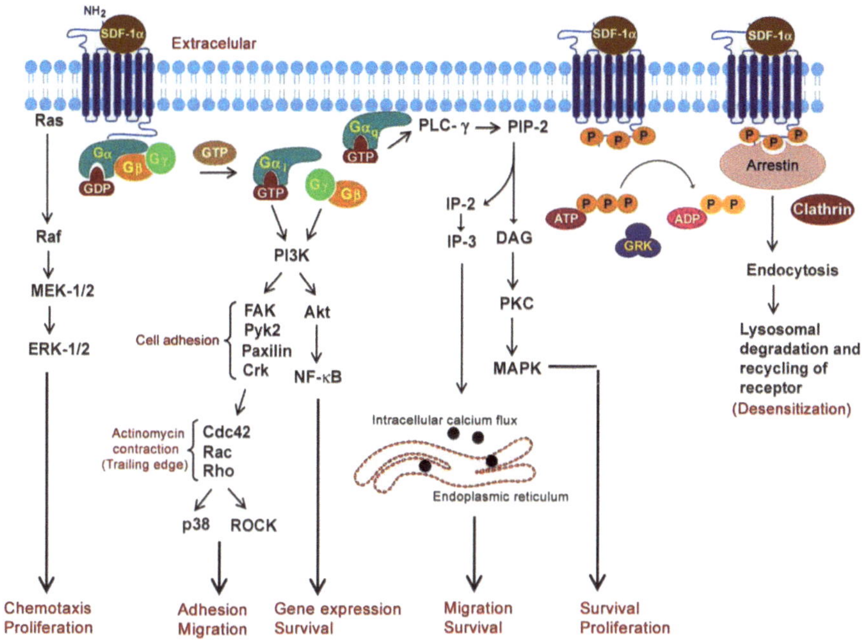

Fig. 1 Schematic overview of CXCR4-SDF-1α-induced intracellular signal transduction pathway and desensitization of activated receptor signaling

cognate receptor CXCR4, but upcoming evidences have shown that SDF-1α also binds with an orphan receptor-CXCR7 but does not activate signaling, instead function as a ligand scavenger or a "decoy receptor." CXCR4 receptor has emerged belonging to large diversity of G-protein coupled receptor (GPCR) superfamily that associates with an intracellular heterotrimeric G-protein, linked to the inner surface of the plasma membrane, which initiates intracellular signaling upon ligand binding. The heterotrimeric G-protein complex is comprised of Gα, Gβ, and Gγ subunits. The Gα subunit remains associated with guanine nucleotide GDP under basal or inactivate state. Canonical signaling upon ligand binding invokes conformational change within Gα subunit that signals replacement of the bound GDP by GTP, cleaving the G subunits into a Gα monomer and a Gβ/Gγ dimer with GTP bound to the Gα monomer; these activated components now interact with various effector substrates mediating intracellular signaling. The Gα subunit has been classified into four families-$G\alpha_s$, $G\alpha_i$, $G\alpha_q$, and $G\alpha_{12}$ exhibiting signaling diversity. Each of these Gα subunits, as well as the Gβγ subunit, activates distinct intracellular signaling cascade associated with migration, transcriptional activation, and proliferation. Despite considerable complexity and discrepancies, CXCR4-SDF-1α signaling seems specifically coupled to $G\alpha_i$ and $G\alpha_q$. After relayof the signal, GTP is rapidly hydrolyzed to GDP, leading to re-association of the CXCR4 receptor complex. Activated $G\alpha_i$ protein plays a dual role to inhibit the intracellular enzyme adenylyl cyclase leading to reduction in cAMP levels and concurrently activates phosphodiesterases and phospholipases; these events result in activation of the enzyme PI3K through Gα_i-coupled Src family of tyrosine kinases (Balkwill 2004; New and Wong 2007). PI3K activation signals survival and proliferation of tumor cells through well-known downstream signaling molecules including protein kinase B (PKB/Akt), mitogen/extracellular signal regulated kinase (MEK-1/2), and extracellular signal regulated kinase (ERK1/2). Gα_q-dependent GPCR signaling pathways activate the enzyme protein kinase C (PKC) and generate a second messenger molecule-inositol-1,4,5-trisphosphate (IP3); the later (IP3) diffuses into endoplasmic reticulum, opens calcium channels, and stimulates their release from intracellular stores into the cytoplasm facilitating cellular chemotaxis by stimulating migration and survival of cells. GPCR signaling by Gβγ dimer activates guanine nucleotide exchange factors for the Rho family of GTPases Rho, Rac, and Cdc42 proteins to regulate cytoskeletal actin dynamics for directed migration. To undertake this intracellular action, active Rho along with its major downstream target Rho-dependent coiled-coil kinase (ROCK) and Dia1—the mammalian ortholog of Drosophila diaphanous 1, initiate contractility through phosphorylation-induced inactivation of myosin light chain phosphatase, while Rac and Cdc42 orchestrate the formation of specialized membrane protrusions - lamellipodia and filopodia (Jaffe and Hall 2005; Ridley et al. 2003). Importantly, in addition to Gα monomer-induced activation of PI3K, direct binding of Gβγ dimer also results in the activation of Akt. Akt contributes an important role in breast cancer chemotaxis to SDF-1α, by phosphorylating the G protein - Girdin, and other downstream targets that modulate reorganization of actin fibers within cell and additionally activates focal adhesion kinase (FAK), which induces migratory activity in different types of cells including tumor cells (Enomoto et al. 2005; Liang and Slingerland 2003; New and Wong 2007; Rozengurt 1998). Hsp90 protects Akt from dephosphorylation and degradation (Ramsey and McAlpine 2013; Zhao et al. 2008). Thus, tumor cells utilize the CXCR4/SDF-1α signaling cascade to precisely coordinate the cytoskeleton remodeling dynamics, and CXCR4-positive cancer cells exploit autocrine and/or paracrine-generated SDF-1α gradient to maintain an altered phenotype enabling them to spread to other tissues.

Since SDF-1α is constitutively expressed, it has been reported that shutting off continuous stimulation of the GPCR signaling is vital to normal tissue homeostasis and depends on the duration of Gα subunit in the GTP-bound state. Studies have shown that hydrolysis of Gα-GTP to GDP inactivates the Gα subunit, permitting it to re-associate with the Gβ/Gγ dimer and recycled back to plasma membrane terminating all effector interactions. Additionally, novel feedback regulatory mechanisms by members of the GPCR kinase (GRK) family desensitizing agonist-bound GPCRs have been reported resulting in downregulation of chemokine signaling (Pitcher et al. 1998; Premont and Gainetdinov 2007; Robinson and Pitcher 2013).

4 Regulation of Expression of CXCR4

The entire transcription unit of the human CXCR4 gene has been characterized for elucidating the presence of potential binding sites for known transcription factors and its regulation. Based on the information available thus far, it is concluded that the local expression of chemokines and chemokine receptors in breast and various cancers are regulated at multiple levels, including transcription, translation, and protein degradation although no CXCR4 specific transcription factor has been reported till date.

Emerging evidence highlights the critical role of Hypoxia-inducible factor-1α (HIF-1α), a central mediator of tissue hypoxia, to induce upregulation in the expression of CXCR4 in MCF-7 and MDA-231 cells (Matteucci et al. 2007; Schioppa et al. 2003). Additionally, HIF-1α also induces SDF-1α expression on endothelial cells enabling their trafficking to distinctive niches of hypoxic regions; in doing so it stimulates recruitment of endothelial cells to the growing tumor along with their colocalization with tumor cells. It has been found that under normal oxygen tension, pVHL, the product of the von Hippel–Lindau tumor suppressor gene (VHL), induces degradation of HIF-1α. However, during hypoxia and circumstances harboring mutations in the VHL gene, HIF-1α degradation is compromised leading to its accumulation and stimulating expression of CXCR4. Notably, it has been shown that the promoter for CXCR4 retains a functional hypoxia response element attesting the regulation of CXCR4 expression by HIF transcription factor (Staller et al. 2003). Patients bearing renal clear cell carcinoma with inactivating mutations in the VHL gene express higher levels of CXCR4 than those without VHL mutations and associated with poor survival (Staller et al. 2003; Zagzag et al. 2005). Importantly, other transcription factors such as NF-kB and YY1 also influence the induction of expression of the chemokine receptor CXCR4 transcription. Nuclear factor-kappa B (NF-κB) is one of the key regulators of proper organogenesis of the mammary gland and plays an important role in the etiology of breast cancer. Constitutively, active NF-κB DNA-binding activity is detected in both mammary carcinoma cell lines and primary human breast cancer tissues and is responsible for overexpression of prometastatic, proangiogenic, and antiapoptotic genes in breast cancer (Badr et al. 2013a). Further CXCR4 expression in breast cancer cells is regulated by NF-κB, as well as by cytokines that induce NF-κB. A number of known activators of NF-κB, including TPA and CD30, have shown to induce CXCR4 (Caruz et al. 1998; Vinante et al. 2002) conveying the message that CXCR4 is one of the NF-κB target genes. Subsequent studies revealed a putative NF-κB binding site (5-GAGGCATTTCC-3, 230–240) within the −66 to +7 region of the CXCR4 promoter, which convey this important message that NF-κB directly regulates the expression of CXCR4 and directly involves in SDF-1α-mediated migration of breast cancer cells (Caruz et al. 1998; Helbig et al. 2003).

Furthermore, within proximal promoter region of CXCR4, consensus sequences complimenting Sp1 and nuclear receptor-1 (NRF-1) binding site have been identified (Moriuchi et al. 1997). It is worth noting NRF-1 binding sites are involved in transcriptional regulation of multiple mitochondrial genes; one may conceptualize that coordinated NRF-1 expression might contribute to cell's increased metabolic demand in response to proliferative signals and cell migration. NRF-1 has been reported to upregulate CXCR4 expression in human rhabdomyosarcoma (Tarnowski et al. 2010), although it remains unknown in breast cancer since no studies have addressed this aspect.

5 Chemokines and Angiogenesis

Empirically, angiogenesis is the process of formation of new blood vessels towards tumor and constitutes an important feature for tumor cells to survive and facilitate growth. It is now widely recognized that breast and many other solid tumors require angiogenesis and fail to grow beyond a few millimeters in diameter in absence of angiogenesis. Vascular endothelial growth factor (VEGF)—a pro-angiogenic molecule—is a critical mediator of this process and potent endothelial mitogen that prompts a rapid and complete angiogenic response in normal and malignant tissues by sprouting new blood vessels. VEGF is secreted by a number of different cancer cell types and overexpressed not only by breast cancer cells but also by activated breast stromal cells suggesting an active role for the latter in tumor growth and angiogenesis (Folkman 1995). Interestingly, chemokines have been suggested to actively participate in the process of angiogenesis by inducing the recruitment and proliferation of endothelial cells to form vessel walls. Corollary to such observations, CXCR4/SDF-1α interaction leading to capillary tube formation of HUVECs in vitro and tumor angiogenesis in vivo has been recorded, and SDF-1α mediates angiogenic effects in part through the induction of VEGF and downregulation of negative regulator of VEGF such as, expression of the glycolytic enzyme phosphoglycerate kinase-1 (PGK1), an ATP-generating glycolytic enzyme that forms part of the glycolytic pathway and directly involved in CXCR4/SDF-1α signaling (Wang et al. 2007). Additionally, it has been shown that VEGF can induce the expression of CXCR4 on breast cancer cells as part of its autocrine function, thus coupling VEGF expression with the migratory potential of cells and to SDF-1α signaling (Bachelder et al. 2002). Moreover, it has been shown that mechanistically CXCR4/SDF-1α signaling cascade can persuade angiogenesis and progression of tumors by increasing expression of VEGF through the activation of PI3K/Akt pathway (Badr et al. 2013b).

6 Chemokine Receptors and Microenvironment

Researchers in molecular pathology over the past decade have shed light to understand the contribution of tissue microenvironment in cancer progression and conceded CXCR4-SDF1α signaling axis as the main driver regulating this interactive function. According to contemporary views, for invasion to proceed, it is important for tumor cells to lose cell-to-cell adhesion properties, reorganize their cytoskeleton, translate into epithelial-to-mesenchymal (EMT) phenotype, and modulate the surrounding extracellular matrix (ECM). To accomplish these physiological alterations, overexpression of proteolytic activities of matrix metalloproteinase (MMPs) assists in the degradation of ECM and basement membrane. In cell culture models, SDF-1α upregulated protein expression and increased the enzymatic activity of MMP-9, while SDF-1α inhibitors abolished this activity. These and other related studies confirm MMP-9 as SDF-1α responsive mediator instigating the degradation of ECM and assists in subsequent steps of cancer invasion and metastasis. Additionally, SDF-1α and CXCR4 expression dictate EMT phenotype characterized by the loss of epithelial markers (E-cadherin, Zeb-1) and gain of mesenchymal surface markers (N-cadherin, vimentin; Fig. 2). Yang and coworkers demonstrated that silencing of CXCR4 was associated with a decrease in the tumorigenic properties of MDA-MB-231 breast cancer cells, with reversion of EMT, and repression of MMP-9 along with reduction in the incidence of lung metastasis in mice (Yang et al. 2014). Furthermore, a permissive tumor microenvironment have been underscored for its vital role in fostering the growth of cancer cells in parallel with the existence of a dynamic reciprocal interaction between

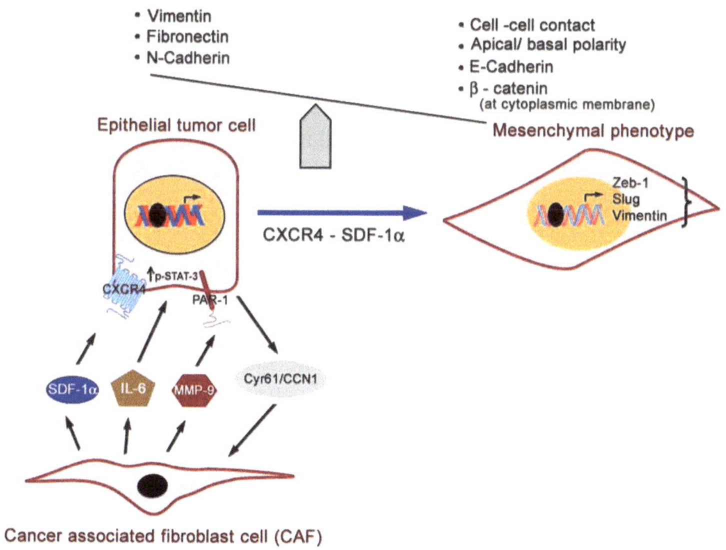

Fig. 2 Epithelial–mesenchymal transition (EMT) events and associated cellular and phenotype alterations and signaling interactions between cancer-associated fibroblasts (CAF) and tumor cells aiding growth and invasion of cancer cells. Cancer-associated fibroblasts secrete SDF-1α and IL-6 for paracrine actions on tumor cells activating CXCR4 and STAT-3 signaling. Matrix metalloproteinases (MMP-9) secreted by CAF cleave and activates protease-activated receptor-1 (PAR1) on the tumor cell surface stimulating growth and invasion pathways, while tumor cells secrete Cyr61/CCN1 stimulating MMP-1 production by adjacent fibroblasts creating a positive feedback loop potentiating tumor invasion

tumor cells and diverse variety of resident cells in stroma, including tissue-associated fibroblasts, inflammatory cells, endothelial cells, adipocytes, and mesenchymal stromal elements. In breast cancer, stromal fibroblasts often constitute a major fraction of the stromal cellular environment and express high levels of CXCL12, but not normal mammary fibroblasts (Allinen et al. 2004). Further, the significance of high-level expression of SDF-1α by carcinoma-associated fibroblasts (CAF) in promoting breast cancer progression has been well illustrated in a co-implantation tumor xenograft model. CAF isolated from surgically resected human breast carcinoma specimens promotes the growth of admixed breast carcinoma cells significantly more than do normal mammary fibroblasts derived from the same patients (Orimo et al. 2005). Of interest, it is only the breast fibroblasts but not skin fibroblasts that enhance the growth rate of primary breast carcinoma xenografts in vivo (Kang et al. 2005b). Further investigations revealed that CAFs, which exhibit the traits of myofibroblasts (as deduced from expression of α-smooth muscle actin- a characteristic marker of myofibroblasts), play a central role in promoting the growth of tumor cells through their ability to secrete SDF-1α and soluble IL-6 (Kang et al. 2005a) (Fig. 2). In addition to direct effects on breast cancer cells, CAFs also promote neo-angiogenesis by trafficking endothelial progenitor cells (EPCs) into tumor stromal microenvironment, an effect mediated again in part, by SDF-1α. Thus, SDF-1α secreted by CAF cells directly stimulates tumor growth interacting directly through the cognate receptor CXCR4 expressed by cancer cells, strengthening the notion that CAFs within invasive breast carcinomas contribute aggressively to tumor promotion in large part through the secretion of SDF-1α. These two major mechanisms by which fibroblast-derived SDF-1α promotes tumorigenesis have been confirmed in other tumor types as well. Another noteworthy feature involving interaction with tumor microenvironment relates to the adhesion receptors present on cell surface. Integrin $\alpha\nu\beta6$ is an important adhesion receptor that results in firm adhesion and transendothelial migration into tissues exhibiting chemokine gradients. Integrin $\alpha\nu\beta6$ has been found reportedly upregulated in SDF-1α/CXCR-induced cell migration.

Mounting evidence suggests the bone microenvironment is critical in supporting the homing of the breast tumor cells into bone marrow similar to hematopoietic stem cells (HSC). Approximately, 65–75 % of patients with advanced breast cancer develop bone metastasis with shorter median survival times compared to those without bone metastasis (Kato et al. 2003). Soluble factors such as osteopontin (OPN) secreted by breast cancer cells mediate cell adhesion to bone matrix and initiate a complex network impairing osteoblast differentiation. Once the circulating tumor cells have embarked inside the bone marrow, the high concentration of SDF-1α therein downregulates CXCR4 expression which prevents these cells from migrating to sites expressing SDF-1α, highlighting specific regulation of CXCR4 expression within bone marrow microenvironment. Combined with SDF-1α-induced adhesion to bone stromal cells and growth factors (Connective tissue growth factor, TGFβ, Interleukin-11)-stimulated proliferation, results in the establishment and persistence of breast cancer bone metastasis. Collectively, the foregoing information provides enough support for the crucial role of microenvironment in maintenance of malignant behavior of tumor cells and consequent progression of the disease state.

Bioactive Natural Products Naturally occurring chemokine antagonists hold prospects in era of drug discovery. Several natural chemopreventive compounds have been evaluated for attributes targeting CXCR4-SDF1α signaling axis leveraging a rationale-based generation of anti-metastatic protocol along with traditional chemo- and radio therapy. Several lines of evidence document anti-metastatic phenomenon of bioactive compounds in breast cancer along with pro-apoptotic activities in tumor cells and tissues. Among class of bioactive natural products, polyphenols constitute a large family of compounds with many component compounds being used to complement cancer therapies in cancer patients. We summarize below some natural plant and nonherbal agents capable of thwarting CXCR4-SDF1α signaling thus providing a window of opportunity to lower the risk of metastasis in women with higher risk and preventive approach through downregulation of this pathway in human. It has been reported that the breast cancer survivors are amongst highest users of dietary supplements some of which helps in delaying comorbid conditions associated with disease progression. Further elucidation of structure–activity relationship may prove useful in new drug design and development based on screening assays in preclinical models of breast diseases including cancer in general and breast cancer in particular.

Omega-3 Polyunsaturated Fatty Acids (n-3 PUFAs) Ever since Endres et al. provided first evidence of optimal health beneficial actions of the key family of Omega-3 PUFA, the effect of n-3 PUFAs in prevention of chronic diseases has received considerable attention. n-3 PUFAs which include eicosapentaenoic acid (EPA) and docosahexaenoic acid (DHA) are biochemically classified as essential fatty acids that cannot be synthesized by mammals and, thus, their source of availability in human are basically through natural dietary sources such as fish, flax seeds, and nuts. In cell culture studies using MDA-MB 231 human breast cancer cell line, the effect of EPA and DHA on expression and activity of CXCR4 has been reported (Altenburg and Siddiqui 2009). n-3 PUFA treatment results in reduced surface expression of CXCR4 corresponding with reduced migration of treated cells. However, in vivo efficacy of n-3 PUFA in preclinical animal models of breast cancer needs to be evaluated before translation into clinical practice.

Tannic Acid Tannins and tannic acid (polymer of gallic acid molecules and glucose) are water soluble polyphenols found widely distributed in plant kingdom including food grains and fruits. Although the mechanism is still being explored, tannins and tannic acid exert chemopreventive action as a result of inducing cellular death- apoptosis resulting in inhibition of tumor growth and antioxidative properties. Tannins and tannic acid have been identified as constituents of a herbal medicine Lianqiao (fruit of *Forsythia suspensa*), and under the laboratory culture conditions using MDA MB-231 cells, these molecules have been considered as a novel selective CXCL12/CXCR4 antagonist inhibiting the migration of CXCL12-

induced migration of breast tumor cells, and prevents bovine aorta endothelial cell capillary tube formation (Chen et al. 2003).

Ginsenoside Rg3 This is the active natural triterpenoid saponin ingredient isolated from *Panax ginseng*. Using indirect investigational techniques, the influence of Rg3 on CXCR4 expression has been reported in cultured MDA-MB-231 breast cancer cell line (Chen et al. 2011). Based on Immunohistochemistry, chemotaxis, and wound healing mobility assays, it has been shown that Rg3 treatment at nontoxic dose range elicits a weak CXCR4 staining indicative of downregulation of the receptor, concomitant with diminutions in the number of migrated cells in CXCL12-elicited chemotaxis, and reduction in the width of the scar in wound healing assay attesting Rg3 efficacy with CXCR4 inhibition (Chen et al. 2011).

Baohuoside-I This flavonoid constituent from *Epimedium koreanum*, an ingredient of Chinese traditional medicine, has the potential to suppress cancer metastasis. Baohuoside-I downregulates CXCR4 expression in a dose- and time-dependent manner in cervical cancer (HeLa) and breast cancer cells at mRNA and protein level, conforming to inhibition of CXCL12-induced invasion of both cervical and breast cancer cells (Kim and Park 2014). Thus, baohuoside-I may exert antimetastatic effect through the downregulation of CXCR4 expression.

Plumbagin This is a bioactive naphthoquinone derived from the roots of plant *Plumbago zeylanica* with validatedanticancer activities documented against a wide variety of cancers. Plumbagin reportedly targets multiple cancer signaling proteins and pathways in breast cancer that plays an important role in cancer cell survival, proliferation, invasion, and metastasis of cancer cells and thus potentially associated with preventative and therapeutic values. Referencing breast cancer, plumbagin downregulates the expression of CXCR4 in breast cancer cells irrespective of their HER2 status (Manu et al. 2011). Further, in depth analysis reveals that plumbagin mediates the downregulation of CXCR4 at the transcriptional level along with inhibition of NF-κB activation. Additional information derived from extrapolative, functional proteomics-based tumor pathway platform confirms that NF-κB inhibition by plumbagin causes decrease in CXCR4 and other metastatic genes which coordinate well with the inhibition of CXCL12-induced migration and invasion of both breast and gastric cancer cells (Manu et al. 2011). This confirms plumbagin as novel blocker of CXCR4 expression and thus has the potential to suppress metastasis of cancer.

Zerumbone This is a bioactive sesquiterpenoid derived from roots of subtropical *Zingiber zerumbet*. Zerumbone has been shown to downregulate chemokine receptor CXCR4 expression on HER2-overexpressing breast cancer cells in a dose- and time-dependent manner including downregulation of mRNA expression and inhibition of NF-κB activity; together these all lead to inhibition of CXCL12-induced invasion of breast tumor cells(Sung et al. 2008). Furthermore, an analogue of zerumbone, alpha-humulene, which lacks the carbonyl group, has been reported to be inactive in inducing CXCR4 downregulation confirming zerumbone as novel inhibitor of CXCR4 expression and has the potential to suppress cancer metastasis.

Celasterol This compound is a pleiotropic natural ingredient of traditional Chinese medicinal plant—*Tripterygium wilfordii*. The antitumor activities of celasterol in different preclinical models of site specific cancers as well as, an anti-inflammatory and a novel HSP inhibitor have been documented. Celasterol can downregulate the CXCR4 expression on breast cancer MCF-7 cells stably transfected with HER2 oncogene which is known to induce the chemokine receptor (Yadav et al. 2010). Quantitative reverse transcription polymerase chain reaction and chromatin immunoprecipitation analysis reveal that downregulation of CXCR4 by celasterol is targeted both at transcription and translational levels, and that abrogation of chemokine receptor by celasterol leads to suppression of invasiveness of cancer cells induced by CXCL12, the ligand for CXCR4.

Xanthohumol This is a polyphenol chalcone (2′, 4′,4-trihydroxy-6′-methoxy-3-′-prenylchalcone) found in hops (*Humulus lupulus*) flower, and associated with multiple pharmacological activities including anticancer effects and suppresses CXCR4 expression in various cell types in dose and time responsive manner. The inhibitory effect of xanthohumol is not due to proteolytic degradation of the receptor, but initiated at the transcriptional level(Wang et al. 2012). At molecular level, xanthohumol blocks endogenous NF-κB activation, thus affecting the expression of CXCR4 in tumor cells. In line with this observation, zanthohumol could effectively abolish cell invasion induced by CXCL12 in breast cancer cells which one may anticipate a promising therapeutic agent in breast cancer treatment. More studies are warranted especially in in vivo model.

Violacein This is a small violet pigment molecule and cytotoxic drug produced by various bacterial strains such as *Chromobacterium violaceum, Janthinobacterium lividum, Chromobacterium lividum,* and *Pseudoalteromonas luteoviolacea*. The antitumor efficacy of violacein has been attributed to downregulation of matrix metalloproteinases (MMP-2 and -9) along with chemokine-receptor ligand interaction (Platt et al. 2014). Violacein has been shown to significantly inhibit the cytokine (TNF-α and TGF-β)-mediated MMP-2 activation in MCF-7 breast cancer cell line, and MMP-2 plays a critical role in the secretion of CXCL12 chemokine involved in cell migration and cancer metastasis. Additionally, violacein downregulates CXCR4 membrane expression; this opens avenue for further exploration of violacein in cancer therapy and as anti-metastasis agent.

Butein 3,4,2′,4′-tetrahydroxy chalone—is the major bioactive polyphenol components of the bark and stems of *Rhus verniciflua* Stokes and traditionally used in many Oriental herbal medicinal formulations, and also as a food additive. Among its many notable pharmacological cffccts, inhibition of protcin tyrosine kinase and antineoplastic actions resulting in inhibition of tumor growth, invasion, metastasis, and angiogenesis has been reported in literature. In HER2 overexpressing breast cancer cells, butein has been shown to downregulate the expression of CXCR4 in dose- and time-dependent manner which parallels with the inhibition of CXCL12-induced migration and invasion of breast cancer cells (Chua et al. 2010). Furthermore, butein-mediated downregulation of CXCR4 correlates with its effect in the inhibition of NF-κB activation and repression of CXCR4 mRNA transcription (Chua et al. 2010). Thus, butein has the propensity to inhibit breast cancer metastasis, which needs further confirmation in in vivo models.

Gallic Acid Chemically identified as 4,5-trihydroxybenzoic acid, it is a naturally occurring polyphenol constituent of gall nuts, sumac, oak bark, tea leaves, green tea, apple peels, grapes, and wine. Recent studies document gallic acid to exert anticancer and antiproliferative activities including proapoptotic activities in animal models as well as, in cells in culture. Additionally, gallic acid has been shown to inhibit cancer cell migration and metastasis, which at molecular level have been encrypted resulting from suppression in the expression of proinflammatory cytokines and chemokines. As a constituent of anti-inflammatory phytomedicine-Vimang, gallic acid inhibits classical NF-κB activation by IKKα/β kinases and IκBα degradation. These actions of gallic acid results in potent inhibition of CXCR4 and other molecules related to anti-apoptosis and anti-angiogenesis phenomenon resulting in loss of cell survival, and significant antitumor and cytotoxic effect have been recorded in MDA MB-231 breast cancer cells(Garcia-Rivera et al. 2011).

Citrus Peel Volatile oil constituent derived from the peel of citrus fruits contain monoterpene hydrocarbons with evidence for potential role in breast cancer prevention and treatment. Species of citrus family such as hassaku (*Citrus hassaku* Hort. ex Tanaka) has thick peel and less juicy flesh. Recently, supercritical extracts of hassaku peel (SEPS) have been shown to inhibit tumor metastasis and invasion which mechanistically corroborate with SEPS-mediated downregulation of constitutive expression of CXCR4 and HER2 in MDA-MB-231 human breast cancer cells and suppression of matrix metalloproteinase-9 (MMP-9) expression and its enzymatic activity under non-cytotoxic concentrations(Kim et al. 2014). Furthermore, the downregulation of CXCR4 by SEPS reportedly occurs at the transcriptional level as concluded from downregulation of mRNA expression. Additionally, suppression of NF-κB activity by SEPS synchronizes with the observed inhibition of CXCL12-stimulated invasion of MDA-MB-231 breast cancer cells. Thus, SEPS by suppressing CXCR4 and MMP-9 expressions through blockade of NF-κB activation has the potential to suppress metastasis of breast cancer.

Nobiletin Is an active bioflavonoid found in citrus fruits such as lemons, oranges, tangerines, and grapefruits. Nobiletin has been screened for its potential to suppress metastasis of breast cancer cells and found to downregulate the constitutive expression of both MMP-9 and CXCR4 in human breast cancer cells along with suppression of the MMP-9 enzymatic activity. Nobiletin effect is at the transcriptional level, as deduced from downregulation of m-RNA expression, and through suppression of the constitutive NF-κB and MAPK activation (Baek et al. 2012).

Curcumin and Demethoxycurcumin These naturally occurring polyphenols are yellow colored pigments present abundantly in rhizomes of *Curcuma longa*. Curcumin and demethoxycurcumin (DMC) have been shown to exert anticancer, antiproliferative, radioprotective, and chemo-sensitizing activities in animal models and in vitro in cell culture. Curcumin and DMC mediate various antitumor activities through suppression of the transcription factor NF-κB. Microarray gene expression analyses upon curcumin treatment in breast cancer cells (MDA MB-231) reveal downregulation of inflammatory cytokines CXCL-1 and -2 and corresponding proteins. Additional experimental strategies involving CXCL1 and -2 silencing led to downregulation of several metastasis-promoting genes including that of cytokine receptor CXCR4 suggestive of its involvement in the inhibition of breast cancer cell metastasis. One amongst us has earlier reported dietary curcumin decreased the incidence of breast to lung cancer metastasis in nude mice (Aggarwal et al. 2005). Furthermore, DMC inhibits adhesion, migration, and invasion of MDA-MB-231 cells concomitant with decrease in the levels of ECM degradation-associated proteins MMP-9, and reduced expression of intercellular adhesion molecule-1 (ICAM-1) and CXCR4, all of these implicated in the tumor metastasis process (Yodkeeree et al. 2010).

Silibinin Is the major bioactive flavano lignan derived from medicinal herb *Silybum marianum* and associated with multi-targeted actions culminating in regulation of cell survival, proliferation, and angiogenesis of various tumor cells. It has also been reported to inhibit migration and adhesion capacity of MDA-MB-231 by regulating β1-integrin and MMP-9 expression and exhibit significant anti-metastatic effects in a variety of in vitro and in vivo breast cancer models (Dastpeyman et al. 2012; Kim et al. 2009, 2011; Lee et al. 2007; Oh et al. 2013). Based on molecular docking studies, silibinin has been categorized as a natural CXCR4 antagonist with potential to inhibit CXCL12-induced intracellular signaling; this action of silibinin results in the inhibition of CXCR4-mediated migration and invasion of breast cancer cells. Silibinin also inhibits MMP-9 expression in breast cancer cells (Kim et al. 2009; Oh et al. 2013).

Indole 3-Carbinol and DIM Indole-3-carbinol (I3C) represents enzymatically hydrolyzed breakdown product of glucobrassicin found abundantly in cruciferous vegetables such as broccoli, Brussels sprouts, kale, and cabbage. It has been hypothesized earlier that increased cabbage intake may prevent or delay metastatic and invasive capacity of breast cancer cells in operable breast cancer patients by inhibiting CXCL12/CXCR4 (Altundag et al. 2006). This was based on earlier report by Fowke et al. showing that Chinese cabbage consumption was associated with significantly reduced breast cancer risk among Chinese women. As an extension to these hypotheses, one of us reported that I3C, the natural compound present in vegetables of the genus *Brassica*, can inhibit NF-κB, CXCR4, and MMP-9 expression in breast cancer cells not only in vitro but also in vivo in a modified severe combined immunodeficient (SCID)-human mouse model of experimental bone metastasis using MDA-MB-231 breast cancer cell line (Rahman et al. 2006). Our findings established that 13C significantly inhibited MDA-MB-231 tumor growth in bone microenvironment. This growth inhibition of tumor in bone microenvironment correlated well with inhibition of the expression of multiple genes involved in the control of metastasis and invasion in vitro and in vivo, especially the expression of CXCR4 and MMP-9 along with pro-MMP-9 and decrease in Bcl-2 and increase in the proapoptotic protein Bax. Based on our findings, one may hypothesize and suggest that I3C could be a promising agent for future implementation in the prevention and/or treatment strategies of breast cancer bone metastasis albeit stabilization of I3C in acid condition of stomach.

Physiologically, in acid environment of the stomach, two molecules of I3C dimerize and form a stable compound- 3,3′-Diindolylmethane (DIM), authenticated to be a chemoprotective compound for breast and prostate cancer. DIM has also been shown to downregulate both CXCR4 and CXCL12 in breast (MCF-7 and MDA-MB-231) and ovarian (BG-1) cancer cells at transcriptional level and in an estrogen-independent manner. Consequently, the potential of these tumor cells for chemotaxis and invasion towards CXCL12 was found inhibited by DIM, strengthening the efficacy of DIM to lower the invasive and metastatic potential of breast and ovarian cancer cells (Hsu et al. 2008). The effect of I3C and DIM as risk factor for human consumption has not been reported in literature.

Breast Defend™ This is a polybotanical natural dietary supplement (BD), containing extracts from medicinal mushrooms (*Coriolus versicolor, Ganoderma lucidum, Phellinus linteus*), medicinal herbs (*Scutellaria barbata, Astragalus membranaceus, Curcuma longa*), and purified biologically active compounds (DIM and quercetin). BD inhibits proliferation and metastatic behavior of MDA-MB-231 invasive human breast cancer cells in vitro and further assessed against suppressing growth and breast-to-lung cancer metastasis in an orthotopic model of human breast cancer in mice (Jiang et al. 2012). Also no adverse effect of oral BD oral treatment (100 mg/kg of body weight for 4 weeks) by intragastric gavage on major organs of mice has been recorded (Jiang et al. 2012). Of clinical interest was the noticeable significant decrease in tumor volume over time, and also markedly decreased incidence of breast-to-lung cancer metastasis from 67% (control) to 20% (BD). The anti-metastatic activity of BD in vivo has been further established due to downregulation of expression of PLAU (urokinase plasminogen activator, uPA) and CXCR4 genes in breast tumors. This supports BD may have biological therapeutic potential for prevention and/or treatment of highly metastatic breast tumors and awaits clinical trial.

7 Conclusion

It is becoming increasingly clear and noteworthy from foregoing presentation and emerging evidence that metastasis of cancer cells is a well-orchestrated phenomenon integrating oncogenic pathways and governed by distinct signaling mechanism. This opens up avenue for therapeutic exploitation of this signaling axis, amid limitations owing to sharing of similar mechanism for homing of hematopoietic stem cells and close association with immune system alerting nontarget effects needs attention for adverse effects. With due advancements, development of small molecule inhibitors of CXCR4 are being examined in preclinical models with successful and promising results and have moved from bench to clinical trials mostly in multiple myeloma and hematological malignancies. Peptide inhibitors of CXCR4 also are showing promise in the clinics (www.http//clinicaltrials.gov). It is suggested that further development and mining of lead compounds with antagonistic functioning from natural products may be effective in minimizing and curtailing the metastatic process. These can further be refined by appropriate modification based on in silico investigations and modeling data. Finally, we conclude by encouraging early diagnosis and preventive measures as key to minimize burden and painful events accompanying cancer metastasis.

References

Aggarwal BB, Shishodia S, Takada Y, Banerjee S, Newman RA, Bueso-Ramos CE et al (2005) Curcumin suppresses the paclitaxel-induced nuclear factor-kappaB pathway in breast cancer cells and inhibits lung metastasis of human breast cancer in nude mice. Clin Cancer Res 11:7490–7498

Allinen M, Beroukhim R, Cai L, Brennan C, Lahti-Domenici J, Huang H et al (2004) Molecular characterization of the tumor microenvironment in breast cancer. Cancer Cell 6:17–32

Altenburg JD, Siddiqui RA (2009) Omega-3 polyunsaturated fatty acids down-modulate CXCR4 expression and function in MDA-MB-231 breast cancer cells. Mol Cancer Res 7:1013–1020

Altundag K, Gundeslioglu O, Altundag O (2006) Increased cabbage intake may inhibit metastatic and invasive capacity of breast cancer cells by inhibiting CXCL12(SDF-1 alpha)/CXCR4. Med Hypotheses 66:672

Bachelder RE, Wendt MA, Mercurio AM (2002) Vascular endothelial growth factor promotes breast carcinoma invasion in an autocrine manner by regulating the chemokine receptor CXCR4. Cancer Res 62:7203–7206

Badr G, Al-Sadoon MK, Rabah DM (2013a) Therapeutic efficacy and molecular mechanisms of snake (Walterinnesia aegyptia) venom-loaded silica nanoparticles in the treatment of breast cancer- and prostate cancer-bearing experimental mouse models. Free Radic Biol Med 65:175–189

Badr G, Al-Sadoon MK, Rabah DM, Sayed D (2013b) Snake (Walterinnesia aegyptia) venom-loaded silica nanoparticles induce apoptosis and growth arrest in human prostate cancer cells. Apoptosis 18:300–314

Baek SH, Kim SM, Nam D, Lee JH, Ahn KS, Choi SH et al (2012) Antimetastatic effect of nobiletin through the down-regulation of CXC chemokine receptor type 4 and matrix metallopeptidase-9. Pharm Biol 50:1210–1218

Balkwill F (2004) The significance of cancer cell expression of the chemokine receptor CXCR4. Semin Cancer Biol 14:171–179

Balkwill FR (2012) The chemokine system and cancer. J Pathol 226:148–157

Bleul CC, Farzan M, Choe H, Parolin C, Clark-Lewis I, Sodroski J et al (1996) The lymphocyte chemoattractant SDF 1 is a ligand for LESTR/fusin and blocks HIV-1 entry. Nature 382:829–833

Caruz A, Samsom M, Alonso JM, Alcami J, Baleux F, Virelizier JL et al (1998) Genomic organization and promoter characterization of human CXCR4 gene. FEBS Lett 426:271–278

Chen X, Beutler JA, McCloud TG, Loehfelm A, Yang L, Dong HF et al (2003) Tannic acid is an inhibitor of CXCL12 (SDF-1alpha)/CXCR4 with antiangiogenic activity. Clin Cancer Res 9:3115–3123

Chen XP, Qian LL, Jiang H, Chen JH (2011) Ginsenoside Rg3 inhibits CXCR4 expression and related migrations in a breast cancer cell line. Int J Clin Oncol 16:519–523

Chua AW, Hay HS, Rajendran P, Shanmugam MK, Li F, Bist P et al (2010) Butein downregulates chemokine receptor CXCR4 expression and function through suppression of NF-kappab activation in breast and pancreatic tumor cells. Biochem Pharmacol 80:1553–1562

Dastpeyman M, Motamed N, Azadmanesh K, Mostafavi E, Kia V, Jahanian-Najafabadi A et al (2012) Inhibition of silibinin on migration and adhesion capacity of human highly metastatic breast cancer cell line, MDA-MB-231, by evaluation of beta1-integrin and downstream molecules, Cdc42, Raf-1 and D4GDI. Med Oncol 29:2512–2518

Dealwis C, Fernandez EJ, Thompson DA, Simon RJ, Siani MA, Lolis E (1998) Crystal structure of chemically synthesized [N33a] stromal cell-derived factor 1alpha, a potent ligand for the HIV-1 "fusin" coreceptor. Proc Natl Acad Sci U S A 95:6941–6946

Enomoto A, Murakami H, Asai N, Morone N, Watanabe T, Kawai K et al (2005) Akt/PKB regulates actin organization and cell motility via Girdin/APE. Dev Cell 9:389–402

Folkman J (1995) Angiogenesis in cancer, vascular, rheumatoid and other disease. Nat Med 1:27–31

Gangadhar T, Nandi S, Salgia R (2010) The role of chemokine receptor CXCR4 in lung cancer. Cancer Biol Ther 9:409–416

Garcia-Rivera D, Delgado R, Bougarne N, Haegeman G, Berghe WV (2011) Gallic acid indanone and mangiferin xanthone are strong determinants of immunosuppressive anti-tumour effects of Mangifera indica L. Bark in MDA-MB231 breast cancer cells. Cancer Lett 305:21–31

Helbig G, Christopherson KW 2nd, Bhat-Nakshatri P, Kumar S, Kishimoto H, Miller KD et al (2003) Nf-kappaB promotes breast cancer cell migration and metastasis by inducing the expression of the chemokine receptor CXCR4. J Biol Chem 278:21631–21638

Hsu EL, Chen N, Westbrook A, Wang F, Zhang R, Taylor RT et al (2008) CXCR4 and CXCL12 down-regulation: a novel mechanism for the chemoprotection of 3,3′-diindolylmethane for breast and ovarian cancers. Cancer Lett 265:113–123

Jaffe AB, Hall A (2005) Rho GTPases: biochemistry and biology. Annu Rev Cell Dev Biol 21:247–269

Janowski M (2009) Functional diversity of SDF-1 splicing variants. Cell Adhes Migr 3:243–249

Jiang J, Thyagarajan-Sahu A, Loganathan J, Eliaz I, Terry C, Sandusky GE et al (2012) BreastDefend™ prevents breast-to-lung cancer metastases in an orthotopic animal model of triple-negative human breast cancer. Oncol Rep 28:1139–1145

Kang Y, Siegel PM, Shu W, Drobnjak M, Kakonen SM, Cordon-Cardo C et al (2003) A multigenic program mediating breast cancer metastasis to bone. Cancer Cell 3:537–549

Kang H, Watkins G, Douglas-Jones A, Mansel RE, Jiang WG (2005a) The elevated level of CXCR4 is correlated with nodal metastasis of human breast cancer. Breast 14:360–367

Kang H, Watkins G, Parr C, Douglas-Jones A, Mansel RE, Jiang WG (2005b) Stromal cell derived factor-1: its influence on invasiveness and migration of breast cancer cells in vitro, and its association with prognosis and survival in human breast cancer. Breast Cancer Res 7:R402–R410

Kato M, Kitayama J, Kazama S, Nagawa H (2003) Expression pattern of CXC chemokine receptor-4 is correlated with lymph node metastasis in human invasive ductal carcinoma. Breast Cancer Res 5:R144–R150

Kelsey JL, Bernstein L (1996) Epidemiology and prevention of breast cancer. Annu Rev Public Health 17:47–67

Kim B, Park B (2014) Baohuoside I suppresses invasion of cervical and breast cancer cells through the downregulation of CXCR4 chemokine receptor expression. Biochemistry 53:7562–7569

Kim S, Kim SH, Hur SM, Lee SK, Kim WW, Kim JS et al (2009) Silibinin prevents TPA-induced MMP-9 expression by down-regulation of COX-2 in human breast cancer cells. J Ethnopharmacol 126:252–257

Kim S, Han J, Kim JS, Kim JH, Choe JH, Yang JH et al (2011) Silibinin suppresses EGFR ligand-induced CD44 expression through inhibition of EGFR activity in breast cancer cells. Anticancer Res 31:3767–3773

Kim C, Kim D, Nam D, Chung WS, Ahn KS, Kim SH et al (2014) Anti-metastatic effect of supercritical extracts from the citrus hassaku pericarp via inhibition of C-X-C chemokine receptor type 4 (CXCR4) and matrix metalloproteinase-9 (MMP-9). Phytother Res 28:1374–1382

Lee SO, Jeong YJ, Im HG, Kim CH, Chang YC, Lee IS (2007) Silibinin suppresses PMA-induced MMP-9 expression by blocking the AP-1 activation via MAPK signaling pathways in MCF-7 human breast carcinoma cells. Biochem Biophys Res Commun 354:165–171

Li YM, Pan Y, Wei Y, Cheng X, Zhou BP, Tan M et al (2004) Upregulation of CXCR4 is essential for HER2-mediated tumor metastasis. Cancer Cell 6:459–469

Liang J, Slingerland JM (2003) Multiple roles of the PI3K/PKB (Akt) pathway in cell cycle progression. Cell Cycle 2:339–345

Liang Z, Yoon Y, Votaw J, Goodman MM, Williams L, Shim H (2005) Silencing of CXCR4 blocks breast cancer metastasis. Cancer Res 65:967–971

Mandawat A, Fiskus W, Buckley KM, Robbins K, Rao R, Balusu R et al (2010) Pan-histone deacetylase inhibitor panobinostat depletes CXCR4 levels and signaling and exerts synergistic antimyeloid activity in combination with CXCR4 antagonists. Blood 116:5306–5315

Manu KA, Shanmugam MK, Rajendran P, Li F, Ramachandran L, Hay HS et al (2011) Plumbagin inhibits invasion and migration of breast and gastric cancer cells by downregulating the expression of chemokine receptor CXCR4. Mol Cancer 10:107

Matteucci E, Ridolfi E, Maroni P, Bendinelli P, Desiderio MA (2007) c-Src/histone deacetylase 3 interaction is crucial for hepatocyte growth factor dependent decrease of CXCR4 expression in highly invasive breast tumor cells. Mol Cancer Res 5:833–845

Moriuchi M, Moriuchi H, Turner W, Fauci AS (1997) Cloning and analysis of the promoter region of CXCR4, a coreceptor for HIV-1 entry. J Immunol 159:4322–4329

Muller A, Homey B, Soto H, Ge N, Catron D, Buchanan ME et al (2001) Involvement of chemokine receptors in breast cancer metastasis. Nature 410:50–56

Nagasawa T, Hirota S, Tachibana K, Takakura N, Nishikawa S, Kitamura Y et al (1996) Defects of B-cell lymphopoiesis and bone-marrow myelopoiesis in mice lacking the CXC chemokine PBSF/SDF-1. Nature 382:635–638

New DC, Wong YH (2007) Molecular mechanisms mediating the g protein-coupled receptor regulation of cell cycle progression. J Mol Signal 2:2

Oh SJ, Jung SP, Han J, Kim S, Kim JS, Nam SJ et al (2013) Silibinin inhibits tpa-induced cell migration and MMP-9 expression in thyroid and breast cancer cells. Oncol Rep 29:1343–1348

Orimo A, Gupta PB, Sgroi DC, Arenzana-Seisdedos F, Delaunay T, Naeem R et al (2005) Stromal fibroblasts present in invasive human breast carcinomas promote tumor growth and angiogenesis through elevated SDF-1/CXCL12 secretion. Cell 121:335–348

Phillips RJ, Burdick MD, Lutz M, Belperio JA, Keane MP, Strieter RM (2003) The stromal derived factor-1/CXCL12-CXC chemokine receptor 4 biological axis in non-small cell lung cancer metastases. Am J Respir Crit Care Med 167:1676–1686

Pitcher JA, Freedman NJ, Lefkowitz RJ (1998) G protein-coupled receptor kinases. Annu Rev Biochem 67:653–692

Platt D, Amara S, Mehta T, Vercuyssee K, Myles EL, Johnson T et al (2014) Violacein inhibits matrix metalloproteinase mediated CXCR4 expression: potential anti-tumor effect in cancer invasion and metastasis. Biochem Biophys Res Commun 455:107–112

Premont RT, Gainetdinov RR (2007) Physiological roles of g protein-coupled receptor kinases and arrestins. Annu Rev Physiol 69:511–534

Rahimi M, George J, Tang C (2010) EGFR variant-mediated invasion by enhanced CXCR4 expression through transcriptional and post-translational mechanisms. Int J Cancer 126:1850–1860

Rahman KM, Sarkar FH, Banerjee S, Wang Z, Liao DJ, Hong X et al (2006) Therapeutic intervention of experimental breast cancer bone metastasis by indole-3-carbinol in SCID-human mouse model. Mol Cancer Ther 5:2747–2756

Ramsey DM, McAlpine SR (2013) Halting metastasis through CXCR4 inhibition. Bioorg Med Chem Lett 23:20–25
Ridley AJ, Schwartz MA, Burridge K, Firtel RA, Ginsberg MH, Borisy G et al (2003) Cell migration: integrating signals from front to back. Science 302:1704–1709
Robinson JD, Pitcher JA (2013) G protein-coupled receptor kinase 2 (GRK2) is a Rho-activated scaffold protein for the ERK MAP kinase cascade. Cell Signal 25:2831–2839
Rollins BJ (1997) Chemokines. Blood 90:909–928
Rozengurt E (1998) Signal transduction pathways in the mitogenic response to g protein-coupled neuropeptide receptor agonists. J Cell Physiol 177:507–517
Schioppa T, Uranchimeg B, Saccani A, Biswas SK, Doni A, Rapisarda A et al (2003) Regulation of the chemokine receptor CXCR4 by hypoxia. J Exp Med 198:1391–1402
Siegel RL, Miller KD, Jemal A (2015) Cancer statistics, 2015. CA Cancer J Clin 65:5–29
Singh AK, Arya RK, Trivedi AK, Sanyal S, Baral R, Dormond O et al (2013) Chemokine receptor trio: CXCR3, CXCR4 and CXCR7 crosstalk via CXCL11 and CXCL12. Cytokine Growth Factor Rev 24:41–49
Smith H, Whittall C, Weksler B, Middleton J (2012) Chemokines stimulate bidirectional migration of human mesenchymal stem cells across bone marrow endothelial cells. Stem Cells Dev 21:476–486
Staller P, Sulitkova J, Lisztwan J, Moch H, Oakeley EJ, Krek W (2003) Chemokine receptor CXCR4 downregulated by von Hippel-Lindau tumour suppressor pVHL. Nature 425:307–311
Steeg PS (2003) Metastasis suppressors alter the signal transduction of cancer cells. Nat Rev Cancer 3:55–63
Sung B, Jhurani S, Ahn KS, Mastuo Y, Yi T, Guha S et al (2008) Zerumbone down-regulates chemokine receptor CXCR4 expression leading to inhibition of CXCL12-induced invasion of breast and pancreatic tumor cells. Cancer Res 68:8938–8944
Tarnowski M, Grymula K, Reca R, Jankowski K, Maksym R, Tarnowska J et al (2010) Regulation of expression of stromal-derived factor-1 receptors: CXCR4 and CXCR7 in human rhabdomyosarcomas. Mol Cancer Res 8:1–14
Tashiro K, Tada H, Heilker R, Shirozu M, Nakano T, Honjo T (1993) Signal sequence trap: a cloning strategy for secreted proteins and type I membrane proteins. Science 261:600–603
Vinante F, Rigo A, Scupoli MT, Pizzolo G (2002) CD30 triggering by agonistic antibodies regulates CXCR4 expression and CXCL12 chemotactic activity in the cell line L540. Blood 99:52–60
Viola A, Luster AD (2008) Chemokines and their receptors: drug targets in immunity and inflammation. Annu Rev Pharmacol Toxicol 48:171–197
Wang J, Wang J, Dai J, Jung Y, Wei CL, Wang Y et al (2007) A glycolytic mechanism regulating an angiogenic switch in prostate cancer. Cancer Res 67:149–159
Wang Y, Chen Y, Wang J, Chen J, Aggarwal BB, Pang X et al (2012) Xanthohumol, a prenylated chalcone derived from hops, suppresses cancer cell invasion through inhibiting the expression of CXCR4 chemokine receptor. Curr Mol Med 12:153–162
Xu TP, Shen H, Liu LX, Shu YQ (2013) The impact of chemokine receptor CXCR4 on breast cancer prognosis: a meta-analysis. Cancer Epidemiol 37:725–731
Yadav VR, Sung B, Prasad S, Kannappan R, Cho SG, Liu M et al (2010) Celastrol suppresses invasion of colon and pancreatic cancer cells through the downregulation of expression of CXCR4 chemokine receptor. J Mol Med 88:1243–1253
Yang P, Liang SX, Huang WH, Zhang HW, Li XL, Xie LH et al (2014) Aberrant expression of CXCR4 significantly contributes to metastasis and predicts poor clinical outcome in breast cancer. Curr Mol Med 14:174–184
Yodkeeree S, Ampasavate C, Sung B, Aggarwal BB, Limtrakul P (2010) Demethoxycurcumin suppresses migration and invasion of MDA-MB-231 human breast cancer cell line. Eur J Pharmacol 627:8–15
Zagzag D, Krishnamachary B, Yee H, Okuyama H, Chiriboga L, Ali MA et al (2005) Stromal cell-derived factor-1alpha and CXCR4 expression in hemangioblastoma and clear cell-renal cell

carcinoma: von Hippel-Lindau loss-of-function induces expression of a ligand and its receptor. Cancer Res 65:6178–6188
Zhang Z, Ni C, Chen W, Wu P, Wang Z, Yin J et al (2014) Expression of CXCR4 and breast cancer prognosis: a systematic review and meta-analysis. BMC Cancer 14:49
Zhao M, Mueller BM, DiScipio RG, Schraufstatter IU (2008) Akt plays an important role in breast cancer cell chemotaxis to CXCL12. Breast Cancer Res Treat 110:211–222
Zou YR, Kottmann AH, Kuroda M, Taniuchi I, Littman DR (1998) Function of the chemokine receptor CXCR4 in haematopoiesis and in cerebellar development. Nature 393:595–599

Dietary Factors May Influence the Clinical Outcome of Chemotherapy in Cancer Multidrug Resistance

Mohammad Fahad Ullah, Showket H. Bhat, and Faisel M. Abuduhier

Abstract A substantive burden of cancer mortality results from poor prognosis of the disease due to the failure of chemotherapeutic regimen under the influence of Multidrug Resistance (MDR). The outcome of chemotherapy which is the most effective treatment for patients with cancer is impeded by the development of drug resistance. Anticancer drugs can fail to kill cancer cells for various reasons that include variations in the absorption, metabolism, and delivery of drug to target tissues and tumor location in parts of the body into which the drugs do not easily penetrate. In addition, certain cancer cells develop resistance by micro-evolutionary means through mutations occurring in the drug target, thus rendering the drugs ineffective. However, the most common of these mechanisms is the efflux of hydrophobic drugs mediated by energy driven ATP-binding cassette (ABC) family of transporters such as P-glycoprotein (P-gp), an integral membrane protein over-expressed in several malignancies. Various generations of MDR modulators have presented novel and improved interventions, though not to the perfection. Studies have shown that natural compounds found in vegetables, fruits, plant-derived beverages, and herbal dietary supplements not only have anticancer properties but may also modulate P-gp activity. P-gp inhibitors found in natural products, especially those found in plants of dietary origin and traditional medicine, have the potential to be developed as MDR reversing agents as adjuvant to chemotherapy leading to better clinical prognosis.

M.F. Ullah (✉)
Laboratory of Phytomedicine & Therapeutics, Prince Fahd Research Chair, Department of Medical Laboratory Technology, Faculty of Applied Medical Science, University of Tabuk-71491, Tabuk, Saudi Arabia
e-mail: m.ullah@ut.edu.sa

S.H. Bhat • F.M. Abuduhier
Prince Fahd Research Chair, Faculty of Applied Medical Sciences, Department of Medical Laboratory Technology, University of Tabuk, Tabuk 71491, Saudi Arabia

M.F. Ullah, A. Ahmad (eds.), *Critical Dietary Factors in Cancer Chemoprevention*,
DOI 10.1007/978-3-319-21461-0_15

1 Introduction

Cancer cells can develop resistance against structurally and mechanistically unrelated chemotherapeutic drugs, a phenomenon termed as multidrug resistance (MDR) (Gottesman and Pastan 1993). This reactive phenomenon developed by cancer cells to counter the effect of various classes of anticancer agents became a hotspot of cancer research after the emergence of a novel type of resistance discovered by Juliano and Ling (1976). It was observed that a glycoprotein of 170 kD, called P-glycoprotein, correlated with the degree of drug resistance in several Chinese hamster ovary cell lines.

There are two factors that are primarily responsible for MDR: (1) Individual specificity with regard to variations in absorption, metabolism, and delivery of drugs to target tissues. This factor is influenced by individual's genetic pattern which generates various cellular responses that obstruct the drug from reaching to threshold levels inside the cells which is required for its pharmacological action (acquired resistance). (2) Tumor specificity in terms of origin, vasculature, and tissue function. Tumors are located in parts of the body where the drug is not accessible or tumors with compromised vasculature often show resistance to chemotherapy (inherent or natural resistance). Intrinsic resistance results in the failure of chemotherapy from the start of the treatment due to presence of resistant phenotype in the tumor cells. However, acquired resistance develops during the course of the treatment when tumor cells showing initial responsiveness towards anticancer drugs are induced to attain resistant phenotype. This renders subsequent therapy ineffective leading to cancer recurrence and progression to metastatic stages (Goldie 2001).

As mentioned above and presented in Fig. 1, MDR can have many causes, but the most commonly encountered mechanism in the laboratory is the increased efflux of cytotoxic drugs by energy-dependent transporters belonging to ATP-binding cassettes (ABC) superfamily. P-glycoprotein was the first member of ABC transporters to be identified as an integral membrane protein overexpressed in many malignancies, conferring resistance to a variety of pharmacologically unrelated anticancer drugs, such as vinblastine, vincristine, daunorubicin, epirubicin, etoposide, imatinib, irinotecan, and paclitaxel (Ambudkar et al. 1999; Szakács et al. 2006; Eckford and Sharom 2009; Holohan et al. 2013).

A large number of chemical agents including calcium blocker, calmodulin inhibitors, coronary vasodilators, indole alkaloids, quinolines, hormones, cyclosporins, surfactants, and antibodies act as modulators of acquired MDR, which have the ability to reverse the drug efflux function of P-gp (Krishna and Mayer 2000). Toxicity is one of the significant issues reported in several clinical studies, as most of these modulators resulted in nonspecific toxic effects which are not considered acceptable during chemotherapy and prevents their safe use during treatment (Shukla et al. 2011). The use of natural agents in the realm of MDR holds potential as these display minimal toxicity to humans compared to conventional chemotherapies and have pleiotropic action mechanism that could target numerous signaling pathways. This is beneficial as malignant transformation and progression are multistage processes caused by gene alterations in more than one signaling pathway. Therefore, the impact of natural agents

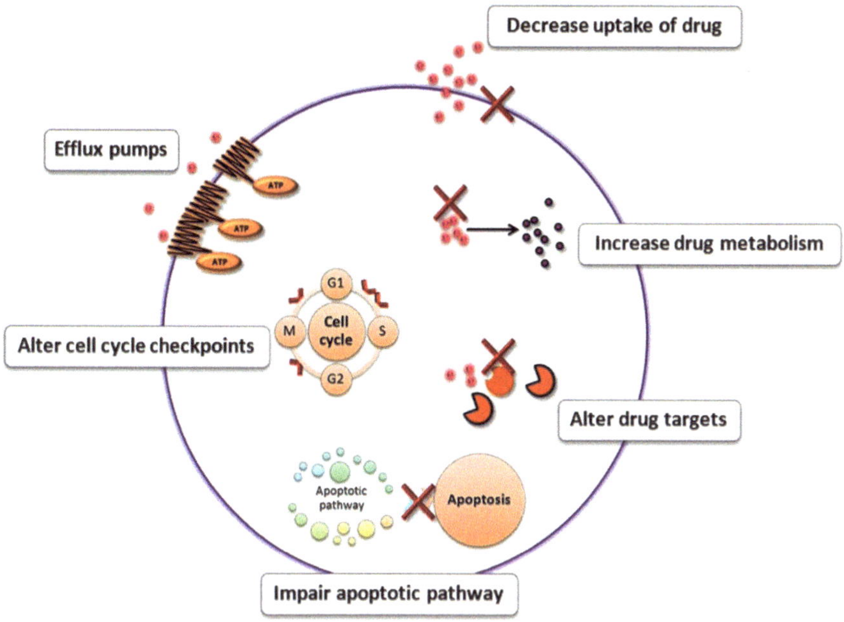

Fig. 1 Mechanisms of MDR towards cancer chemotherapeutic drugs. Cancer cells can develop resistance to multiple drugs by various mechanisms as depicted. Mechanisms include (**a**) decreased uptake of drug, (**b**) reduced intracellular drug concentration by efflux pumps, (**c**) altered cell cycle checkpoints, (**d**) altered drug targets, (**e**) increased metabolism of drug, and (**f**) induced emergency response genes to impair apoptotic pathway [Reproduced from Chai et al. (2010) under the terms of Creative Common Attribution License]

on cancer treatment could be more efficacious, as they can be used alone or as an adjuvant in standard chemotherapy to counter cancer cells' defense mechanisms such as MDR (Abdallah et al. 2015). The present chapter provides a brief overview of the potential the natural compounds of dietary and herbal origin hold as promising candidates in overcoming drug resistance in cancer disease.

2 Mechanisms of MDR

A diverse range of molecular mechanisms have been implicated in drug resistance; these include reduced cellular uptake of drug, increased rates of drug efflux, alterations in drug metabolism (drug inactivation and elimination), altered expression of drug targets, epigenetic events, activation of survival signaling pathways, inhibition of downstream death signaling pathways, and the influence of the local tumor microenvironment (Fig. 2). Recently, the failure of chemotherapy in certain cases has been attributed to the presence of cancer stem cells, which are intrinsically highly resistant to many therapeutic approaches (Valent et al. 2012).

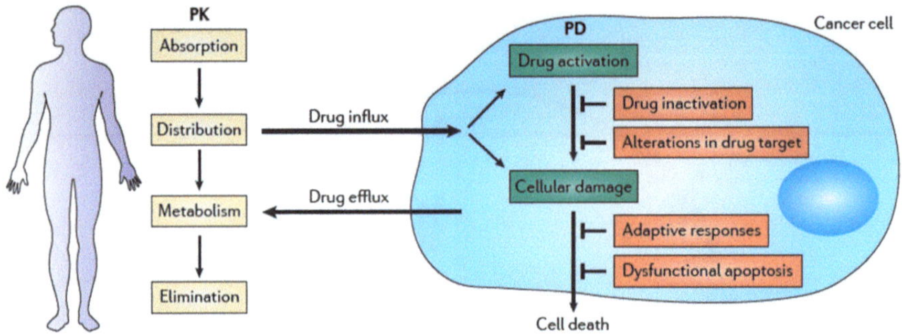

Fig. 2 General principles of drug resistance. Pharmacokinetic (PK) factors such as drug absorption, distribution, metabolism, and elimination (ADME) limit the amount of a systemically administered drug that reaches the tumor. In the tumor, the effects of the drug on the cancer cell are collectively termed its pharmacodynamic (PD) properties. The anticancer activity of a drug can be limited by poor drug influx or excessive efflux; drug inactivation or lack of activation; alterations such as changes in expression levels of the drug target; activation of adaptive prosurvival responses; and a lack of cell death induction due to dysfunctional apoptosis, which is a hallmark of cancer [Reproduced from Holohan et al. (2013) with permission of Macmillan Publishers Limited]

In case of certain solid tumors, angiogenesis is compromised (Jain 1987) leading to poor vasculatures that hinder the accessibility of the drug to the cancer cells thereby limiting the drug-induced cytotoxicity. The growth environment in which cancer cells proliferate is markedly different from that of the normal cells. Obstructed access of nutrition and hypoxia due to poor vasculature and the resultant lactic acid accumulation could confer resistance to cancer cells against drugs that act on actively dividing cells or the cellular uptake of which requires a pH gradient (Demant et al. 1990). However, the major factor observed to be responsible for multi drug resistance is the efflux of drugs across the plasma membrane by the ATP-binding (ABC) transporter family of transmembrane proteins. These are multidrug resistance protein-1 (MDR1) also known as P-glycoprotein and breast cancer resistance protein (BRCP). MDR1 over-expression has been associated with chemotherapy failure in many cancers, including kidney, colon, liver, prostate, lung, and breast cancers as well as in leukaemias and lymphomas (Holohan et al. 2013).

Drug inactivation is another mechanism of drug resistance induced by cellular xenobiotic metabolism, for example, inactivation of platinum drugs by thiol glutathione (Meijer et al. 1992). Epigenetic events that silence gene of key enzyme required for the activation of pro-drug such as methylation of gene encoding thymidine phosphorylase have also been attributed to drug resistance. An example of this kind is the resistance to capecitabine which is a prodrug that needs thymidine phosphorylase for conversion to active drug 5-FU (Kosuri et al. 2009). Alteration in drug targets such as increased expression of target proteins reduces the efficacy of inhibitors of these targets as more target molecule must be inhibited to have an effective outcome (Palmberg et al. 1997). Most of the anticancer chemotherapeutic drugs act to damage DNA in cancer cells in order to direct these cells to apoptosis.

However, cancer cells have evolved mechanisms that alter the normal cell cycle and DNA repair machinery enhancing its repair capacity and also evade the phenomenon of apoptosis thereby rendering the drug ineffective (Bouwman and Jonkers 2012). The target-associated resistance has also been observed such as gatekeeper mutations in oncogenic kinases such as that of BCR-ABL1 and T315, associated with imatinib resistance in chronic myeloid leukemia (Weisberg et al. 2005). Furthermore, recent studies have shown that cancer stem cells which might be contributing to the majority of the incidence of relapse are armed with several of these critical features responsible for drug resistance and projects emerging challenge in the premises of multidrug resistance in cancer (Holohan et al. 2013). Thus, drug resistance may be regarded as a multifaceted and dynamic phenotype which ultimately results in enhanced tumor cell survival and reduced chemo-responsiveness, regardless of the specific mechanism(s) involved.

3 Pharmacological Modulators of MDR

The pharmaceutical agents that posses the ability to reverse the resistance against anticancer drugs are called MDR inhibitors, chemosensitizers, or MDR modulators (Kellen 2003). Most of these inhibitors are targeted against P-gp transporters which were considered to be the principal factor responsible for the multidrug resistance. Accordingly, they are classified as the first, second and third generation of MDR reversal agents (Ullah 2008), with the fourth generation modulators still in infancy.

First Generation MDR Agents First-generation modulators include verapamil (calcium channel blocker), quinine (antimalarial), cyclosporine A (immunosuppressant), tamoxifen (anti-steroid), and erythromycin (Ford and Hait 1990). These drugs were not specifically developed for MDR inhibition but were used for other pharmacological interventions and coincidentally found to be effective in sensitizing the drug-resistant tumors towards chemotherapy. However, their low affinity for the transporter proteins required high doses to achieve the desired effect, which resulted in adverse effects due to enhanced toxicity to normal cells, thus undermining the overall impact on clinical management (Lampidis et al. 1986).

Second Generation MDR Agents The second generation drugs included valspodar (a non-immunosuppressive analogue of cyclosporine A) and R verapamil (R-enantiomer of verapamil, a weaker calcium channel blocker) (Hollt et al. 1992), which were designed by modification of the first generation modulators. The modifications were aimed at reducing their adverse effects by eliminating their non-MDR pharmacological action, thereby making them specific for MDR. However, within few years, the need for better MDR drug candidates arise as second generation drugs also failed to deliver the desired range of efficacy due to their low affinity for their target transporter proteins.

Third Generation MDR Agents The third generation inhibitors are designed specifically for high transport affinity and low pharmacokinetic interaction. These include tariquidar (anthranilamide derivative), biricodar (pipecolinate derivative), Annamycin (anthracycline derivative), mitotane (2,4-dichloro-diphenyldichloroethane derivative), zosuquidar (dibenzosuberane derivative), and laniquidar (benzazepine derivative) (Liscovitch and Lavie 2002). These compounds exhibit effective MDR modulatory potency, high affinity, and selectivity for target MDR transporter(s) at low nanomolar range and subsequently low toxicity towards normal cells.

It may be mentioned that first- and second-generation modulators compete as a substrate with the cytotoxic agent for transport by the P-gp pump. This limits the efflux of the cytotoxic agent, increasing its intracellular concentration. However, third-generation inhibitors of P-gp, such as tariquidar, are noncompetitive inhibitors that bind with high affinity to the pump but are not themselves substrates. This induces a conformational change in the protein, thereby preventing ATP hydrolysis and transport of the cytotoxic agent out of the cell, resulting in an increased intracellular concentration. Moreover, in response to cytotoxic agents, cytochrome P450 enzymes are also induced and aid in drug metabolism and clearance. Several of the second-generation P-gp modulators, including valspodar and biricodar, are substrates for this enzyme. These partially impair drug metabolism and elimination, significantly reduce the systemic clearance of anticancer drugs, and consequently elevate toxicity. The competition between cytotoxic drug and these P-gp modulators for cytochrome P450 3A4 activity has resulted in unpredictable pharmacokinetic interactions. MDR inhibitors such as valspodar block the cytochrome P450 3A4-mediated metabolism of paclitaxel and vinblastine resulting in increased serum concentrations of the cytotoxic agents and potentially placing patients at risk of cytotoxic drug overexposure (Thomas and Coley 2003). Third generation agents do not affect cytochrome P450 3A4 at relevant concentrations and therefore do not alter the plasma pharmacokinetics of the cytotoxic drug.

It is to be noted that an array of novel approaches are being conceived to circumvent MDR including inhibition of expression of ABC transporter by targeting mRNA through antisense oligonucleotides, hammerhead ribozymes, and siRNA in addition to transcriptional regulation, plasma membrane alteration, drug encapsulation, and antibodies (Wu et al. 2008). Novel strategy using improvised nanoparticle-based drug delivery system (DDS) has also been suggested to reverse the MDR in resistant phenotype (Fig. 3). As the cancer cells continuously evolve novel mechanisms of drug resistance which might impede the conventional therapy, a proactive approach is warranted to explore large number of MDR modulators with elevated margin of safety and desired range of efficacy. Many natural products of dietary and non-dietary origin have shown promising chemosensitizing effects on ABC drug transporters demonstrating broad-spectrum modulatory effects on more than one ABC drug transporter (Wu et al. 2008).

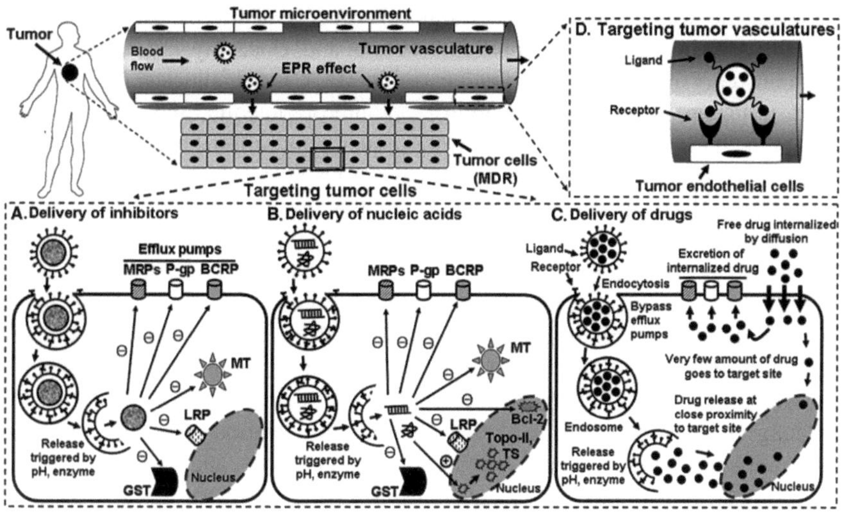

Fig. 3 Schematic representation of the application of a DDS for reversing cancer MDR. The expression of proteins or enzymes, responsible for MDR in cancer cells, can be controlled by delivering either a specific inhibitor or nucleic acids followed by the delivery of cytotoxic drug (either concurrently or separately) via a nanoparticle. The free drug, internalized by diffusion, can easily be detected by the ABC transporters and excreted out before going to the depth of the cells. Nanoparticles loaded with free drug can be endocytosed, thus permitting them to bypass the ABC transporters and deliver their payload to the target organelle where the drug exerts it action. These delivery approaches would reverse the MDR of cancer cells by making them chemosensitive [Reproduced from Kibria et al. (2014) with permission of Springer Science & Business Media]

4 Diet-Derived Factors as Potential MDR Modulators

Clinical experiences from the past have demonstrated that most of the agents from the first, second, or third generation of MDR modulators suffer clinically from their intrinsic toxicity or from undesired effects on the pharmacokinetics of the accompanying anticancer drugs (Holohan et al. 2013). These limitations have lead to continuous efforts to search for new and more productive compounds that could be effective at tolerable doses without any adverse effect. It is understood that on account of their routine intake and least toxicity, many of the natural products from fruits, vegetable, spices, and other dietary supplements are currently being investigated for their anticancer activities and their role as MDR modulators is thought to augment their efficacy against cancer (Ullah 2008). Furthermore, the enormous diversity of compounds derived from natural resources such as plants provide chemical scaffolds as lead compounds suitable for development of novel inhibitors.

The earliest observation that elicited great interest in studies related to dietary modulation of drug transporters originated from study that reported the impact of active components of fruit extracts on the outcome of clinical treatment using P-gp drug substrates (Bailey et al. 1991). Since then a large number of dietary and non-dietary plant products have been the subject of MDR studies. Flavonoids, which are the widely distributed natural constituents of human diet, have been reported as drug transporters inhibitors (Yarla and Ganapaty 2013). Apigenin, biochanin, chrysin, daidzein, epigallocatechin (EGC), epigallocatechin-3-gallate (EGCG), fisetin, genistein, hesperetin, kaempferol, luteolin, morin, myricetin, naringenin, naringin, phloretin, phloridzin, quercetin, silibin, and silymarin are the different kinds of flavonoids which have been reported as BCRP inhibitors. Among these Chrysin and biochanin A are the most potent BCRP inhibitors, producing significant increases in mitoxantrone accumulation in BCRP over-expressing cancer cell lines (Zhang et al. 2004). The diverse structure of flavonoids has been subjected to various chemical modifications in order to obtain better P-glycoprotein inhibitors. In general, it was found that modifications that increased hydrophobicity of the molecule such as prenylation or geranylation significantly increased the modulatory activity of flavonoids (Kitagawa et al. 2005).

Chung et al. (2005) have examined the effects of various flavonoids such as biochanin A, diadzein, fisetin, morin, naringenin, quercetin, and silymarin on P-gp function in human breast cancer cell lines, MCF-7 (sensitive) and MCF-7/ADR (resistant). The accumulation of daunomycin (DNM), a Pgp substrate, was greater in the sensitive cells compared to the resistant cells, while the efflux of DNM was higher in the resistant cells compared to the sensitive cells over a period of 2 h. The IC_{50} value of DNM in the resistant cells was about 22 times higher than that in the sensitive cells, indicating an over-expression of P-gp in the resistant cells, MCF-7/ ADR. Biochanin A exhibited the greatest increase in DNM accumulation while DNM accumulation with quercetin and silymarin was similar to that of a well-known P-gp inhibitor, verapamil. Biochanin A and silymarin significantly decreased the IC_{50} value of DNM, potentiating the cytotoxicity of DNM. The observation suggests that biochanin A and silymarin appear to be potent and safe P-gp inhibitors that can increase the efficacy of chemotherapeutic agents when administered concomitantly.

In a number of studies, Nabekura and coworkers have implicated the inhibitory effects of dietary nutraceuticals on the function of P-glycoprotein using multidrug-resistant human carcinoma cell line, KB-C2 (Nabekura 2010). It was shown that tea catechins (10–100 μM) increased the cellular accumulation of daunorubicin and rhodamine 123 in the order of (−)-epigallocatechin < (−)-epicatechin gallate < EGCG. Similar observation was made for curcumin which increased the accumulation of daunorubicin in KB-C2 cells in a concentration-dependant manner, induced by the inhibition of the efflux transporter (Nabekura et al. 2005). Moreover, the major metabolite of curcumin, tetrahydrocurcumin was also reported to restore drug sensitivity in cancer cells over-expressing the MDR-linked ABC transporters Pgp, MRP1, and ABCG2 (Limtrakul et al. 2007) by directly inhibiting their functions. In addition, phytochemicals like capsaicin and [6]-gingerol enhanced the susceptibility of KB-C2 cells to the cytotoxic effect of anticancer drug vinblastine by inhibiting P-glycoprotein (Nabekura et al. 2005). Citrus phytochemicals, auraptene and nobiletin at concentrations present in grapefruit and valencia orange juice, are also considered promising agents against multidrug-resistant cancer (Nabekura et al. 2008). Another citrus derived flavonoid, tangeretin, was shown to inhibit P-glycoprotein, as demonstrated by a rhodamine 123 accumulation assay and doxorubicin accumulation in multidrug-resistant (LoVo/Dx) human colon adenocarcinoma cells sensitizing them to doxorubicin (Wesołowska et al. 2012).

As described previously, many flavonoids are excellent modulators of major ABC drug transporters; these can change the overall pharmacokinetics, including drug absorption, penetration, and elimination (Yarla and Ganapaty 2013; Cermak and Wolffram 2006; Brand et al. 2006). Thus in addition to direct inhibition, many natural products overcome ABC transporter-mediated MDR by altering the bioavailability of various therapeutic drugs upon oral uptake. Transporters such as P-gp and ABCG2 are both expressed at the apical or luminal membrane of enterocytes in the intestine, which are involved in the elimination of substrate drugs and food components from inside to the outside (lumen) of the cells. Although the elimination of substrates is a physiological role of ABC transporters expressed in the intestine, this function limits the absorption of substrate drugs and food components (Wu et al. 2011). Flavonoids have the ability to modulate intestinal ABC transporters as demonstrated by the coadministration of isoflavone biochanin A with anticancer drug paclitaxel which enhanced the oral bioavailabilty and peak plasma concentration of the drug by 3.7- to 2-fold in a rat model (Peng et al. 2006). Quercetin and flavone were also shown to increase the bioavailability of paclitaxel in male SD rats (Choi et al. 2004a, b). In similar context, although apigenin is not a substrate of P-glycoprotein, it is able to inhibit the transport of other P-glycoprotein substrates and modulate drug resistance (Hadjeri et al. 2003). Apigenin may bind to P-glycoprotein without being transported. Binding of apigenin disturbs the outward transport of substrates, leading to increased intracellular accumulation of anticancer drugs and improved cell killing as shown for doxorubicin in resistant uterine sarcoma cells (MES-SA/Dx5) (Angelini et al. 2010) and resistant leukemia cells CEM/ADR5000 (Saeed et al. 2015). Furthermore, apigenin inhibited ABCB1 expression and resensitized resistant prostate cancer cells to docetaxel treatment (Zhu et al. 2013).

Resveratrol (200 nM) was also demonstrated to sensitize resistant human oral epidermoid carcinoma cell line KBv200 to vincristine, doxorubicin, and paclitaxel (Quan et al. 2008; Wesołowska 2011). Its influence on P-gp transport function and the MDR reversing activity was attributed to inhibition of *MDR1* gene expression as well as to promotion of cell apoptosis. One of the derivatives of piceatannol, 3,5,3′,4′-tetramethoxy-*trans*-stilbene, turned out to be a potent inhibitor of rhodamine 123 efflux carried out by P-gp. It also sensitized an *MDR1* gene-transfected mouse T lymphoma cell line as well as resistant human breast cancer cell line MCF-7/KCR to doxorubicin (Ferreira et al. 2006). The MDR-reversing activity of resveratrol, piceatannol, and its two synthetic derivatives has additionally been studied in drug-sensitive and doxorubicin-resistant human adenocarcinoma cell lines, LoVo and LoVo/Dx (Wesolowska et al. 2010). One MDR modulator that was effective in the resistant cell line was identified—3,5,3′,4′-tetramethoxy-*trans*-stilbene which not only inhibited P-gp-mediated rhodamine 123 transport but also significantly increased doxorubicin accumulation inside resistant cells and

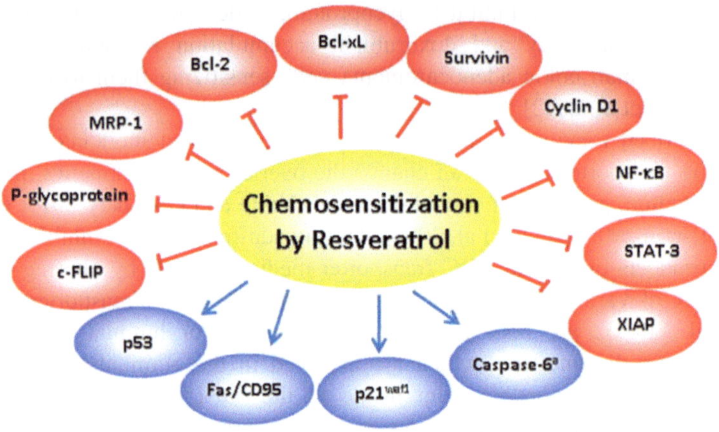

Fig. 4 Mechanism of chemosensitization of tumors by resveratrol. Resveratrol sensitizes tumor cells to chemotherapeutic agents by targeting proteins involved in cell survival, cell proliferation, and drug transport [Reproduced from Gupta et al. (2011) with permission of John Wiley and Sons]

sensitized them to the anticancer drug. Moreover, Kweon et al. (2010) have demonstrated the ability of resveratrol to reverse the resistance to doxorubicin in an MRP1-expressing acute myeloid leukemia cell line. However, this effect was attributed to resveratrol-induced downregulation of MRP1 expression and not to the interference of the stilbene with the protein's transport function. In a similar study, resveratrol was observed to reverse the MDR of resistant breast cancer cell MCF7/DOX by downregulation of MDR1 gene and P-glycoprotein expression levels (Huang et al. 2014). Interestingly, in vivo experiments in the xenograft model of MCF-7/adr revealed that treatment with a combination of resveratrol and Dox significantly inhibited tumor volume by 60 %, relative to the control group (Kim et al. 2014). The tumors shown to be sensitized by resveratrol include lung carcinoma, acute myeloid leukemia, promyelocytic leukemia, multiple myeloma, prostate cancer, oral epidermoid carcinoma, and pancreatic cancer (Gupta et al. 2011). The chemosensitization of these tumor cells by resveratrol appears to be mediated through its ability to modulate multiple cell-signaling molecules, including drug transporters, cell survival proteins, cell proliferative proteins, and members of the NF-κB and STAT3 signaling pathways (Fig. 4).

5 Conclusion

In the context of MDR, it needs to be mentioned that ABC transporters are only partial determinants of drug resistance phenotype that develops as an outcome of multicomponent system and therefore agents with multi-target efficacy are considered more significant in the queue as candidates for MDR modulator. Moreover, physiologically these transporters play a vital role in protecting the cells from xenobiotics. Altering the function of these transporters may lead to a severe physiological imbalance resulting in high toxicity which has been clinically witnessed with conventional inhibitors. The three major advantages associated with natural product derived MDR modulators particularly those of dietary origin are their diverse chemical structure (to act as lead compounds), pleiotropic (multi-target) action mechanisms, and tolerance (high index of safety) which make them suitable candidates worthy of extensive research in the premises of cancer multidrug resistance.

References

Abdallah HM, Al-Abd AM, El-Dine RS, El-Halawany AM (2015) P-glycoprotein inhibitors of natural origin as potential tumor chemosensitizers: a review. J Adv Res 6:45–62

Ambudkar S, Dey S, Hrycyna CA et al (1999) Biochemical, cellular, and pharmacological aspects of the multidrug transporter. Annu Rev Pharmacol Toxicol 39:361–398

Angelini A, Di Ilio C, Castellani ML, Conti P, Cuccurullo F (2010) Modulation of multidrug resistance p-glycoprotein activity by flavonoids and honokiol in human doxorubicin- resistant sarcoma cells (MES-SA/DX-5): implications for natural sedatives as chemosensitizing agents in cancer therapy. J Biol Regul Homeost Agents 24:197–205

Bailey DG, Spence JD, Munoz C, Arnold JM (1991) Interaction of citrus juices with felodipine and nifedipine. Lancet 337:268–269

Bouwman P, Jonkers J (2012) The effects of deregulated DNA damage signalling on cancer chemotherapy response and resistance. Nat Rev Cancer 12:587–598

Brand W, Schutte ME, Williamson G et al (2006) Flavonoid-mediated inhibition of intestinal ABC transporters may affect the oral bioavailability of drugs, food-borne toxic compounds and bioactive ingredients. Biomed Pharmacother 60:508–519

Cermak R, Wolffram S (2006) The potential of flavonoids to influence drug metabolism and pharmacokinetics by local gastrointestinal mechanisms. Curr Drug Metab 7:729–744

Chai S, To KW, Lin G (2010) Circumvention of multi-drug resistance of cancer cells by Chinese herbal medicines. Chin Med 5:26

Choi JS, Choi HK, Shin SC (2004a) Enhanced bioavailability of paclitaxel after oral co-administration with flavone in rats. Int J Pharm 275:165–170

Choi JS, Jo BW, Kim YC (2004b) Enhanced paclitaxel bioavailability after oral administration of paclitaxel or prodrug to rats pretreated with quercetin. Eur J Pharm Biopharm 57:313–318

Chung SY, Sung MK, Kim NH et al (2005) Inhibition of P-glycoprotein by natural products in human breast cancer cells. Arch Pharm Res 28:823–828

Demant EJ, Sehested M, Jensen PB (1990) A model for computer simulation of P-glycoprotein and transmembrane delta pH-mediated anthracycline transport in multi drug resistant tumor cells. Biochim Biophys Acta 1055:117–125

Eckford PDW, Sharom FJ (2009) ABC efflux pump-based resistance to chemotherapy drugs. Chem Rev 109:2989–3011

Ferreira MJ, Duarte N, Gyemant N et al (2006) Interaction between doxorubicin and the resistance modifier stilbene on multidrug resistant mouse lymphoma and human breast cancer cells. Anticancer Res 26:3541–3546

Ford JM, Hait WN (1990) Pharmacology of drugs that alter multidrug resistance in cancer. Pharmacol Rev 42:155–199

Goldie JH (2001) Drug resistance in cancer: a perspective. Cancer Metastasis Rev 20:63–68

Gottesman MM, Pastan I (1993) Biochemistry of multidrug resistance mediated by the multidrug transporter. Annu Rev Biochem 62:385–427

Gupta SC, Kannappan R, Reuter S, Kim JH, Aggarwal BB (2011) Chemosensitization of tumors by resveratrol. Ann N Y Acad Sci 1215:150–160

Hadjeri M, Barbier M, Ronot X, Mariotte AM, Boumendjel A, Boutonnat J (2003) Modulation of P-glycoprotein-mediated multidrug resistance by flavonoid derivatives and analogues. J Med Chem 46:2125–2131

Hollt V, Kouba M, Dietel M et al (1992) Stereoisomers of calcium antagonists which differ markedly in their potencies as calcium blockers are equally effective in modulating drug transport by P-glycoprotein. Biochem Pharmacol 43:2601–2608

Holohan C, Schaeybroeck SV, Longley DB, Johnston PG (2013) Cancer drug resistance: an evolving paradigm. Nat Rev Cancer 13:714–726

Huang F, Wu XN, Chen J, Wang WX, Lu ZF (2014) Resveratrol reverses multidrug resistance in human breast cancer doxorubicin-resistant cells. Exp Ther Med 7:1611–1616

Jain RK (1987) Transport of molecules in the tumour interstitium: a review. Cancer Res 47:3039–3051

Juliano RL, Ling V (1976) A surface glycoprotein modulating drug permeability in Chinese hamster ovary cell mutants. Biochim Biophys Acta 455:152–162

Kellen JA (2003) The reversal of multidrug resistance: an update. J Exp Ther Oncol 3:5–13

Kibria G, Hatakeyama H, Harashima H (2014) Cancer multidrug resistance: mechanisms involved and strategies for circumvention using a drug delivery system. Arch Pharm Res 37:4–15

Kim TH, Shin YJ, Won AJ, Lee BM, Choi WS, Jung JH, Chung HY, Kim HS (2014) Resveratrol enhances chemosensitivity of doxorubicin in multidrug-resistant human breast cancer cells via increased cellular influx of doxorubicin. Biochim Biophys Acta 1840:615–625

Kitagawa S, Nabekura T, Takahashi T, Nakamura Y, Sakamoto H (2005) Structure-activity relationship of the inhibitory effects of flavonoids on P-glycoprotein-mediated transport in KB-C2 cells. Biol Pharm Bull 28:2274–2278

Kosuri KV, Wu X, Wang L, Villalona-Calero MA, Otterson GA (2009) An epigenetic mechanism for capecitabine resistance in mesothelioma. Biochem Biophys Res Commun 391:1465–1470

Krishna R, Mayer LD (2000) Multidrug resistance (MDR) in cancer. Mechanisms, reversal using modulators of MDR and the role of MDR modulators in influencing the pharmacokinetics of anticancer drugs. Eur J Pharm Sci 11:265–283

Kweon SH, Song JH, Kim TS (2010) Resveratrol-mediated reversal of doxorubicin resistance in acute myeloid leukemia cells via downregulation of MRP1 expression. Biochem Biophys Res Commun 395:104–110

Lampidis TJ, Krishan A, Planas L et al (1986) Reversal of intrinsic resistance to adriamycin in normal cells by verapamil. Cancer Drug Deliv 3:251–259

Limtrakul P, Chearwae W, Shukla S, Phisalphong C, Ambudkar SV (2007) Modulation of function of three ABC drug transporters, P-glycoprotein (ABCB1), mitoxantrone resistance protein (ABCG2) and multidrug resistance protein 1 (ABCC1) by tetrahydrocurcumin, a major metabolite of curcumin. Mol Cell Biochem 296:85–95

Liscovitch M, Lavie Y (2002) Cancer multidrug resistance: a review of recent drug discovery research. Drugs 5:349–355

Meijer C et al (1992) Relationship of cellular glutathione to the cytotoxicity and resistance of seven platinum compounds. Cancer Res 52:6885–6889

Nabekura T (2010) Overcoming multidrug resistance in human cancer cells by natural compounds. Toxins (Basel) 2:1207–1224

Nabekura T, Kamiyama S, Kitagawa S (2005) Effects of dietary chemopreventive phytochemicals on P-glycoprotein function. Biochem Biophys Res Commun 327:866–870

Nabekura T, Yamaki T, Kitagawa S (2008) Effects of chemopreventive citrus phytochemicals on human P-glycoprotein and multidrug resistance protein 1. Eur J Pharmacol 600:45–49

Palmberg C et al (1997) Androgen receptor gene amplification in a recurrent prostate cancer after monotherapy with the nonsteroidal potent antiandrogen Casodex (bicalutamide) with a subsequent favorable response to maximal androgen blockade. Eur Urol 31:216–219
Peng SX, Ritchie DM, Cousineau M, Danser E, Dewire R, Floden J (2006) Altered oral bioavailability and pharmacokinetics of P-glycoprotein substrates by co-administration of biochanin A. J Pharm Sci 95:1984–1993
Quan F, Pan C, Ma Q, Zhang S, Yan L (2008) Reversal effect of resveratrol on multidrug resistance in KBv200 cell line. Biomed Pharmacother 62:622–629
Saeed M, Kadioglu O, Khalid H, Sugimoto Y, Efferth T (2015) Activity of the dietary flavonoid, apigenin, against multidrug-resistant tumor cells as determined by pharmacogenomics and molecular docking. J Nutr Biochem 26:44–56
Shukla S, Ohnuma S, Ambudkar SV (2011) Improving cancer chemotherapy with modulators of ABC drug transporters. Curr Drug Targets 12:621–630
Szakács G, Paterson JK, Ludwig JA, Genthe C, Gottesman MM (2006) Targeting multidrug resistance in cancer. Nat Rev Drug Discov 5:219–234
Thomas H, Coley HM (2003) Overcoming multidrug resistance in cancer: an update on the clinical strategy of inhibiting P-glycoprotein. Cancer Control 10:159–165
Ullah MF (2008) Cancer multidrug resistance (MDR): a major impediment to effective chemotherapy. Asian Pac J Cancer Prev 9:1–6
Valent P et al (2012) Cancer stem cell definitions and terminology: the devil is in the details. Nat Rev Cancer 12:767–775
Weisberg E et al (2005) Characterization of AMN107, a selective inhibitor of native and mutant Bcr-Abl. Cancer Cell 7:129–141
Wesołowska O (2011) Interaction of phenothiazines, stilbenes and flavonoids with multidrug resistance-associated transporters, P-glycoprotein and MRP1. Acta Biochim Pol 58:433–448
Wesolowska O, Wisniewski J, Bielawska-Pohl A et al (2010) Stilbenes as multidrug resistance modulators and apoptosis inducers in human adenocarcinoma cells. Anticancer Res 30:4587–4593
Wesołowska O, Wiśniewski J, Sroda-Pomianek K (2012) Multidrug resistance reversal and apoptosis induction in human colon cancer cells by some flavonoids present in citrus plants. J Nat Prod 75:1896–1902
Wu CP, Calcagno AM, Ambudkar SV (2008) Reversal of ABC drug transporter-mediated multidrug resistance in cancer cells: evaluation of current strategies. Curr Mol Pharmacol 1:93–105
Wu CP, Ohnuma S, Ambudkar SV (2011) Discovering natural product modulators to overcome multidrug resistance in cancer chemotherapy. Curr Pharm Biotechnol 12:609–620
Yarla NS, Ganapaty S (2013) Bioactive flavonoids as ABC transporters inhibitors for reversion of multidrug resistance in cancer. J Mar Sci Res Dev 4:e123
Zhang S, Yang X, Morris ME (2004) Flavonoids are inhibitors of breast cancer resistance protein (ABCG2)-mediated transport. Mol Pharmacol 65:1208–1216
Zhu Y, Liu C, Nadiminty N et al (2013) Inhibition of ABCB1 expression overcomes acquired docetaxel resistance in prostate cancer. Mol Cancer Ther 12:1829–1836

The Role of Energy Balance in Cancer Prevention

Suzanne L. Doyle, Claire L. Donohoe, and John V. Reynolds

Abstract There is a well established link between obesity and cancer. Emerging research is characterising this relationship further and delineating the specific role of excess visceral adiposity, as opposed to simple obesity, in promoting tumourigenesis. This chapter summarises the evidence from an epidemiological and pathophysiological perspective. Numerous epidemiological studies consistently identify an increased risk of developing carcinoma in the obese. Adipose tissue, particularly viscerally located fat, is metabolically active and exerts systemic endocrine effects. Putative pathophysiological mechanisms linking obesity and carcinogenesis include the paracrine effects of adipose tissue and systemic alterations associated with obesity. Systemic changes in the obese state include chronic inflammation and alterations in adipokines and sex steroids. Insulin and the insulin-like growth factor axis influence tumourigenesis and also have a complex relationship with adiposity. There is evidence to suggest that insulin and the IGF axis play an important role in mediating obesity-associated malignancy. There is much evidence to support a role for obesity in cancer progression; however, further research is warranted to determine the specific effect of excess visceral adipose tissue on tumourigenesis. Investigation of the potential mechanisms underpinning the association, including the role of insulin and the IGF axis, will improve understanding of the obesity and cancer link and may uncover targets for intervention.

S.L. Doyle • C.L. Donohoe • J.V. Reynolds (✉)
Department of Surgery, Trinity Centre for Health Sciences, St James' Hospital, Dublin 8, Ireland

Trinity College Dublin, Dublin 2, Ireland
e-mail: reynoljv@tcd.ie

M.F. Ullah, A. Ahmad (eds.), *Critical Dietary Factors in Cancer Chemoprevention*,
DOI 10.1007/978-3-319-21461-0_16

1 Epidemiology of Obesity and Cancer

Lifestyle and environmental factors affect the development of cancer (Parkin et al. 2005). The most compelling evidence to support this comes from the study of migrant populations, where cancer incidence within the population can be altered within one generation. Since not enough time has elapsed in order for significant genetic changes to account for the increased cancer incidence, it has to be attributed to environmental factors (Jemal et al. 2011). Our environment has evolved to an urban-industrialised society and with this there have been a number of inter-related changes to body composition, physical activity levels, energy balance and diet. It is these lifestyle and environmental changes which are thought to be the cause of the alteration in cancer epidemiology (Cordain et al. 2005; Eaton et al. 1988).

Worldwide, the prevalence of overweight and obesity combined rose by 27.5 % for adults between 1980 and 2013 with an estimated 2.1 billion adults currently overweight or obese (Ng et al. 2014). This pattern shows no signs of abating as obesity rates are also increasing amongst children (Ng et al. 2014), and overweight children tend to become overweight adults. Epidemiological studies have demonstrated a robust link between obesity and cancer development at numerous sites, in particular the oesophagus, pancreas, colorectum, breast (postmenopausal), endometrium and kidney (Renehan et al. 2008). The World Cancer Research Fund estimates up to 28 % of gallbladder cancers, 35 % of pancreatic, 16 % of colorectal, 17 % of breast, 49 % of endometrial, 28 % of kidney and 35 % of oesophageal cancers are attributable to obesity (World Cancer Research Fund / American Institute for Cancer Research. Food, Nutrition, Physical Activity, and the Prevention of Cancer: a Global Perspective 2007). This association carries relative risk (RR) estimates of 1.1–1.6 per 5 kg/m^2 incremental increase in BMI (Renehan et al. 2008). Obesity also increases cancer-related mortality with studies reporting that obesity could account for 14 % of all deaths from cancer in men and 20 % in women (Calle et al. 2003). Thus, the potential mechanisms by which obesity increases both the incidence of certain malignancies as well as death from malignancy have become the focus of considerable research. In addition, the quantity and location of adipose, as opposed to overall body mass, has emerged as an essential factor in the study of obesity-associated pathologies.

2 Lifestyle Factors Fuelling Obesity and Cancer

It has been estimated that ingestion of 5 % more calories than expended may result in an accumulation of 5 kg of adipose tissue in a single year (Klein et al. 2002). In developed countries where sedentary lifestyles and high energy foods are abundant, it is easy to see how energy intake exceeds that expended.

Dietary energy density describes the energy content per unit weight of food, e.g. kcal/100 g. In an age of mass production and availability of high fat, high sugar, inexpensive food, the energy density of our diets has increased (Drewnowski 2000). It has been reported that the average energy density of a typical western diet is 27 % greater (not inclusive of beverages) than the energy density of a diet adherent to healthy eating guidelines (Prentice and Jebb 2003). There is strong evidence that these convenience or "fast foods" are a cause of obesity. Increased energy density does not equal increased satiety, and it has been demonstrated that humans possess a weak innate ability to recognise foods with a high energy density and to appropriately down-regulate the bulk of food eaten in order to maintain energy homeostasis. Consequently, there is passive over-consumption of calories leading to positive energy balance (World Cancer Research Fund / American Institute for Cancer Research. Food, Nutrition, Physical Activity, and the Prevention of Cancer: a Global Perspective 2007; Prentice and Jebb 2003; Pérez-Escamilla et al. 2012; Viskaal-van Dongen et al. 2009).

This positive energy balance, if persistent, results in accumulation of adipose tissue and the development of obesity which in turn increases cancer risk. Conversely, dietary energy restriction has consistently been shown to be anti-tumourigenic. Studies of populations that engage in fasting practices have shown that it reduces oxidative damage, inflammation and levels of glucose, insulin and IGF-1, factors which all play an important role in cancer progression. The association between energy intake and cancer is further strengthened by research in animal models which demonstrates that restricted caloric intake decreases spontaneous tumour occurrence (Calle et al. 2003; Dirx et al. 2003; Hursting et al. 2013; Longo Valter and Mattson 2014).

In its comprehensive report on cancer prevention, the World Cancer Research Fund recommends limiting the consumption of energy-dense foods and avoiding sugary drinks. The public health goal is to reduce the average energy density of the diet to 125 kcal per 100 g and to reduce by half every 10 years the population average consumption of sugary drinks. Personal recommendations are to consume energy-dense foods sparingly, avoid sugary drinks and consume "fast foods" sparingly, if at all (World Cancer Research Fund / American Institute for Cancer Research. Food, Nutrition, Physical Activity, and the Prevention of Cancer: a Global Perspective 2007).

Physical inactivity is the fourth greatest contributor to mortality worldwide (Kohl et al. 2012). Occupational physical activity levels have decreased overtime, and there has been an increase in the amount of time spent in sedentary activities (Hallal et al. 2012). There is convincing evidence that physical activity reduces cancer risk, particularly breast and colorectal cancer (World Cancer Research Fund / American Institute for Cancer Research. Food, Nutrition, Physical Activity, and the Prevention of Cancer: a Global Perspective 2007; Yang and Colditz 2014). This can be attributed largely through its impact on energy expenditure and thus negative correlation with obesity. However, physical activity has also been purported to reduce cancer risk through regulation of sex hormones, insulin, and prostaglandins and reduction in pro-inflammatory markers (Kushi et al. 2012; Hamer et al. 2012).

The World Cancer Research Fund advises individuals to be physically active as part of everyday life. The public health goals are to reduce by half every 10 years the proportion of the population that is sedentary and for average physical activity levels to be above 1.6. The personal recommendations are to be moderately physically active, equivalent to brisk walking, for at least 30 min every day and to limit sedentary habits (World Cancer Research Fund / American Institute for Cancer Research. Food, Nutrition, Physical Activity, and the Prevention of Cancer: a Global Perspective 2007).

3 Adipose Tissue, the Metabolic Syndrome and Cancer

It is now well established that adipose tissue is not simply an inert energy store, but rather a metabolically active organ (Galic et al. 2010). Adipose tissue can be classified based on its location within the body. Subcutaneous adipose tissue is found under the skin, and visceral adipose tissue, which is largely comprised of omental adipose tissue but also includes other intra-abdominal fat sources such as mesenteric fat, is located within the peritoneal cavity. The different patterns in fat distribution were the first indication that adipose tissue may play a role in disease. In 1947, Jean Vague described two distinct types of fat deposition: upper-body, male-type fat (visceral) and lower-body, female-type fat (subcutaneous), and the association of visceral fat with type 2 diabetes, atherosclerosis and gout (Vague 1947, 1956). Visceral adipose tissue is more metabolically active than subcutaneous adipose tissue (Fox et al. 2007) and has multiple endocrine, metabolic and immunological functions which have been shown to be central to the pathogenesis of the metabolic syndrome (MetSyn), a pro-inflammatory, pro-coagulant state associated with insulin resistance (Galic et al. 2010). The multiple risk factors that commonly appear together as the MetSyn include abdominal obesity, atherogenic dyslipidaemia (raised triglycerides and reduced high-density lipoprotein cholesterol), elevated fasting plasma glucose and hypertension (Alberti et al. 2006). The distinct role of excess visceral adiposity in dysmetabolism is further evidenced by the observation that an increased ratio of visceral fat area to subcutaneous fat area is strongly related with disorders of glucose and lipid metabolism in obese subjects (Fujioka et al. 1987). Furthermore, visceral obesity is more strongly associated with increased risk of insulin resistance, the MetSyn and cardiovascular diseases than BMI alone (Nedungadi and Clegg 2009).

Visceral fat has been identified as an independent risk factor for breast cancer (Schapira et al. 1994), oesophageal adenocarcinoma (Beddy et al. 2010), colorectal adenocarcinoma (Schoen et al. 1999) and colorectal adenomas (Yamaji et al. 2009; Nam et al. 2010). The other elements of the MetSyn, i.e. dyslipidaemia, hypertension and insulin resistance, have also been independently linked with increased cancer risk (Cowey and Hardy 2006; Giovannucci 2007; Bowers et al. 2006; Colangelo et al. 2002). The Me-Can Study, a prospective international population-based study of 580,000 people, examined the impact of MetSyn on various cancer types (Stocks et al. 2010) and reported that it was associated with increased relative risk of colorectal cancer (Stocks et al. 2011), endometrial cancer

(Bjørge et al. 2010), oesophageal adenocarinoma (Lindkvist et al. 2014), bladder cancer (Häggström et al. 2011) and pancreatic cancer (Johansen et al. 2010). Similarly, in studies of pancreatic and colorectal cancer, a high prevalence of MetSyn, central obesity and systemic inflammation has been identified (Russo et al. 2008; Kang et al. 2009; Siegel et al. 2010) and has been shown to be associated with advanced tumour stage and reduced survival (Healy et al. 2010, 2012; Shen et al. 2010; Moon et al. 2008).

4 Mechanisms Underlying Obesity and Tumourigenesis

4.1 Altered Adipokine Production

Since the 1980s, it has been hypothesised that adipose tissue secretes factors that influence metabolism (Cook et al. 1987; Flier et al. 1987). With the discovery of the adipokines leptin (Zhang et al. 1994) and adiponectin (Scherer et al. 1995), the concept of adipose tissue as an endocrine organ was confirmed. Subsequently, a plethora of adipokines have been identified such as resistin, plasminogen activator inhibitor-1, tumour necrosis factor-α (TNF-α) and IL-6 (Ouchi et al. 2011). The altered secretion of these and other adipokines in obesity has been implicated in the pathogenesis of obesity-associated pathologies, including cancer (Ouchi et al. 2011).

Adiponectin demonstrates both anti-angiogenic and anti-inflammatory properties, and it has been shown to inhibit tumour growth in animal models (Dalamaga et al. 2012). Furthermore, studies in cancer patients have demonstrated reduced circulating levels (Rose et al. 2004) and a negative correlation with survival (Siegel et al. 2015; Duggan et al. 2011; Guadagni et al. 2009). Whilst adiponectin is the most abundant adipokine and is secreted mainly from adipocytes in visceral fat, levels are inversely correlated with obesity (Kadowaki and Yamauchi 2005). Leptin may be considered the antithesis of adiponectin. In vitro and animal studies confirm promotion of cancer cell proliferation, angiogenesis, migration and invasion (VanSaun 2013). Furthermore, in contrast to adiponectin, serum levels of leptin are positively correlated with obesity, although the relationship between circulating levels of leptin and cancer risk is not clear (Garofalo and Surmacz 2006; Grossmann and Cleary 2012; Aleksandrova et al. 2012). It is hypothesised that it is the deleterious combination of decreased production of adiponectin and increased production of leptin, in the context of visceral adiposity and the MetSyn, that drives cancer-promoting pathways including cellular proliferation, angiogenesis and metalloproteinase expression across a wide variety of cancer subtypes (Kadowaki and Yamauchi 2005; VanSaun 2013; Grossmann and Cleary 2012; Somasundar et al. 2004; Howard et al. 2010).

4.2 Visceral Obesity-Associated Inflammation and Cancer

In 1863, Virchow first hypothesised that the origin of cancer was at sites of chronic inflammation. Today we know that there is an increased risk of malignancy associated with chronic inflammation arising from carcinogenic agents (tobacco and lung cancer), autoimmune and inflammatory reactions of uncertain aetiology (ulcerative colitis and colon cancer) and infectious agents (*Helicobacter pylori* and gastrointestinal cancer, hepatitis C and liver cancer) (Balkwill and Mantovani 2001). In chronic inflammation, repeated tissue damage and regeneration in the presence of highly reactive nitrogen and oxygen species released from inflammatory cells leads to permanent genomic alterations in proliferating epithelium (Coussens and Werb 2002). Key features of cancer-related inflammation include the infiltration of immune cells and the presence of cytokines and chemokines, such as TNF-α, IL-1β, IL-6, monocyte chemotactic protein-1 (MCP-1) and IL-8 (Colotta et al. 2009). Thus, cancer-related inflammation is a key component of the tumourigenic process and is increasingly referred to as the seventh hallmark of cancer.

Excess adiposity, in particular visceral obesity, results in a state of chronic systemic low-grade inflammation, attributed to production of these inflammatory cytokines by both adipocytes and infiltrating immune cells creating a pro-tumourigenic environment (Harvey et al. 2011). Viscerally obese individuals demonstrate higher circulating levels of pro-inflammatory mediators such as C-reactive protein (CRP), TNF-α, IL-6 and MCP-1 (Fried et al. 1998; Visser et al. 1999; Weyer et al. 2002; Hotamisligil et al. 1995; Kern et al. 1995; Kim et al. 2006), and the level of this adipocytokine release is strongly influenced by immune cell populations present in adipose tissue (Schaffler et al. 2006; Xu et al. 2003; Weisberg et al. 2003; Kershaw and Flier 2004). With the expansion of adipose tissue in obesity, there is a proportional increase in the infiltration of immune cells. The recruitment of monocytes to adipose tissue is stimulated through TNF-α and MCP-1, levels of which positively correlate with obesity (Neels and Olefsky 2006). The monocytes then differentiate into activated macrophages, with a predominance of the pro-inflammatory M1 macrophage phenotype (Curat et al. 2004; Morris et al. 2011). It is this vicious cycle of adipocytokine production and immune cell infiltration that is believed to drive metabolic dysfunction, insulin resistance and inflammation in obese individuals (Sartipy and Loskutoff 2003; Wellen and Hotamisligil 2003). Research has shown that co-culture of adipocytes with macrophage-conditioned media causes increased adipokine and inflammatory cytokine production by adipocytes (Bassols et al. 2009), further supporting this hypothesis.

Whilst the majority of studies to date evaluating the immune cell properties of visceral adipose tissue have predominantly focused on macrophages, emerging research has suggested a role for T cells as key regulators of adipose tissue inflammation. Nishimura et al. reported in a murine model of diet induced obesity that there was a significant increase in $CD8^+$ T cell infiltration in expanding visceral adipose tissue, and this preceded macrophage infiltration. Furthermore, depletion of $CD8^+$ T cells lead to a reduction in macrophage infiltration (M1 phenotype) and a reduction in inflammatory mediators in visceral adipose tissue (Nishimura et al. 2009). Research has demonstrated that visceral adipose tissue is a rich source of $CD8^+$ T cells and in a study of oesophageal adenocarcinoma patients, a higher percentage of $CD4^+$ and $CD8^+$ omental T cells were found to be activated with an inflammatory T helper (Th)-1 phenotype (Lysaght et al. 2011). These findings suggest that visceral adipose tissue is a reservoir of activated T cells in cancer patients, promoting inflammation and possibly influencing cancer progression.

Recently, the role of invariant natural killer (iNKT) cells in obesity has been investigated by Lynch et al. in both human and murine studies (Lynch et al. 2009, 2012). Upon activation, iNKT cells rapidly release Th1- and Th2-type cytokines and can demonstrate cytotoxic activity (Matsuda et al. 2008). Research in human visceral adipose tissue samples demonstrated that it is a rich source of iNKT cells but levels inversely correlated with BMI. Interestingly, following weight loss, circulating levels of iNKT rise (Lynch et al. 2009). In a further study, iNKT depleted mice demonstrated enhanced weight gain and dysmetabolism, with increased adipose tissue infiltration of M1-type macrophages. To further confirm the association between iNKT cells and visceral obesity, adoptive transfer of iNKT cells into obese mice was performed, and this resulted in weight loss and improved metabolic function. Furthermore, injection of the iNKT agonist alpha-galactocylceramide into wild-type obese mice resulted in weight loss, decreased fasting glucose and decreased circulating levels of pro-inflammatory cytokines (Lynch et al. 2012).

The findings of these studies and others investigating immune cell activity in visceral obesity confirm the absolute association between excess visceral adiposity and inflammation. Chronic inflammation is a hallmark of cancer, and it may be deduced that visceral obesity increases cancer risk by creating a state of systemic inflammation that is pro-tumourigenic.

4.3 *Hyperinsulinaemia and Insulin-Like Growth Factor Axis*

A large amount of adipose tissue is associated with raised free fatty acids and insulin. Insulin can act as a mitogen and has been associated with several cancers. Epidemiological evidence has implicated colorectal cancer and insulin resistance. Colon cancer risk is increased in those who consume a diet low in fruit, vegetables and fibre and high in refined carbohydrates. It was thus proposed that this effect was mediated by insulinaemia. Specifically, it was proposed that high levels of insulin, such as in those with insulin resistance and type 2 diabetes mellitus, were related to the development of cancer (Giovannucci 1995). Cohort studies have demonstrated increased risk of colorectal cancer in those with insulin resistance (Schoen et al. 1999; Colangelo et al. 2002; Trevisan et al. 2001), the metabolic syndrome (Ahmed et al. 2006) and type 2 diabetics (Larsson et al. 2005). Interestingly, the risk of colorectal cancer in type 2 diabetes treated with insulin appears to be even higher (Yang et al. 2004).

Insulin resistance is a pre-diabetes state which is strongly related to obesity. The development of insulin resistance increases as body weight increases and is reversed with weight loss (Despres 2006). The mechanisms whereby obesity causes insulin resistance are not fully elucidated but it appears that inflammatory events are of central importance. Raised circulating free fatty acids, due to increased lipolysis in obese subjects, are a factor in the development of insulin resistance as they affect hepatic glucose production (Despres and Lemieux 2006).

The ability of a carbohydrate containing food to cause an increase in blood glucose and thus hyperinsulinaemia is measured by the glycaemic index(GI)—defined as the incremental area under the blood glucose response curve of a 50 g pure glucose load. High GI foods have been linked to excess weight gain which may be explained by a combination of factors, including a higher rate of digestion of high versus low GI foods (Brand-Miller et al. 2002). High GI foods are palatable which may lead to excess consumption. The resulting hyperinsulinaemia may promote lipogenesis, inhibit lipolysis and increase appetite (Kopp 2003). Case control studies have implicated a diet high in glycaemic index foods and a sedentary lifestyle with the risk of developing colorectal (Franceschi et al. 2001; McCarl et al. 2006; Hu et al. 1999; Higginbotham et al. 2004) and breast cancer (Augustin et al. 2001).

Although supra-physiological doses of insulin promote tumourigenesis in animal studies, these doses are not clinically relevant in humans. Epidemiological studies examining the role of type 2 Diabetes in carcinogenesis report consistent increases in cancer incidence at certain sites (liver, pancreas, endometrium, breast, colorectal, bladder, non-Hodgkin's lymphoma and kidney) (Johnson et al. 2012). Insulin acts as a growth promoter via insulin receptor signalling but whether the level of hyperinsulinaemia in patients with type 2 diabetes alone is sufficient to account for this increase in cancer incidence is not clear. There are numerous confounding factors in patients with type 2 diabetes including obesity, diet, socio-economic status, physical activity and smoking making it difficult to decipher the mechanism of carcinogenesis in these patients.

It has been proposed that some of the adverse effects of hyperinsulinaemia are mediated via activation of the insulin-like growth factor axis. Putative cancer-promoting effects of activation of the IGF axis include protection against apoptosis and increased invasiveness when the IGF1 receptor is activated (Frasca et al. 2008; Samani et al. 2007). Little direct evidence exists to support this hypothesis, however, and a large systematic review and meta-analysis of studies of serum concentrations of IGF-1 and insulin as biomarkers reveal there to be significant bias found in the studies which have been published in the literature (Tsilidis et al. 2012). Once-off serum concentrations can be highly variable between different times of the day as well as different assay types and are unlikely to meaningfully reflect activation of the IGF axis over time in individuals (Coe et al. 2014). However, increased expression of the IGF1 receptor (IGF1R) is reported in a number of cancer subtypes (Hellawell et al. 2002; Law et al. 2008; Donohoe et al. 2012). In a study of patients with oesophageal adenocarcinoma, viscerally obese patients were also more likely to have increased IGF1R mRNA expression and protein expression in their tumours, and tumour IGF1R expression correlated more strongly with waist circumference than with BMI (Donohoe et al. 2012). These data may indicate differential expression of this growth factor receptor in tumour tissue influenced by the patient's obesity status.

4.4 Obesity and Pathway Addiction

Eukaryotic cells coordinate cell growth in line with the availability of nutrients in their environment (Shaw and Cantley 2006). Obesity as a condition of both systemic insulin resistance and nutrient excess may lead to activation of intracellular pathways that promote tumour growth and progression. The systemic alterations associated with obesity include a change in inflammatory, sex hormone, insulin and adipokine secretion which may directly influence the tumour microenvironment (Donohoe et al. 2010). Cancers which arise in this environment may go on to develop progressive mutations and epigenetic alterations which are influenced by this obese milieu.

The concept of oncogene addiction describes the apparent dependency of some tumours on one or a few genes to maintain the malignant phenotype (Weinstein 2002). Clinical evidence of this is cited as the ability of therapies targeting specific genes or pathways to inhibit cancer cell growth or improve survival rates (Weinstein and Joe 2006). Whole genome arrays have demonstrated that breast cancer may be subdivided into a number of types based on the genes over-expressed in certain subtypes and that targeting these predominant pathways provides avenues for chemotherapy treatment for each subtype (Perou et al. 2000; Sørlie et al. 2003; Sawyers 2004). Molecular characterisation of tumours has been exploited to develop assays to predict subgroups of patients with poorer prognosis who may benefit from adjuvant therapy (Paik et al. 2004).

Cancers which develop within an obese environment may become selectively altered to signal via specific pathways. For examples, in patients with non-small cell lung cancer, only a subset (approximately 10–20 %) respond to the EGFR targeted therapy gefitinib—and these patients often have an activating mutation of EGFR (Lynch et al. 2004). Patients with activating mutations are more likely to have adenocarcinomas, and to be female, non-smokers and Japanese (Taron et al. 2005). Similarly, obesity-related cancers may have a specific set of targets (malfunctioning molecules or pathways) which may be exploitable in clinical practice. Certainly, a number of the putatively dysregulated adipokines and growth factors in obesity do signal via the same intracellular signalling pathways.

Candidate pathways include the phosphoinositide 3-kinase (PI3K), mitogen-activated protein kinase (MAPK) and signal transducer and activator of transcription 3 (STAT3) pathways. Activation of these pathways leads to multiple downstream effects which underpin cancer progression and metastasis (Huang et al. 2010; Yu et al. 2009; Aggarwal et al. 2009). Importantly, inhibitors of these pathways are under development at present in order to provide new therapeutic avenues (Sebolt-Leopold and Herrera 2004; Liu et al. 2009; Jing and Tweardy 2005). Resistance to targeted therapies is an ongoing issue in translational oncology (Ellis and Hicklin 2009) and the mechanisms underpinning resistance to targeted therapies will require detailed insights into the molecular signalling events associated with their use. Bypassing tyrosine kinases and instead focusing on inhibiting pathways downstream from them may be the next logical step in developing new therapeutic targets. For this strategy to be successful, biomarkers of pathway activity will need to be developed.

One hypothesised pathway which is strongly implicated in mediating the effect of the obese environment is the PI3K pathway. Many of the factors upregulated in the obese state signal via the PI3K pathway. These include leptin, IL-6, insulin, tumour necrosis factor and IGF-1. Is there any evidence that cancers which develop within the obese milieu are “addicted to” or preferentially signal via these pathways?

Whole genome analysis of breast cancer tumours divided according to body mass index demonstrates that an obesity-associated gene signature pattern is associated with a shorter time to metastasis and is associated with IGF signalling signature in multiple publically available breast cancer genome arrays (Creighton et al. 2012).

Most data to support this hypothesis are derived from mouse models. PI3K activity (measured by pAkt and mTOR protein levels) is increased in diet induced obesity in mice and is associated with an increased level of circulating IGF-1 compared to controls (Moore et al. 2008). Mice fed a high energy diet have twice the volume of tumours 17 days after colon cancer cell injection versus controls. PI3K pathway activity was demonstrated by increased phosphorylated Akt protein levels. The tumour growth effect was abrogated by metformin treatment, which led to decreased pAkt levels (Algire et al. 2010). In a mouse model of obesity-related skin cancer, obese mice had higher PI3K activity after UV exposure than lean mice (Sharma and Katiyar 2010). Activity of MAPK phosphorylation and NF-kB signalling were also higher following UVB irradiation in the leptin-deficient mice (Katiyar and Meeran 2007). In an obesity associated hepatoma model, IL-6 and TNF-alpha induce the development of cancer via activation of STAT3 pathway (Park et al. 2010). Excess energy balance associated with the obese state may influence tumour growth. Mouse tumour xenografts have decreased incidence and slower growth in mice that are fed a calorie restricted diet. Tumours which are resistant to dietary restriction have constitutive activation of the PI3K pathway (Kalaany and Sabatini 2009).

4.5 Cell Energy and Metabolism

At the cellular level, cancer cells are characterised by a change in energy production to anaerobic glycolysis which is directed by oncogenes and enhances the ability of cancer cells to proliferate (Ward and Thompson 2012). This change in metabolism represents an adaptation to the cellular environment where oxygen availability may be poor and the end products of this metabolic path can alter cell signalling and block cellular differentiation. Adipose conditioned media derived from the adipose tissue of patients with visceral obesity can induce altered mitochondrial function indicating the factors produced by the expanded fat mass in obese patients may play a role in this key characteristic of cancer cells (Lynam-Lennon et al. 2014).

References

Aggarwal BB, Kunnumakkara AB, Harikumar KB, Gupta SR, Tharakan ST, Koca C et al (2009) Signal transducer and activator of transcription-3, inflammation, and cancer. Ann N Y Acad Sci 1171:59–76

Ahmed RL, Schmitz KH, Anderson KE, Rosamond WD, Folsom AR (2006) The metabolic syndrome and risk of incident colorectal cancer. Cancer 107:28–36

Alberti KGMM, Zimmet P, Shaw J (2006) Metabolic syndrome—a new world-wide definition. A consensus statement from the international diabetes federation. Diabet Med 23:469–480

Aleksandrova K, Boeing H, Jenab M, Bueno-de-Mesquita HB, Jansen E, van Duijnhoven FJB et al (2012) Leptin and soluble leptin receptor in risk of colorectal cancer in the European prospective investigation into cancer and nutrition cohort. Cancer Res 72:5328–5337

Algire C, Amrein L, Zakikhani M, Panasci L, Pollak M (2010) Metformin blocks the stimulative effect of a high-energy diet on colon carcinoma growth in vivo and is associated with reduced expression of fatty acid synthase. Endocr Relat Cancer 17:351–360

Augustin LS, Dal Maso L, La Vecchia C, Parpinel M, Negri E, Vaccarella S et al (2001) Dietary glycemic index and glycemic load, and breast cancer risk: a case-control study. Ann Oncol 12:1533–1538

Balkwill F, Mantovani A (2001) Inflammation and cancer: back to Virchow? Lancet 357:539–545

Bassols J, Ortega FJ, Moreno-Navarrete JM, Peral B, Ricart W, Fernandez-Real JM (2009) Study of the proinflammatory role of human differentiated omental adipocytes. J Cell Biochem 107:1107–1117

Beddy P, Howard J, McMahon C, Knox M, de Blacam C, Ravi N et al (2010) Association of visceral adiposity with oesophageal and junctional adenocarcinomas. Br J Surg 97:1028–1034

Bjørge T, Stocks T, Lukanova A, Tretli S, Selmer R, Manjer J et al (2010) Metabolic syndrome and endometrial carcinoma. Am J Epidemiol 171:892–902

Bowers K, Albanes D, Limburg P, Pietinen P, Taylor PR, Virtamo J et al (2006) A prospective study of anthropometric and clinical measurements associated with insulin resistance syndrome and colorectal cancer in male smokers. Am J Epidemiol 164:652–664

Brand-Miller JC, Holt SH, Pawlak DB, McMillan J (2002) Glycemic index and obesity. Am J Clin Nutr 76:281S–285S

Calle EE, Rodriguez C, Walker-Thurmond K, Thun MJ (2003) Overweight, obesity, and mortality from cancer in a prospectively studied cohort of U.S. adults. N Engl J Med 348:1625–1638

Coe PO, O'Reilly DA, Renehan AG (2014) Excess adiposity and gastrointestinal cancer. Br J Surg 101:1518–1531

Colangelo LA, Gapstur SM, Gann PH, Dyer AR, Liu K (2002) Colorectal cancer mortality and factors related to the insulin resistance syndrome. Cancer Epidemiol Biomarkers Prev 11:385–391
Colotta F, Allavena P, Sica A, Garlanda C, Mantovani A (2009) Cancer-related inflammation, the seventh hallmark of cancer: links to genetic instability. Carcinogenesis 30:1073–1081
Cook KS, Min HY, Johnson D, Chaplinsky RJ, Flier JS, Hunt CR et al (1987) Adipsin: a circulating serine protease homolog secreted by adipose tissue and sciatic nerve. Science 237:402–405
Cordain L, Eaton SB, Sebastian A, Mann N, Lindeberg S, Watkins BA et al (2005) Origins and evolution of the Western diet: health implications for the 21st century. Am J Clin Nutr 81:341–354
Coussens LM, Werb Z (2002) Inflammation and cancer. Nature 420:860–867
Cowey S, Hardy RW (2006) The metabolic syndrome: a high-risk state for cancer? Am J Pathol 169:1505–1522
Creighton CJ, Sada YH, Zhang Y, Tsimelzon A, Wong H, Dave B et al (2012) A gene transcription signature of obesity in breast cancer. Breast Cancer Res Treat 132(3):993–1000
Curat CA, Miranville A, Sengenes C, Diehl M, Tonus C, Busse R et al (2004) From blood monocytes to adipose tissue-resident macrophages: induction of diapedesis by human mature adipocytes. Diabetes 53:1285–1292
Dalamaga M, Diakopoulos KN, Mantzoros CS (2012) The role of adiponectin in cancer: a review of current evidence. Endocr Rev 33:547–594
Despres JP (2006) Is visceral obesity the cause of the metabolic syndrome? Ann Med 38:52–63
Despres JP, Lemieux I (2006) Abdominal obesity and metabolic syndrome. Nature 444:881–887
Dirx MJM, Zeegers MPA, Dagnelie PC, van den Bogaard T, van den Brandt PA (2003) Energy restriction and the risk of spontaneous mammary tumors in mice: a meta-analysis. Int J Cancer 106:766–770
Donohoe CL, Pidgeon GP, Lysaght J, Reynolds JV (2010) Obesity and gastrointestinal cancer. B J Surg 97:628–642
Donohoe CL, Doyle SL, McGarrigle S, Cathcart MC, Daly E, O'Grady A et al (2012) Role of the insulin-like growth factor 1 axis and visceral adiposity in oesophageal adenocarcinoma. Br J Surg 99:387–396
Drewnowski A (2000) Nutrition transition and global dietary trends. Nutrition 16:486–487
Duggan C, Irwin ML, Xiao L, Henderson KD, Smith AW, Baumgartner RN et al (2011) Associations of insulin resistance and adiponectin with mortality in women with breast cancer. J Clin Oncol 29:32–39
Eaton SB, Konner M, Shostak M (1988) Stone agers in the fast lane: chronic degenerative diseases in evolutionary perspective. Am J Med 84:739–749
Ellis LM, Hicklin DJ (2009) Resistance to targeted therapies: refining anticancer therapy in the era of molecular oncology. Clin Cancer Res 15:7471–7478
Flier JS, Cook KS, Usher P, Spiegelman BM (1987) Severely impaired adipsin expression in genetic and acquired obesity. Science 237:405–408
Fox CS, Massaro JM, Hoffmann U, Pou KM, Maurovich-Horvat P, Liu C-Y et al (2007) Abdominal visceral and subcutaneous adipose tissue compartments. Circulation 116:39–48
Franceschi S, Dal Maso L, Augustin L, Negri E, Parpinel M, Boyle P et al (2001) Dietary glycemic load and colorectal cancer risk. Ann Oncol 12:173–178
Frasca F, Pandini G, Sciacca L, Pezzino V, Squatrito S, Belfiore A et al (2008) The role of insulin receptors and IGF-I receptors in cancer and other diseases. Arch Physiol Biochem 114:23–37
Fried SK, Bunkin DA, Greenberg AS (1998) Omental and subcutaneous adipose tissues of obese subjects release interleukin-6: depot difference and regulation by glucocorticoid. J Clin Endocrinol Metab 83:847–850
Fujioka S, Matsuzawa Y, Tokunaga K, Tarui S (1987) Contribution of intra-abdominal fat accumulation to the impairment of glucose and lipid metabolism in human obesity. Metabolism 36:54–59

Galic S, Oakhill JS, Steinberg GR (2010) Adipose tissue as an endocrine organ. Mol Cell Endocrinol 316:129–139
Garofalo C, Surmacz E (2006) Leptin and cancer. J Cell Physiol 207:12–22
Giovannucci E (1995) Insulin and colon cancer. Cancer Causes Control 6:164–179
Giovannucci E (2007) Metabolic syndrome, hyperinsulinemia, and colon cancer: a review. Am J Clin Nutr 86:836S–842S
Grossmann ME, Cleary MP (2012) The balance between leptin and adiponectin in the control of carcinogenesis—focus on mammary tumorigenesis. Biochimie 94:2164–2171
Guadagni F, Roselli M, Martini F, Spila A, Riondino S, D'Alessandro R et al (2009) Prognostic significance of serum adipokine levels in colorectal cancer patients. Anticancer Res 29:3321–3327
Häggström C, Stocks T, Rapp K, Bjørge T, Lindkvist B, Concin H et al (2011) Metabolic syndrome and risk of bladder cancer: prospective cohort study in the metabolic syndrome and cancer project (Me-Can). Int J Cancer 128:1890–1898
Hallal PC, Andersen LB, Bull FC, Guthold R, Haskell W, Ekelund U (2012) Global physical activity levels: surveillance progress, pitfalls, and prospects. Lancet 380:247–257
Hamer M, Sabia S, Batty GD, Shipley MJ, Tabák AG, Singh-Manoux A et al (2012) Physical activity and inflammatory markers over 10 years: follow-up in men and women from the Whitehall II Cohort Study. Circulation 126:928–933
Harvey AE, Lashinger LM, Hursting SD (2011) The growing challenge of obesity and cancer: an inflammatory issue. Ann N Y Acad Sci 1229:45–52
Healy LA, Ryan AM, Carroll P, Ennis D, Crowley V, Boyle T et al (2010) Metabolic syndrome, central obesity and insulin resistance are associated with adverse pathological features in postmenopausal breast cancer. Clin Oncol (R Coll Radiol) 22:281–288
Healy L, Howard J, Ryan A, Beddy P, Mehigan B, Stephens R et al (2012) Metabolic syndrome and leptin are associated with adverse pathological features in male colorectal cancer patients. Colorectal Dis 14:157–165
Hellawell GO, Turner GDH, Davies DR, Poulsom R, Brewster SF, Macaulay VM (2002) Expression of the type 1 insulin-like growth factor receptor is up-regulated in primary prostate cancer and commonly persists in metastatic disease. Cancer Res 62:2942–2950
Higginbotham S, Zhang ZF, Lee IM, Cook NR, Giovannucci E, Buring JE et al (2004) Dietary glycemic load and risk of colorectal cancer in the Women's Health Study. J Natl Cancer Inst 96:229–233
Hotamisligil GS, Arner P, Caro JF, Atkinson RL, Spiegelman BM (1995) Increased adipose tissue expression of tumor necrosis factor-alpha in human obesity and insulin resistance. J Clin Invest 95:2409–2415
Howard JM, Beddy P, Ennis D, Keogan M, Pidgeon GP, Reynolds JV (2010) Associations between leptin and adiponectin receptor upregulation, visceral obesity and tumour stage in oesophageal and junctional adenocarcinoma. Br J Surg 97:1020–1027
Hu FB, Manson JE, Liu S, Hunter D, Colditz GA, Michels KB et al (1999) Prospective study of adult onset diabetes mellitus (type 2) and risk of colorectal cancer in women. J Natl Cancer Inst 91:542–547
Huang P, Han J, Hui L (2010) MAPK signaling in inflammation-associated cancer development. Protein Cell 1:218–226
Hursting SD, Dunlap SM, Ford NA, Hursting MJ, Lashinger LM (2013) Calorie restriction and cancer prevention: a mechanistic perspective. Cancer Metab 1:10
Jemal A, Bray F, Center MM, Ferlay J, Ward E, Forman D (2011) Global cancer statistics. CA Cancer J Clin 61:69–90
Jing N, Tweardy DJ (2005) Targeting Stat3 in cancer therapy. Anticancer Drugs 16:601–607
Johansen D, Stocks T, Hk J, Br L, Bjørge T, Concin H et al (2010) Metabolic factors and the risk of pancreatic cancer: a prospective analysis of almost 580,000 men and women in the metabolic syndrome and cancer project. Cancer Epidemiol Biomarkers Prev 19:2307–2317

Johnson JA, Carstensen B, Witte D, Bowker SL, Lipscombe L, Renehan AG (2012) Diabetes and cancer (1): evaluating the temporal relationship between type 2 diabetes and cancer incidence. Diabetologia 55:1607–1618

Kadowaki T, Yamauchi T (2005) Adiponectin and adiponectin receptors. Endocr Rev 26:439–451

Kalaany NY, Sabatini DM (2009) Tumours with PI3K activation are resistant to dietary restriction. Nature 458:725–731

Kang HW, Kim D, Kim HJ, Kim CH, Kim YS, Park MJ et al (2009) Visceral obesity and insulin resistance as risk factors for colorectal adenoma: a cross-sectional, case-control study. Am J Gastroenterol 105:178–187

Katiyar SK, Meeran SM (2007) Obesity increases the risk of UV radiation-induced oxidative stress and activation of MAPK and NF-kappaB signaling. Free Radic Biol Med 42:299–310

Kern PA, Saghizadeh M, Ong JM, Bosch RJ, Deem R, Simsolo RB (1995) The expression of tumor necrosis factor in human adipose tissue. Regulation by obesity, weight loss, and relationship to lipoprotein lipase. J Clin Invest 95:2111–2119

Kershaw EE, Flier JS (2004) Adipose tissue as an endocrine organ. J Clin Endocrinol Metab 89:2548–2556

Kim CS, Park HS, Kawada T, Kim JH, Lim D, Hubbard NE et al (2006) Circulating levels of MCP-1 and IL-8 are elevated in human obese subjects and associated with obesity-related parameters. Int J Obes (Lond) 30:1347–1355

Klein S, Wadden T, Sugerman HJ (2002) AGA technical review on obesity. Gastroenterology 123:882–932

Kohl HW 3rd, Craig CL, Lambert EV, Inoue S, Alkandari JR, Leetongin G et al (2012) The pandemic of physical inactivity: global action for public health. Lancet 380:294–305

Kopp W (2003) High-insulinogenic nutrition—an etiologic factor for obesity and the metabolic syndrome? Metabolism 52:840–844

Kushi LH, Doyle C, McCullough M, Rock CL, Demark-Wahnefried W, Bandera EV et al (2012) American Cancer Society guidelines on nutrition and physical activity for cancer prevention. CA Cancer J Clin 62:30–67

Larsson SC, Orsini N, Wolk A (2005) Diabetes mellitus and risk of colorectal cancer: a meta-analysis. J Natl Cancer Inst 97:1679–1687

Law JH, Habibi G, Hu K, Masoudi H, Wang MYC, Stratford AL et al (2008) Phosphorylated insulin-like growth factor-1/insulin receptor is present in all breast cancer subtypes and is related to poor survival. Cancer Res 68:10238–10246

Lindkvist B, Johansen D, Stocks T, Concin H, Bjørge T, Almquist M et al (2014) Metabolic risk factors for esophageal squamous cell carcinoma and adenocarcinoma: a prospective study of 580,000 subjects within the Me-Can project. BMC Cancer 14:103

Liu P, Cheng H, Roberts TM, Zhao JJ (2009) Targeting the phosphoinositide 3-kinase pathway in cancer. Nat Rev Drug Discov 8:627–644

Longo Valter D, Mattson MP (2014) Fasting: molecular mechanisms and clinical applications. Cell Metab 19:181–192

Lynam-Lennon N, Connaughton R, Carr E, Mongan AM, O'Farrell NJ, Porter RK et al (2014) Excess visceral adiposity induces alterations in mitochondrial function and energy metabolism in esophageal adenocarcinoma. BMC Cancer 14:907

Lynch TJ, Bell DW, Sordella R, Gurubhagavatula S, Okimoto RA, Brannigan BW et al (2004) Activating mutations in the epidermal growth factor receptor underlying responsiveness of non-small-cell lung cancer to gefitinib. N Engl J Med 350:2129–2139

Lynch L, O'Shea D, Winter DC, Geoghegan J, Doherty DG, O'Farrelly C (2009) Invariant NKT cells and CD1d(+) cells amass in human omentum and are depleted in patients with cancer and obesity. Eur J Immunol 39:1893–1901

Lynch L, Nowak M, Varghese B, Clark J, Hogan AE, Toxavidis V et al (2012) Adipose tissue invariant NKT cells protect against diet-induced obesity and metabolic disorder through regulatory cytokine production. Immunity 37:574–587

Lysaght J, Allott EH, Donohoe CL, Howard JM, Pidgeon GP, Reynolds JV (2011) T lymphocyte activation in visceral adipose tissue of patients with oesophageal adenocarcinoma. Br J Surg 98:964–974
Matsuda JL, Mallevaey T, Scott-Browne J, Gapin L (2008) CD1d-restricted iNKT cells, the 'Swiss-Army knife' of the immune system. Curr Opin Immunol 20:358–368
McCarl M, Harnack L, Limburg PJ, Anderson KE, Folsom AR (2006) Incidence of colorectal cancer in relation to glycemic index and load in a cohort of women. Cancer Epidemiol Biomarkers Prev 15:892–896
Moon H-G, Ju Y-T, Jeong C-Y, Jung E-J, Lee Y-J, Hong S-C et al (2008) Visceral obesity may affect oncologic outcome in patients with colorectal cancer. Ann Surg Oncol 15:1918–1922
Moore T, Beltran L, Carbajal S, Strom S, Traag J, Hursting SD et al (2008) Dietary energy balance modulates signaling through the Akt/mammalian target of rapamycin pathways in multiple epithelial tissues. Cancer Prev Res 1:65–76
Morris DL, Singer K, Lumeng CN (2011) Adipose tissue macrophages: phenotypic plasticity and diversity in lean and obese states. Curr Opin Clin Nutr Metab Care 14:341–346
Nam SY, Kim BC, Han KS, Ryu KH, Park BJ, Kim HB et al (2010) Abdominal visceral adipose tissue predicts risk of colorectal adenoma in both sexes. Clinical Gastroenterology and Hepatology 8:443.e2–450.e2
Nedungadi TP, Clegg DJ (2009) Sexual dimorphism in body fat distribution and risk for cardiovascular diseases. J Cardiovasc Transl Res 2:321–327
Neels JG, Olefsky JM (2006) Inflamed fat: what starts the fire? J Clin Invest 116:33–35
Ng M, Fleming T, Robinson M, Thomson B, Graetz N, Margono C et al (2014) Global, regional, and national prevalence of overweight and obesity in children and adults during 1980–2013: a systematic analysis for the Global Burden of Disease Study 2013. Lancet 384:766–781
Nishimura S, Manabe I, Nagasaki M, Eto K, Yamashita H, Ohsugi M et al (2009) CD8+ effector T cells contribute to macrophage recruitment and adipose tissue inflammation in obesity. Nat Med 15:914–920
Ouchi N, Parker JL, Lugus JJ, Walsh K (2011) Adipokines in inflammation and metabolic disease. Nat Rev Immunol 11:85–97
Paik S, Shak S, Tang G, Kim C, Baker J, Cronin M et al (2004) A multigene assay to predict recurrence of tamoxifen-treated, node-negative breast cancer. N Engl J Med 351:2817–2826
Park EJ, Lee JH, Yu G-Y, He G, Ali SR, Holzer RG et al (2010) Dietary and genetic obesity promote liver inflammation and tumorigenesis by enhancing IL-6 and TNF expression. Cell 140:197–208
Parkin DM, Bray F, Ferlay J, Pisani P (2005) Global cancer statistics, 2002. CA Cancer J Clin 55:74–108
Pérez-Escamilla R, Obbagy JE, Altman JM, Essery EV, McGrane MM, Wong YP et al (2012) Dietary energy density and body weight in adults and children: a systematic review. J Acad Nutr Diet 112:671–684
Perou CM, Sorlie T, Eisen MB, van de Rijn M, Jeffrey SS, Rees CA et al (2000) Molecular portraits of human breast tumours. Nature 406:747–752
Prentice AM, Jebb SA (2003) Fast foods, energy density and obesity: a possible mechanistic link. Obes Rev 4:187–194
Renehan AG, Tyson M, Egger M, Heller RF, Zwahlen M (2008) Body-mass index and incidence of cancer: a systematic review and meta-analysis of prospective observational studies. Lancet 371:569–578
Rose DP, Komninou D, Stephenson GD (2004) Obesity, adipocytokines, and insulin resistance in breast cancer. Obes Rev 5:153–165
Russo A, Autelitano M, Bisanti L (2008) Metabolic syndrome and cancer risk. Eur J Cancer 44:293–297
Samani AA, Yakar S, LeRoith D, Brodt P (2007) The role of the IGF system in cancer growth and metastasis: overview and recent insights. Endocr Rev 28:20–47

Sartipy P, Loskutoff DJ (2003) Monocyte chemoattractant protein 1 in obesity and insulin resistance. Proc Natl Acad Sci U S A 100:7265–7270
Sawyers C (2004) Targeted cancer therapy. Nature 432:294–297
Schaffler A, Muller-Ladner U, Scholmerich J, Buchler C (2006) Role of adipose tissue as an inflammatory organ in human diseases. Endocr Rev 27:449–467
Schapira DV, Clark RA, Wolff PA, Jarrett AR, Kumar NB, Aziz NM (1994) Visceral obesity and breast cancer risk. Cancer 74:632–639
Scherer PE, Williams S, Fogliano M, Baldini G, Lodish HF (1995) A novel serum protein similar to c1q, produced exclusively in adipocytes. J Biol Chem 270:26746–26749
Schoen RE, Tangen CM, Kuller LH, Burke GL, Cushman M, Tracy RP et al (1999) Increased blood glucose and insulin, body size, and incident colorectal cancer. J Natl Cancer Inst 91:1147–1154
Sebolt-Leopold JS, Herrera R (2004) Targeting the mitogen-activated protein kinase cascade to treat cancer. Nat Rev Cancer 4:937–947
Sharma SD, Katiyar SK (2010) Leptin deficiency-induced obesity exacerbates ultraviolet B radiation-induced cyclooxygenase-2 expression and cell survival signals in ultraviolet B-irradiated mouse skin. Toxicol Appl Pharmacol 244:328–335
Shaw RJ, Cantley LC (2006) Ras, PI(3)K and mTOR signalling controls tumour cell growth. Nature 441:424–430
Shen Z, Wang S, Ye Y, Yin M, Yang X, Jiang K et al (2010) Clinical study on the correlation between metabolic syndrome and colorectal carcinoma. ANZ J Surg 80:331–336
Siegel EM, Ulrich CM, Poole EM, Holmes RS, Jacobsen PB, Shibata D (2010) The effects of obesity and obesity-related conditions on colorectal cancer prognosis. Cancer Control 17:52–57
Siegel AB, Goyal A, Salomao M, Wang S, Lee V, Hsu C et al (2015) Serum adiponectin is associated with worsened overall survival in a prospective cohort of hepatocellular carcinoma patients. Oncology 88:57–68
Somasundar P, McFadden DW, Hileman SM, Vona-Davis L (2004) Leptin is a growth factor in cancer. J Surg Res 116:337–349
Sørlie T, Tibshirani R, Parker J, Hastie T, Marron JS, Nobel A et al (2003) Repeated observation of breast tumor subtypes in independent gene expression data sets. Proc Natl Acad Sci 100:8418–8423
Stocks T, Borena W, Strohmaier S, Bjørge T, Manjer J, Engeland A et al (2010) Cohort profile: the metabolic syndrome and cancer project (Me-Can). Int J Epidemiol 39:660–667
Stocks T, Lukanova A, Bjørge T, Ulmer H, Manjer J, Almquist M et al (2011) Metabolic factors and the risk of colorectal cancer in 580,000 men and women in the metabolic syndrome and cancer project (Me-Can). Cancer 117:2398–2407
Taron M, Ichinose Y, Rosell R, Mok T, Massuti B, Zamora L et al (2005) Activating mutations in the tyrosine kinase domain of the epidermal growth factor receptor are associated with improved survival in gefitinib-treated chemorefractory lung adenocarcinomas. Clin Cancer Res 11:5878–5885
Trevisan M, Liu J, Muti P, Misciagna G, Menotti A, Fucci F (2001) Markers of insulin resistance and colorectal cancer mortality. Cancer Epidemiol Biomarkers Prev 10:937–941
Tsilidis KK, Papatheodorou SI, Evangelou E, Ioannidis JPA (2012) Evaluation of excess statistical significance in meta-analyses of 98 biomarker associations with cancer risk. J Natl Cancer Inst 104:1867–1878
Vague J (1947) La differenciation sexuelle, facteur determinant des formes de l'obesité. Presse Med 53:339–340
Vague J (1956) The degree of masculine differentiation of obesities: a factor determining predisposition to diabetes, atherosclerosis, gout, and uric calculous disease. Obes Res 4:204–212
VanSaun MN (2013) Molecular pathways: adiponectin and leptin signaling in cancer. Clin Cancer Res 19:1926–1932

Viskaal-van Dongen M, de Graaf C, Siebelink E, Kok FJ (2009) Hidden fat facilitates passive overconsumption. J Nutr 139:394–399

Visser M, Bouter LM, McQuillan GM, Wener MH, Harris TB (1999) Elevated C-reactive protein levels in overweight and obese adults. JAMA 282:2131–2135

Ward PS, Thompson CB (2012) Metabolic reprogramming: a cancer hallmark even Warburg did not anticipate. Cancer Cell 21:297–308

Weinstein IB (2002) Addiction to oncogenes—the Achilles heal of cancer. Science 297:63–64

Weinstein IB, Joe AK (2006) Mechanisms of Disease: oncogene addiction—a rationale for molecular targeting in cancer therapy. Nat Clin Pract Oncol 3:448–457

Weisberg SP, McCann D, Desai M, Rosenbaum M, Leibel RL, Ferrante AW Jr (2003) Obesity is associated with macrophage accumulation in adipose tissue. J Clin Invest 112:1796–1808

Wellen KE, Hotamisligil GS (2003) Obesity-induced inflammatory changes in adipose tissue. J Clin Invest 112:1785–1788

Weyer C, Yudkin JS, Stehouwer CD, Schalkwijk CG, Pratley RE, Tataranni PA (2002) Humoral markers of inflammation and endothelial dysfunction in relation to adiposity and in vivo insulin action in Pima Indians. Atherosclerosis 161:233–242

World Cancer Research Fund / American Institute for Cancer Research (2007). Food, Nutrition, Physical Activity, and the Prevention of Cancer: a Global Perspective. Washington DC: AICR

Xu H, Barnes GT, Yang Q, Tan G, Yang D, Chou CJ et al (2003) Chronic inflammation in fat plays a crucial role in the development of obesity-related insulin resistance. J Clin Invest 112:1821–1830

Yamaji T, Iwasaki M, Sasazuki S, Kurahashi N, Mutoh M, Yamamoto S et al (2009) Visceral fat volume and the prevalence of colorectal adenoma. Am J Epidemiol 170:1502–1511

Yang L, Colditz GA (2014) An active lifestyle for cancer prevention. J Natl Cancer Inst 106: dju135

Yang YX, Hennessy S, Lewis JD (2004) Insulin therapy and colorectal cancer risk among type 2 diabetes mellitus patients. Gastroenterology 127:1044–1050

Yu H, Pardoll D, Jove R (2009) STATs in cancer inflammation and immunity: a leading role for STAT3. Nat Rev Cancer 9:798–809

Zhang Y, Proenca R, Maffei M, Barone M, Leopold L, Friedman JM (1994) Positional cloning of the mouse obese gene and its human homologue. Nature 372:425–432

Dietary/Environmental Factors and Breast Cancer

Michel de Lorgeril and Patricia Salen

Abstract Adhering to a healthy dietary pattern—specifically the modernized Mediterranean diet—may be critical to reduce breast cancer (BC) risk in high-risk women and in women who wish to decrease their BC risk. In the context of the Mediterranean diet, it is important to increase plant and marine n-3 and decrease plant and animal n-6. High flavonoid intake—which increases n-3—should be encouraged as it is associated with lower BC risk. To reduce insulin resistance and diabetes—which are associated with an increased BC risk—women should increase fiber consumption and favor low-GI foods. Women should choose organic foods because of their effect on the n-3/n-6 ratio and because they contain fewer contaminants—and lower levels of each contaminant—in particular endocrine disruptors. Finally, any drug thought to increase diabetes and/or BC risk—in particular, the statins and certain antihypertensive medications—should be prohibited. To lower blood pressure or to decrease the risk of cardiovascular disease, physicians do have lifestyle strategies, and it would be tragically unwise to persist in prescribing anticholesterol statins and antihypertensive drugs in women wishing to decrease their BC risk.

Abbreviations

BC	Breast cancer
n-3	Omega-3 fatty acids
n-6	Omega-6 fatty acids
GI	Glycemic index

M. de Lorgeril (✉) • P. Salen
Laboratoire TIMC-IMAG, CNRS UMR 5525, PRETA Cœur & Nutrition, and Faculté de Médecine, Université Joseph Fourier, Grenoble, France
e-mail: michel.delorgeril@ujf-grenoble.fr; patricia.salen@ujf-grenoble.fr

M.F. Ullah, A. Ahmad (eds.), *Critical Dietary Factors in Cancer Chemoprevention*,
DOI 10.1007/978-3-319-21461-0_17

1 Introduction

Breast cancer (BC) is the most frequent cancer in women and a leading cause of death from cancer (Matsen and Neumayer 2013). A critical issue is to implement a preventive strategy (Eccles et al. 2013). Genetic predisposition cannot be modified but other factors—unhealthy diet, sedentary lifestyle for instance—can be avoided (http://www.cancer.gov/bcrisktool/ (Assessed April 8 2014). Other strategies—for instance decreasing estrogen exposition—may help prevent BC but is difficult to implement (http://www.cancer.gov/cancertopics/pdq/prevention/breast/patient (Assessed April 8 2014). Increasing protective factors, such as dietary factors, is also critical, in particular among high-risk women (http://www.cancer.gov/bcrisktool/ (Assessed April 8 2014).

2 Dietary Fats, Omega-6, Omega-3, and Their Ratio

Dietary fats have been studied in the prevention of BC (Khaw 2013; Alexander et al. 2010; Prentice et al. 2006) but only marine omega-3 fatty acids (n-3) seem to be protective (Khaw 2013). In a meta-analysis of more than 20 cohort studies, a significant reduction of BC risk was found with n-3 (Zheng et al. 2013) whereas omega-6 fatty acids (n-6) may increase risk (Zock and Katan 1998; de Lorgeril and Salen 2012). The carcinogenetic effect of n-6 was also suggested in controlled trials where n-6 intakes were modified (Pearce and Dayton 1971; de Lorgeril et al. 1998). These trials were too small to analyze specific cancers (such as BC) rather the incidence of cancers in general. However, in the same way as smoking increases the risk of several cancers—lung and bladder for instance—these trials indicate that n-6 may increase the risk of several cancers, and it is reasonable to think that n-6 increases BC risk as epidemiological studies did suggest (de Lorgeril and Salen 2012).

It means that both n-6 and n-3 may contribute to BC risk but in opposite directions. As these fatty acids are both present in various oils and foods, their opposite effects may introduce confusion in the analyses. Thus, when analyzing the associations between n-3 and BC risk, it is critical that n-6 is included in the analyses as Yang et al. did (Yang et al. 2014). They used the ratio of n-3/n-6 in a meta-analysis including 274,135 women from 11 prospective studies. Women with a higher n-3/n-6 ratio had a significantly lower risk of BC compared to women with low n-3/n-6 ratio (Yang et al. 2014).

This means that all the factors (including medical drug) influencing the n-3/n-6 ratio are critical in BC risk (de Lorgeril and Salen 2014). Increased intake of n-3 and decreased intake of n-6 through consumption of foods rich in n-3 and poor in n-6 (de Lorgeril and Salen 2012; Meyer et al. 2003)—resulting in higher n-3/n-6 ratio—are therefore important to decrease BC risk (Yang et al. 2014; de Lorgeril and Salen 2014).

In the same way, it has been shown that polyphenol flavonoids increase n-3 by about 30 % without increasing n-6 (Toufektsian et al. 2011; di Giuseppe et al. 2009; de Lorgeril et al. 2008). This results in a significant increase in the n-3/n-6 ratio. As expected on the basis of that polyphenol/fat interaction, consumption of flavonoids was shown to be associated with a decreased BC risk (Hui et al. 2013; Bosetti et al. 2005).

Organic plant foods contain more polyphenols than similar conventional foods (Dangour et al. 2009; Benbrook et al. 2008, 2009; Hallmann et al. 2013), which suggests that organic foods may contribute to decrease BC risk through an effect on the n-3/n-6 ratio. In the same way, organic animal fat—for instance milk and milk products (Benbrook et al. 2013; Ellis et al. 2006; Tsiplakou et al. 2010)—does have a higher n-3/n-6 ratio compared with conventional products. Thus, women who wish to decrease their BC risk should select plant and animal organic foods.

Conventional foods contain more contaminants than organic foods. Do food contaminants increase BC risk? A report from the American Institute of Medicine states that none of the potentially carcinogenetic contaminants, including organochlorine pesticides and polychlorinated biphenyls (PCBs), is linked to BC risk (Smith-Bindman 2012). However, recent studies showing strong association between estrogenic-like PCB congeners or dioxin and BC risk (Recio-Vega et al. 2011; Cohn et al. 2012; Warner et al. 2011) do not confirm that statement. While further studies are needed, including studies of polymorphisms in the cytochrome P450 1A1 (CYP1A1) gene (Sergentanis and Economopoulos 2010)—a confounding factor when studying the associations between PCBs and BC risk—these data are not reassuring. Actually CYP1A1 is a member of the CYP1 family and is involved in the metabolism of many xenobiotics including PCBs and dioxin. The study pointed to the A2455G allele as a risk factor of BC among Caucasian women (Sergentanis and Economopoulos 2010). Further analyses of the relations between estrogenic PCB congeners and BC risk should include CYP1A1 polymorphisms as a potential marker of predisposition to BC.

In this context, it is critical to recall that endocrine disruptors—such as phthalates—increase insulin resistance, diabetes, and obesity (Lind et al. 2012; Stahlhut et al. 2007; Hatch et al. 2010), all of which increase BC risk (see below).

Other substances that influence both n-3/n-6 ratio and BC risk are the cholesterol-lowering statins. The effect of statins on cancer risk is a long and controversial story (Bonovas et al. 2005; Ravnskov et al. 2012; Alsheikh-Ali et al. 2007). It began in 1996 with the publication of the CARE trial, a trial evaluating (vs. a placebo) the effects of a statin against cardiac and cerebral ischemic complications (Sacks et al. 1996). Unexpectedly, 12 out of 286 women in the statin group but only 1 out of 290 in the placebo group had BC at follow-up (Sacks et al. 1996). The difference was statistically significant but curiously attributed to chance.

After that, however, most statin investigators took care not to include high-risk women in their trials (Ravnskov et al. 2012) and carefully monitored them through repeated interim analyses for early detection of intergroup difference trends in cancer incidence. To further confuse the data, many statin trials were prematurely terminated—not all have been published—without valid justification raising the possibility that they did so to mask the reality. Cancers diagnosed during short-term drug trials are more likely to be dormant cancers that are "invited" to clinically surface under the effect of the treatment. As the process requires a minimal length of exposure, premature termination is the best way of avoiding the cancer issue in relation to any investigated drug. In that context, premature termination seems to be an intentional flaw that leads to confusion and prevents clarification of whether the investigated drug may increase cancer risk in the nonselected general population in whom the drug is then prescribed without precaution by unaware physicians. Despite this, a meta-analysis published in 2006 found a (nonsignificant) 33 % increase in BC incidence with statins compared with a placebo (Dale et al. 2006). We note that confidence intervals were large in that meta-analysis, that there was a great heterogeneity between trials (which may reduce statistical significance), and that curiously only 5 of the 26 trials included in the analysis reported BC data (Dale et al. 2006) suggesting a lack of completeness of reporting harm effect, a well-known source of bias (Song et al. 2010). In view of the inherent limitations of randomized trials discussed above, in particular premature termination and short follow-up, data from observational studies are critical to examine the statin/BC relations.

In fact, meta-analyses of epidemiological studies reported no significant association between statin use and BC risk. However, since high cholesterol may reduce cancer risk, and as patients taking statins have spent most of their lives with high cholesterol—which is thought to lower cancer risk (Ravnskov et al. 2012)—observational epidemiology is also facing difficulty in identifying statin cancer signals. Thus, even a lack of difference in BC risk between statin users and nonusers in observational studies may suggest that statins actually increase BC risk. The demonstration that long-term (10-year) statin use is associated with a twofold increase in BC risk among postmenopausal women (McDougall et al. 2013) confirms the previous data (Bonovas et al. 2005; Ravnskov et al. 2012; Alsheikh-Ali et al. 2007; Sacks et al. 1996; Dale et al. 2006) and strongly suggests that statins and cholesterol lowering increase BC risk.

Regarding statins and BC recurrence, a recent study suggests that one particular highly lipophilic statin (simvastatin) may be associated with a reduced risk (Ahern et al. 2011). However, the study suffers major limitations: the duration of exposure was short (a median of 4 years), the numbers of recurrences were small ($n = 249$ among statin users) and statin users and non-users were very different at baseline, rendering adjustments and between-group comparison problematic. Still more important [as discussed above and admitted by the authors (Ahern et al. 2011)], confounding by indication likely explains their data (Bosco et al. 2010): the major indication for statin therapy is hypercholesterolemia which is inherently associated with lower risk of BC recurrence (Ozdemir et al. 2004).

2.1 What About the Biological Mechanisms to Explain the Cancer Effect of Statins?

Statins are known to interfere with the metabolism of n-3 and n-6—i.e., statins decrease the n-3/n-6 ratio (Jula et al. 2005; de Lorgeril et al. 2005; Harris et al. 2004)—which may in turn increase BC risk (Yang et al. 2014; de Lorgeril and Salen 2014). Statins lower blood cholesterol, and low blood cholesterol is often (but not always) associated with a high cancer rate (Ravnskov et al. 2012). Inconsistency in the blood cholesterol-cancer data likely reflects the existence of confounding factors. One of these factors could be insulin resistance (Osaki et al. 2012; Strohmaier et al. 2013). The *Metabolic Syndrome and Cancer Project* (Me-Can)—with more than 577,000 participants and a follow-up of 12 years—reported that cholesterol is negatively associated with BC risk (Strohmaier et al. 2013) confirming the low cholesterol–cancer relation. Also, it has been shown that a substance arising from cholesterol (dendrogenin A) is a key factor in the development of human BC (de Medina et al. 2013) reinforcing the theory that high cholesterol may be protective. Statins are toxic to mitochondria (Sirvent et al. 2012; Kaufmann et al. 2006), and mitochondrial dysfunction contributes to tumorigenesis and cancer progression (Wallace 2012; Cuezva et al. 2002). Converging evidence supports that statins increase insulin resistance and new-onset diabetes possibly (but not only) through mitochondrial toxicity in the muscles and other tissues (Golomb et al. 2012; Larsen et al. 2013; Bouitbir et al. 2011; Koh et al. 2010). This side effect of statins is usually underestimated (Ridker et al. 2012), and trials upon which this underestimation is based are flawed (de Lorgeril et al. 2010, 2013). Other studies indicate significant increases of diabetes risk among statin users (Carter et al. 2013; Zaharan et al. 2013), culminating in a 70 % increase among women (Culver et al. 2012). At the same time, it was learned that diabetes increases BC risk (Boyle et al. 2012; Redaniel et al. 2012) as well as the overall risk of cancers and cancer death (Collaboration et al. 2011). As statins increases insulin resistance, it is critical that metabolic syndromes are associated with BC risk (Gunter et al. 2009; Rosato et al. 2011; Minicozzi et al. 2013; Agnoli et al. 2010).

Recently, investigators curiously claimed that hypercholesterolemia is a risk factor for BC and that lowering cholesterol in animals is a useful strategy to prevent BC (Nelson et al. 2013). Studies using more humanized models are required before these data could have any clinical impact. Finally, statins were shown to increase immune regulatory T cells (Tregs) which in turn may hinder the antitumor defenses and increase BC risk (Goldstein et al. 2009).

Thus, through increased insulin resistance and new-onset diabetes, decreased n-3/n-6 ratio, cholesterol lowering, mitochondrial toxicity, and immunomodulatory effect, statins may increase BC risk. Statin use results in skeletal muscle toxicity and decreased physical activity (Golomb et al. 2012; Larsen et al. 2013; Bouitbir et al. 2011). In the same time, international Guidelines (Matsen and Neumayer 2013; Eccles et al. 2013; http://www.cancer.gov/bcrisktool/ (Assessed April

8 2014) recommend that women should try having optimal physical activity which is known to decrease both diabetes (Dengel et al. 1998; Smutok et al. 1993) and BC (Matsen and Neumayer 2013; Eccles et al. 2013; http://www.cancer.gov/bcrisktool/ (Assessed April 8 2014; http://www.cancer.gov/cancertopics/pdq/prevention/ breast/patient (Assessed April 8 2014) risks.

Guidelines to prevent BC also recommend that women limit weight gain (Matsen and Neumayer 2013; Eccles et al. 2013; http://www.cancer.gov/bcrisktool/ (Assessed April 8 2014). The report showing a rapid increase in body mass index among statin users compared with nonusers is of concern (Sugiyama et al. 2014). Whatever the cause of weight gain—reduced physical activity in relation with the statin-induced muscle toxicity (Golomb et al. 2012; Larsen et al. 2013; Bouitbir et al. 2011), increased insulin resistance, or increased energy intake (Sugiyama et al. 2014)—this may contribute to the increased risk of BC with statins.

3 Other Lifestyle Factors and BC Risk

As diabetes increases BC risk, all factors that increase diabetes risk are important. Increased fiber intake, consumption of flavonoids, and n-3 are all inversely associated with diabetes risk (Yao et al. 2014; Zamora-Ros et al. 2014; Zheng et al. 2012; Djoussé et al. 2011; Brostow et al. 2011). Not surprisingly, fiber intake (Suzuki et al. 2008; Zhang et al. 2011; Ferrari et al. 2013; Park et al. 2009), flavonoids (Hui et al. 2013; Bosetti et al. 2005), and n-3 (Zheng et al. 2013; de Lorgeril and Salen 2012, 2014; Yang et al. 2014) have all been shown inversely associated with BC risk.

In the same way of reasoning, consumption of foods with a low glycemic index (GI) is associated with both lower diabetes (Oba et al. 2013; Salmerón et al. 1997) and BC (Choi et al. 2012; Dong and Qin 2011; Lajous et al. 2008; Sieri et al. 2007) risks.

The Mediterranean diet, the traditional dietary habits of people living around the Mediterranean Sea, is a well-known healthy dietary pattern (de Lorgeril 2013). A modernized version of that dietary pattern has been tested in randomized trials and was shown to result in health benefits (de Lorgeril 2013; de Lorgeril et al. 1999). The combination of high fiber, high n-3/n-6 ratio, high polyphenols, and low-GI foods definitely represents a healthy dietary pattern. Adoption of such a healthy diet is associated with lower BC risk (Brennan et al. 2010; Männistö et al. 2005; Cottet et al. 2009; Link et al. 2013; Sieri et al. 2004). Among women with early-stage breast cancer, adoption of such a healthy diet was associated with lower risk of mortality and lower non-breast cancer causes of death (Kwan et al. 2009).

More specifically, increased adherence to the Mediterranean diet pattern is also clearly associated with fewer cancers (Grosso et al. 2013), specifically fewer pancreatic (Bosetti et al. 2013), gastric (Praud et al. 2014), colorectal (Bamia et al. 2013), hepatocellular (Turati et al. 2014), prostate (Kenfield et al. 2014), and breast (Buckland et al. 2013; Demetriou et al. 2012; Trichopoulou et al. 2010) cancers. This is not surprising as the Mediterranean diet increases the n-3/n-6 ratio on the one hand (de Lorgeril and Salen 2012; de Lorgeril 2013) and on the other hand decreases the risk of metabolic syndrome (Kastorini et al. 2011; Esposito et al. 2004) and diabetes (Martínez-González et al. 2008; Salas-Salvadó et al. 2014), both of which increase the risk of many cancers—including BC—and cancer deaths (Boyle et al. 2012; Redaniel et al. 2012; Collaboration et al. 2011; Gunter et al. 2009; Rosato et al. 2011; Minicozzi et al. 2013; Agnoli et al. 2010).

Also polyphenols of olive oil—a typical ingredient of the Mediterranean diet—were shown to lower body iron stores which in turn lower the risk of metabolic syndrome (Mascitelli and Goldstein 2011).

Finally, the Mediterranean diet was shown effective for obtaining statistically and clinically significant weight loss (Shai et al. 2008; Richard et al. 2013; Ryan et al. 2013) which is considered a valuable strategy to reduce BC risk (Matsen and Neumayer 2013; Eccles et al. 2013; http://www.cancer.gov/bcrisktool/ (Assessed April 8 2014; http://www.cancer.gov/cancertopics/pdq/prevention/breast/patient (Assessed April 8 2014).

The only limitation regarding adherence to the Mediterranean diet to prevent BC risk regards alcohol consumption. Wine drinking during meals is indeed a major component of the Mediterranean diet (de Lorgeril 2013). Alcohol consumption increases BC risk (Zhang et al. 2007), while the specific effect of wine—and of wine drinking in the context of the Mediterranean diet—is unclear. The usual estimate for postmenopausal women who consume no more than one alcoholic drink per day is about a 7 % risk increase in comparison with nondrinkers (Matsen and Neumayer 2013; Eccles et al. 2013). This is small but significant. Alcohol consumption may also increase BC recurrence (Kwan et al. 2010). In some (Tjønneland et al. 2006; Baglietto et al. 2005) but not all (Stolzenberg-Solomon et al. 2006) studies, the excess BC risk with alcohol (not wine) consumption is reduced by increasing folate intake while folate consumption is high in the Mediterranean diet. Thus, experts have stated that the Mediterranean way of drinking alcohol—chronic moderate consumption of polyphenol-rich wine mainly with folate-rich foods—should not appreciably influence BC risk (Giacosa et al. 2013). Given that moderate alcohol consumption also reduces the risk of cardiovascular disease (Costanzo et al. 2010), it appears that consuming one alcoholic drink per day on average is likely associated with optimal life expectancy without compromising BC-specific survival (Newcomb et al. 2013; Demark-Wahnefried and Goodwin 2013; Arranz et al. 2012).

4 Conclusions

Adhering to a healthy dietary pattern—specifically the modernized Mediterranean diet (de Lorgeril 2013; de Lorgeril et al. 1999)—may be critical to reduce BC risk in high-risk women and in women who wish to decrease their BC risk.

In the context of the Mediterranean diet, it is important to increase plant and marine n-3 and decrease plant and animal n-6. High flavonoid intake—which increases n-3 (Toufektsian et al. 2011; di Giuseppe et al. 2009; de Lorgeril et al. 2008)—should be encouraged as it is associated with lower BC risk. To reduce insulin resistance and diabetes—which are associated with an increased BC risk—women should increase fiber consumption and favor low-GI foods. Women should choose organic foods because of their effect on the n-3/n-6 ratio and because they contain fewer contaminants—and lower levels of each contaminant—in particular endocrine disruptors. Finally, any drug thought to increase diabetes and/or BC risk—in particular, the statins and certain antihypertensive medications (Li et al. 2013; Bhaskaran et al. 2012)—should be prohibited. To lower blood pressure or to decrease the risk of cardiovascular disease, physicians do have lifestyle strategies, and it would be tragically unwise to persist in prescribing anticholesterol statins and antihypertensive drugs in women wishing to decrease their BC risk.

National and international guidelines recommend healthy diet and physical activity to decrease BC risk (Kushi et al. 2012). It is time however to go further and be more specific. A specific dietary pattern such as the modernized Mediterranean diet, and not simply "*consuming a diet rich in vegetables and fruits*," should be adopted to decrease BC risk. This is also an effective way of maintaining a healthy weight and preventing diabetes and cardiovascular disease. This also applies to BC survivors to prevent recurrence and improve survival (Rock et al. 2012; Wolin and Colditz 2013).

Acknowledgements MdeL and PS receive research grants (through Grenoble University School of Medicine) from the European Community and from the Barilla G&R F.lli Company.

References

Agnoli C, Berrino F, Abagnato CA et al (2010) Metabolic syndrome and postmenopausal breast cancer in the ORDET cohort: a nested case–control study. Nutr Metab Cardiovasc Dis 20:41–48

Ahern TP, Pedersen L, Tarp M et al (2011) Statin prescriptions and breast cancer recurrence risk: a Danish nationwide prospective cohort study. J Natl Cancer Inst 103:1461–1468

Alexander DD, Morimoto LM, Mink PJ, Lowe KA (2010) Summary and meta-analysis of prospective studies of animal fat intake and breast cancer. Nutr Res Rev 23:169–179

Alsheikh-Ali AA, Maddukuri PV, Han H, Karas RH (2007) Effect of the magnitude of lipid lowering on risk of elevated liver enzymes, rhabdomyolysis, and cancer: insights from large randomized statin trials. J Am Coll Cardiol 50:409–418

Arranz S, Chiva-Blanch G, Valderas-Martínez P et al (2012) Wine, beer, alcohol and polyphenols on cardiovascular disease and cancer. Nutrients 4:759–781

Baglietto L, English DR, Gertig DM, Hopper JL, Giles GG (2005) Does dietary folate intake modify effect of alcohol consumption on breast cancer risk? Prospective cohort study. BMJ 331:807

Bamia C, Lagiou P, Buckland G et al (2013) Mediterranean diet and colorectal cancer risk: results from a European cohort. Eur J Epidemiol 28:317–328

Benbrook C, Zhao X, Yanez J, Davies N, Andrews P (2008) New evidence confirms the nutritional superiority of plant-based organic foods. An Organic Center State of Science Review. Available from http://www.organic-center.org/science.nutri.php?action = view&report_id = 126. Accessed 7 April 2014

Benbrook C, Davis DR, Andrews PK (2009) Methodologic flaws in selecting studies and comparing nutrient concentrations led Dangour et al. to miss the emerging forest amid the trees. Am J Clin Nutr 90:1700–1701, Author reply 1701

Benbrook CM, Butler G, Latif MA, Leifert C, Davis DR (2013) Organic production enhances milk nutritional quality by shifting fatty acid composition: a United States-wide, 18-month study. PLoS One 8:e82429

Bhaskaran K, Douglas I, Evans S, van Staa T, Smeeth L (2012) Angiotensin receptor blockers and risk of cancer: cohort study among people receiving antihypertensive drugs in UK General Practice Research Database. BMJ 344:e2697

Bonovas S, Filioussi K, Tsavaris N, Sitaras NM (2005) Use of statins and breast cancer: a meta-analysis of seven randomized clinical trials and nine observational studies. J Clin Oncol 23:8606–8612

Bosco JL, Silliman RA, Thwin SS et al (2010) A most stubborn bias: no adjustment method fully resolves confounding by indication in observational studies. J Clin Epidemiol 63:64–74

Bosetti C, Spertini L, Parpinel M, Gnagnarella P, Lagiou P, Negri E, Franceschi S, Montella M, Peterson J, Dwyer J, Giacosa A, La Vecchia C (2005) Flavonoids and breast cancer risk in Italy. Cancer Epidemiol Biomarkers Prev 14:805–808

Bosetti C, Turati F, Dal Pont A et al (2013) The role of Mediterranean diet on the risk of pancreatic cancer. Br J Cancer 109:1360–1366

Bouitbir J, Charles AL, Rasseneur L et al (2011) Atorvastatin treatment reduces exercise capacities in rats: involvement of mitochondrial impairments and oxidative stress. J Appl Physiol 111:1477–1483

Boyle P, Boniol M, Koechlin A et al (2012) Diabetes and breast cancer risk: a meta-analysis. Br J Cancer 107:1608–1617

Brennan SF, Cantwell MM, Cardwell CR, Velentzis LS, Woodside JV (2010) Dietary patterns and breast cancer risk: a systematic review and meta-analysis. Am J Clin Nutr 91:1294–1302

Brostow DP, Odegaard AO, Koh WP et al (2011) Omega-3 fatty acids and incident type 2 diabetes: the Singapore Chinese Health Study. Am J Clin Nutr 94:520–526

Buckland G, Travier N, Cottet V et al (2013) Adherence to the Mediterranean diet and risk of breast cancer in the European prospective investigation into cancer and nutrition cohort study. Int J Cancer 132:2918–2927

Carter AA, Gomes T, Camacho X, Juurlink DN, Shah BR, Mamdani MM (2013) Risk of incident diabetes among patients treated with statins: population based study. BMJ 346:f2610

Choi Y, Giovannucci E, Lee JE (2012) Glycaemic index and glycaemic load in relation to risk of diabetes-related cancers: a meta-analysis. Br J Nutr 108:1934–1947

Cohn BA, Terry MB, Plumb M, Cirillo PM (2012) Exposure to polychlorinated biphenyl (PCB) congeners measured shortly after giving birth and subsequent risk of maternal breast cancer before age 50. Breast Cancer Res Treat 136:267–275

Collaboration ERF, Seshasai SR, Kaptoge S, Thompson A et al (2011) Diabetes mellitus, fasting glucose, and risk of cause-specific death. N Engl J Med 364:829–841

Costanzo S, Di Castelnuovo A, Donati MB, Iacoviello L, de Gaetano G (2010) Cardiovascular and overall mortality risk in relation to alcohol consumption in patients with cardiovascular disease. Circulation 121:1951–1959

Cottet V, Touvier M, Fournier A et al (2009) Postmenopausal breast cancer risk and dietary patterns in the E3N-EPIC prospective cohort study. Am J Epidemiol 170:1257–1267

Cuezva JM, Krajewska M, de Heredia ML et al (2002) The bioenergetic signature of cancer: a marker of tumor progression. Cancer Res 62:6674–6681

Culver AL, Ockene IS, Balasubramanian R et al (2012) Statin use and risk of diabetes mellitus in postmenopausal women in the Women's Health Initiative. Arch Intern Med 172:144–152

Dale KM, Coleman CI, Henyan NN, Kluger J, White CM (2006) Statins and cancer risk: a meta-analysis. JAMA 295:74–80

Dangour AD, Dodhia SK, Hayter A et al. (2009) Comparison of composition (nutrients and other substances) of organically and conventionally produced foodstuffs: a systematic review of the available literature. Report for the Food Standards Agency, July 2009, contract number: PAU221. Available from http://webarchive.nationalarchives.gov.uk/20120206100416/http://food.gov.uk/multimedia/pdfs/organicreviewappendices.pdf. Accessed 7 April 2014

de Lorgeril M (2013) Mediterranean diet and cardiovascular disease: historical perspective and latest evidence. Curr Atheroscler Rep 15:370

de Lorgeril M, Salen P (2012) New insights into the health effects of dietary saturated and omega-6 and omega-3 polyunsaturated fatty acids. BMC Med 10:50

de Lorgeril M, Salen P (2014) Helping women to good health: breast cancer, omega-3/omega-6 lipids and related lifestyle factors. BMC Med 12:54

de Lorgeril M, Salen P, Martin JL, Monjaud I, Boucher P, Mamelle N (1998) Mediterranean dietary pattern in a randomized trial: prolonged survival and possible reduced cancer rate. Arch Intern Med 158:1181–1187

de Lorgeril M, Salen P, Martin JL, Monjaud I, Delaye J, Mamelle N (1999) Mediterranean diet, traditional risk factors, and the rate of cardiovascular complications after myocardial infarction: final report of the Lyon Diet Heart Study. Circulation 99:779–785

de Lorgeril M, Salen P, Guiraud A et al (2005) Lipid-lowering drugs and essential omega-6 and omega-3 fatty acids in patients with coronary heart disease. Nutr Metab Cardiovasc Dis 15:36–41

de Lorgeril M, Salen P, Martin JL et al (2008) Interactions of wine drinking with omega-3 fatty acids in patients with coronary heart disease: a fish-like effect of moderate wine drinking. Am Heart J 155:175–181

de Lorgeril M, Salen P, Abramson J et al (2010) Cholesterol lowering, cardiovascular diseases, and the rosuvastatin-JUPITER controversy: a critical reappraisal. Arch Intern Med 170:1032–1036

de Lorgeril M, Salen P, Defaye P, Rabaeus M (2013) Recent findings on the health effects of omega-3 fatty acids and statins, and their interactions: do statins inhibit omega-3? BMC Med 11:5

de Medina P, Paillasse MR, Segala G et al (2013) Dendrogenin A arises from cholesterol and histamine metabolism and shows cell differentiation and anti-tumour properties. Nat Commun 4:1840

Demark-Wahnefried W, Goodwin PJ (2013) To your health: how does the latest research on alcohol and breast cancer inform clinical practice? J Clin Oncol 31:1917–1919

Demetriou CA, Hadjisavvas A, Loizidou MA et al (2012) The Mediterranean dietary pattern and breast cancer risk in Greek-Cypriot women: a case–control study. BMC Cancer 12:113

Dengel DR, Hagberg JM, Pratley RE, Rogus EM, Goldberg AP (1998) Improvements in blood pressure, glucose metabolism, and lipoprotein lipids after aerobic exercise plus weight loss in obese, hypertensive middle-aged men. Metabolism 47:1075–1082

di Giuseppe R, de Lorgeril M, Salen P, European Collaborative Group of the IMMIDIET Project et al (2009) Alcohol consumption and n-3 polyunsaturated fatty acids in healthy men and women from 3 European populations. Am J Clin Nutr 89:354–362

Djoussé L, Biggs ML, Lemaitre RN et al (2011) Plasma omega-3 fatty acids and incident diabetes in older adults. Am J Clin Nutr 94:527–533

Dong JY, Qin LQ (2011) Dietary glycemic index, glycemic load, and risk of breast cancer: meta-analysis of prospective cohort studies. Breast Cancer Res Treat 126:287–294

Eccles SA, Aboagye EO, Ali S, Anderson AS et al (2013) Critical research gaps and translational priorities for the successful prevention and treatment of breast cancer. Breast Cancer Res 15:R92

Ellis KA, Innocent G, Grove-White D et al (2006) Comparing the fatty acid composition of organic and conventional milk. J Dairy Sci 89:1938–1950

Esposito K, Marfella R, Ciotola M et al (2004) Effect of a Mediterranean-style diet on endothelial dysfunction and markers of vascular inflammation in the metabolic syndrome: a randomized trial. JAMA 292:1440–1446

Ferrari P, Rinaldi S, Jenab M et al (2013) Dietary fiber intake and risk of hormonal receptor-defined breast cancer in the European Prospective Investigation into Cancer and Nutrition study. Am J Clin Nutr 97:344–353

Giacosa A, Barale R, Bavaresco L et al (2013) Cancer prevention in Europe: the Mediterranean diet as a protective choice. Eur J Cancer Prev 22:90–95

Goldstein MR, Mascitelli L, Pezzetta F (2009) The double-edged sword of statin immunomodulation. Int J Cardiol 135:128–130

Golomb BA, Evans MA, Dimsdale JE, White HL (2012) Effects of statins on energy and fatigue with exertion: results from a randomized controlled trial. Arch Intern Med 172:1180–1182

Grosso G, Buscemi S, Galvano F et al (2013) Mediterranean diet and cancer: epidemiological evidence and mechanism of selected aspects. BMC Surg 13(Suppl 2):S14

Gunter MJ, Hoover DR, Yu H et al (2009) Insulin, insulin-like growth factor-I, and risk of breast cancer in postmenopausal women. J Natl Cancer Inst 101:48–60

Hallmann E, Lipowski J, Marszałek K, Rembiałkowska E (2013) The seasonal variation in bioactive compounds content in juice from organic and non-organic tomatoes. Plant Foods Hum Nutr 68:171–176

Harris JI, Hibbeln JR, Mackey RH, Muldoon MF (2004) Statin treatment alters serum n-3 and n-6 fatty acids in hypercholesterolemic patients. Prostaglandins Leukot Essent Fatty Acids 71:263–269

Hatch EE, Nelson JW, Stahlhut RW, Webster TF (2010) Association of endocrine disruptors and obesity: perspectives from epidemiological studies. Int J Androl 33:324–332

Hui C, Qi X, Qianyong Z, Xiaoli P, Jundong Z, Mantian M (2013) Flavonoids, flavonoid subclasses and breast cancer risk: a meta-analysis of epidemiologic studies. PLoS One 8:e54318

Jula A, Marniemi J, Rönnemaa T, Virtanen A, Huupponen R (2005) Effects of diet and simvastatin on fatty acid composition in hypercholesterolemic men: a randomized controlled trial. Arterioscler Thromb Vasc Biol 25:1952–1959

Kastorini CM, Milionis HJ, Esposito K, Giugliano D, Goudevenos JA, Panagiotakos DB (2011) The effect of Mediterranean diet on metabolic syndrome and its components: a meta-analysis of 50 studies and 534,906 individuals. J Am Coll Cardiol 57:1299–1313

Kaufmann P, Török M, Zahno A et al (2006) Toxicity of statins on rat skeletal muscle mitochondria. Cell Mol Life Sci 63:2415–2425

Kenfield SA, Dupre N, Richman EL, Stampfer MJ, Chan JM, Giovannucci EL (2014) Mediterranean diet and prostate cancer risk and mortality in the Health Professionals Follow-up Study. Eur Urol 65(5):887–894

Khaw KT (2013) Dietary fats and breast cancer risk. BMJ 347:f4518

Koh KK, Quon MJ, Han SH, Lee Y, Kim SJ, Shin EK (2010) Atorvastatin causes insulin resistance and increases ambient glycemia in hypercholesterolemic patients. J Am Coll Cardiol 55:1209–1216

Kushi LH, Doyle C, McCullough M, American Cancer Society 2010 Nutrition and Physical Activity Guidelines Advisory Committee et al (2012) American Cancer Society Guidelines on nutrition and physical activity for cancer prevention: reducing the risk of cancer with healthy food choices and physical activity. CA Cancer J Clin 62:30–67

Kwan ML, Weltzien E, Kushi LH, Castillo A, Slattery ML, Caan BJ (2009) Dietary patterns and breast cancer recurrence and survival among women with early-stage breast cancer. J Clin Oncol 27:919–926

Kwan ML, Kushi LH, Weltzien E et al (2010) Alcohol consumption and breast cancer recurrence and survival among women with early-stage breast cancer: the life after cancer epidemiology study. J Clin Oncol 28:4410–4416

Lajous M, Boutron-Ruault MC, Fabre A, Clavel-Chapelon F, Romieu I (2008) Carbohydrate intake, glycemic index, glycemic load, and risk of postmenopausal breast cancer in a prospective study of French women. Am J Clin Nutr 87:1384–1391

Larsen S, Stride N, Hey-Mogensen M et al (2013) Simvastatin effects on skeletal muscle: relation to decreased mitochondrial function and glucose intolerance. J Am Coll Cardiol 61:44–53

Li CI, Daling JR, Tang MT, Haugen KL, Porter PL, Malone KE (2013) Use of antihypertensive medications and breast cancer risk among women aged 55 to 74 years. JAMA Intern Med 173:1629–1637

Lind PM, Zethelius B, Lind L (2012) Circulating levels of phthalate metabolites are associated with prevalent diabetes in the elderly. Diabetes Care 35:1519–1524

Link LB, Canchola AJ, Bernstein L et al (2013) Dietary patterns and breast cancer risk in the California Teachers Study cohort. Am J Clin Nutr 98:1524–1532

Männistö S, Dixon LB, Balder HF et al (2005) Dietary patterns and breast cancer risk: results from three cohort studies in the DIETSCAN project. Cancer Causes Control 16:725–733

Martínez-González MA, de la Fuente-Arrillaga C, Nunez-Cordoba JM et al (2008) Adherence to Mediterranean diet and risk of developing diabetes: prospective cohort study. BMJ 336:1348–1351

Mascitelli L, Goldstein MR (2011) Mediterranean diet, lower body iron stores and metabolic syndrome. Int J Clin Pract 65:1110

Matsen CB, Neumayer LA (2013) Breast cancer: a review for the general surgeon. JAMA Surg 148:971–979

McDougall JA, Malone KE, Daling JR et al (2013) Long-term statin use and risk of ductal and lobular breast cancer among women 55 to 74 years of age. Cancer Epidemiol Biomarkers Prev 22:1529–1537

Meyer BJ, Mann NJ, Lewis JL, Milligan GC, Sinclair AJ, Howe PR (2003) Dietary intakes and food sources of omega-6 and omega-3 polyunsaturated fatty acids. Lipids 38:391–398

Minicozzi P, Berrino F, Sebastiani F et al (2013) High fasting blood glucose and obesity significantly and independently increase risk of breast cancer death in hormone receptor-positive disease. Eur J Cancer 49:3881–3888

Nelson ER, Wardell SE, Jasper JS et al (2013) 27-Hydroxycholesterol links hypercholesterolemia and breast cancer pathophysiology. Science 342:1094–1098

Newcomb PA, Kampman E, Trentham-Dietz A et al (2013) Alcohol consumption before and after breast cancer diagnosis: associations with survival from breast cancer, cardiovascular disease, and other causes. J Clin Oncol 31:1939–1946

Oba S, Nanri A, Kurotani K et al (2013) Japan Public Health Center-based Prospective Study Group. Dietary glycemic index, glycemic load and incidence of type 2 diabetes in Japanese men and women: the Japan public health center-based prospective study. Nutr J 2:165

Osaki Y, Taniguchi S, Tahara A, Okamoto M, Kishimoto T (2012) Metabolic syndrome and incidence of liver and breast cancers in Japan. Cancer Epidemiol 36:141–147

Ozdemir BH, Akcali Z, Haberal M (2004) Hypercholesterolemia impairs angiogenesis in patients with breast carcinoma, and therefore, lowers the risk of metastases. Am J Clin Pathol 122:696–703

Park Y, Brinton LA, Subar AF, Hollenbeck A, Schatzkin A (2009) Dietary fiber intake and risk of breast cancer in postmenopausal women: the National Institutes of Health-AARP Diet and Health Study. Am J Clin Nutr 90:664–671

Pearce ML, Dayton S (1971) Incidence of cancer in men on a diet high in polyunsaturated fat. Lancet 1:464–467

Praud D, Bertuccio P, Bosetti C, Turati F, Ferraroni M, La Vecchia C (2014) Adherence to the Mediterranean diet and gastric cancer risk in Italy. Int J Cancer 134(12):2935–2941

Prentice RL, Caan B, Chlebowski RT et al (2006) Low-fat dietary pattern and risk of invasive breast cancer: the Women's Health Initiative Randomized Controlled Dietary Modification Trial. JAMA 295:629–642

Ravnskov U, McCully KS, Rosch PJ (2012) The statin-low cholesterol-cancer conundrum. QJM 105:383–388
Recio-Vega R, Velazco-Rodriguez V, Ocampo-Gómez G et al (2011) Serum levels of polychlorinated biphenyls in Mexican women and breast cancer risk. J Appl Toxicol 31:270–278
Redaniel MT, Jeffreys M, May MT, Ben-Shlomo Y, Martin RM (2012) Associations of type 2 diabetes and diabetes treatment with breast cancer risk and mortality: a population-based cohort study among British women. Cancer Causes Control 23:1785–1795
Richard C, Royer MM, Couture P et al (2013) Effect of the Mediterranean diet on plasma adipokine concentrations in men with metabolic syndrome. Metabolism 62:1803–1810
Ridker PM, Pradhan A, MacFadyen JG, Libby P, Glynn RJ (2012) Cardiovascular benefits and diabetes risks of statin therapy in primary prevention: an analysis from the JUPITER trial. Lancet 380:565–571
Rock CL, Doyle C, Demark-Wahnefried W et al (2012) Nutrition and physical activity guidelines for cancer survivors. CA Cancer J Clin 62:243–274
Rosato V, Bosetti C, Talamini R et al (2011) Metabolic syndrome and the risk of breast cancer in postmenopausal women. Ann Oncol 22:2687–2692
Ryan MC, Itsiopoulos C, Thodis T et al (2013) The Mediterranean diet improves hepatic steatosis and insulin sensitivity in individuals with non-alcoholic fatty liver disease. J Hepatol 59:138–143
Sacks FM, Pfeffer MA, Moye LA et al (1996) The effect of pravastatin on coronary events after myocardial infarction in patients with average cholesterol levels. Cholesterol and Recurrent Events Trial investigators. N Engl J Med 335:1001–1009
Salas-Salvadó J, Bullo M, Estruch R et al (2014) Prevention of diabetes with Mediterranean diets: a subgroup analysis of a randomized trial. Ann Intern Med 160:1–10
Salmerón J, Manson JE, Stampfer MJ et al (1997) Dietary fiber, glycemic load, and risk of non-insulin-dependent diabetes mellitus in women. JAMA 277:472–477
Sergentanis TN, Economopoulos KP (2010) Four polymorphisms in cytochrome P450 1A1 (CYP1A1) gene and breast cancer risk: a meta-analysis. Breast Cancer Res Treat 122:459–469
Shai I, Schwarzfuchs D, Henkin Y et al (2008) Dietary Intervention Randomized Controlled Trial (DIRECT) Group: weight loss with a low-carbohydrate, Mediterranean, or low-fat diet. N Engl J Med 359:229–241
Sieri S, Krogh V, Pala V et al (2004) Dietary patterns and risk of breast cancer in the ORDET cohort. Cancer Epidemiol Biomarkers Prev 13:567–572
Sieri S, Pala V, Brighenti F, Pellegrini N et al (2007) Dietary glycemic index, glycemic load, and the risk of breast cancer in an Italian prospective cohort study. Am J Clin Nutr 86:1160–1166
Sirvent P, Fabre O, Bordenave S et al (2012) Muscle mitochondrial metabolism and calcium signaling impairment in patients treated with statins. Toxicol Appl Pharmacol 259:263–268
Smith-Bindman R (2012) Environmental causes of breast cancer and radiation from medical imaging: findings from the Institute of Medicine report. Arch Intern Med 172:1023–1027
Smutok MA, Reece C, Kokkinos PF (1993) Aerobic versus strength training for risk factor intervention in middle-aged men at high risk for coronary heart disease. Metabolism 42:177–184
Song F, Parekh S, Hooper L et al (2010) Dissemination and publication of research findings: an updated review of related biases. Health Technol Assess 14:1–193
Stahlhut RW, van Wijngaarden E, Dye TD, Cook S, Swan SH (2007) Concentrations of urinary phthalate metabolites are associated with increased waist circumference and insulin resistance in adult U.S. males. Environ Health Perspect 115:876–882
Stolzenberg-Solomon RZ, Chang SC, Leitzmann MF et al (2006) Folate intake, alcohol use, and postmenopausal breast cancer risk in the Prostate, Lung, Colorectal, and Ovarian Cancer Screening Trial. Am J Clin Nutr 83:895–904
Strohmaier S, Edlinger M, Manjer J et al (2013) Total serum cholesterol and cancer incidence in the Metabolic syndrome and Cancer Project (Me-Can). PLoS One 8:e54242

Sugiyama T, Tsugawa Y, Tseng CH, Kobayashi Y, Shapiro MF (2014) Different time trends of caloric and fat intake between statin users and nonusers among US adults: gluttony in the time of statins? JAMA Intern Med 174(7):1038–1045
Suzuki R, Rylander-Rudqvist T, Ye W et al (2008) Dietary fiber intake and risk of postmenopausal breast cancer defined by estrogen and progesterone receptor status—a prospective cohort study among Swedish women. Int J Cancer 122:403–412
Tjønneland A, Christensen J, Olsen A et al (2006) Folate intake, alcohol and risk of breast cancer among postmenopausal women in Denmark. Eur J Clin Nutr 60:280–286
Toufektsian MC, Salen P, Laporte F, Tonelli C, de Lorgeril M (2011) Dietary flavonoids increase plasma very long-chain (n-3) fatty acids in rats. J Nutr 141:37–41
Trichopoulou A, Bamia C, Lagiou P, Trichopoulos D (2010) Conformity to traditional Mediterranean diet and breast cancer risk in the Greek EPIC (European Prospective Investigation into Cancer and Nutrition) cohort. Am J Clin Nutr 92:620–625
Tsiplakou E, Kotrotsios V, Hadjigeorgiou I, Zervas G (2010) Differences in sheep and goats milk fatty acid profile between conventional and organic farming systems. J Dairy Res 77:343–349
Turati F, Trichopoulos D, Polesel J et al (2014) Mediterranean diet and hepatocellular carcinoma. J Hepatol 60(3):606–611
Wallace DC (2012) Mitochondria and cancer. Nat Rev Cancer 12:685–698
Warner M, Mocarelli P, Samuels S, Needham L, Brambilla P, Eskenazi B (2011) Dioxin exposure and cancer risk in the Seveso Women's Health Study. Environ Health Perspect 119:1700–1705
Wolin KY, Colditz GA (2013) Cancer and beyond: healthy lifestyle choices for cancer survivors. J Natl Cancer Inst 105:593–594
Yang B, Ren XL, Fu YQ, Gao JL, Duo L (2014) Ratio of n-3/n-6 PUFAs and risk of breast cancer: a meta-analysis of 274,135 adult females from 11 independent prospective studies. BMC Cancer 14:105
Yao B, Fang H, Xu W et al (2014) Dietary fiber intake and risk of type 2 diabetes: a dose–response analysis of prospective studies. Eur J Epidemiol 29:79–88
Zaharan NL, Williams D, Bennett K (2013) Statins and risk of treated incident diabetes in a primary care population. Br J Clin Pharmacol 75:1118–1124
Zamora-Ros R, Forouhi NG, Sharp SJ et al (2014) Dietary intakes of individual flavanols and flavonols are inversely associated with incident type 2 diabetes in European populations. J Nutr 144:335–343
Zhang SM, Lee IM, Manson JE et al (2007) Alcohol consumption and breast cancer risk in the Women's Health Study. Am J Epidemiol 165:667–676
Zhang CX, Ho SC, Cheng SZ et al (2011) Effect of dietary fiber intake on breast cancer risk according to estrogen and progesterone receptor status. Eur J Clin Nutr 65:929–936
Zheng JS, Huang T, Yang J, Fu YQ, Li D (2012) Marine N-3 polyunsaturated fatty acids are inversely associated with risk of type 2 diabetes in Asians: a systematic review and meta-analysis. PLoS One 7:e44525
Zheng JS, Hu XJ, Zhao YM, Yang J, Li D (2013) Intake of fish and marine n-3 polyunsaturated fatty acids and risk of breast cancer: meta-analysis of data from 21 independent prospective cohort studies. BMJ 346:f3706
Zock PL, Katan MB (1998) Linoleic acid intake and cancer risk: a review and meta-analysis. Am J Clin Nutr 68:142–153

Probiotic Bacteria in Patients Treated with Chemotherapy and Radiation Therapy

Michal Mego, Sona Ciernikova, Martin Razus, Lubos Drgona, and Vladimir Zajac

Abstract Probiotics are live microorganisms, which as drugs or food supplements help to maintain health beneficial microbial balance in the digestive tract of a human or other host. Probiotics by their properties may help strengthen homeostasis and thus reduce side effects associated with cancer treatment. Experimental evidence suggest that probiotics might have beneficial effect on the toxicity of anticancer therapy. Probiotics might have beneficial effects on some aspects of toxicity related to anticancer treatment especially radiation therapy. However, reported trial varies in utilized probiotic strains and dose of probiotics, and vast majority of them are small trials with substantial risk of bias. Despite limited data, it seems that probiotic bacteria as live microorganisms could be safely administered even in setting of prolonged neutropenia. Current evidence supporting probiotic use as adjunctive therapy to anticancer treatment is limited, especially in cancer patients treated with chemotherapy. Well designed clinical trials are needed to find true role of probiotics in oncology.

1 Introduction

More than 80 % of cancer patients are supposed to use complementary and alternative medicine, like vitamins, minerals, herbs, and other dietary supplements including probiotics (Richardson et al. 2000). Probiotics are live microorganisms, which as drugs or food supplements help to maintain health beneficial microbial balance in the digestive tract of a human or other host (Fuller 1989; Joint FAO/WHO Working Group 2002). Increasing number of research studies reflects a rising interest and shows their multiple indications including gastrointestinal disorders like prevention and treatment of infectious and antibiotic-induced diarrhea, treatment of liver insufficiency, lactose intolerance, inflammatory bowel disease, irritable bowel syndrome. Probiotics are also evaluated in rheumatic and

M. Mego (✉) • M. Razus • L. Drgona
Second Department of Oncology and National Cancer Institute, Comenius University, Klenova 1, 833 10 Bratislava, Slovakia
e-mail: misomego@gmail.com

S. Ciernikova • V. Zajac
Department of Cancer Genetics, Cancer Research Institute, Bratislava, Slovakia

M.F. Ullah, A. Ahmad (eds.), *Critical Dietary Factors in Cancer Chemoprevention*,
DOI 10.1007/978-3-319-21461-0_18

allergic diseases, in the prevention of urogenital infections, or in cardiology based on their effect on serum cholesterol, lipids, or hypertension (Girardin and Seidman 2011; Goldin and Gorbach 2008; Ferenčík et al. 1999).

Prevention of colorectal cancer represents the main interest in use of probiotics in oncology as an adjunctive therapy to anticancer treatment (Fotiadis et al. 2008). However, current evidence is still limited mainly because of the risk of inducing iatrogenic infection in immunocompromised cancer patients and lack of robust efficacy data. On the other hand, damage in natural protective barriers, due to the frequent use of chemotherapy, radiation therapy, and especially antibiotics, leads to colonization by pathogenic microorganisms and the emergence of multiresistant strains. Probiotics by their properties may help strengthen homeostasis and thus reduce side effects associated with cancer treatment. Experimental and some clinical evidence suggest that lactic acid bacteria might have beneficial effect on the toxicity of anticancer therapy (Mego et al. 2005, 2006; Fuccio et al. 2009).

Disrupting the microbial balance in the gut through the use of antibiotics can affect the response to cancer therapy. According to currently released ASCO report, Clinical Cancer Advances 2015: An Annual Report on Progress Against Cancer (Masters et al. 2015), two recent studies in mice confirmed the protective role of gut bacteria in cancer (Iida et al. 2013; Viaud et al. 2013). The results showed that gut bacteria enhance the body's immune response to cancer and mobilizing immunity throughout the body to kill cancer cells. Further confirmation in human studies might bring the possibility to manipulate the microflora for improving the immune response to cancer and increasing the efficacy of certain cancer therapies.

Many cancer patients suppose to use probiotics during course of their disease due to the availability without prescription restriction and relative cheapness. However, exact epidemiological data are lacking. Probiotics are live organisms, and there is still limited evidence for their effectivity and safety in cancer patients treated with chemotherapy or radiation therapy.

Here we present current evidence of the status of probiotics in clinical oncology, their potential clinical position as a part of anticancer treatment, and safety concerns associated with their application.

2 Changes of Gut Bacteria Composition due to Chemotherapy Treatment and Radiation Therapy

Intestinal microbiota interacts with the host's immune system, and wide bacterial enzymatic activity can affect the intestinal homeostasis in many ways. The majority of studies dealing with the effect of chemotherapy on human fecal microbiota used standard microbiological culture techniques. Conversely, a combination of molecular methods including high-throughput sequencing to compare diversity (PCR-DGGE) and abundance (qPCR) of 16S rRNA genes in all bacteria, *Bacteroides*, bifidobacteria, *Clostridium* cluster IV and XIVa, as well as

Clostridium difficile, pointed out the significant decrease in total microbiota ($p = 0.037$) after various regimes of chemotherapy. In particular, declining levels of *Bifidobacterium* spp., *Lactobacillus* spp., and *Faecalibacterium prausnitzii* have been detected. On the other hand, changes in the human gut microbiota have favored colonization with *C. difficile* and *Enterococcus faecium* following chemotherapy (Zwielehner et al. 2011).

Intestinal microbiota disruption after chemotherapy treatment leads to mucositis and microfloral dysbiosis. These phenomenons are also associated with various mucositis-related diseases, including inflammatory bowel disease (Marteau and Chaput, 2011), irritable bowel syndrome (Malinen et al. 2005), and colorectal cancer (Azcárate-Peril et al. (2011)).

2.1 Mucositis

Mucosal barrier injury, mucositis, is characterized by both inflammation and cell loss in the epithelial barrier lining the gastrointestinal tract. It is associated with bacteremia, malnutrition, an increment in the use of intravenous analgesics, and represents a serious side effect of radiotherapy and chemotherapy treatment. All these complications often led to reduction of chemotherapeutics' dosages and deferred radiotherapy, resulting in a higher mortality (Blijlevens et al. 2000; Sonis et al. 2001). Intestinal mucositis includes the clinical symptoms like nausea, bloating, vomiting, abdominal pain, diarrhea, constipation, and subsequent weight loss. Mucositis is tightly connected with chemotherapy-induced diarrhea and has severe impact on quality of life of cancer patients.

Although no role of gut microflora was described in five-phase model of mucositis pathophysiology introduced by Sonis (Sonis 2004), recent studies point to the effects of microfloral changes to development and severity of mucositis. Moreover, it has been shown that bacteria play a role in the metabolism of certain chemotherapeutics.

2.2 Studies of Irinotecan and 5-FU Effect on Gut Microflora Changes

The most investigated chemotherapeutic agent interacting with patients' microbiota is irinotecan, a potent drug used in the treatment of metastatic colorectal cancer. Irinotecan is a topoisomerase-I inhibitor converted to active toxic metabolite SN-38, which is in liver glucuronidated (SN-38G) and subsequently expelled into the intestine. Afterwards, the cleavage by bacterial enzyme β-D-glucuronidase rendering it to re-activated and toxic form representing the main cause of diarrhea in irinotecan-treated patients (Takasuna et al. 1996). Diarrhea is one of the most important factors in morbidity and mortality during irinotecan-based chemotherapy with an incidence ranging between 60 and 90 %. In addition, severe diarrhea has been reported in 20–40 % of irinotecan-treated patients (Michael et al. 2004).

Intestinal microbiota interacts with both the host digestive and immune systems. Members of the TLR signaling pathway were also heavily upregulated after irinotecan treatment (Bowen et al. 2007a; Bowen et al. 2007b). TLR signaling has been shown to be upregulated in response to increased bacterial ligands, resulting in further downstream upregulation of NFκB and pro-inflammatory cytokines. In this way, TLR signaling may contribute to pathophysiology of mucositis (Cario 2005). In both studies by Logan and colleagues (Logan et al. 2008a; Logan et al. 2008b), intestinal serum level of NF-kb was significantly increased 6–12 h following administration of irinotecan ($p < 0.05$). Increased level and upregulation of these cytokines probably resulted from goblet cells' activity, which might have a downstream effect of intestinal microbiota, due to the subsequently altered environmental conditions in the intestinal mucosa and lumen.

Changes in microflora composition according to irinotecan treatment have been detected in various studies. A significant increase in β-D-glucuronidase-producing Gram-negative bacteria *E. coli* has been detected in rats that received a single dose irinotecan. In addition, the levels of nonproducing species *Bifidobacterium* spp. and *Lactobacillus* spp. after treatment were significantly lower (Stringer et al. 2007, 2008, 2009). The study by Lin et al. on tumor bearing rats showed increased abundance of intestinal *Enterobacteriaceae* and *Clostridium* cluster XI after the dose-intensive irinotecan-based therapy (Lin et al. 2012). This observation might reflect intestinal dysbiosis (Marteau and Chaput 2011) as a result of altered function of the intestinal mucosa and the gut-associated immune system. Changes in fecal microbiota were less pronounced compared to changes in cecal microbiota, which agreed with the observation that gut injury induced by irinotecan chemotherapy was observed mostly in the cecum (Takasuna et al. 1996; Yang et al. 2006).

Recently, the role of bacterial β-D-glucuronidase in irinotecan toxicity was confirmed by Lin XB and colleagues (Lin et al. 2014). Rats bearing a Ward colon carcinoma received two cycles of irinotecan/5-FU treatment. To ensure a higher butyrate production, rats were fed with different dietary fibres (isomalto-oligosaccharides, fructooligosaccharides, inulin, and mixture of fructooligosaccharides and inulin). Butyrate promotes the condition of cecal and colonic mucosa and improves immune and barrier function of intestines. The results showed that SN-38G metabolite was mainly presented in the jejunum. Conversely, deconjugated SN-38 was most abundant in cecum. On the other hand, the study indicated that dietary intervention does not significantly reduce the conversion of SN-38G to toxic SN-38 (Lin et al. 2014).

In addition to irinotecan, antimetabolite 5-Fluorouracil (5-FU), used to treat colorectal, breast, and liver cancers, has also been associated with modification of microbiota composition in Lewis rats given 50 mg/kg 5-FU i.v. for 6 days. 5-FU treatment shifted the composition of microbiota from predominantly Gram-positive to Gram-negative bacteria in biopsies from both the oral cavity and intestine (Von Bultzingslowen et al. 2003).

2.3 The Impact of Radiation Therapy on Intestinal Microbiota

Many cancer patients undergoing radiotherapy period suffer from diarrhea, mucus discharge, rectal bleeding, tenesmus, and fecal incontinence. These radiation-induced complications assumed to be a result of gut microbial dysbiosis in cancer patients. Nevertheless, clinical or experimental data on the impact of radiation on gut microbiota are not sufficient. Elucidation of human–microbiome interactions may provide the insight into potential therapeutics.

Crawford and Gordon revealed the importance of gut microbiota in the occurrence of radiation injury. Comparing to conventional mice with commensal gut microbial flora, germ-free mice were resistant to lethal radiation injury and had less radiation-induced epithelial cell damage (Crawford and Gordon 2005). The study comprising 41 consecutive female patients with symptoms of late radiation enteropathy has showed that the overgrowth of gram-negative bacilli corresponding to the severity of disease was essential in the pathogenesis of radiation enteropathy (Husebye et al. 1995). Bowel irradiation led to a general decrease of gut microbiota, imbalance of the gut bacterial community structure, and subsequent pathogenic effects on the epithelial mucosa of experimental mice (Johnson et al. 2004). In addition, a prospective observational study of gut microbiota using 454 pyrosequencing in gynecological cancer patients receiving pelvic radiotherapy showed significant differences in the overall gut microbial composition ($p < 0.001$) between cancer patients and healthy individuals. Radiotherapy severely reduced the numbers of species-level taxa ($p < 0.045$), and the abundance of each community largely changed. In particular, the phyla *Firmicutes* and *Fusobacterium* were significantly decreased by 10 % and increased by 3 % after radiation therapy, respectively (Nam et al. 2013).

3 Probiotics and Chemotherapy

3.1 Augmentation of Colonization Resistance in Cancer Patients by Probiotics

Infections in cancer patients are often preceded by bowel colonization with pathogenic bacteria followed by translocation across the gut mucosa and systemic dissemination (Schimpff et al. 1972; Marshall 1999). Chemotherapy and particularly the use of broad-spectrum antibiotics result in bowel flora alteration suppressing the growth of normal anaerobic microflora leading to diminishing of colonization resistance. Maintenance of the natural commensal flora provides a potent barrier to acquisition of pathogenic aerobic gram-negative rods (Buck and Cooke 1969). Competitive inhibition of bowel colonization by pathogenic microorganisms with probiotic strains might represent a useful prevention of infections in cancer patients (Mego et al. 2006).

Beneficial effect of probiotic bacteria consists of increased transepithelial resistance by stimulation of the immune system, competition for nutrition with pathogenic bacteria, competitive inhibition of bacterial adhesion sites, and in the production of bacteriocins (Marin et al. 1998; Neumann et al. 1998; Perdigon et al. 1995; Resta-Lenert and Barrett 2003; Vandenplas 1999). Lactic acid bacteria could be involved in treatment of dysbiosis after antibiotics use. Moreover, their enzymatic activity affects the activation or deactivation of metabolites inducing diarrhea. Production of short-chain fatty acids, mainly butyrate, during lactic acid bacteria fermentation, provides nutrition for colonocytes and participates in the restitution of colonocytes after chemotherapy.

Germ-free environment was considered to be an important tool for reduction of infections by gut colonization with virulent bacteria in neutropenic patients. Paradoxically, the comparison of protective isolation with standard hospital care in neutropenic patients with acute leukemia uncovered the higher rate of bacteremia in patients randomized to protective isolation (Nauseef and Maki 1981). This finding was in accordance with animal models pointing at higher rates of infection and susceptibility to infection among germ-free animals in comparison to normal animals (Baba et al. 1991; Taguchi et al. 2002). Therefore, augmentation of colonization resistance by lactic acid bacteria might represent an effective and unexpensive way for infection prevention in granulocytopenic patients. This hypothesis was tested in animal models and small clinical trials.

In experimental animal model, administration of heat inactivated strain *Enterococcus faecalis* FK-23 in cyclophosphamide-induced neutropenic dogs led to shortening of duration of neutropenia and to augmentation of leukocyte reconstituting capacity (Hasegawa et al. 1996). In addition, oral or intraperitoneal prophylactic administration of FK-23 preparation to mice infected by *Candida albicans* significantly prolonged survival periods of mice and decreased viable counts of *C. albicans* recovered from their kidneys (Satonaka et al. 1996).

There are only anecdotal reports in the literature concerning the use of probiotics in granulocytopenic patients. In a small study comprising five granulocytopenic patients with intestinal flora suppressed by antibiotics, administration of lactobacilli strains was not successful in spontaneous recolonization of bowel by enteric bacteria. However, significant number of lactobacilli in stool was detected only in two patients (Hengens and Klastersky 1976). In randomized study performed by Eker and coauthors, 33 children with leukemia and solid tumors received framycetin, colimycin, nystatin, and metronidazol in 35 neutropenic episodes, while 35 children received co-trimoxazole with lactobacilli in 35 episodes. There were not significant differences in incidence of infections during neutropenia nor in duration of neutropenia. Combination of co-trimoxazole with lactobacilli was considerably better tolerated (Eker et al. 1980). Nevertheless, small number of participants and the dose of the probiotics insufficient for colonization resistance were the main limitations of these studies.

Efficacy and safety of the probiotic strain *E. faecium* M74 in neutropenic patients with solid and hematological malignancies were evaluated in two small studies (Mego et al. 2005; Mego et al. 2006). In phase I study, the probiotics were administered to six patients with testicular cancer treated with chemotherapy. The febrile episode was not observed in any of the patients. Then *E. faecium* M-74 was administered to five patients with relapsed acute leukemia. During 127 days of severe neutropenia, 12 febrile episodes occurred. No any febrile episode or infection provoked by the tested strain was noted (Mego et al. 2005).

Subsequently an open-label, nonrandomized, phase II study was performed. The primary end point of the study was the prevention of febrile neutropenia by probiotic strain *E. faecium* M-74 during the induction and consolidation chemotherapy in patients with acute and chronic myelogenous leukemia. Fourteen patients were included in the study. Patients received prophylaxis with *E. faecium* M-74 during one cycle of chemotherapy. The daily dose was 36×10^9 CFU (colony forming units) tid. All patients experienced febrile neutropenia. During 231 days of severe neutropenia, 30 febrile episodes occurred, but none of them was provoked by the study strain. However, administration of this bacterial strain was not effective in the prevention of febrile neutropenia, but this does not preclude the protective effect of other probiotic strains. Moreover, tolerance of therapy was excellent without significant adverse effects in both studies (Mego et al. 2006).

Based on our previous experience, double-blinded, randomized, multicentric, placebo controlled phase III study was designed, aimed to reduce incidence of febrile neutropenia and gastrointestinal complications by symbiotic preparation in children after chemotherapy. Patients in active group receive mixture of two probiotic strains (*Lactobacillus rhamnosus* LGG and *Bifidobacterium animalis* subsp. *lactis*, BB-12) together with oligofructose-enriched inulin. Final data are awaited by the end of 2015.

Another similar randomized placebo-controlled trial aimed to evaluate the effects of the enteral administration of the probiotic, *Bifidobacterium breve* strain Yakult, on its ability to prevent infection, fecal micro flora, and intestinal environments in cancer patients receiving chemotherapy ($N = 42$). The study product contained 10^9 freeze-dried, living BBG-01, cornstarch, and hydroxypropyl cellulose. The results showed lower frequency of fever and use of intravenous antibiotics in the active group and also enhanced habitation of anaerobes after probiotic administration. On the other hand, increased levels of *Enterobacteriaceae*, one of the facultative anaerobes, were more striking in the placebo group (Wada et al. 2010). The concentration of organic acids produced by anaerobes maintains the intestinal acidity and inhibits the colonization of pathogenic organisms (Asahara et al. 2001, 2004). Normal levels of total organic acids detected most of the study duration maintained the pH below 7.0 only in the probiotic group (Wada et al. 2010).

3.2 Prevention and Treatment of Anticancer Therapy-Related Diarrhea by Probiotics

Diarrhea is a common complication of anticancer therapy. Several mechanisms play role in the development of diarrhea including malabsorption due to mucositis induced by chemotherapy, dysmicrobia induced by broad-spectrum antibiotics, and predisposition to infectious diarrhea in immunocompromised patients. Some cytostatics and their metabolites induce diarrhea through direct effects on the intestinal mucosa (Michael et al. 2004).

Cancer patients treated with chemotherapy are often exposed to antibiotic treatment during treatment of febrile neutropenia or other infections associated with cancer-induced immunosupression (Gafter-Gvili et al. 2005). Effects of probiotics on antibiotic-induced diarrhea is well established. Several single trials as well as meta-analysis support the beneficial role of lactic acid bacteria in this setting, including immunocompromised patients (Born et al. 1993; McFarland 2006; Kale-Pradhan et al. 2010). Meta-analyses confirmed efficacy of probiotics in prevention of antibiotic-induced diarrhea including *Clostridium difficile* infection in adults (McFarland 2006; Kale-Pradhan et al. 2010; Hempel et al. 2012) and suggest their beneficial role in children, especially when higher doses of probiotics are administered (Johnston et al. 2011; D'souza et al. 2002).

Higher incidence of diarrhea was recorded in patients with hematological malignancies with prolonged neutropenia after chemotherapy or patients treated with anticancer drugs with direct diarrhea inducing effects. There is limited experience with probiotics in the prevention and treatment of diarrhea related to chemotherapy; however, several trials are ongoing (Table 1). The incidence of diarrhea during the treatment of acute leukemia ranges between 15 and 80 % (Wiernik et al. 1992; Camera et al. 2003). Severe diarrhea grade 3–4 occurring in 8–20 % is more frequent during the induction phase of chemotherapy. In a phase II trial, preventive administration of probiotic strain *E. faecium* M-74 with selenium was associated with a low incidence (14 %) and severity (all grade 1) of diarrhea, despite the fact that half of the patients received induction therapy (Mego et al. 2006).

Irinotecan is one of key drug used in the treatment of colorectal cancer, but its toxic metabolite is associated with malabsorption and the development of diarrhea (Michael et al. 2004). It is known that probiotic bacteria reduce activity of intestinal beta-D-glucuronidase, and therefore these bacteria could be applied in the prevention of diarrhea in patients treated by this food supplement. Given their low toxicity and good tolerability, probiotics may be an important part of supportive therapy.

Randomized, double blind, placebo controlled pilot study suggest that administration of probiotic formula Colon DophilusTM compared to placebo is associated with reduction of gastrointestinal toxicity of irinotecan-based chemotherapy, and these results were consistent for all types of recorded gastrointestinal toxicity. Administration of probiotics compared to placebo led to a reduction in the incidence of severe diarrhea of grade 3 or 4 [0 % for probiotics vs. 17.4 % (95% CI 1.9–32.9 %), for placebo, $p = 0.11$], as well as reduction of the overall incidence of

Table 1 Selected ongoing trials investigating probiotics in clinical oncology

Trial number[a]	Objectives	Patient population	Intervention	Stage of trial	Country
NCT01473290	Prevention of gastrointestinal complication	Cancer patients treated by chemotherapy or radiation therapy to pelvic region	VSL#3 (mixture of probiotic strains)	Phase III	USA
NCT01723592	Improvement of the quality of the vaginal flora	Women with breast cancer treated with chemotherapy	Mixture of probiotic strains of *L. rhamnosus, L. jensenii, L. crispatus, L. gasseri*	Phase II	Austria
NCT00197873	Prevention of chemotherapy-related diarrhea	Patients on first-line CAPOX treatment for metastatic colorectal cancer	*L. rhamnosus* GG	Phase II	Finland
NCT01579591	Pathological major response rate in patients with rectal cancer	Rectal cancer patients undergoing concurrent chemotherapy and radiation therapy	VSL#3 (mixture of probiotic strains)	Phase III	Italy
NCT01480011	Prevention of high-dose chemotherapy-induced oral mucositis	Cancer patients treated with high dose chemotherapy with autologous stem cell transplantation	*Lactobacillus* CD2 Lozenges	Phase II	India
NCT01706393	Prevention of radiation-induced enteropathy	Cancer patients treated with abdominal/pelvic radiation therapy	(mixture of several probiotic strains)	Phase II	South Korea
NCT01790035	Acute treatment-related GI toxicity	Cancer patients with GI malignancy	Probiotic LGG	Phase III	USA
NCT02144701	Reduction of incidence of Graft-Versus-Host disease	Patients who have undergone donor stem cell transplant	*Lactobacillus Rhamnosus* GG	Pilot study	USA

[a]ClinicalTrials.gov identifier
CAPOX Capecitabine and Oxaliplatin

diarrhea [39.1 % (95 % CI 19.2–59.0 %) for probiotics vs. 60.9 % (95 % CI 41.0–80.8 %) for placebo, $p = 0.24$] and incidence of enterocolitis (0 % for probiotics vs. 8.7 % for placebo). Patients on placebo arm reported more often bloating compared to probiotic arm. Moreover, no infection caused by probiotic strains used in this study was observed. Although limited statistical power caused by lower sample size than expected, these data suggest probiotics could be simple, effective, and nontoxic approach to reduce gastrointestinal toxicity of irinotecan-based chemotherapy (Mego et al. 2015) (Table 1).

Administration of 5-fluorouracil, one of the key anticancer drugs in treatment of colorectal cancer, is associated not only with direct mucosal damage but also with development of lactose intolerance and diarrhea in duration-dependent manner. *Lactobacillus rhamnosus* GG supplementation reduced the frequency of severe diarrhea and abdominal discomfort related to 5-FU-based chemotherapy in the study with 150 colorectal cancer patients. Moreover, the probiotic administration was well tolerated, and none *L. rhamnosus* was identified in the blood cultures during the study (Osterlund et al. 2007).

Recently, the results from 11 randomized, controlled trials concerning on the efficacy of probiotics in people with cancer ($N = 1557$ participants) displayed reducing the severity and frequency of diarrhea in patients with cancer and the requirement for antidiarrheal medication, respectively. Meta-analysis found that probiotics significantly reduced incidence of CTC (Common Terminology Criteria for Adverse Events) grade ≥ 2 diarrhea (odds ratio 0.32, 95 % confidence interval, 0.13–0.79, PI 0.11–0.97, $p = 0.01$), but was unclear for CTC grade ≥ 3 diarrhea (odds ratio 0.72, 95 % CI of 0.42–1.25, 95 % PI of 0.41–1.27, $p = 0.24$) (Redman et al. 2014).

4 Probiotics and Radiation Therapy

Radiation therapy is an inherent part of anticancer treatment; however, it is associated with several adverse effects. Some of them are related to mucosal damage by ionizing radiation, with subsequent alterations in intestinal flora, accelerated small and large bowel transit, malabsorption of bile salts, and development of gastrointestinal toxicity manifested in the form of diarrhea, nausea, or loss of appetite (Ludgate and Merrick 1985; Gami et al. 2003). Diarrhea is the most significant toxicity of patients undergoing radiation therapy to the area of the abdomen and pelvis. The incidence of diarrhea ranges from 50 to 90 % when total tumoricidal dose of 45 Gy is administered (Andreyev et al. 2005). While chemotherapy is mostly associated with the development of neutropenia, administration of radiotherapy alone is usually not associated with severe hematological toxicity, and therefore the risk of iatrogenic infection caused by probiotics is very low. This is the reason for relatively more experience with probiotics in patients treated with radiation therapy.

Experimental animal models have shown that intestinal microbiota play a role in the development of radiation-induced intestinal damage, while germ-free animals were more resistant to lethal radiation enteritis (Crawford and Gordon 2005). Radiation reduces the intestinal motility (Husebye et al. 1995; Summers et al. 1991), and consecutive slower stool transit can lead to bacterial overgrowth, especially from gram-negative bacteria (Husebye et al. 1995), described in up to

45 % of patients with postradiation diarrhea (Danielsson et al. 1991). This imbalance together with inflammatory response could increase the permeability of the mucosa barrier and promote the bacterial translocation (Berg 1999), which can subsequently lead to development of pelvic sepsis described in 3–4 % of patients during treatment (Andreyev et al. 2005; Ludgate and Merrick 1985).

Two animal studies investigated the effect of probiotic supplementation in irradiated male Wistar rats. The first study supported the potential of *Lactobacillus delbrueckii* subsp. *Bulgaricus* B3 strain, in the prevention of postradiation intestinal damage as well as in prevention of gastrointestinal toxicity (Demirer et al. 2006). In the other study, animals received probiotic mixture containing *Lactobacillus acidophilus, Lactobacillus helveticus* and *Bifidobacterium* sp. to evaluate bacterial translocation and endotoxinemia after abdominal irradiation. Rats receiving probiotic supplementation presented a statistically significant reduction of endotoxin levels and bacterial translocation. Probiotics administration was associated with qualitative change in bacterial translocation. Gram-negative bacteria were predominant in blood cultures of rats fed with placebo, while gram-positive bacteria were more common in blood samples from probiotic group (Seal et al. 2007). Recent animal study showed a protective effect of probiotics on intestinal epithelium from radiation injury in a TLR-2/cyclo-oxygenase-2-dependent manner (Ciorba et al. 2012).

Several, randomized clinical trials and one meta-analysis examined preventive and therapeutic role of probiotics in patients treated with radiation therapy and some are ongoing (Tables 1 and 2). Three trials focused on prevention of radiation-related diarrhea (Salminen et al. 1988; Delia et al. 2007; Giralt et al. 2008).

The pilot controlled trial included only 21 patients with cervical or uterine carcinoma treated with radiotherapy. This trial showed beneficial effect of probiotics in this patients' population; however, this study had several weaknesses including a small sample size and lack of double-blinded placebo-controlled design (Salminen et al. 1988).

The efficacy of probiotic *Lactobacillus case*i DN-114 001 to reduce the incidence of radiation-induced diarrhea in patients with advanced cervical and/or endometrial carcinoma undergoing pelvic radiotherapy or chemoradiotherapy was investigated in large trial. Although 115 patients were randomized at the beginning; only 85 patients were included to final analysis. This trial was double blind; placebo controlled study, and didn't show statistically significant differences between two randomized arms. This study had some limitation as well, including insufficient statistical power, relatively low dose of utilized probiotic strain, and heterogeneity of treatment populations, when some patients underwent only radiation while some were treated with concomitant chemo-radiotherapy (Giralt et al. 2008).

The largest of these trials included 482 patients. This was a double-blinded, randomized, placebo-controlled study. The study investigated probiotic formula VSL#3, containing viable lyophilized bacteria from several different strains of lactobacilli (*L. casei, L. plantarum, L. acidophilus, L. delbrueckii* subsp. *bulgaricus*), bifidobacteria (*B. longum, B. breve, B. infantis*) and one strain of *Streptococcus salivarius* subsp. *thermophilus*. This study conclusively confirmed

Table 2 Clinical trials evaluating preventive and therapeutic role of probiotics in patients treated with radiation therapy

Study aim	Patient population	Randomized patients (patients in analysis)	Study arms	Study outcome	Author
Prevention	Cervical and uterine cancer treated with radiotherapy	24 (21)	*Lactobacillus acidophilus* vs. no intervention	Diarrhea Probiotics: 27 % Control: 90 % $p<0.05$ Rescue medication for diarrhea Probiotics: 9 % Control: 60 % $p<0.05$	Salminen et al. (1988)
Treatment	Mixture of cancer in lower abdomen treated with postoperative radiotherapy	205 (205)	*Lactobacillus rhamnosus* vs. placebo	Need for rescue medication for diarrhea Probiotics: 35 % Placebo: 48 % $p=\text{NS}$	Urbancsek et al. (2001)
Prevention	Cervical, sigmoid or rectal cancer treated with postoperative radiation therapy	490 (482)	VSL#3 (mixture of probiotic strains) vs. placebo	Diarrhea (all grades) Probiotics: 31.6 % Placebo: 51.8 % $p<0.001$	Delia et al. (2007)
Prevention	Cervical cancer treated with chemoradiation therapy or endometrial cancer treated with radiotherapy	118 (85)	*Lactobacillus casei* DN-114 001 vs. placebo	Co-primary endpoint defined as: At least four or more bowel movements, need for rescue medication, or premature withdrawal because of lack of efficacy. Probiotics: 68.2 % Placebo: 58.5 % $p=\text{NS}$	Giralt et al. (2008)

(continued)

Table 2 (continued)

Study aim	Patient population	Randomized patients (patients in analysis)	Study arms	Study outcome	Author
Prevention	Head and neck cancer treated with chemo-radiotherapy	200 (188)	*Lactobacillus brevis* CD2 *lozenges* vs. placebo	Grade III and IV mucositis: Probiotics: 52 % Placebo: 77 % $p < 0.001$ Anticancer treatment completion rates: Probiotics: 92 % Placebo: 70 % $p = 0.001$	Sharma et al. (2012)

NS nonsignificant

that VSL#3 is an effective and safe preventive therapy. Patients receiving probiotics had significantly lower incidence (31.6 % vs. 51.8 %, $p < 0.001$) and also severity of diarrhea compared to placebo. Authors also reported significantly lower mean daily number of bowel movements and shorter time of rescue medication use (loperamide) in probiotic group (Delia et al. 2007).

Meta-analysis of these three preventive trials included 632 patients did not show significant benefit of probiotics compared to placebo in prevention of radiation-induced diarrhea (odds ratio = 0.47, 95 % confidence interval: 0.13–1.67). However, the few available trials and the presence of significant clinical and statistical heterogeneity limited the analysis (Fuccio et al. 2009). No major adverse events owing to probiotic supplementation were reported in any study. However, the few available clinical studies do not allow firm conclusions (Fuccio et al. 2009). In addition to these mentioned results, one case study suggested that probiotics can be used effectively in the management of chemotherapy-induced diarrhea in patients with advanced breast cancer (Abd et al. 2009).

Only one clinical trial evaluated probiotic supplementation as a treatment for acute radiation-induced diarrhea. This randomized, placebo-controlled, double-blinded trial investigated the treatment efficacy of 1-week supplementation with *Lactobacillus rhamnosus* based on the need of rescue medication per patient. This study included 202 patients. Authors observed trend for beneficial effect of probiotics compared to placebo in the treatment of radiation-related diarrhea; however, the differences didn't reach statistical significance. Patients' rating of diarrhea and feces consistency was in favor of probiotic supplementation (Urbancsek et al. 2001).

Oral mucositis is a frequent and serious complication in patients receiving chemo-radiotherapy for head and neck cancer. Recently published study evaluated the effects of administering *Lactobacillus brevis* CD2 lozenges on the incidence and severity of mucositis and tolerance to chemo-radiotherapy. This randomized, double-blind study included 200 patients, who were treated with chemoradiation. The efficacy analysis included the 188 patients who received $\geq$1 week of study treatment. This study showed beneficial effect of probiotic supplementation on primary endpoints (Table 2). Moreover, a larger proportion of patients remained free of mucositis when treated with *L. brevis* CD2 compared to the placebo (28 % vs. 7 %). This study suggests that beneficial role of probiotics in prevention of radiation-induced toxicity is not restricted only to prevention of diarrhea (Sharma et al. 2012).

5 Safety of Probiotic Administration

Decreasing the toxicity related to anticancer chemotherapy or radiation treatment by probiotics represent a possible trend. However, safety of probiotic use in immunocompromised cancer patients became an essential issue of the research these days. Probiotics fall into the category of organisms classified as "generally regarded as safe"—GRAS (Vanderhoof and Young 2008). The safety concerns with probiotic administration in cancer patients are related mainly to risk of infection caused by probiotic bacteria and transfer of antibiotics resistance.

Many probiotic strains are naturally resistant to antibiotics, but majority of this resistance is intrinsic (chromosomally encoded) and therefore nontransmissible (Swenson et al. 1990; Handwerger et al. 1994; Klein et al. 1998; Charteris et al. 1998). This could be a danger, when probiotics become infectious agents; on the other hand probiotic strains with intrinsically antibiotic resistance may benefit patients, whose normal intestinal microflora has become greatly reduced or unbalanced due to the administration of various antimicrobial agents (Salminen et al. 1998). For some strains (e.g., *Lactobacillus* GG), the plasmid-free status was proven (Tynkkynen et al. 1998), but at the same time it was shown that some strains may carry potentially transmissible plasmid-encoded antibiotic resistance genes (Gevers et al. 2003; Ishiwa and Iwata 1980; Ahn et al. 1992; Tannock et al. 1994; Fons et al. 1997). So there exists a possible risk with respect to the development and transfer of antibiotic resistance between probiotic strain and endogenous flora, which could lead to the formation of new antibiotic-resistant pathogens (Morelli and Wright 1997; Salminen et al. 1998; Saarela et al. 2000; Mathur and Singh 2005; Salyers et al. 2004). Therefore, one of the key requirement for probiotic strains is that they should not carry transmissible antibiotic resistance genes (Morelli and Wright 1997; Salminen et al. 1998; Saarela et al. 2000).

Incidence of infection caused by lactic acid bacteria is extremely low. Despite that fact, there exists certain risk of their pathogenic shift especially in immunocompromised patients (Gasser 1994). Therefore, experience with administration of probiotics in granulocytopenic patients is limited. In addition, bacterial translocation from gastrointestinal tract to extraintestinal sites may result in the transfer of viable indigenous bacteria to other organs, thereby potentially causing bacteremia, septicemia, and multiple organ failure (Berg 1992, 1995).

Some case reports described the local infections of chest, digestive and urinary tract, and meningitis caused by lactic acid bacteria (Fruchart et al. 1997; Gasser 1994). *Lactobacillus* spp. is probably most common probiotics associated with bacteremia, characterized by a very low mortality rate (Olano et al. 2001). Reported in severely sick patients, *Bacillus subtilis* bacteremia also occurred in 4 of 20 oncologic patients (Richard et al. 1998). Our hospital's experience confirms this finding too. Fungemia caused by *Saccharomyces* was reported in 6-month-old neutropenic patient with acute leukemia receiving diarrhea prophylaxis by *Saccharomyces boulardii* (Cesaro et al. 2000). A similar infection was also noted in two other immunocompromised persons with *Saccharomyces boulardii* prophylaxis (Riquelme et al. 2003).

Systematic review concerning on safety of probiotic use has identified 11,977 publications, of which 622 studies were included in the review. Based on reported adverse events, randomized controlled trials showed no statistically significantly increased relative risk (RR) of the overall number of experienced adverse events (RR = 1.00; 95 % CI: 0.93, 1.07, $p = 0.999$), gastrointestinal, infections, or other adverse events, including serious adverse events (RR = 1.06; 95 % CI: 0.97, 1.16; $p = 0.201$), associated with short-term probiotic use compared to control group participants; long-term effects are largely unknown. Case studies suggested that adverse events are associated with probiotics most likely between participants with compromised health. However, RCTs in medium-risk and critically ill participants did not report a statistically significantly increased risk of adverse events compared to control group of participants (Hempel et al. 2011). Authors of this analysis concluded that the available evidence in RCTs did not indicate an increased risk; however, rare adverse events were difficult to assess. Despite the substantial number of publications, it was not well equipped to answer questions on the safety of probiotic interventions with confidence (Hempel et al. 2011).

More recently, analysis of 17 studies ($N = 1530$ participants) selected under strict criteria aimed to asses the safety of probiotic administration in oncologic patients. Participants consuming probiotics displayed 105 adverse events compared to 145 adverse events in patients without probiotic supplementation. Five case reports showed probiotic-related bacteraemia, fungaemia, or positive blood tests. Due to the heterogeneity of probiotic supplements, treatment regimes, and patients' diagnosis, infectious potential of various probiotics could not be established. However, no deaths attributed to probiotic-associated infection was recorded (Redman et al. 2014). Current dietary advice for neutropenic patients is to avoid the products containing probiotics (Beckerson et al. 2012). Nevertheless, this statement is not based on critical, large-scale scientific reports, and further analyses need to be evaluated.

6 Conclusions and Future Directions

In conclusion, current evidence supporting probiotic use as adjunctive therapy to anticancer treatment is limited, especially in cancer patients treated with chemotherapy. The reported trial varies in utilized probiotic strains, dose of probiotics and vast majority of them are small trials with substantial risk of bias. Some of the reports support their beneficial effects on certain aspects of toxicity related to chemotherapy and radiation therapy; however, large, properly designed clinical trials are needed to assess their real position as a part of anticancer treatment. Despite limited data, it seems that probiotic bacteria as live microorganisms could be safely administered even in setting of prolonged neutropenia. Future research should focus on selection of most effective and safe probiotic strains and their combinations, and/or administration of probiotics with prebiotics to increase their success in maintaining colonization resistance and in prevention of the adverse events of anticancer treatment. Accurate determination of bacterial species responsible for improved cancer treatment responses and boosting immune system attacks on cancer is highly desirable.

Acknowledgement This work was supported by Grant of Slovak Ministry of Education VEGA 1/0722/11 and by the Slovak Research and Development Agency under the contract No. APVV-0646-11.

References

Abd El-Atti S, Wasicek K, Mark S, Hegazi R (2009) Use of probiotics in the management of chemotherapy-induced diarrhea: a case study. J Parenter Enteral Nutr 33:569–570

Ahn C, Thompson DC, Duncan C, Stiles ME (1992) Mobilization and location of the genetic determinant of chloramphenicol resistance from Lactobacillus plantarum ca TC2R. Plasmid 27:169–176

Andreyev HJ, Vlavianos P, Blake P et al (2005) Gastrointestinal symptoms after pelvic radiotherapy: role for the gastroenterologist? Int J Radiat Oncol Biol Phys 62:1464–1471

Asahara T, Nomoto K, Shimizu K, Watanuki M, Tanaka R (2001) Increased resistance of mice to Salmonella enterica serovar Typhimurium infection by synbiotic administration of Bifidobacteria and transgalactosylated oligosaccharides. J Appl Microbiol 91:985–996

Asahara T, Shimizu K, Nomoto K, Hamabata T, Ozawa A, Takeda Y (2004) Probiotic Bifidobacteria protect mice from lethal infection with Shiga toxin-producing Escherichia coli O157:H7. Infect Immun 72:2240–2247

Azcárate-Peril MA, Sikes M, Bruno-Bárcena JM (2011) The intestinal microbiota, gastrointestinal environment and colorectal cancer: a putative role for probiotics in prevention of colorectal cancer? Am J Physiol Gastrointest Liver Physiol 301:G401–G424

Baba E, Nagaishi M, Fukata T, Arakawa A (1991) The role of intestinal microflora on the prevention of Salmonella colonization in gnotobiotic chickens. Poult Sci 70:1902–1907

Beckerson J, Jones N, Lodhia S et al (2012) Dietary advice during neutropenia. An update and consensus from the Haematology subgroup of the BDA Oncology Group. Complete Nutr 12:40–42

Berg RD (1992) Translocation and the indigenous gut flora. In: Fuller R (ed) Probiotics: the scientific basis. Chapman & Hall, London, pp 55–85

Berg RD (1995) Bacterial translocation from the gastrointestinal tract. Trends Microbiol 3:149–154
Berg RD (1999) Bacterial translocation from the gastrointestinal tract. Adv Exp Med Biol 473:11–30
Blijlevens NM, Donnelly JP, De Pauw BE (2000) Mucosal barrier injury: biology, pathology, clinical counterparts and consequences of intensive treatment for haematological malignancy: an overview. Bone Marrow Transplant 25:1269–1278
Born P, Lersch C, Zimmerhackl B, Classen M (1993) The *Saccharomyces boulardii* therapy of HIV-associated diarrhoea (letter). Dtsch Med Wochenschr 118:765
Bowen JM, Gibson RJ, Cummins AG, Tyskin A, Keefe DM (2007a) Irinotecan changes gene expression in the small intestine of the rat with breast cancer. Cancer Chemother Pharmacol 59:337–348
Bowen JM, Gibson RJ, Tsykin A, Stringer AM, Logan RM, Keefe DM (2007b) Gene expression analysis of multiple gastrointestinal regions reveals activation of common cell regulatory pathways following cytotoxic chemotherapy. Int J Cancer 121:1847–1856
Buck AC, Cooke EM (1969) The fate of ingested Pseudomonas aeruginosa in normal persons. J Med Microbiol 2:521–525
Camera A, Andretta C, Villa MR, Volpicelli M, Picardi M, Rossi M, Rinaldi CR, Della Cioppa P, Ciancia R, Selleri C, Rotoli B (2003) Intestinal toxicity during induction chemotherapy with cytarabine-based regimens in adult acute myeloid leukemia. Hematol J 4:346–350
Cario E (2005) Bacterial interactions with cells of the intestinal mucosa: toll-like receptors and Nnod2. Gut 54:1182–1193
Cesaro S, Chinello P, Rossi L, Zanesco L (2000) Saccharomyces cerevisiae fungemia in a neutropenic patient treated with Saccharomyces boulardii. Support Care Cancer 8:504–505
Charteris WP, Kelly PM, Morelli L, Collins JK (1998) Antibiotic susceptibility of potentially probiotic Lactobacillus species. J Food Prot 61:1636–1643
Ciorba MA, Riehl TE, Rao MS, Moon C, Ee X, Nava GM, Walker MR, Marinshaw JM, Stappenbeck TS, Stenson WF (2012) Lactobacillus probiotic protects intestinal epithelium from radiation injury in a TLR-2/cyclo-oxygenase-2-dependent manner. Gut 61:829–838
Crawford PA, Gordon JI (2005) Microbial regulation of intestinal radiosensitivity. Proc Natl Acad Sci U S A 102:13254–13259
D'souza AL, Rajkumar CH, Cooke J, Bulpitt CHJ (2002) Probiotics in prevention of antibiotic associated diarrhoe: meta-analysis. BMJ 324:1361–1366
Danielsson A, Nyhlin H, Persson H et al (1991) Chronic diarrhea after radiotherapy for gynaecological cancer: occurrence and aetiology. Gut 32:1180–1187
Delia P, Sansotta G, Donato V et al (2007) Use of probiotics for prevention of radiation-induced diarrhea. World J Gastroenterol 13:912–915
Demirer S, Aydintug S, Aslim B et al (2006) Effects of probiotics on radiation-induced intestinal injury in rats. Nutrition 22:179–186
Eker H, Jurk IH, Waters KD, Tiedemann K (1980) Prophylactic co-trimoxazole and lactobacilli preparation in neutropenic patients. Med Pediatr Oncol 8:47–51
Ferenčík M, Ebringer L, Mikeš Z, Jahnová E, Čiznár I (1999) Beneficial modification of the human intestinal microflora using orally administered lactic acid bacteria. Bratisl Lek Listy 100:238–245
Fons M, Hege T, Ladire M, Raibaud P, Ducluzeau R, Maguin E (1997) Isolation and characterization of a plasmid from Lactobacillus fermentum conferring erythromycin resistance. Plasmid 37:199–203
Fotiadis CI, Stoidis CN, Spyropoulos BG, Zografos ED (2008) Role of probiotics, prebiotics and synbiotics in chemoprevention for colorectal cancer. World J Gastroenterol 14:6453–6457
Fruchart C, Salah A, Gray C, Martin E, Stamatoullas A et al (1997) Lactobacillus species as emerging pathogens in neutropenic patients. Eur J Clin Microbiol Infect Dis 16:681–684
Fuccio L, Guido A, Eusebi LH, Laterza L, Grilli D, Cennamo V, Ceroni L, Barbieri E, Bazzoli F (2009) Effects of probiotics for the prevention and treatment of radiation-induced diarrhea. J Clin Gastroenterol 43:506–513

Fuller R (1989) Probiotics in man and animals. J Appl Bacteriol 66:365–378

Gafter-Gvili A, Fraser A, Paul M, Leibovici L (2005) Meta-analysis: antibiotic prophylaxis reduces mortality in neutropenic patients. Ann Intern Med 142:979–995

Gami B, Harrington K, Blake P et al (2003) How patients manage gastrointestinal symptoms after pelvic radiotherapy. Aliment Pharmacol Ther 18:987–994

Gasser S (1994) Safety of lactic acid bacteria and their occurrence in human clinical infection. Bull Inst Pasteur 92:45–67

Gevers D, Danielsen M, Huys G, Swings J (2003) Molecular characterization of tet(M) genes in Lactobacillus isolates from different types of fermented dry sausage. Appl Environ Microbiol 69:1270–1275

Giralt J, Regadera JP, Verges R et al (2008) Effects of probiotic Lactobacillus casei DN-114 001 in prevention of radiationinduced diarrhea: results from multicenter, randomized, placebo-controlled nutritional trial. Int J Radiat Oncol Biol Phys 71:1213–1219

Girardin M, Seidman EG (2011) Indications for the use of probiotics in gastrointestinal diseases. Dig Dis 29:574–587

Goldin BR, Gorbach SL (2008) Clinical indications for probiotics: an overview. Clin Infect Dis 46 (Suppl 2):S96–S100, Discussion S144–S151

Handwerger S, Pucci MJ, Volk KJ, Liu JP, Lee MS (1994) Vancomycin-resistant Leuconostoc mesenteroides and Lactobacillus casei synthesize cytoplasmic peptidoglycan precursors that terminate in lactate. J Bacteriol 176:260–264

Hasegawa T, Kanasugu H, Hidaka M, Yamamoto T, Abe S, Yamaguchi H (1996) Effect of orally administered heat-killed Enterococcus faecalis FK-23 preparation on neutropenia in dogs treated with cyclophosphamide. Int Immunopharmacol 18:103–112

Hempel S, Newberry S, Ruelaz A, Wang Z, Miles JNV, Suttorp MJ, Johnsen B, Shanman R, Slusser W, Fu N, Smith A, Roth E, Polak J, Motala A, Perry T, Shekelle PG (2011) Safety of probiotics to reduce risk and prevent or treat disease. Evidence Report/Technology Assessment No. 200 (Prepared by the Southern California Evidence-based Practice Center under Contract No. 290-2007-10062-I.), AHRQ Publication No. 11-E007. Agency for Healthcare Research and Quality, Rockville, MD, April 2011. Available at www.ahrq.gov/clinic/tp/probiotictp.htm

Hempel S, Newberry SJ, Maher AR, Wang Z, Miles JN, Shanman R, Johnsen B, Shekelle PG (2012) Probiotics for the prevention and treatment of antibiotic-associated diarrhea: a systematic review and meta-analysis. JAMA 307:1959

Hengens C, Klastersky J (1976) Intestinal colonization with lactobacilli strains in neutropenic patients. Biomedicine 25:11–15

Husebye E, Skar V, Hoverstad T et al (1995) Abnormal intestinal motor patterns explain enteric colonization with gram-negative bacilli in late radiation enteropathy. Gastroenterology 109:1078–1089

Iida N, Dzutsev A, Stewart CA, Smith L, Bouladoux N, Weingarten RA, Molina DA, Salcedo R, Back T, Cramer S, Dai RM, Kiu H, Cardone M, Naik S, Patri AK, Wang E, Marincola FM, Frank KM, Belkaid Y, Trinchieri G, Goldszmid RS (2013) Commensal bacteria control cancer response to therapy by modulating the tumor microenvironment. Science 342:967–970

Ishiwa H, Iwata S (1980) Drug resistance plasmids in Lactobacillus fermentum. J Gen Appl Microbiol 26:71–74

Johnson LB, Riaz AA, Adawi D, Wittgren L, Bäck S, Thornberg C, Osman N, Gadaleanu V, Thorlacius H, Jeppsson B (2004) Radiation enteropathy and leucocyte-endothelial cell reactions in a refined small bowel model. BMC Surg 4:10

Johnston BC, Goldenberg JZ, Vandvik PO, Sun X, Guyatt GH (2011) Probiotics for the prevention of pediatric antibiotic-associated diarrhea. Cochrane Database Syst Rev 9:CD004827

Joint FAO/WHO Working Group on Drafting Guidelines for the Evaluation of Probiotics in Food. London, Ontario, Canada, April 30 and May 1, 2002

Kale-Pradhan PB, Jassal HK, Wilhelm SM (2010) Role of Lactobacillus in the prevention of antibiotic-associated diarrhea: a meta-analysis. Pharmacotherapy 30:119–126

Klein G, Pack A, Bonaparte C, Reuter G (1998) Taxonomy and physiology of probiotic lactic acid bacteria. Int J Food Microbiol 41:103–105

Lin XB, Dieleman LA, Ketabi A, Bibova I, Sawyer MB, Xue H, Field CJ, Baracos VE, Ganzle MG (2012) Irinotecan (CPT-11) chemotherapy alters intestinal microbiota in tumour bearing rats. PLoS One 7:e39764

Lin XB, Farhangfar A, Valcheva R, Sawyer MB, Dieleman L, Schieber A, Gänzle MG, Baracos V (2014) The role of intestinal microbiota in development of irinotecan toxicity and in toxicity reduction through dietary fibres in rats. PLoS One 9:e83644

Logan RM, Gibson RJ, Bowen JM, Stringer AM, Sonis ST, Keefe DM (2008a) Characterisation of mucosal changes in the alimentary tract following administration of irinotecan: implications for the pathobiology of mucositis. Cancer Chemother Pharmacol 62:33–41

Logan RM, Stringer AM, Bowen JM, Gibson RJ, Sonis ST, Keefe DM (2008b) Serum levels of NFkappaB and pro-inflammatory cytokines following administration of mucotoxic drugs. Cancer Biol Ther 7:1139–1145

Ludgate SM, Merrick MV (1985) The pathogenesis of post-irradiation chronic diarrhoea: measurement of SeHCAT and B12 absorption for differential diagnosis determines treatment. Clin Radiol 36:275–278

Malinen E, Rinttilä T, Kajander K, Mättö J, Kassinen A et al (2005) Analysis of the fecal microbiota of irritable bowel syndrome patients and healthy controls with real-time PCR. Am J Gastroenterol 100:373–382

Marin ML, Tejada-Simon MV, Lee JH, Murtha J, Ustunol Z, Pestka JJ (1998) Stimulation of cytokine production in clonal macrophage and T-cell models by Streptococcus thermophilus: comparison with Bifidobacterium sp. and Lactobacillus bulgaricus. J Food Prot 61:859–864

Marshall JC (1999) Gastrointestinal flora and its alterations in critical illness. Curr Opin Clin Nutr Metab Care 2:405–411

Marteau P, Chaput U (2011) Bacteria as trigger for chronic gastrointestinal disorders. Dig Dis 29:166–171

Masters GA, Krilov L, Bailey HH, Brose MS, Burstein H, Diller LR, Dizon DS, Fine HA, Kalemkerian GP, Moasser M, Neuss MN, O'Day SJ, Odenike O, Ryan CJ, Schilsky RL, Schwartz GK, Venook AP, Wong SL, Patel JD (2015) Clinical cancer advances 2015: annual report on progress against cancer from the American Society of Clinical Oncology. J Clin Oncol 33(7):786–809, pii: JCO.2014.59.9746

Mathur S, Singh R (2005) Antibiotic resistance in food lactic acid bacteria—a review. Int J Food Microbiol 105:281–295

McFarland LV (2006) Meta-analysis of probiotics for the prevention of antibiotic associated diarrhea and the treatment of Clostridium difficile disease. Am J Gastroenterol 101:812–822

Mego M, Ebringer L, Koza I et al (2005) Prevention of febrile neutropenia in cancer patients by probiotic strain Enterococcus faecium M -74. Pilot study phase I. Neoplasma 52:159–164

Mego M, Koncekova R, Mikuskova E, Drgona L, Ebringer L, Demitrovicova L, Nemova I, Trupl J, Mardiak J, Koza I, Zajac V (2006) Prevention of febrile neutropenia in cancer patients by probiotic strain Enterococcus faecium M-74. Phase II study. Support Care Cancer 14:285–290

Mego M, Chovanec J, Vochyanova-Andrezalova I, Konkolovsky P, Mikulova M, Reckova M, Miskovska V, Bystricky B, Beniak J, Medvecova L, Lagin A, Svetlovska D, Spanik S, Zajac V, Mardiak J, Drgona L (2015) Prevention of irinotecan induced diarrhea by probiotics: a randomized double blind, placebo controlled pilot study. Complement Ther Med 23(3):356–62

Michael M, Brittain MA, Nagai J, Feld R, Hedley D, Oza A, Siu L, Moore M (2004) Phase II study of activated charcoal to prevent irinotecan-induced diarrhea. J Clin Oncol 22:4410–4417

Morelli L, Wright AV (1997) Probiotic bacteria and transferable antibiotic resistance-safety aspects. Demonstration Nutr Functionality Probiotic Foods News Lett 2:9–14

Nam YD, Kim HJ, Seo JG, Kang SW, Bae JW (2013) Impact of pelvic radiotherapy on gut microbiota of gynecological cancer patients revealed by massive pyrosequencing. PLoS One 8 (12):e82659

Nauseef WM, Maki DG (1981) A study of the value of simple protective isolation in patients with granulocytopenia. N Engl J Med 304:448–453

Neumann E, Oliveira MA, Cabral CM, Moural N, Nicoli JR et al (1998) Monoassociation with Lactobacillus acidophilus UFV-H2b20 stimulates the immune defense mechanisms of germ free mice. Braz J Med Biol Res 31:1565–1573

Olano A, Chua J, Schroeder S, Minari A, La Salvia M, Hall G (2001) Weissella confusa (Basonym: Lactobacillus confusus) bacteremia: a case report. J Clin Microbiol 39:1604–1607

Osterlund P, Ruotsalainen T, Korpela R, Saxelin M, Ollus A, Valta P, Kouri M, Elomaa I, Joensuu H (2007) Lactobacillus supplementation for diarrhoea related to chemotherapy of colorectal cancer: a randomised study. Br J Cancer 97:1028–1034

Perdigon G, Alvarez S, Rachid M, Aguero G, Gobbato N (1995) Immune system stimulation by probiotics. J Dairy Sci 78:1597–1606

Redman MG, Ward EJ, Phillips RS (2014) The efficacy and safety of probiotics in people with cancer: a systematic review. Ann Oncol 25:1919–1929

Resta-Lenert S, Barrett KE (2003) Live probiotics protect intestinal epithelial cells from the effects of infection with enteroinvasive Escherichia coli (EIEC). Gut 52:988–997

Richard V, Van Der Auwera P, Snoeck R, Daneau D, Meunier F (1998) Nosocomial bacteremia caused by Bacillus species. Eur J Microbiol Infect Dis 7:783–785

Richardson MA, Sanders T, Palmer JL et al (2000) Complementary/alternative medicine use in a comprehensive cancer center and the implications for oncology. J Clin Oncol 18:2505–2514

Riquelme AJ, Calvo MA, Guzman AM, Depix MS, Garcia P et al (2003) Saccharomyces cerevisiae fungemia after Saccharomyces boulardii treatment in immunocompromised patients. J Clin Gastroenterol 36:41–43

Saarela M, Mogensen G, Fonden R, Matto J, Mattila-Sandholm T (2000) Probiotic bacteria: safety, functional and technological properties. J Biotechnol 84:197–215

Salminen E, Elomaa I, Minkkinen J et al (1988) Preservation of intestinal integrity during radiotherapy using live Lactobacillus acidophilus cultures. Clin Radiol 39:435–437

Salminen S, von Wright A, Morelli L, Marteau P, Brassart D, de Vos WM, Fonde'n R, Saxelin M, Collins K, Mogensen G, Birkeland SE, Sandholm TM (1998) Demonstration of safety of probiotics- a review. Int J Food Microbiol 44:93–106

Salyers AA, Gupta A, Wang Y (2004) Human intestinal bacteria as reservoirs for antibiotic resistance genes. Trends Microbiol 12:412–416

Satonaka K, Ohashi K, Nohmi T, Yamamoto T, Abe S et al (1996) Prophylactic effect of Enterococcus faecalis FK-23 preparation on experimental candidiasis in mice. Microbiol Immunol 40:217–222

Schimpff SC, Young VM, Green WH (1972) Origin of infection in acute lymphocytic leukemia: significance of hospital acquisition of potential pathogens. Ann Intern Med 77:707–714

Seal M, Naito Y, Barreto R et al (2007) Experimental radiotherapyinduced enteritis: a probiotic interventional study. J Dig Dis 8:143–147

Sharma A, Rath GK, Chaudhary SP, Thakar A, Mohanti BK, Bahadur S (2012) Lactobacillus brevis CD2 lozenges reduce radiation- and chemotherapy-induced mucositis in patients with head and neck cancer: a randomized double-blind placebo-controlled study. Eur J Cancer 48:875–881

Sonis ST (2004) A biological approach to mucositis. J Support Oncol 2:21–32, Discussion 35–36

Sonis ST, Oster G, Fuchs H, Bellm L, Bradford WZ et al (2001) Oral mucositis and the clinical and economic outcomes of hematopoietic stem-cell transplantation. J Clin Oncol 19:2201–2205

Stringer AM, Gibson RJ, Logan RM, Bowen JM, Yeoh AS, Burns J, Keefe DM (2007) Chemotherapy-induced diarrhea is associated with changes in the luminal environment in the da rat. Exp Biol Med (Maywood) 232:96–106

Stringer AM, Gibson RJ, Logan RM, Bowen JM, Yeoh AS, Keefe DM (2008) Faecal microflora and beta-glucuronidase expression are altered in an irinotecan-induced diarrhea model in rats. Cancer Biol Ther 7:1919–1925

Stringer AM, Gibson RJ, Bowen JM, Logan RM, Ashton K, Yeoh AS, Al-Dasooqi N, Keefe DM (2009) Irinotecan-induced mucositis manifesting as diarrhoea corresponds with an amended intestinal flora and mucin profile. Int J Exp Pathol 90:489–499

Summers RW, Glenn CE, Flatt AJ et al (1991) Radiation and indomethacin effects on morphology, prostaglandins, and motility in dog jejunum. Am J Physiol 261:G145–G151

Swenson JM, Facklamand RR, Thornsberry C (1990) Antimicrobial susceptibility of vancomycin-resistant Leuconostoc, Pediococcus, and Lactobacillus species. Antimicrob Agents Chemother 34:543–549

Taguchi H, Takahashi M, Yamaguchi H et al (2002) Experimental infection of germ-free mice with hyper-toxigenic enterohemorrhagic Escherichia coli O157:H7, strain 6. J Med Microbiol 51:336–343

Takasuna K, Hagiwara T, Hirohashi M, Kato M, Nomura M, Nagai E, Yokoi T, Kamataki T (1996) Involvement of β-glucuronidase in intestinal microflora in the intestinal toxicity of the antitumor camptothecin derivative irinotecan hydrochloride (CPT-11) in rats. Cancer Res 56:3752–3757

Tannock GW, Luchansky JB, Miller L, Connell H, Thode-Andersen S, Mercer AA, Klaenhammer TR (1994) Molecular characterization of a plasmid-borne (pGT633) erythromycin resistance determinant (ermGT) from Lactobacillus reuteri 100-63. Plasmid 31:60–71

Tynkkynen S, Singh KV, Varmanen P (1998) Vancomycin resistance factor of Lactobacillus rhamnosus GG in relation to enterococcal vancomycin resistance (van) genes. Int J Food Microbiol 41:195–204

Urbancsek H, Kazar T, Mezes I et al (2001) Results of a doubleblind, randomized study to evaluate the efficacy and safety of Antibiophilus in patients with radiation-induced diarrhoea. Eur J Gastroenterol Hepatol 13:391–396

Vandenplas Y (1999) Bacteria and yeast in the treatment of acuta and chronic infectious diarrhea. Part I. Bacteria. Clin Microbiol Infect 5:299–307

Vanderhoof JA, Young R (2008) Probiotics in the United States. Clin Infect Dis 46(Suppl 2):S67–S72, Discussion S144–S151

Viaud S, Saccheri F, Mignot G, Yamazaki T, Daillère R, Hannani D, Enot DP, Pfirschke C, Engblom C, Pittet MJ, Schlitzer A, Ginhoux F, Apetoh L, Chachaty E, Woerther PL, Eberl G, Bérard M, Ecobichon C, Clermont D, Bizet C, Gaboriau-Routhiau V, Cerf-Bensussan N, Opolon P, Yessaad N, Vivier E, Ryffel B, Elson CO, Doré J, Kroemer G, Lepage P, Boneca IG, Ghiringhelli F, Zitvogel L (2013) The intestinal microbiota modulates the anticancer immune effects of cyclophosphamide. Science 342:971–976

Von Bultzingslowen I, Adlerberth I, Wold AE, Dahlen G, Jontel M (2003) Oral and intestinal microflora in 5-fluorouracil treated rats, translocation to cervical and mesenteric lymph nodes and effects of probiotic bacteria. Oral Microbiol Immunol 18:278–284

Wada M, Nagata S, Saito M, Shimizu T, Yamashiro Y, Matsuki T, Asahara T, Nomoto K (2010) Effects of the enteral administration of Bifidobacterium breve on patients undergoing chemotherapy for pediatric malignancies. Support Care Cancer 18:751–759

Wiernik PH, Bansks PLC, Case DC, Arlin ZA, Periman PO, Todd MB, RitchPS ERE, Weitberg AB (1992) Cytarabine plus idarubicine or daunorubicine as induction and consolidation therapy for previously untreated adult patients with acute myeloid leukemia. Blood 79:313–319

Yang XX, Hu ZP, Xu AL, Duan W, Zhu YZ et al (2006) A mechanistic study on reduced toxicity of irinotecan by coadministered thalidomide, a tumor necrosis factor alpha inhibitor. J Pharmacol Exp Ther 319:82–104

Zwielehner J, Lassl C, Hippe B, Pointner A, Switzeny OJ, Remely M, Kitzweger E, Ruckser R, Haslberger AG (2011) Changes in human fecal microbiota due to chemotherapy analyzed by TaqMan-PCR, 454 sequencing and PCR-DGGE fingerprinting. PLoS One 6:e28654

MIX
Papier aus verantwortungsvollen Quellen
Paper from responsible sources
FSC® C105338
www.fsc.org

If you have any concerns about our products,
you can contact us on
ProductSafety@springernature.com

In case Publisher is established outside the EU,
the EU authorized representative is:
Springer Nature Customer Service Center GmbH
Europaplatz 3, 69115 Heidelberg, Germany

Printed by Libri Plureos GmbH
in Hamburg, Germany